Vascular Nursing

Fourth Edition

Victora A. Fahey, RN, MSN, CVN
Advanced Practice Nurse: Vascular Surgery
Division of Surgical Nursing
Northwestern Memorial Hospital
Chicago, Illinois

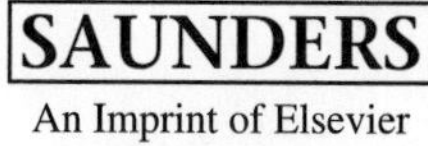

An Imprint of Elsevier

SAUNDERS
An Imprint of Elsevier

11830 Westline Industrial Drive
St. Louis, Missouri 63146

VASCULAR NURSING ISBN 0-7216-9567-1

NOTICE

Vascular nursing is an ever-changing field. Standard safety precautions must be followed, but as new research and clinical experience broaden our knowledge, changes in treatment and drug therapy may become necessary or appropriate. Readers are advised to check the most current product information provided by the manufacturer of each drug to be administered to verify the recommended dose, the method and duration of administration, and contraindications. It is the responsibility of the licensed health care provider, relying on experience and knowledge of the patient, to determine dosages and the best treatment for each individual patient. Neither the publisher nor the editor assumes any liability for any injury and/or damage to persons or property arising from this publication.

Previous editions copyrighted 1999, 1994, 1988

International Standard Book Number 0-7216-9567-1

Acquisitions Editor: Sandra Brown
Developmental Editor: Cindi Anderson
Publishing Services Manager: John Rogers
Project Manager: Helen Hudlin
Design Coordinator: Teresa McBryan Breckwoldt

Printed in USA

Last digit is the print number: 9 8 7 6 5 4 3 2 1

Contributors

Louise Anderson, RN, MS
Patient Care Resource Manager
Division of Vascular Surgery
The Ohio State University Medical Center
Columbus, Ohio

B. Timothy Baxter, MD
Professor of Surgery
Department of Surgery
The University of Nebraska Medical Center
Omaha, Nebraska

Marshall E. Benjamin, MD
Associate Professor of Surgery
Division of Vascular Surgery
University of Maryland School of Medicine
Baltimore, Maryland

Donna Blackburn, RN, MS, RVT
Clinical Instructor
Vascular Laboratory
Northwestern Memorial Hospital
Chicago, Illinois

Lisa Boggio, MS, MD
Instructor in Medicine
Division of Hematology/Oncology
Feinberg School of Medicine
Northwestern University
Chicago, Illinois

Lynn M. Borgini, RN
Staff Nurse
Vascular/Thoracic Operating Room
Northwestern Memorial Hospital
Chicago, Illinois

Karen Bruni RN, MSN, NP, CVN
Nurse Practitioner
The Vascular Institute
Albany Medical Center
Albany, New York

Carol N. Cox, RN
Nurse Specialist
Vascular/Thoracic Operating Room
Northwestern Memorial Hospital
Chicago, Illinois

Michael C. Dalsing, MD
Professor of Surgery
Director of Vascular Surgery
Department of Surgery
Indiana University Medical School
Indianapolis, Indiana

Diana Eastridge, RN, MS, CNP, CCRN
Nurse Practitoner
Department of Vascular Surgery
Northwestern Memorial Hospital
Chicago, Illionos

Mitzi Ekers, RN, MS, ARNP
Vascular Nurse Practitioner
Department of Surgery
Division of Vascular Surgery
University of South Florida College of Medicine
Tampa, Florida

Mark Eskandari, MD
Assistant Professor of Surgery
Division of Vascular Surgery
Feinberg School of Medicine
Northwestern University
Chicago, Illinois

Victora A. Fahey, RN, MSN, CVN
Advanced Practice Nurse: Vascular Surgery
Division of Surgical Nursing
Northwestern Memorial Hospital
Chicago, Illinois

Cindy L. Felty, RN, CNP, CWS
Dirictor, Vascular Ulcer/Wound Healing Clinic
Gonda Vascular Center
Mayo Clinic
Rochester, Minnesota

Michael A. Fotis, RPh
Manager, Drug Information
Pharmacy Department
Northwestern Memorial Hospital
Chicago, Illinois

Linda M. Graham, MD
Staff Surgeon
Department of Vascular Surgery
Cleveland Clinic Foundation
Cleveland, Ohio

David Green, MD, PhD
Professor of Medicine
Department of Medicine
Hematology/Oncology Division
Feinberg School of Medicine
Northwestern University
Chicago, Illinois

Alan T. Hirsch, MD
Associate Professor of Medicine and Radiology
Director, Vascular Medicine Program
Cardiovascular Division, Department of Medicine
University of Minnesota Medical School
Minneapolis, Minnesota

Mark E. Huang, MD
Assistant Professor
Physical Medicine and Rehabilitation
Feinberg School of Medicine
Northwestern University
Rehabilitation Institute of Chicago
Chicago, Illinois

Joan Jacobsen, RN, MSN, CVN
Clinical Nurse Specialist/Case Manager
Department of Case Management
Meriter Hospital
Madison, Wisconsin

Richard R. Keen, MD
Associate Chair of Surgery
Chief of Vascular Surgery
Department of Surgery
Cook County Hospital
Chicago, Illinois

Kimberly A. Kerr, MD
Department of Surgery
Indiana University School of Medicine
Indianapolis, Indiana

Todd Kuiken, MD, PhD
Assistant Professor
Physical Medicine and Rehabilitation
Feinberg School of Medicine
Northwestern University
Rehabilitation Institute of Chicago
Chicago, Illinois

Jon S. Matsumura, MD
Associate Professor of Surgery
Division of Vascular Surgery
Feinberg School of Medicine
Northwestern University
Chicago, Illinois

Mark D. Morasch, MD
Assistant Professor of Surgery
Division of Vascular Surgery
Feinberg School of Medicine
Northwestern University
Chicago, Illinois

Kim Mulkay, RN, MSN, ACNP
Division of Vascular Surgery
University of Maryland Medical Center
Baltimore, Maryland

Janice Nunnelee, RN, PhD, ANP, CVN
Nurse Practitioner, Clinical Associate Professor of Nursing
College of Nursing
University of Missouri—St. Louis
St. Louis, Missouri

William Oppat, MD
Attending Vascular Surgeon
Associate Program Director of Surgery
Department of Surgery
Providence Hospital and Medical Centers
Novi, Michigan

Peter J. Pappas, MD
Associate Professor of Surgery
Director, Division of Vasular Surgery
New Jersey Medical School
University of Medicine and Dentistry of New Jersey
Newark, New Jersey

William H. Pearce, MD
Violet R. and Charles A. Baldwin Professor of Vascular Surgery
Chief, Division of Surgery
Feinberg School of Medicine
Northwestern University
Chicago, Illinois

Linda Peterson-Kennedy, RN, RVT
Vascular Technologist
Northwestern Memorial Hospital
Chicago, Illinois

Karen L. Rice, MSN, APRN, BC
Adult Nurse Practitioner/Geriatric Resource Nurse
Department of Nursing Administration
Ochsner Clinic Foundation
New Orleans, Louisiana

Heron Rodriguez, MD
Assistant Professor of Surgery
Division of Vascular Surgery
Stitch School of Medicine
Loyola University Medical Center
Maywood, Illinois

Thom W. Rooke, MD
Section Head, Vascular Center, Mayo Clinic
John and Posy Krehbiel Professor of Vascular Medicine
Department of Vascular Medicine
Mayo Clinic
Rochester, Minnesota

Nancy Schindler, MD, FACS
Assistant Professor of Surgery
Department of Surgery
Feinberg School of Medicine
Northwestern University
Chicago, Illinois

Kelli J. Stott, RN, BS
Nurse Coordinator, Vascular Surgery
Department of Surgery
The University of Nebraska Medical Center
Omaha, Nebraska

Shubha Varma, MD
Department of Surgery
Columbia Presbyterian Hospital
New York, New York

Robert L. Vogelzang, MD
Professor of Radiology
Chief, Division of Vascular and Interventional Radiology
Feinberg School of Medicine
Northwestern University
Chicago, Illinois

M. Eileen Walsh, RN, PhD, CVN
Advanced Practice Nurse, Vascular Clinical Nurse Specialist
Jobst Vascular Center
The Toledo Hospital
Toledo, Ohio

William C. Watson, MD
Department of Surgery
Indiana University School of Medicine
Indianapolis, Indiana

Reviewers

Kim Cantwell-Gab, RN, BSN, RVT, CVN, RDMS
Nurse Coordinator, Vascular Division
Department of Surgery
University of Washington Medical Center
Seattle, Washington

Cynthia Natiello, RNC, BSN
Research Nurse—Vascular Surgery
University of Washington
Harborview Medical Center
Seattle, Washington

Foreword

Vascular patients are among the most critically ill patients in our hospitals. They are elderly with a devastating systemic disease (atherosclerosis or diabetes mellitus) that has weakened or damaged multiple organ systems. They, then, undergo a major operative or endovascular procedure, which further stresses their weakened resources. However, with careful preoperative evaluation and meticulous intraoperative management and postoperative care, perioperative mortality for all vascular patients undergoing major vascular procedures has fallen dramatically. The perioperative death rate for carotid endarterectomy is less than 1%, for open aneurysm repair less than 2%, and for lower-extremity bypass procedures less than 5%.

Despite these excellent results, we should not remain complacent. We must reevaluate clinical protocols and operative procedures to maximize the health and well-being of our patients. Many times we have the opportunity to offer less invasive procedures with excellent short-term results but unknown long-term benefits. Even though these procedures are less invasive, attention to detail and the reduction of errors must remain our constant priority.

Vascular nurses and physicians are facing additional challenges in the next 5 years. The elderly population is rapidly expanding during a time when resources are limited. The nursing shortage will continue and grow worse. Resident hours will decrease. And physician numbers will decrease given the increasingly hostile environment of rising malpractice rates and declining reimbursements. We must maintain high-quality patient outcomes and patient safety while streamlining care in a cost-effective manner.

There are national efforts, led by industry, to establish quality markers of excellent care for vascular surgery, such as the Leapfrog Initiative Project. However, vascular nurses and surgeons working together must assume a leadership role in creating the practice guidelines for vascular disease rather than have these imposed on us by the business community. Hopefully, from this edition, the reader will be able to develop and defend practice guidelines.

In the last 5 years, the rate of change in knowledge and technology in vascular disease has accelerated. As can be seen from the Table of Contents, this fourth edition of *Vascular Nursing* attempts to be the single source for the latest in the care of the patients with vascular disease. The health and well-being of our patients is our primary concern; thus, this text is an important resource for all who care for the vascular patient, including nurses in all clinical settings, physical and occupational therapists, dietitians, and physicians.

William Pearce, MD

Preface

Vascular disease encompass a wide array of arterial and venous problems, including stroke, abdominal aortic aneurysm, and peripheral arterial disease, as well as acute and chronic venous disease. As life expectancy increases, there will be more patients with vascular disease. Stroke is the third leading cause of death and the primary cause of adult disability in the United States. Over 600,000 people suffer new or recurrent strokes each year with 4,400,000 stroke survivors alive today. Carotid artery disease is the single most important risk factor in the development of stroke. Abdominal aortic aneurysms are the 15th leading cause of death overall and the 10th leading cause of death in men over 55 years of age. Peripheral arterial disease (PAD) affects 12% of the general population and 20% of persons older than 70 years. Although few people die of PAD, it has been identified as a marker for systemic atherosclerosis and, thus, is associated with increased risk of cardiovascular events.

Trends in health care are changing as a result of a number of factors, including new technology, an increase in life expectancy worldwide, alternative health care delivery systems, economic factors forcing abbreviated hospital stays and early discharge of patients with increased acuity in the community, and a health-conscious population interested in health promotion and quality care. In addition, the high cost of health care is demanding a focus on health promotion and prevention. Competition between organizations has heightened pressure on institutions to ensure patient satisfaction with services.

These trends have had a profound impact on nursing. As vascular nurses, we must identify ways to meet the needs and influence the health care of our patients through education, health promotion, and research. Because of the systemic nature of vascular diseases, nurses must take an active role in primary and secondary risk-reduction education to reduce risks of cardiovascular morbidity and mortality. By participation in community awareness programs (educational and screening), we can promote early recognition and prevention of vascular disease. Nurses have additional opportunities to improve clinical outcomes, decrease complications and readmission rates, improve community-based care, and improve care of vascular patients in long-term care facilities.

Since the third edition of this book, significant advancements have occurred in the treatment of vascular disease through improved technology in vascular imaging, endovascular intervention, a renewed interest in venous disease, newly available anticoagulants, a better understanding of hematologic and biochemical factors, and the expanded role of vascular medicine in the treatment of arterial disease.

Patients with vascular disease present with complex nursing problems because of advanced age, associated medical conditions such as hypertension or diabetes, and the fact that multiple organ systems are affected by atherosclerosis.

Because of significant strides in the diagnosis and treatment of vascular disease as well as the increased responsibility of nurses caring for vascular patients, the vascular nurse must have a thorough understanding of vascular disease to deliver optimal care. As can be seen from the Table of Contents, this fourth edition provides a comprehensive overview of vascular disease, current treatment, and nursing management. This text is designed to encourage excellence in vascular nursing by establishing standards of vascular nursing practice, ultimately resulting in quality patient care, which must remain our highest priority.

Victora A. Fahey, RN, MSN, CVN

Acknowledgments and Dedication

I would like to express my graditude and sincere appreciation to the dedicated authors for their professional expertise and time. This book would not have been possible without their chapter contributions. I would also like to acknowledge John J. Bergan, MD; Mark Eskandari, MD; William Flinn, MD; Jon Matsumura, MD; Mark Morasch, MD; Walter J McCarthy, MD; William H. Pearce, MD; and James Yao, MD, for their mentorship; my nursing colleagues for their support and friendship; Northwestern Memorial Hospital Division of Patient Care and the Division of Vascular Surgery, Northwestern University Medical School, for their support; Lynnette Dangerfield, Janet Goldstein, and Sarah Minton for their assistance in manuscript preparation; the staff at Elsevier Science; and my family and friends for their constant presence and encouragement.

I dedicate this book to my patients with vascular disease who have taught me valuable lessons in facing life's many challenges.

Contents

PART ONE
BASIC CONSIDERATIONS

PART TWO
PERIOPERATIVE EVALUATION AND MANAGEMENT

PART THREE
ARTERIAL DISEASES

PART ONE

Basic Considerations

1

The Arterial System

WILLIAM OPPAT □ LINDA M. GRAHAM

The blood vessels that constitute the circulatory system not only are responsible for circulating nutrients and oxygen throughout the body but also are involved in complex homeostatic mechanisms such as coagulation, inflammation, and healing. Until recently the circulatory system was considered a passive conduit without significant biologic function. The simple observation of the endothelium-denuded blood vessel that behaved differently when exposed to pressor agents initiated research investigations that have described their biologic behavior and function, both in healthy and diseased states.[1] Before the pathophysiology of blood vessels was understood, treatment of most clinical illnesses focused on end-organ damage. However, we now realize the central role diseased blood vessels can contribute to organ injury. Much interest has accompanied the recent elucidation of capillary growth into tissues; it has been extended into fields as diverse as cancer ablation and organ regeneration.

Despite significant advances in public awareness, preventative medicine, diagnosis, and treatment, atherosclerosis remains the most common cause of death in the United States.[2] Its many clinical manifestations, including strokes, myocardial infarctions, and extremity arterial occlusive disease, inconvenience or incapacitate countless others. As the post–World War II baby boomers enter their sixth and seventh decades of life, it is expected that many more people will seek medical care for the complications of atherosclerosis.

Equipped with the common goal of providing ever increasingly focused and specific care for vascular patients, the pathobiology of the vascular tree will be reviewed. It is our hope that with an increased understanding of arterial disease, quality nursing care and patient education will result. To understand the biologic nature of atherosclerosis, healthy arteries will be described.

ANATOMY AND PHYSIOLOGY OF BLOOD VESSELS AND LYMPHATICS

The circulatory system is comprised of arteries, arterioles, capillaries, venules, veins, and lymphatics. In each instance the architectural organization of a particular vessel is adapted to the vessel's function. For example, the aorta is a large tapering tube that begins at the aortic root of the heart and ends at the aortic bifurcation in the abdomen. It is an elastic artery that not only conducts blood, but also stores fluid energy as a result of its elastic composition. During systole the aorta expands, storing energy; in diastole the artery recoils, providing both continuous forward and reverse blood flow, thereby augmenting both distal perfusion and coronary artery blood flow. Capillaries, important for the delivery of nutrients to individual tissues, are thin and permeable to facilitate passive diffusion of molecules to their intended destinations. Veins serve as reservoirs of ever-increasing size that collect and return the nutrient-extracted blood to the right side of the heart for reoxygenation through the lungs and to the left side of the heart for systemic recirculation.

Arteries are composed of three histologic and functional layers: the intima, the media, and the adventitia (Figs. 1-1 and 1-2). The innermost layer, the intima, consists of a single layer of endothelial cells resting on a connective tissue layer. The endothelium (the collective term of endothelial cells) is the layer of cells that actually lines the blood vessel and interfaces with the

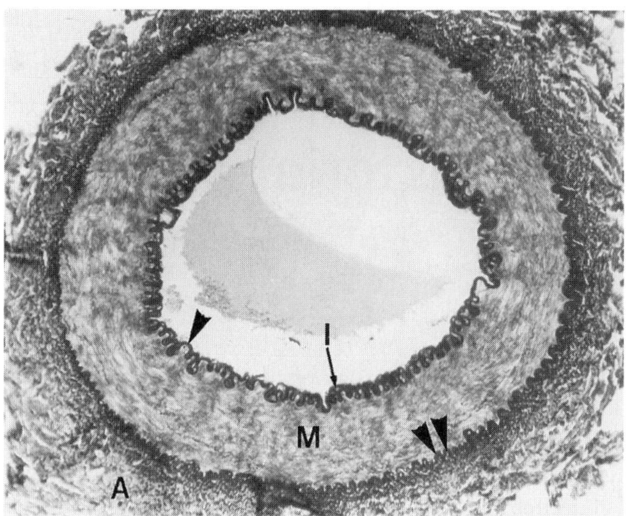

FIG. 1–1. Light micrograph of a normal artery. The intima *(I)* contains a single layer of endothelial cells lining the lumen of the artery. The internal elastic membrane *(single arrowhead)* separates the intima from the media *(M)*. The external elastic membrane *(double arrowheads)* separates the media from the adventitia *(A)*. (Aldehyde fuchsin, ×73.)

moving blood. Its biologic properties are immense and complex. It prevents the contained blood from clotting under normal conditions by providing a barrier to the underlying connective tissue. Heparan sulfate, a negatively charged glycoprotein that is found on the endothelial cell surface, inhibits platelet aggregation. Conversely, thrombomodulin, a receptor for thrombin on the endothelial cell surface, forms a complex on the endothelial cell surface that both localizes platelet aggregation and limits local clot formation. The endothelium responds to changes in shear force, cyclic strain, circulating factors, and oxygen tension. It releases factors, such as nitric oxide, that regulate the function of other cells within the vessel wall. It expresses signaling molecules on its surface and releases cytokines that attract and allow white blood cells to migrate from within the vessel lumen into the surrounding tissues. High shear stress upregulates the endothelial cell production of many factors such as prostacyclin, which limits vasoconstriction, and transforming growth factor, which may be responsible for smooth muscle cell migration to the endothelial layer of the vessel wall. As the interface between blood and the body's tissues, the endothelium serves a number of important roles.

The media is separated from the intima by the internal elastic lamina. The media is composed mainly of vascular smooth muscle cells and structural proteins such as collagen and

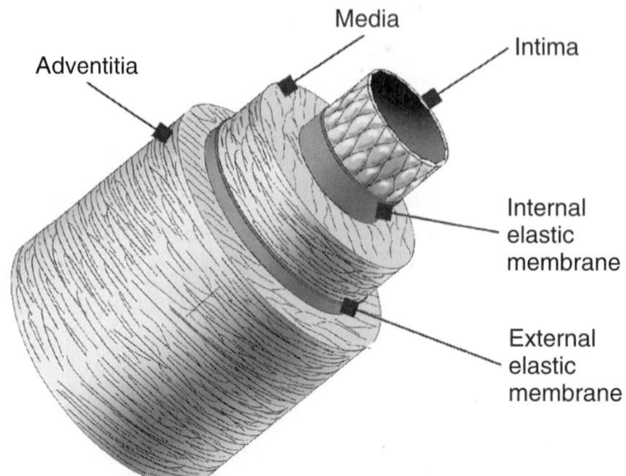

FIG. 1–2. Schematic drawing of artery wall layers.

elastin. Elastin content is greatest in the proximal aorta, where it constitutes 30 percent of the protein content of the aortic wall and decreases to less than 20 percent in the infrarenal aorta.[3] Current research suggests that the loss of elastin formation over time may contribute to aneurysm formation in the abdominal aorta.[4] Vascular smooth muscle cells in the media can manipulate the diameter of a blood vessel depending upon their contractile state. The sum of the contractile states of all arterioles throughout the body contributes to the total peripheral vascular resistance that is clinically observed when blood pressure is measured. Locally secreted endothelial cell factors and products of activated macrophages can cause vascular smooth muscle cells to transform from contractile cells to secretory cells. The secretory smooth muscle cells have a number of complex biologic functions. These cells are responsible for the production of the extracellular matrix proteins such as collagen, fibrillin, and elastin. Under the influence of locally released cytokines, they accumulate lipids and contribute to atherosclerotic plaque formation. The external elastic lamina separates the media from the adventitia.

The adventitia forms the outer layer of the blood vessel and provides the majority of its strength. The strength of this layer results from its high collagen content, although elastin is also found within this layer. In the inner layers of the adventitia, elastin and collagen are tightly compacted; they are more loosely associated in the outer layers. As in the media, the adventitia consists of lamellar units of elastin and collagen arranged into sheets. Generally, the intima and the inner one third of the media receive the majority of their nutrients by diffusion from the blood vessel lumen. The outer portion of the media and the adventitia depend upon the vasa vasorum, small blood vessels that penetrate the vessel wall, for their nutrients.

Arteries (Fig. 1-3) are classified by size, the composition of the wall, their function or biologic behavior, or by their propensity to accumulate disease. Simplest conceptually, conductive arteries generally carry blood over distances and give few branches. The aorta and iliac vessels are clear examples of conductive arteries. Conversely, distributive arteries originate from the conductive vessels, branch frequently, and supply nutrients locally to the capillaries of individual tissues. Common examples of distributive vessels include the external carotid arteries, the internal iliac arteries, and the profunda femoris arteries. Vessels such as the tibial arteries of the legs have properties of both.

PERIPHERAL RESISTANCE AND BLOOD PRESSURE

The contractile state of vascular smooth muscle cells contained within the media is manipulated both locally within the tissues (by nitric oxide [NO], prostaglandins, oxygen and carbon dioxide tension, potassium, and lactic acid) and systemically by circulating factors found in the blood (such as epinephrine and angiotensin II).[5]

In addition to local and systemic control of peripheral vascular resistance, neural control of blood flow is accomplished via resistance blood vessels named arterioles. The arterioles are the smallest arteries and provide the greatest component of resistance to blood flow and regulate regional tissue perfusion. Arterioles contained in the skin (important for temperature regulation) and in the viscera (for increasing blood flow after eating or shunting blood away from the intestines after acute hemorrhage) are innervated by both the sympathetic and parasympathetic neural fibers of the autonomic nervous system. The release of the neurotransmitter epinephrine from sympathetic nerve fibers causes contraction of smooth muscle cells, narrowing of the vessel lumen, and ultimately vasoconstriction. Conversely, sympathetic denervation, a technique seldom used today, increases blood flow to the limbs mainly by increasing perfusion of the skin and the nonnutritive arteriovenous shunts within it.

Blood flow to specific regions of the body is easily controlled by manipulating the resistance of individual vascular beds. The normal resting vascular resistance is relatively high, but it can be rapidly decreased locally by the response of the arterioles to both local and systemic factors. At rest, skeletal muscle requires relatively little blood flow, but exercising muscles can increase their need for blood (and its contained nutrients, including oxygen) twentyfold to

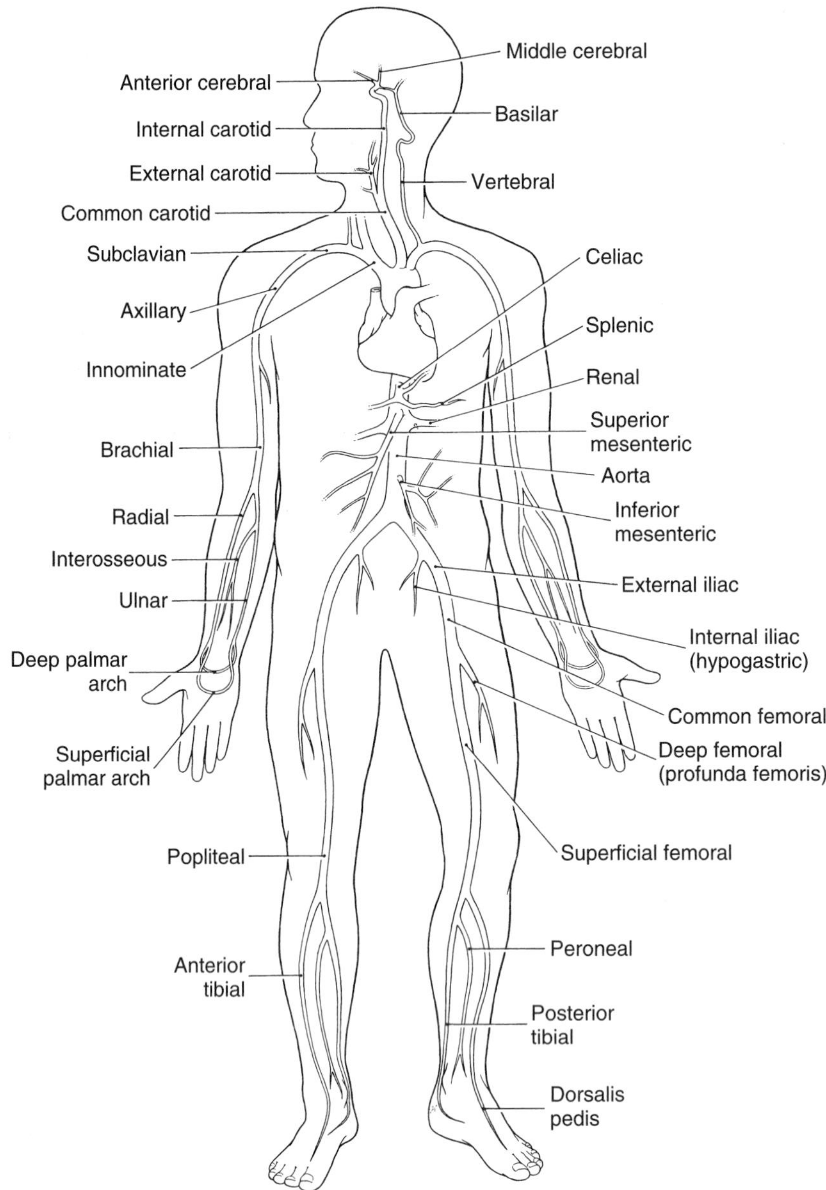

FIG. 1–3. Arterial anatomy.

thirtyfold. Locally produced by-products of actively metabolizing muscle, such as carbon dioxide, lactic acid, and extracellular potassium, are potent vasorelaxing agents; their presence will contribute to arteriolar smooth muscle relaxation and increased blood flow to active muscle.

Circulating factors in the blood also affect individual vascular beds by the presence of specific membrane receptors present on the cell surface. Hormones, such as epinephrine, angiotensin II, and even the thyroid hormones, regulate systemic vascular tone. The hormones have regional regulatory control if specific receptors are present and interface with the individual molecules or hormones.

The ability of the vascular tree to regulate vascular resistance is lost as occlusive diseases, such as atherosclerosis, accumulate within the vessel wall. Intrinsic arterial narrowing from disease and the inability to increase blood flow to the extremities clinically is manifested by symptoms of claudication or in the most extreme cases, rest pain and tissue loss (gangrene).

ARTERIAL OCCLUSIVE DISEASE

Although arterial occlusive disease has many causes, such as embolism, thrombosis, arteritis, and fibromuscular dysplasia, arteriosclerosis is the most common. Despite its cause, the clinical presentation of occlusive disease generally manifests in three ways in the lower extremities: claudication, rest pain, and ulceration.

Claudication, from the Latin *claudios* (to limp), refers to symptoms of muscle cramping when the exercised muscle's requirements for oxygen and nutrients exceed what the circulatory system is capable of delivering. Characteristically, the symptoms of claudication are readily repeatable (the distance at which claudication occurs is consistent), and patients will state that a given distance will precipitate the tiredness in the affected muscle group. Generally, a single level of occlusive disease is demonstrated by angiography. Careful history will reveal that usually one of three muscle groups is predominantly affected: the buttocks, the thighs, or the calves, depending upon the level of arterial obstruction in the vascular tree. The afflicted muscle group is one level below the obstruction. For buttock claudication, patients generally have distal aortic or common iliac arterial obstruction. When symptoms are localized to the thigh, the external iliac artery is involved. Most common is superficial femoral artery occlusion, which results in calf claudication. It is important to realize that the symptoms readily predict the level of obstruction. Furthermore, symptoms of claudication have prognostic significance. Patients with claudication who participate in appropriate risk factor modification and exercise can avoid the need for amputation, even without surgical intervention.

The symptom of rest pain presents when the blood supply to a given vascular bed, mainly the foot, lacks adequate tissue perfusion even with little or no activity. Because sensory nerves have the highest resting metabolic rate, these are the first tissues affected by the diminished blood flow. This causes pain or burning across the dorsum of the foot, which is called rest pain. Classically the pain occurs at night (when the cardiac output drops) and responds to dependency such as dangling the affected leg over the bedside to overcome the pain. Rest pain is a sign of severe circulatory compromise, and the patient may develop gangrene if blood flow is not improved. Typically two or more levels of the vascular tree are disrupted before the symptoms of rest pain are realized. An example of an angiogram finding in patients with rest pain would demonstrate not only occlusion of the superficial femoral artery but also the tibial vessels.

As with rest pain, patients with ulceration, gangrene, and other forms of tissue loss suffer from multilevel occlusive disease. However, diabetic patients complicate these generalized clinical scenarios. The peripheral neuropathy associated with diabetes renders this subset of patients susceptible to more advanced infection and ulceration at presentation. The lack of sensation limits the pain experience. Unlike other patients with ischemic gangrene, diabetics form ulcers at pressure points on the foot where poorly fitted shoes erode the skin. In addition, the insensate foot may harbor foreign bodies that can progress rapidly into foot abscesses.[6] Diabetics do not experience the agonizing pain that other patients experience that forces early medical attention.

ANEURYSM DISEASE

Unlike those with occlusive vascular disease, patients with arterial aneurysms are unaware of their presence until symptoms are severe. Generally, aneurysms force emergent presentation both when they rupture and hemorrhage internally and when they thrombose and occlude blood flow to the tissues distal to the aneurysm.

Aortic aneurysms are the most deadly aneurysms. Affecting men almost five times more commonly than women, 5 percent of Americans over age 55 are believed to have abdominal aortic aneurysms.[7] Risk factors for aortic aneurysm development include smoking, hypertension, and a family history of aneurysms. Most patients have no symptoms attributable to an aortic aneurysm until they rupture. The sudden onset of severe abdominal or back pain, coupled with hypotension, syncope, and a pulsatile abdominal mass, is assumed to be a ruptured aortic aneurysm and these patients are taken emergently to surgery. Fifty percent of patients with these symptoms and signs never present to the hospital (they arrest from internal bleeding); of those patients who do make it to the hospital, 50 percent do not survive surgery or the postoperative complications (they suffer from a host of underlying comorbidities). Therefore, only 10-20 percent of patients with ruptured aneurysms survive emergent management. With such a high mortality from aortic rupture, aortic aneurysms generally are electively repaired in selected patients. Without symptoms, the aneurysms may be detected by screening programs in susceptible populations. The backbone of appropriate screening begins with the identification of risk factors and the palpation of a pulsatile mass in the abdomen. Much debate has centered on the routine use of ultrasonography in all patients over age 55 years for analyzing aortic aneurysms, an effective but somewhat expensive tool, which may be cost prohibitive if universally applied.

Unlike aortic aneurysms, which tend to rupture (even when they accumulate thrombus) as they grow, aneurysms of the popliteal artery do not burst. As these aneurysms grow, they accumulate thrombus within the sac of the aneurysm. Eventually, the organized material becomes unstable and tends to embolize into the distal vessels. Over time, the distal runoff vessels to the foot fill with the debris and render the affected foot ischemic. Except in the acute setting, the embolic debris cannot be extracted from the occluded vessels. Frequently, an amputation is necessary to overcome the ischemic rest pain and gangrene.

PATHOBIOLOGY OF ARTERIAL DISEASE

The understanding of atherosclerosis remains in a state of evolution because active research is expanding our insight into the pathophysiology of the disease complex. The clinical observation that atherosclerotic vessels may become aneurysmal has lead to the conclusion that both aneurysmal and occlusive disease can develop from atherosclerosis. As the molecular mechanisms of occlusive atherosclerosis and aneurysms are elucidated, it becomes increasingly clear that a relationship between the two disease complexes does exist. However, current theories cannot explain all of the observations at the molecular level. For instance, why some patients develop aneurysms and others progress to occlusive disease cannot be explained by current theories.[8] Nevertheless, the molecular models of atherosclerosis and aneurysms provide not only insight into the disease but also potential implications for medical and surgical intervention and, therefore, are worth reviewing.

Arteries that are susceptible to aneurysm formation tend to have the tunica media as their predominant layer. Vessels such as the aorta and other large- to medium-sized arteries make up this subset of arteries. The media is comprised of lamellar units formed by repeating layers of smooth muscle cells and elastic fibers. This design provides the elasticity in the vessel wall needed to accommodate the repeated expansion and contraction with each heartbeat. In additional to elastin, collagen fibrils are also present in the media, although they are the major structural protein of the adventitia and are believed to provide the major component of tensile strength of the aortic wall. Heritable forms of aneurysms, such as Marfan's syndrome and Ehlers-Danlos syndrome, result from abnormalities in the collagen or its ability to properly cross-link. The aortic wall is dependent upon the diffusion of nutrients from the vessel lumen and the vasovasorum to address its metabolic needs. Early hypotheses suggested that the obliteration of the microvascular blood supply or the overt thickening of the vessel wall prevents the delivery of nutrients to the cellular constituents of the wall and ultimately precipitate its destruction. This hypothesis has been difficult to prove clinically. More current theories center on the imbalance of elastin and the relative paucity of collagen in the vessel wall as the aneurysm grows. With aging, the structural proteins slowly diminish from the vessel wall. In patients with aneurysms, however, the collagen and elastin appear to be enzymatically degraded at a rate that far exceeds the expected turnover rate of these proteins in healthy vessels. The role of inflammatory cells and their mediators in the removal of the structural proteins from the vessel wall remains under intense investigation.

Unlike aneurysms, early histopathologic observations have revealed that the atherosclerotic process begins primarily in the intima of the arterial wall. Initially, macrophages are found in these layers and are thought to accumulate lipids within their cytoplasmic inclusions. As the number of lipid-laden macrophages increases, connective tissue matrix and smooth muscle cells proliferate. It is believed that the cells responsible for manufacturing of the extracellular matrix, which consists of collagen and other complex proteins, are actually smooth muscle cells, recruited from the tunica media that have transformed from a contractile to a secretory phenotype under the presence of various growth factors and inflammatory mediators present in the local environment. The secretory smooth muscle cells also manufacture the fibrous cap, the covering that contains and stabilizes the underlying atherosclerotic plaque.

Theories of Atherogenesis

Early anatomic, pathologic, and histologic observations revealed that atherosclerosis seems to accumulate at major arterial branch points. The injury hypothesis initially proposed that atherosclerosis begins with localized endothelial injury or denudation from the vessel wall; the theory now focuses upon endothelial cell dysfunction.[9] It was assumed that the high shear stresses of the moving blood upon the arterial wall caused damage and the atherosclerosis resulted from years of constant repair of the injured vessel. Once there was a realization that the endothelium was more than a passive conduit, investigators focused on its properties in the healthy and diseased states. The endothelium is capable of expression of both cell surface receptors and cytokine chemoattractants, which aid in the attachment of platelets and leukocytes, which then contribute to the proliferation of the atherosclerotic plaque. Disruption of the localized hormonal environment leads to the expression of surface markers and the release of cytokines that promote the development of atherosclerosis. Injury increases the adhesiveness of the endothelium to leukocytes and platelets and increases its permeability. The normal anticoagulant properties of the endothelium, important for blood flow at low rates, are diminished. Elegant blood flow studies have demonstrated that the accumulation of plaque and the migration of leukocytes from the blood actually occur at regions of low shear stress and turbulence, which casts some doubt on the injury hypothesis as the sole explanation of the pathobiology of atherosclerosis.[10] However, the atherosclerotic plaque is found in many susceptible vessels: coronary arteries, carotid arteries, the aortic bifurcation, and the femoral arteries.

Although the exact cause of atherosclerosis remains under intense investigation, many theories, in addition to the injury model, have been proposed. The high saturated fat diet of Americans and the accumulation of oxidized lipids within the vessel wall have suggested a relationship of serum lipid levels and susceptibility to atherosclerosis. Many researchers believe that high circulating cholesterol levels promote the deposition of lipids into the arterial wall. In the presence of inflammatory mediators, they are oxidized by macrophages and perpetuate the inflammatory state. Cytokines and growth factors that are believed to originate from the activated macrophage initiate the transformation of smooth muscle cells from a contractile to a secretory cell. In its secretory state, the smooth muscle cell produces matrix proteins that form the basis for atherosclerotic plaque formation. The oxidized lipids also inhibit normal endothelial cell function and interfere with its ability to regulate vessel tone, repair denuded subendothelial tissues, and ultimately lead to increased thrombogenicity at a site of endothelial injury. Despite changes in the American lifestyle and diet, cardiovascular disease continues to be the principal cause of death in the United States and other nations. Diets rich in fats and cholesterol are not enough alone to explain the diffuse nature of atherosclerosis.

The lesions of atherosclerosis accumulate in large- and medium-sized arteries and seem best described by an inflammatory process that comprises a series of highly specific cellular and molecular reactions that lead to the accumulation of atherosclerotic plaque. Possible causes of inflammation are free radicals formed as by-products of smoking and diabetes, genetic malfunction of healing as might be seen in hyperhomocystinemia, or even infectious agents such as *Chlamydia* or other yet-to-be-discovered organisms. The persistent inflammation within the vessel wall results in the accumulation of macrophages and lymphocytes in the vessel wall at the site of a fatty streak. Activation of the inflammatory cells locally leads to the release of enzymes, cytokines, and numerous growth factors, which are believed to perpetuate the inflammatory state. Ultimately, the local damage progresses into focal necrosis and plaque formation. Initially, the thickening of the vessel wall is overcome by the remodeling of the vessel to increase its diameter and limit the constricting effects of the plaque in the vessel lumen. However, the vessel can only double its diameter before the lumen is compromised. The fibrous cap covers over the lesion in the vessel wall and is believed to stabilize the contents of the plaque beneath it. The fibrous cap is manufactured by the smooth muscle cells within the plaque, and any disruption in smooth muscle cell synthesis can lead to breakdown in the fibrous cap. Most evidence suggests that the actual fibrous plaque rupture presents clinically as a myocardial infarction, stroke, renal failure, or failure of whatever organ is supplied by the offending vessel. It is likely that a plaque begins early in life as a fatty streak, which can be seen in babies; the clinical manifestations of infarction and ischemia of the end organs (heart, brain, or lower extremities) represent the late clinical findings.

The observation that many of the cells that constitute a fibrous plaque are monoclonal has lead to the hypothesis that atherosclerosis arises from a single tumor cell that uncontrollably replicates. The analogy of atherosclerotic plaque development to cancer cell growth does make it easier to explain the chronic, persistent nature of the disease. Another equally plausible explanation is the infiltration of cells within the vessel wall by a viral pathogen that then takes over the cell's replication process. The expression of viral proteins on the endothelial cell surface would initiate and perpetuate the observed inflammatory process.

Current evidence suggests that the atherosclerosis of diabetes is no different than atherosclerosis associated with other diseases but its distribution in the peripheral circulation is different; the tibial vessels seem most susceptible to occlusive atherosclerosis in diabetics. In addition, diabetics develop clinically recognizable occlusive disease at a younger age in the lower extremities. More than 80 percent of patients afflicted with diabetes longer than 20 years will have arterial occlusive disease. Clinically, coronary artery disease and cerebral vascular disease constitute the majority of deaths in diabetic patients. The limited blood supply to the feet, coupled with a peripheral neuropathy and diminished sensation, explains why diabetic patients are so susceptible to foot infections. Furthermore, as the diabetes progresses, the architecture of the foot changes and the body weight is no longer evenly distributed on the foot. Pressure-sensitive areas develop calluses initially, which eventually ulcerate as the blood supply is further diminished.

Risk Factors

Epidemiologic studies have identified a number of risk factors associated with the development of atherosclerosis. In addition to diabetes, cigarettes, hypertension, and hypercholesterolemia have all been implicated in initiating the disease process. Certainly, a family history of vascular disease leaves one more likely to develop similar problems. Heart attacks, strokes, and limb amputations commonly occur in multiple generations. A number of clinical studies have implicated elevations in the serum cholesterol, or specifically low-density lipoproteins (LDL), and atherosclerosis. Conversely, an inverse relationship exists between high-density lipoproteins (HDL) and atherosclerosis. The HDL transport cholesterol to the liver, where it is metabolized. Despite the amount of research that has been performed regarding the role of cigarettes and atherosclerosis, no individual molecule in the smoke has been identified. Cigarette smoke and the by-products of tobacco combustion cause vasoconstriction, hypertension, endothelial cell dysfunction, platelet dysfunction, and increased circulating cholesterol. Even secondhand smoke manifests these harmful effects. Hypertension, in addition to its directly harmful effects, also acts synergistically with other risk factors in the development of atherosclerosis.

By identifying risk factors for the development of peripheral arterial disease, options for modification in dietary habits (low calorie and cholesterol), cessation of offending agents (such as cigarettes), and behavioral modification (exercise and stress reduction) form the basis for medical management of atherosclerosis. Through proper management of diabetes and hypertension, the next level of medical management is achieved. Surgical intervention is reserved for the irreversible manifestations of atherosclerosis such as rest pain or gangrene.

The use of a surgical intervention must always be balanced against the risks of the procedure. Occlusive atherosclerosis is a systemic disease and affects all vascular beds to varying degrees. The clinical presentation for most patients represents progression of occlusive disease to its end stage. For example, if a patient's initial presenting complaint is gangrene of the foot, the coronary arteries of the heart or the carotid arteries leading to the brain are not spared of atherosclerotic occlusive disease. Occlusive disease of the lower extremity only progressed at a faster pace and resulted in complications that precipitated further evaluation. It is not unusual to uncover significant occlusive atherosclerosis to other organs during preoperative surgical risk assessment.

NONATHEROSCLEROTIC ETIOLOGIES

Atherosclerosis makes up the overwhelming majority of occlusive disease seen in humans. Some estimates claim as high as 95 percent of arterial occlusive disease results from atherosclerosis. However, other forms of occlusive disease do exist. Although these diseases afflict all age groups, typically these forms of occlusive disease are observed in younger patients.

Arteritis

Immune arteritis is an inflammatory disease of the arterial vessel wall, but the pathophysiology is much different than atherosclerosis (Fig. 1-4). Like atherosclerosis, it is mediated by leukocytes and macrophages, but unlike atherosclerosis, lipids do not play a dominant role in the initiation or the perpetuation of the inflammatory state. It is hypothesized that the immune system recognizes a portion of the vessel wall as a foreign protein and slowly attacks it. The actual causative antigen responsible for perpetuating a chronic inflammatory response remains elusive. Although many classifications for arteritis exist, the one most commonly used is based upon the afflicted vessel size. Using the Porter classification, four groups exist:

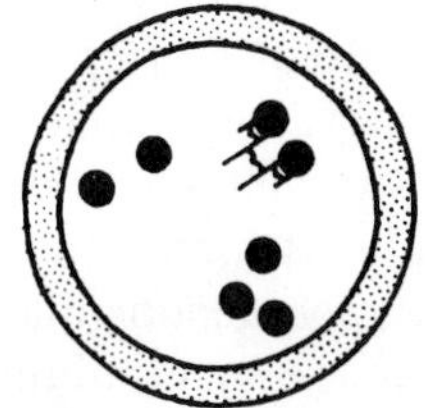

1) Circulating soluble immune complexes in antigen excess

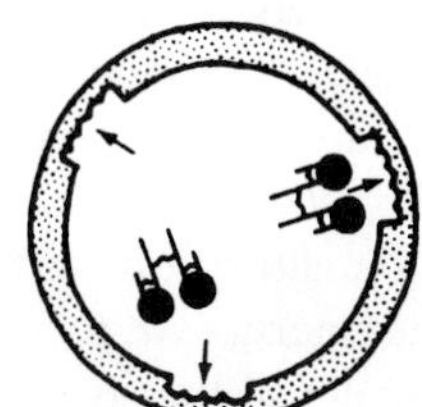

2) Increased vascular permeability via platelet derived vasoactive amines and IgE mediated reactions

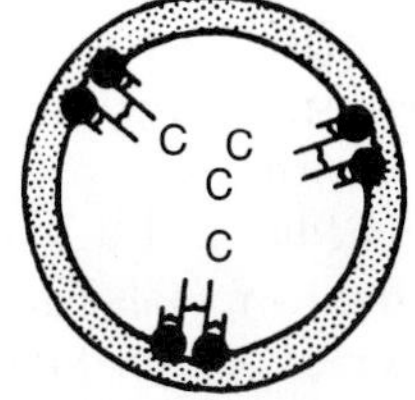

3) Trapping of immune complexes along basement membrane of vessel wall and activation of complement components (C)

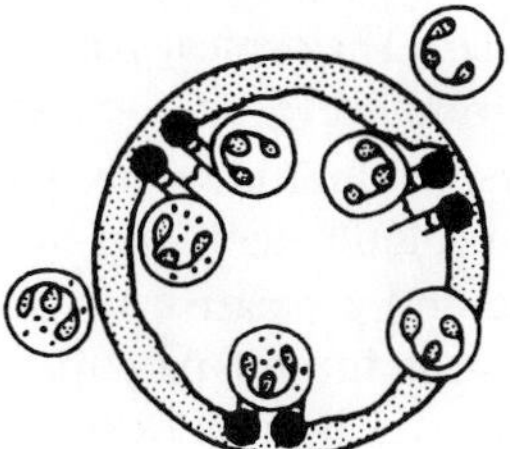

4) Complement derived chemotactic factors (C3a, C5a, C567) cause accumulation of PMNs

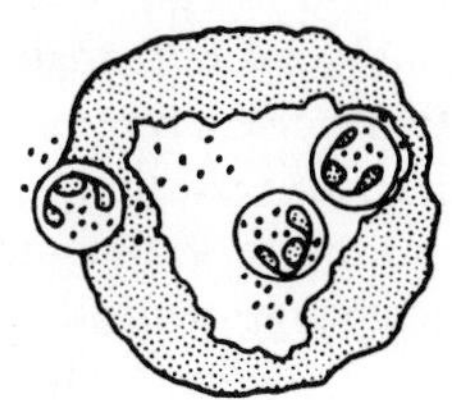

5) PMNs release lysosomal enzymes (collagenase, elastase)

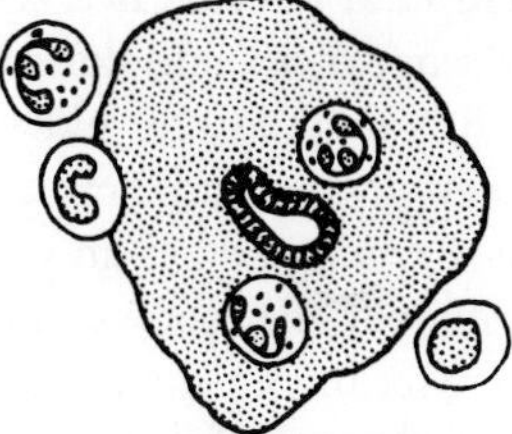

6) Damage and necrosis of vessel wall, thrombosis, occlusion, hemorrhage

FIG. 1–4. Mechanism of arterial damage due to immune arteritis. *PMNs,* polymorphonuclear leukocytes. (From Faci AS, Hayes BF, Katz P: The spectrum of vasculitis, *Ann Intern Med* 89:660-676, 1978.)

Buerger's disease, granulomatous/giant-cell arteritis, polyarteritis nodosa, and hypersensitivity arteritis, and the clinical presentations correspond to the affected vessels.

Buerger's Disease

Buerger's disease, also known as thromboangiitis obliterans, appears to be a unique clinical and pathologic disease entity associated with heavy cigarette smoking. It occurs primarily in men less than 40 years of age, but approximately 20 percent of the patients with Buerger's disease are women.[11] Patients present with occlusions of the distal arteries of the upper and lower extremities. Rest pain and ischemic ulceration occur early in the course of the disease, and patients have a higher incidence of subsequent limb loss than do patients with atherosclerosis. The survival rate of patients with thromboangiitis obliterans, however, is distinctly better than that of patients with atherosclerosis.[12,13]

Histologic studies demonstrate preservation of the general architecture of the vessel wall with a segmental transmural inflammatory process involving small- and medium-sized arteries as well as adjacent veins and nerves.[2] The infiltration of lymphocytes and, occasionally, giant cells is accompanied by fibroblast proliferation. This inflammatory process is often followed by thrombosis, with fibrotic obliteration of the vessels and fibrotic encasement of the adjacent nerve. An arteriogram will show segmental occlusion of the smaller arteries. Treatment consists of abstinence from tobacco in any form. The distal vessel involvement in this disease process usually precludes bypass surgery, but regional sympathectomy is sometimes of benefit in healing superficial ulcerations.

Giant-Cell Arteritis

Giant-cell arteritis includes Takayasu's arteritis and temporal arteritis. Takayasu's disease most commonly affects young women between the ages of 10 and 30.[14] The majority of cases occur in Asia, but many cases have also been reported in the United States, Mexico, and Europe. The typical patient has malaise, fever, night sweats, anorexia, and weight loss. The transmural inflammatory process involves the aortic arch and the vessels arising from the arch (type I—8 percent), the abdominal aorta and visceral vessels (type II—11 percent), both the arch and the abdominal aorta (type III—65 percent), or the pulmonary arteries (type IV—15 percent).[15] Cardiovascular symptoms may develop, and hypertension occurs in up to 70 percent of the cases, with resulting heart failure not unusual. Neurologic symptoms frequently accompany involvement of the aortic arch vessels, but cerebrovascular accidents are unusual. Arterial biopsy reveals diffuse sclerosis, with extensive destruction of elastic fibers of the media, and a transmural inflammatory process with lymphocytes and giant cells. Angiography reveals irregularity of the artery, with areas of stenosis, poststenotic dilatation, occlusion of proximal portions of branches of the aorta, and saccular aneurysms of the aorta and its branches in 10-15 percent of the cases.[16] Active arteritis may continue for years after the onset of the disease. Often steroids are effective in decreasing the activity of the disease process, but bypass surgery is frequently necessary to control hypertension and improve cerebral or visceral perfusion.

Temporal arteritis is a second disease in the giant-cell arteritides. The typical patient is over the age of 50, and the ratio of affected females to males ranges from 2:1 to 4:1. Symptoms frequently include a flu-like illness with malaise, fever, polymyalgias, stiffness of the neck and shoulder girdle, and headache with tenderness along the course of the temporal artery. Diagnosis is based on an elevated erythrocyte sedimentation rate and a positive temporal artery biopsy that shows inflammatory changes with thickening of the intima, patchy areas of necrosis in the media, and infiltration of the media and adventitia by monocytes and eosinophils as well as giant cells.[17] In most cases, the inflammatory process subsides in less than 1 year, but in others it lasts several years.

The major complication of this disease is visual changes or permanent visual loss secondary to ischemic optic neuritis or central retinal artery occlusion, which occurs approximately 3 months after onset. Other complications, including stenosis or aneurysms of the aorta or its main branches, occur about 8 months after onset. Prompt steroid therapy may control the inflammatory response, thereby improving blood flow through the affected vessels. Furthermore, surgical therapy often fails unless high-dose steroids are administered concomitantly. Death is rare but may occur after aortic dissection, rupture of the aorta, myocardial infarction, or cerebral infarction.

Polyarteritis Nodosa

The polyarteritis nodosa group of vasculitides includes classic polyarteritis nodosa, Kawasaki disease, Cogan's syndrome, Behçet's disease, and drug abuse arteritis.[18] Polyarteritis nodosa is a systemic disease that causes fibrinoid necrosis of small- and medium-sized arteries; it afflicts males twice as frequently as females, with a peak incidence in the fifth decade of life. Renal involvement occurs in more than 80 percent of the cases.[19] Visceral ischemia as well as aneurysmal disease may occur as a result of polyarteritis nodosa. Histologic examination reveals a transmural inflammatory process, with destruction of the media causing aneurysm formation.

Kawasaki disease is an acute, febrile, mucocutaneous condition with an associated arteritis similar to polyarteritis nodosa, except that it occurs in young children.[20] Coronary artery involvement leads to cardiac arrhythmias or infarcts, which are the usual cause of death.

Cogan's syndrome is a rare condition manifested as interstitial keratitis, bilateral deafness, and systemic vasculitis similar to polyarteritis nodosa, with focal degeneration, fibrosis, and inflammatory infiltration of large veins and muscular arteries.[21] Systemic manifestations include congestive heart failure, gastrointestinal hemorrhage, adenopathy, splenomegaly, hypertension, musculoskeletal involvement, and eosinophilia.

Behçet's disease, originally described as relapsing iridocyclitis with ulcers of the mouth and genitalia, is a systemic vasculitis that affects both arteries and veins.[22] Superficial or deep venous thrombosis is common. Although aneurysms of large arteries have been reported, thrombosis of small arteries causing involvement of multiple organ systems is more common.

Drug abusers may develop a necrotizing arteritis similar to polyarteritis nodosa, or they may sustain arterial damage secondary to inadvertent intra-arterial injection of drugs.[23] The necrotizing angiitis can lead to aneurysm formation or to stenosis and occlusion secondary to intimal proliferation and medial fibrosis. Patients present with renal failure, hypersensitivity, pulmonary edema, or pancreatitis.

Hypersensitivity Arteritis

Hypersensitivity angiitis is the name applied to a variety of vasculitides involving small arteries. These include classic hypersensitivity angiitis, arteritis of collagen vascular diseases, mixed cryoglobulinemia arteritis, and arteritis associated with malignancy. These conditions appear to result from arterial damage secondary to the formation of antigen-antibody complexes within small arteries, although the cause is never identified in some patients. The typical patient develops a skin rash, fever, and evidence of organ dysfunction.

Vasospastic Phenomenon

Raynaud's syndrome is the classic vasospastic disorder in which the vast majority of patients affected are women. The term *Raynaud's disease* has been used to imply a benign syndrome without demonstrable cause, whereas *Raynaud's phenomenon* is used when there is an underlying immunologic basis for Raynaud's syndrome. The distinction is not always clear, however. Raynaud's syndrome is characterized by episodic digital vasospasm precipitated by cold or emotional stress.[24] The classic Raynaud's attack consists of profound blanching of the digits accompanied by numbness but little pain, followed by cyanosis after prolonged warming, and finally by reactive hyperemia with intense erythema and burning pain. Patients may have normal vessels but an exaggerated vasoconstrictive response to stimuli; however, approximately 60 percent have a normal vasoconstrictive response with underlying digital artery occlusion.[25] Of these latter patients, more than half have an immunologic or connective tissue disorder, most commonly scleroderma. Approximately 10 percent of patients with occlusive disease eventually develop digital gangrene. Treatment is primarily palliative, with blocking agents (most recently calcium channel blockers) being of some benefit.

Vasospasm may also be drug-induced through excessive use of ergotamine tartrate for the treatment of migraine headaches. Ergot-induced vasospasm usually involves the lower extremities, beginning in the superficial femoral arteries and becoming more severe distally.[26] Isolated upper-extremity vasospasm secondary to ergotism is rare. Angiography demonstrates bilateral symmetric arterial spasm, sometimes accompanied by thrombus formation. Treatment consists of withdrawal of ergotamine preparations, hydration, heparinization, and administration of vasodilators. Oral nifedipine has been used with excellent results, and intravenous nitroprusside is effective.

Fibromuscular Dysplasia

Fibromuscular dysplasia is a heterogeneous group of arterial occlusive diseases characterized by abnormalities in the mesenchymal cells and fibrous connective tissue of the arterial wall. Most patients with fibromuscular dysplasia are women under the age of 40. The renal arteries are affected more commonly than any other artery in the body. Fibromuscular dysplasia is the second most common type of renal artery disease causing renovascular hypertension. Arterial fibrodysplasia less commonly affects the internal carotid arteries, vertebral arteries, and external iliac arteries. Fewer than 1 percent of patients undergoing carotid arteriography have fibromuscular dysplasia of the internal carotid or vertebral artery,[27] but this can cause neurologic symptoms identical to those of atherosclerotic disease. When the disease causes symptoms, surgical treatment with gradual dilation is recommended. Renal and iliac lesions are amenable to treatment by percutaneous transluminal angioplasty or surgery.

Four types of renal fibromuscular dysplasia are recognized: intimal fibroplasia, medial hyperplasia, medial fibroplasia, and perimedial dysplasia.[28] Intimal fibroplasia, accounting for 5 percent of fibromuscular disease, is most frequently encountered in infants and young adults. Angiographically, it appears as long, tubular stenoses and is characterized by subendothelial accumulations of mesenchymal cells in fibrous connective tissue. Medial hyperplasia is seen in 1 percent of cases and is characterized by an excess of medial smooth muscle cells without fibrosis. Medial fibroplasia accounts for 85 percent of dysplastic lesions and appears angiographically as a "string of beads." Disorganization of smooth muscle cells, appearance of myofibroblasts, and accumulations of excessive ground substance in the media characterize these stenotic lesions. Adjacent to such narrowings are often areas of marked medial thinning that can progress to macroaneurysms. Perimedial dysplasia makes up 10 percent of dysplastic lesions and appears as a series of stenoses without intervening aneurysms. Excessive accumulation of elastic tissue in the inner adventitia is characteristic of this lesion.

Trauma

Arterial injuries can result from penetrating or blunt trauma. Penetrating trauma includes stab wounds, gunshot wounds, or iatrogenic injuries from vessel catheterization. Blunt trauma may result in direct injury of vessels, but it commonly results in fractures or dislocations of long bones, which secondarily injure vessels. The vessels of the extremities are the most commonly injured because they are long and superficially located. When trauma occurs adjacent to a joint, vascular damage is particularly common because vessels are in a relatively fixed position and thus vulnerable to injury.

Compartment Syndrome

Compartment syndromes are due to swelling within the osteofascial compartments of the leg or arm, which causes increased intracompartmental pressure and results in decreased vascular perfusion. This most commonly occurs with revascularization after prolonged ischemia, particularly that subsequent to arterial trauma or emboli. However, compartment syndromes may develop spontaneously or as a result of external compression or bleeding within the compartment. When the pressure of the compartment exceeds capillary perfusion pressure, nutritive blood flow to the tissues is compromised. This usually occurs with intracompartmental pressures over 30-40 mm Hg, but it may occur at lower intracompartmental pressures in the face of hypotension. Nerves appear to be most susceptible to ischemia-induced injury, with muscle necrosis occurring later. Clinical findings include paresthesias, pain (especially with passive movement of the muscle), weakness of the involved muscle, and tenseness of the compartment. Loss of pulses is a very late sign. The diagnosis is made on clinical grounds, but it may be confirmed by measuring compartment pressures. Fasciotomy is the appropriate treatment.

Arterial Infection

Arterial infection may result from a variety of processes.[29] Bacterial endocarditis may produce septic emboli that can lodge in normal arteries, resulting in infection followed by weakening of the arterial wall and aneurysm formation. A local abscess may spread to an adjacent arterial wall, causing its destruction and pseudoaneurysm formation. Trauma to the artery with concomitant contamination may also result in an infected pseudoaneurysm. Finally, during an episode of bacteremia, microorganisms may lodge in an atherosclerotic plaque or aneurysm, where they begin to multiply.

The bacteriology of arterial infections varies with the type of process. Cultures of arterial lesions secondary to bacterial endocarditis most often grow pneumococci or *Streptococcus*, *Enterococcus*, *Staphylococcus*, *Escherichia coli*, or *Proteus* organisms.[30] *Staphylococcus* and members of the family Enterobacteriaceae are the bacteria encountered most commonly in peripheral mycotic aneurysms that are not associated with bacterial endocarditis. Infected aortic aneurysms most frequently grow staphylococci or salmonella.[31,32] *Salmonella* appears to have a predilection for atherosclerotic arterial walls, particularly in the abdominal aorta. Syphilitic aneurysms and tuberculous aneurysms were common before antibiotic therapy but are rarely seen today.

Compression Syndrome

Several arterial compression syndromes in which the artery is compressed by an abnormal muscle or fibrous band have been described. The most common is the thoracic outlet syndrome, in which the brachial plexus, subclavian artery, or subclavian vein is compressed or irritated as it passes between the first rib and the clavicle. Patients who develop this syndrome often have congenital anomalies, such as a cervical rib or an abnormal fibrous band resulting in a narrow thoracic outlet. Callus formation after clavicular fracture may also result in narrowing of the thoracic outlet with resultant compression syndrome. Symptoms most commonly result from irritation of the brachial plexus (90-95 percent of cases), and less often from compression of the artery or vein (less than 5 percent of cases).[33] Physical therapy and other conservative treatments should be tried before operative intervention in patients with neurogenic symptoms only.

A second compression syndrome is popliteal artery entrapment, in which the artery is compressed by the medial head of the gastrocnemius muscle or by fibrous bands. The popliteal artery may have an abnormal location, deviating medially around a normal medial head of the gastrocnemius muscle (50 percent); the attachment of the medial head of the gastrocnemius muscle may be lateral to its normal location (25 percent); or muscle slips of the medial head of the gastrocnemius muscle may compress the artery. Popliteal entrapment syndrome is most commonly encountered in young men, but it has been diagnosed in older patients and is bilateral in approximately one third of the cases. Repeated trauma to the popliteal artery may result in the development of atherosclerosis, aneurysms, or thrombus and embolization.

Patients with popliteal entrapment present with symptomatic arterial occlusion or intermittent claudication. Active plantar flexion of the foot while the knee is extended, or passive dorsiflexion of the foot, may diminish pulses or alter waveforms. The diagnosis is confirmed on angiography by medial deviation of the popliteal artery or at the time of surgical intervention. In any patient in whom the diagnosis is made, operative therapy should be undertaken to divide the offending muscle band if the artery is patent and free of disease or to bypass the artery if stenosis, occlusion, or aneurysm is present.

Another arterial compression syndrome has been called the adductor canal compression syndrome. The distal superficial femoral artery is compressed by the tendinous insertion of the adductor magnus onto the femur or by an abnormal musculotendinous band arising from the adductor magnus.[34] Treatment involves division of the tendon, with arterial reconstruction if necessary.

Radiation Arteritis

Irradiation of vascular tissue in the treatment of malignant disease causes endothelial damage, with altered permeability, inflammatory changes, and thrombosis of small vessels.[35] Larger vessels develop intimal thickening, proliferation of smooth muscle cells, degenerative changes in the media, and inflammatory infiltration of the adventitia. Segmental or diffuse narrowing, fibrotic occlusion, and atherosclerotic changes are common consequences of radiation therapy and may develop years after irradiation. Surgical therapy is complicated by the dense periarterial fibrous tissue.

Cystic Adventitial Disease

Cystic adventitial disease is an unusual condition in which a cyst filled with mucinous material forms in the adventitia or subadventitial layer of the vessel wall. The condition most commonly affects males and most frequently involves the popliteal artery, but it may occur in other arteries and even in veins.[36] The cause of adventitial cystic disease is not known, but the condition may represent a true ganglion or result from mucin-secreting cells retained within the arterial wall. Treatment by evacuation or enucleation of the cyst is effective.

Congenital Conditions

Congenital anomalies of the arterial system are many and varied and include duplication anomalies, agenesis, hypoplasia, and anomalous courses. An abnormal origin of the right subclavian artery is the most common congenital anomaly of the aortic arch, and such anomalous arteries seem to have an increased incidence of aneurysm formation.[37] Aortic coarctation, a congenital narrowing or stricture of the aorta, most commonly affects a short segment of the thoracic aorta in the region of the isthmus but may involve the abdominal aorta. Patients with aortic coarctation may have hypertension or manifestations of lower-extremity ischemia.

Hypoplasia of the aortoiliac system, characterized by an unusually small caliber of these arteries, is occasionally encountered in patients with lower-extremity ischemic symptoms and seems to have a particular predilection for women.[38] These women are frequently heavy smokers and present at a relatively early age, usually in their early 40s.

Arteriomegaly, an unusual form of arterial disease characterized by excessively large arteries, is identified in 5 percent of arteriograms.[39] The cause and natural history are poorly understood, but arteriomegaly seems to represent a variant of atherosclerosis that appears at an earlier age. Histologic examination of the arterial wall shows fragmentation of the internal elastic membrane and loss of elastic tissue in the media. Arteriography demonstrates large, tortuous arteries, with associated aneurysm formation in 30-66 percent of the patients. The high incidence of thrombotic and embolic complications justifies surgical treatment of these aneurysms, although reconstructive procedures are often complex.

Fetal arteries may persist into adulthood. For example, the sciatic artery, which is present in the embryo but is normally replaced by the femoral artery, may persist into adulthood, traveling through the sciatic foramen and connecting distally to the popliteal artery. The superficial femoral artery may be normal or hypoplastic in such patients, whereas the persistent sciatic artery seems to have a propensity for aneurysmal degeneration.[40]

Congenital arteriovenous fistulae and malformations range from capillary hemangiomas, which usually regress in early childhood, to large arteriovenous connections, causing bony and soft-tissue hypertrophy, distal ischemic changes, and varicosities and ulceration secondary to chronic venous insufficiency. Congenital arteriovenous fistulae are equally distributed between men and women and affect the lower extremity more frequently than the upper extremity. Treatment of simple cutaneous hemangiomas consists of observation because most will regress. Conservative therapy is advocated for large congenital arteriovenous fistulae because of the low incidence of cardiac problems and because of their refractoriness to surgical therapy, which is due to the multitude of arteriovenous connections.

Other congenital arterial disorders include isolated aneurysms caused by a localized defect in the elastic tissue and aneurysms associated with disorders of connective tissue metabolism. Cystic medial necrosis, a condition characterized by hyaline degeneration of the media and manifested by aortic dissection and spontaneous arterial rupture, may result from a variety of metabolic conditions that alter the composition and structure of collagen, elastin, or mucopolysaccharide ground substance, causing a generalized weakening of the arterial wall. Patients with Marfan's syndrome have premature degeneration of vascular elastic tissue, manifested by mitral valvular insufficiency, aortic dissection, and aortic aneurysms. These complications lead to death by the age of 32 in 50 percent of the patients.[41] Another group of disorders affecting vessel wall strength is Ehlers-Danlos syndrome, which is characterized by defects in collagen production. The type IV variety is known as the "arterial" type because defective synthesis of one type of collagen causes decreased strength of major vessels, resulting in the formation of true and false aneurysms and arteriovenous fistulae, spontaneous arterial ruptures, and dissections. Neurofibromatosis has been associated with a variety of vascular disorders, including renal artery stenosis, abdominal aortic coarctation, and aneurysm formation.

Homocystinemia is an inborn error of metabolism with a deficiency of the enzyme cystathionine synthetase, which results in elevated blood levels of homocystine. These patients have rapidly progressive atherosclerosis.

Inherited deficiencies of certain circulating inhibitors of clotting factors may result in repeated episodes of arterial and, particularly, venous thromboses. A deficiency of antithrombin III has been related to recurrent episodes of venous thromboembolism and arterial thromboses. A deficiency of protein C, an enzyme that, when activated, functions as an anticoagulant by inactivating factors V and VIII, is also associated with recurrent thromboses.[42] A deficiency in protein S, another antithrombotic plasma protein that serves as a cofactor for protein C, predisposes to recurrent venous thromboses.

Hyperviscosity Syndromes

A variety of conditions can cause increased blood viscosity, which may lead to venous thrombosis or occlusion of digital vessels. These include polycythemia vera with an increased hematocrit value, elevated fibrinogen levels, myeloma, cryoglobulinemia, myeloid metaplasia, macroglobulinemia, and leukemia.

CONCLUSION

Blood vessels, once believed to passively carry blood to the various organs and collect it for redistribution, are now recognized as a separate organ system. The arteries are susceptible to diseases, like other organs, but given their ubiquitous nature, the clinical presentations are quite varied. Atherosclerotic occlusive disease and aneurysmal disease make up the largest group of arteriopathies, but many other less common forms of vessel disease exist. With a clearer understanding of the various diseases, we will be more effective at managing and treating patients who suffer from arterial disease.

REFERENCES

1. Furchgott RF, Zawadzki JV: The obligatory role of endothelial cells in the relaxation of arterial smooth muscle by acetylcholine, *Nature* 288(5798):373-376, 1980.
2. Braunwald E: Shattuck lecture—cardiovascular medicine at the turn of the millennium: triumphs, concerns, and opportunities, *N Engl J Med* 337(19):1360-1369, 1997.
3. Wolinsky H, Glagov S: Comparison of abdominal and thoracic aorta medial structure in mammals: deviation of man from the usual pattern, *Circ Res* 25:677-686, 1969.
4. Dobrin PB, Mrkvicka R: Failure of elastin or collagen as possible critical connective tissue alterations underlying aneurysmal dilation, *Cardiovasc Surg* 2(4):484-488, 1994.

5. McGrath MA, Verhaeghe RH, Shepherd JT: The physiology of limb blood flow. In Juergens JL, Spittell JA Jr, Fairbairn JF II, eds: *Peripheral vascular diseases*, Philadelphia, 1980, WB Saunders, pp 83-105.
6. Allen BT, Anderson CB, Walker WB et al: Vascular surgery. In Levin ME, O'Neal LW et al, eds: *The diabetic foot*, ed 5, St Louis, 1993, Mosby, pp 385-422.
7. Lederle FA, Johnson GR, Wilson SE et al: Prevalence and associations of abdominal aortic aneurysm detected through screening, *Ann Intern Med* 126:441-449, 1997.
8. Zarins CK, Glagov S: Aneurysms and obstructive plaques: differing local response to atherosclerosis. In Bergan JJ, Yao JST, eds: *Aneurysms: diagnosis and treatment*, New York, 1982, Grune and Stratton, pp 61-82.
9. Oluwole BO, Du W, Mills I et al: Gene regulation by mechanical forces, *Endothelium* 5:85-93, 1997.
10. Gimbrone MA Jr, Resnick N, Nagel T et al: Hemodynamics, endothelial gene expression, and atherogenesis, *Ann N Y Acad Sci* 811:1-10, 1997.
11. Olin JW, Young JR, Graor RA et al: The changing clinical spectrum of thromboangiitis obliterans (Buerger's disease), *Circulation* 82(suppl IV):IV3-IV8, 1990.
12. Abou-Zamzam AM, Edwards JM, Porter JM: Nonatherosclerotic vascular disease. In Moore WS, ed: *Vascular surgery: a comprehensive review*, ed 5, Philadelphia, 1998, WB Saunders, pp 111-145.
13. McPherson JR, Juergens JL, Gifford RW Jr: Thromboangiitis obliterans and arteriosclerosis obliterans: clinical and prognostic differences, *Ann Intern Med* 59:288-296, 1963.
14. Joyce JW, Hollier LH: The giant cell arteritides: temporal and Takayasu's arteritis. In Bergan JJ, Yao JST, eds: *Evaluation and treatment of upper and lower extremity circulatory disorders,* New York, 1984, Grune & Stratton, pp 465-481.
15. Lupi-Herrera E, Torres GS, Marcushamer J et al: Takayasu's arteritis: clinical study of 107 cases, *Am Heart J* 93(1):94-103, 1977.
16. Joyce JW: The giant cell arteritides: diagnosis and the role of surgery, *J Vasc Surg* 3(5):827-833, 1986.
17. Fortner GS, Thiele BL: Giant cell arteritis involving the carotid artery, *Surgery* 95(6):759-762, 1985.
18. Abou-Zamzam AM, Edwards JM, Porter JM: Nonatherosclerotic vascular disease. In Moore WS, ed: *Vascular surgery: a comprehensive review*, ed 5, Philadelphia, 1998, WB Saunders, pp 111-145.
19. Vazquez JJ, San Martin P, Barbado FJ et al: Angiographic findings in systemic necrotizing vasculitis, *Angiology* 32(11):773-779, 1981.
20. Kawasaki T, Kosaki F, Okawa S et al: A new infantile acute febrile mucocutaneous lymph node syndrome (MLNS) prevailing in Japan, *Pediatrics* 54(3):271-276, 1974.
21. Cogan DG: Syndrome of nonsyphilitic interstitial keratitis and vestibuloauditory symptoms, *Arch Ophthalmol* 33:144-149, 1945.
22. Little AG, Zarins CK: Abdominal aortic aneurysm and Behçet's disease, *Surgery* 91(3):359-362, 1982.
23. Citron BP, Halpern M, McCarron M et al: Necrotizing angiitis associated with drug abuse, *N Engl J Med* 283(19):1003-1011, 1970.
24. Porter JM, Edwards JM: Occlusive and vasospastic diseases involving distal upper extremity arteries—Raynaud's syndrome. In Rutherford RB, ed: *Vascular surgery*, ed 4, Philadelphia, 1995, WB Saunders, pp 961-976.
25. Porter JM, Taylor LM: Limb ischemia caused by small artery disease, *World J Surg* 7(3):326-333, 1983.
26. Dagher FJ, Pais SO, Richards W et al: Severe unilateral ischemia of the lower extremity caused by ergotamine: treatment with nifedipine, *Surgery* 97(3):369-373, 1985.
27. Corrin LS, Sadok BA, Houser OW: Cerebral ischemic events in patients with carotid artery fibromuscular dysplasia, *Arch Neurol* 38(10):616-618, 1981.
28. Stanley JC, Gewertz BL, Bove EL et al: Arterial fibrodysplasia: histopathologic character and current etiologic concepts, *Arch Surg* 110(5):561-566, 1975.
29. Anderson CB, Butcher HR Jr, Ballinger WF: Mycotic aneurysms, *Arch Surg* 109(5):712-717, 1974.
30. Brown SL, Busuttil RW, Baker D et al: Bacteriologic and surgical determinants of survival in patients with mycotic aneurysms, *J Vasc Surg* 1(4):541-547, 1984.
31. Bennett DE, Cherry JK: Bacterial infection of aortic aneurysms: a clinicopathologic study, *Am J Surg* 113(3):321-326, 1967.
32. Jarrett F, Darling RC, Mundth ED et al: Experience with infected aneurysms of the abdominal aorta, *Arch Surg* 110(11):1281-1286, 1975.
33. Stoney RJ, Cheng SWK: Neurogenic thoracic outlet syndrome. In Rutherford RB, ed: *Vascular surgery*, ed 4, Philadelphia, 1995, WB Saunders, pp 976-992.
34. Verta MJ Jr, Vitello J, Fuller J: Adductor canal compression syndrome, *Arch Surg* 119(3):345-346, 1984.
35. Lawson JA: Surgical treatment of radiation induced atherosclerotic disease of the iliac and femoral arteries, *J Cardiovasc Surg (Torino)* 26(2):151-156, 1985.
36. Flanigan DP, Burnham SJ, Goodreau JJ et al: Summary of cases of adventitial cystic disease of the popliteal artery, *Ann Surg* 189(2):165-175, 1979.

37. Schmidt FE, Hewitt RL, Flores AA Jr: Aneurysms of anomalous right subclavian artery, *South Med J* 73(2):255-256, 1980.
38. DeLaurentis DA, Friedmann P, Wolferth CC Jr et al: Atherosclerosis and the hypoplastic aortoiliac system, *Surgery* 83(1):27-37, 1978.
39. Hollier LH, Stanson AW, Gloviczi P et al: Arteriomegaly: classification and morbid implications of diffuse aneurysmal disease, *Surgery* 93(5):700-708, 1983.
40. Williams LR, Flanigan DP, O'Connor RJA et al: Persistent sciatic artery: clinical aspects and operative management, *Am J Surg* 145(5):687-693, 1983.
41. Crawford ES: Marfan's syndrome: broad spectral surgical treatment of cardiovascular manifestations, *Ann Surg* 198(4):487-505, 1983.
42. Kakkar VV: Pathophysiologic characteristics of venous thrombosis, *Am J Surg* 150(4A):1-6, 1985.

2

The Venous System

SHUBHA VARMA □ PETER J. PAPPAS

In human beings, the venous system is anatomically and functionally very different from the arterial system. Anatomically, veins in the lower extremities are part of the superficial or deep venous system. Superficial veins consist of the greater (or long) and lesser (or short) saphenous veins and are located beneath the skin and above the muscles. Deep veins consist of the common femoral, femoral, profunda femoris, popliteal, three paired tibial veins (anterior, posterior, and peroneal), and communicating veins. They are surrounded by the muscles of the lower extremity and constitute the main venous outflow of the legs. Blood from the superficial veins drains into the deep veins via communicating veins known as perforators.

Unlike arteries, veins are thin-walled, low-pressure conduits whose function is to return blood from the periphery to the heart. Venous flow depends upon vein collapsibility, pressure variations with respiration, gravitational effects, and the transmitted retrograde flow due to right atrial contraction.[1] Muscular contractions in the upper and lower extremities propel blood forward, and a series of intraluminal valves prevent retrograde flow or reflux (Fig. 2-1). Venous reflux is observed when valvular destruction or dysfunction occurs. Valvular reflux causes an increase in ambulatory venous pressure and a cascade of pathologic events that manifest themselves clinically as lower-extremity edema, pain, itching, skin discoloration, varicose veins, venous ulceration, and in its severest form, limb loss. These clinical symptoms collectively refer to the disorder known as chronic venous insufficiency (CVI). Venous insufficiency affects about 15 percent of the adult population.[2]

CVI is caused by either venous outflow obstruction or valvular reflux. The most common cause of outflow obstruction is a venous thrombosis of the deep venous system. The inflammatory reaction associated with the presence of a deep vein thrombosis (DVT) causes fibrosis of the vein wall and destruction of valve leaflets. Vein wall fibrosis narrows the venous flow channel and can lead to outflow obstruction. Although lower-extremity DVTs destroy valve leaflets and can be a cause of venous reflux, over 70 percent of venous valvular dysfunction is secondary to unknown causes. Pulmonary embolism that may result from migration of the clot from the deep veins to the pulmonary artery could be fatal and is the leading cause of respiratory deaths in the United States.[3] Increasing use of subclavian vein catheterization for invasive hemodynamic monitoring, hemodialysis access, hyperalimentation, and intravenous access are common causes for upper-extremity venous thrombosis leading to swelling, pain, and extremity dysfunction.[4-7]

VENOUS ANATOMY

Microscopic Anatomy

Unlike arteries, veins are collapsible thin-walled tubes that have a circular cross section when distended and an elliptical configuration when collapsed. As in the arterial system, the vein wall is composed of a luminal intima, thin layer muscular media, and adventitia composed of loose connective tissue. The intima is lined by a single layer of endothelial cells that are in contact with the circulating blood. Production of metabolically active inhibitors of

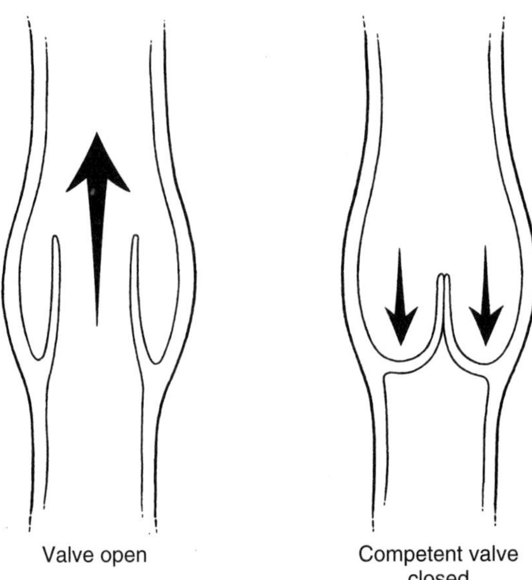

FIG. 2–1. Schematic diagram of normal venous valve in the open *(left)* and closed *(right)* positions.

coagulation such as prostacyclin, plasmin, and nitric oxide by the endothelium maintains the tone and patency of the venular system.[8]

The histologic appearance of veins depends to a large extent upon the location of the vein. Superficial veins are relatively thick walled, large, and muscular. The media is composed primarily of smooth muscle that provides architectural support and contractile properties. However, compared to the arterial system, the media of veins demonstrates fewer numbers of smooth muscle cells and fewer muscular layers. Arteries are, therefore, more contractile and function to regulate blood pressure, whereas veins are primarily capacitance vessels and sites of nutrient exchange. However, when used as a conduit for arterial bypass surgery or dialysis access, the media of veins are able to hypertrophy and develop an arterial phenotype.[9] Examples of the superficial veins are the external jugular vein of the neck, cephalic and basilic veins in the arm, and the greater and lesser saphenous veins in the leg.

Deep veins are located within the intramuscular compartments of the upper and lower extremities. They are thin walled and usually run parallel to named arteries. In the forearm and calf, these veins usually form two venous comites that lie alongside named arteries. The large spindle-shaped veins that drain blood from the calf muscle are often referred to as sinusoids because of the large lumen and almost complete absence of the smooth muscle layer.[10] These sinusoids are important physiologically as a major component of the calf muscle pump mechanism and an important storage site for blood within the body.

The most important difference between arteries and veins in addition to the composition of the media is the presence of valves in the veins. Valves are delicate bicuspid structures that are usually present at an area in the vein that is widened into a sinus. This dilated area facilitates complete opening of the valve leaflets and prompt closure of the valve when blood flow changes direction. This allows only unidirectional flow of blood back to the heart. Because flow is slower in these small recesses, most venous thrombi originate in the base of these sinuses.[11]

Generally, the more distal the vein, the greater the number of valves it contains. The iliac veins and the vena cava are valveless.[12] Valves are occasionally found in the external iliac veins and occur with increasing frequency in the common femoral, superficial femoral, popliteal, and tibial veins. In the greater saphenous vein, there are 10-20 valves, most of which are below the knee. One or two valves are present constantly at the terminal end of the greater saphenous vein just proximal to the saphenofemoral junction. The lesser saphenous vein has 6-12 valves and enters at the saphenopopliteal junction at the posterior knee crease.

Gross Anatomy (Fig. 2-2)

Deep veins usually run adjacent to the arterial circulation. The superficial veins course in the subcutaneous tissue of the extremity and have no arterial analogues. A series of veins known as communicating or perforating veins function to channel blood flow from the superficial to the deep veins.

The Lower Extremity

The thin-walled deep veins of the lower extremities begin as sinusoids within the muscles of the calf. There are two anterior tibial, posterior tibial, and peroneal veins that accompany each similarly named artery (Fig. 2-3). These veins converge at the popliteal vein. The popliteal vein becomes the femoral vein in the adductor canal of the lower thigh. The profunda femoris vein, which drains muscular branches from the thigh, joins with the superficial

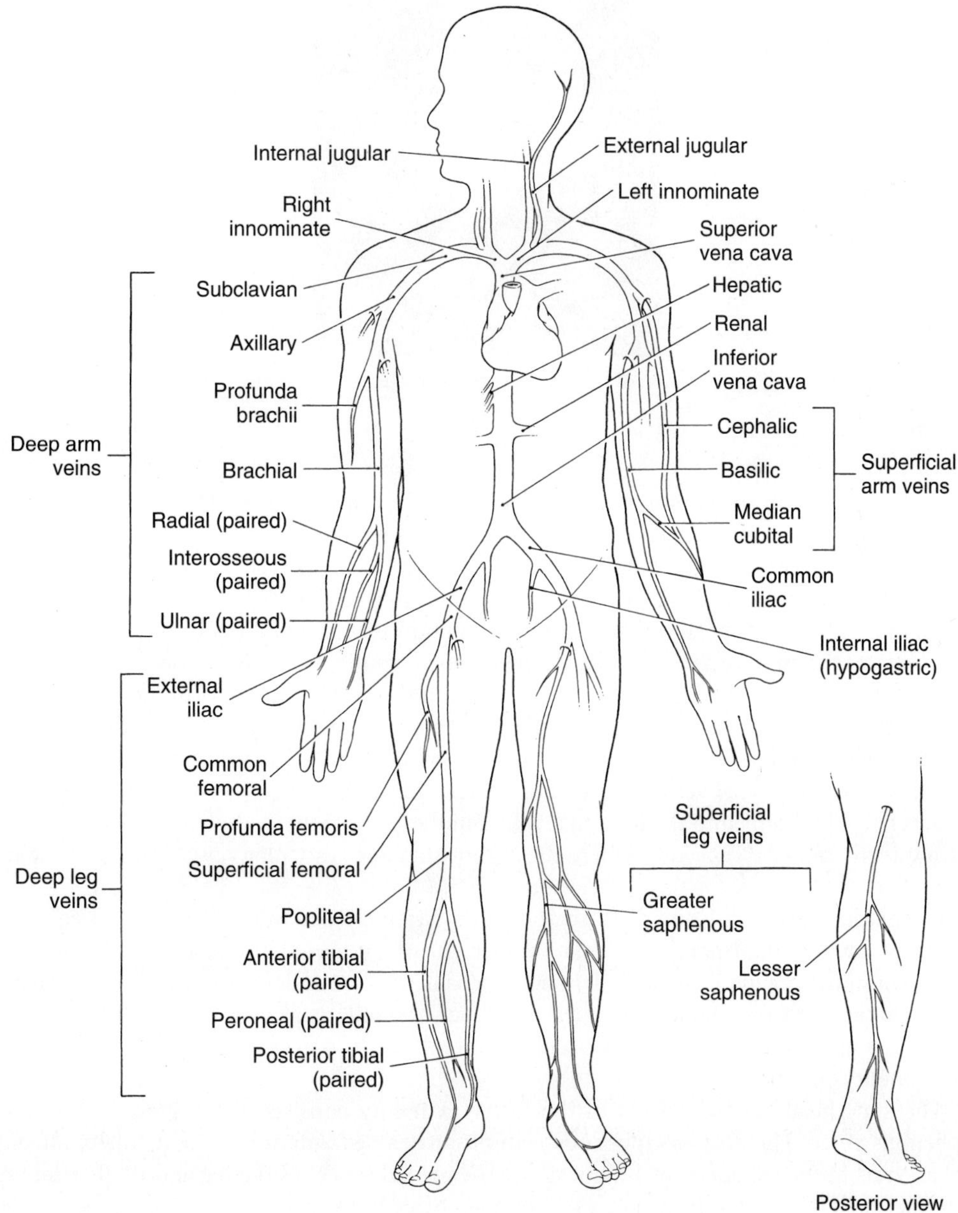

FIG. 2–2. Gross anatomy of the venous system.

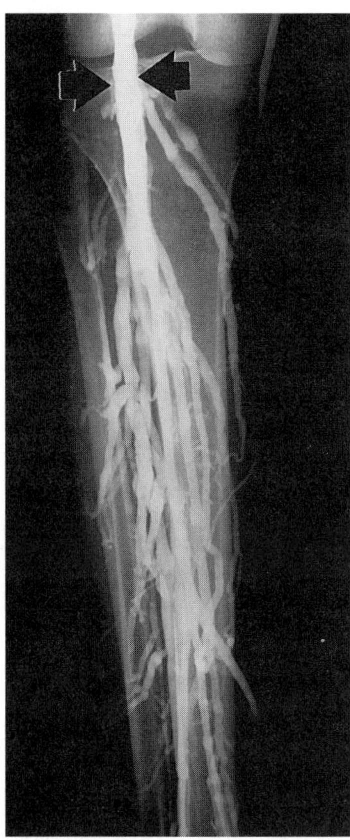

FIG. 2–3. Normal ascending venogram of the leg. The paired tibial veins empty into a single popliteal vein at the level of the knee *(arrows)*.

femoral vein to form the common femoral vein at the groin (Fig. 2-4). The common femoral vein becomes the external iliac vein above the inguinal ligament. The internal iliac vein (also called the hypogastric vein) provides venous drainage for the pelvis. The common iliac vein is formed by the confluence of the internal and the external iliac veins in the pelvis. The left common iliac vein lies posterior to the right common iliac artery. This is an area of venous compression and may be a reason why deep venous thromboses are more common on the left than on the right.[13,14] The right and the left common iliac veins join to form the inferior vena cava (Fig. 2-5). The vena cava drains numerous lumbar veins from the spine, the right and left renal veins, and several hepatic veins within the abdomen before it ascends to the right atrium. The right adrenal vein usually drains directly into the inferior vena cava, whereas the left adrenal vein drains into the left renal vein. Similarly, the right ovarian and testicular veins drain directly into the vena cava where the left ovarian and testicular veins drain into the left renal vein.

Congenital variations in venous anatomy are extremely common. Examples of common variations include dual popliteal veins (10 percent of the population), a double vena cava (1 percent of the population), and a left-sided vena cava.[14,15] Similarly, the renal vein normally crosses anterior to the abdominal aorta. However, the left renal vein can cross behind the aorta. This anatomic variation is particularly important to surgeons performing abdominal aortic aneurysm repairs.

The superficial venous system of the lower extremity consists of the greater and lesser saphenous veins. The greater saphenous vein originates just anterior to the medial malleolus and ascends in the subcutaneous tissue along the medial aspect of the leg and thigh, draining multiple small tributaries. It traverses the foramen ovale in the deep fascia of the upper medial thigh to join the common femoral vein at the saphenofemoral junction. Its subcutaneous

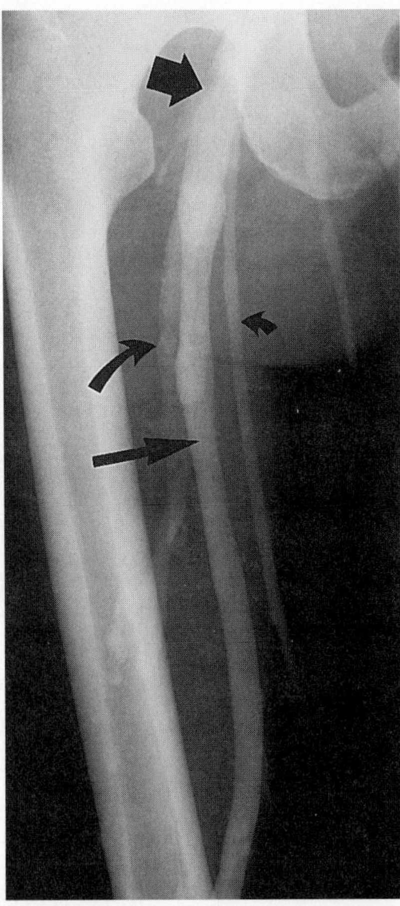

FIG. 2–4. The profunda femoris vein *(long curved arrow)* and the superficial femoral vein *(long straight arrow)* converge to create the common femoral vein *(short thick arrow)*. The greater saphenous vein is imaged medially *(small curved arrow)*.

location, exceptional length, and strong muscular wall make it an ideal conduit for coronary artery and lower-extremity arterial bypass procedures.

The lesser saphenous vein originates at the posterior border of the lateral malleolus and drains into the popliteal vein behind the knee at the saphenopopliteal junction. As with the greater saphenous vein, the lesser saphenous vein may be used as a conduit for arterial bypass. Its posterior location in the calf makes it the second conduit of choice if the greater saphenous vein is not available.

The Upper Extremity

The paired deep veins of the forearm are the radial, the ulnar, and the interosseous veins, which join to form the brachial vein at the elbow. The brachial vein becomes the axillary vein at the border of the pectoralis minor muscle in the upper arm. The axillary vein becomes the subclavian vein at the lateral border of the first rib. The subclavian vein and the internal jugular vein on the left join within the thorax to form the innominate vein. The subclavian vein on the right joins with the innominate vein on the left to form the superior vena cava (Fig. 2-6).

The primary superficial veins of the upper extremity are the cephalic and the basilic veins. The cephalic vein runs along the lateral aspect of the forearm and joins the subclavian vein after coursing through the deltopectoral groove. The basilic vein ascends medially and joins the axillary vein. A median cubital vein is a consistent large branch between the basilic and cephalic veins that runs across the antecubital fossa and is a common site of venipuncture.

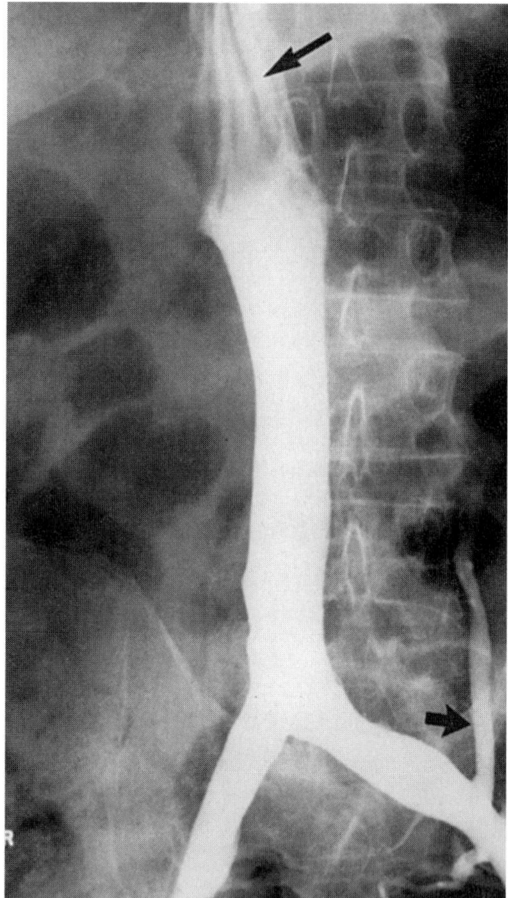

FIG. 2–5. Confluence of two common iliac arteries into the vena cava. Nonopacified blood entering from the two renal veins creates the streaming effect imaged in the suprarenal cava *(long arrow)*. Prominent left gonadal vein is also imaged *(short arrow)*.

VENOUS PHYSIOLOGY

Venous Pressure

The generally perceived notion that veins are low-pressure conduits that return blood to the heart is misleading because it does not take into account the effect of hydrostatic pressure, which may be significant at the ankle in the upright position. The dynamic pressure responsible for the forward flow of blood in the veins comes mainly from left ventricular contraction, in addition to contributions from the calf muscle pump and respiratory mechanisms. At any given site in the venous system, the pressure is equal to the sum of the dynamic pressure and the hydrostatic pressure—the pressure of a column of blood due to gravity. Consequently, in the standing position, hydrostatic pressure greatly exceeds dynamic pressure and acts to impede venous return. Because the hydrostatic pressure is equal on the arteries and the veins, the pressure differential across the capillary remains the same and blood continues to flow towards the heart.

With the supine position, gravitational forces are eliminated and venous flow primarily changes in response to abdominal and thoracic pressure variations induced by respiratory effort.[16] During inspiration, the abdominal pressure is increased by the flattening of the abdominal wall muscles and the downward movement of the diaphragm. This decreases blood return from the lower extremities. Lower-extremity flow is augmented during exhalation, when abdominal muscles relax and intra-abdominal pressure is lowered.[11] These phasic changes are easily detected with a Doppler ultrasound device at the level of the femoral vein.

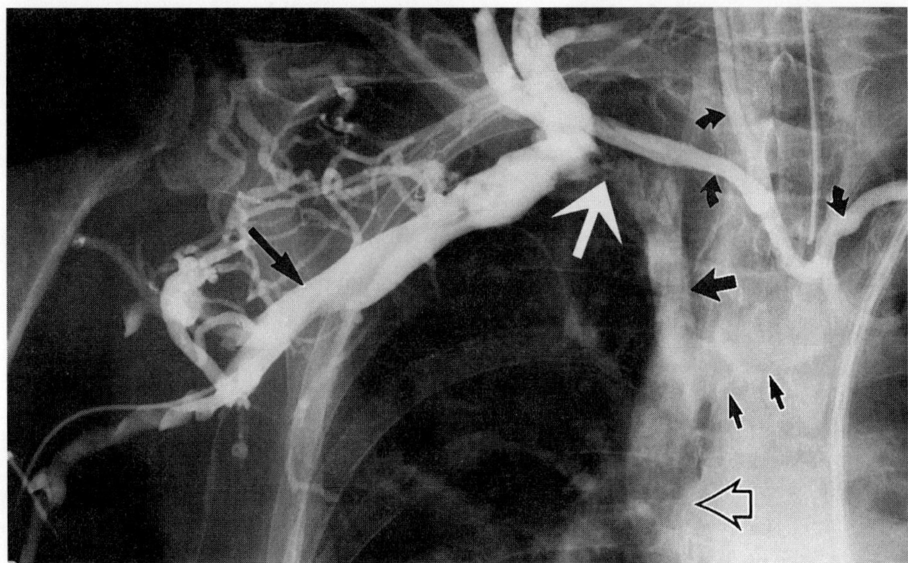

FIG. 2–6. Right upper extremity venogram. The axillary vein *(long thin arrow)*, subclavian vein *(white arrow)*, and right innominate vein *(heaviest arrow)* are imaged. The obstruction in the right subclavian vein (imaged at the tip of the white arrow) has resulted in the filling of collateral veins *(small curved arrows)*, which cross the midline to fill the left innominate vein *(two small arrows)*. The superior vena cava is formed by confluence of two innominate veins *(open arrow)*.

With the increased resistance associated with venous obstruction, venous pressure rises above the intra-abdominal pressure, and flow becomes continuous. This is one of the criteria by which deep venous thrombosis may be detected.

Venous Volume and Compliance

The volume of blood contained in a venous segment is controlled by the transmural pressure. Transmural pressure refers to the pressure difference between the lumen and the interstitium. When the transmural pressure is low, the veins are nearly collapsed and assume an elliptical cross section. At higher pressures, the vein becomes full and the cross section becomes circular. When an individual shifts to a standing position from a supine position, the increased hydrostatic pressure causes the transmural pressure to rise from about 10 mm Hg to about 100 mm Hg in the lower leg. Venous volume increases by about 2-3 percent, reflecting a transfer of about 500 ml of blood from the central circulation to the legs. This is the basis on which orthostatic hypotension occurs in patients who are hypovolemic. This is also the reason why simple maneuvers, such as raising the legs in a patient with hypovolemic shock, result in a significant increase in circulating blood volume. In the supine postoperative patient, the application of antiembolism stockings increases tissue pressures by about 15 mm Hg and decreases transmural pressures. This results in a decrease in venous volume, collapse of the underlying veins, and an increased flow velocity with a theoretical reduction in the incidence of venous thrombosis. This also explains the usefulness of antiembolism stockings in the supine patient and not in patients who are sitting or standing.

Even though the veins and the arteries are charged with carrying the same volume of blood, the cross sectional area of the veins is potentially three to four times that of the arteries. Another difference between the veins and the arteries is that the pressure and volume of a venous segment decrease when the flow is increased and increase when there is venous stasis. In arteries, pressure volume and flow change in the same direction. In a recumbent patient at rest, the pressure difference between the venules and the right atrium is the same as the pressure difference between aortic root and the terminal arteries, which is about 15 mm Hg. This peripheral venous pressure stays relatively stable despite wide fluctuations in venous volume, as seen with massive intravenous transfusions, or severe volume depletion, as in dehydration. However, with calf muscle contraction, pressures in excess of 200 mm Hg can be generated, which provide sufficient driving force for venous return.[17] This is because of its high compliance, a property that enables the vein to increase intravascular volume with minimal changes in venous pressure.[18]

Control of Venous Capacitance

The venous system is richly supplied with sympathetic nerves that constrict with adrenergic stimuli.[19] This facilitates thermoregulation by allowing the hypothalamus to direct sympathetic stimulation to the cutaneous veins, which constrict and redirect blood flow into the deep venous system and reduce heat loss to the environment. However, under comfortable ambient temperatures the resting tone of the veins is minimal as compared with arteries and arterioles, which always remain partially constricted.

The deep veins within skeletal muscle have no sympathetic innervation and play no role in thermoregulation. The splanchnic venous bed and the cutaneous veins can be constricted by circulating catecholamines.[19] Generally, veins constrict in response to all stimuli that increase cardiac output such as epinephrine, norepinephrine, phenylephrine, serotonin, and histamine.[16,19] Pain, emotion, deep breathing, hyperventilation exercise, and hemorrhage are some of the other stimuli that may cause venous constriction. This decrease in venous volume after a deep breath is the basis for assessing the function of the sympathetic nerve supply of an extremity by plethysmography. Exercise-induced venoconstriction aids the calf pump in shifting the blood to the central circulation, where it is needed to maintain a higher cardiac output. The intramuscular sinusoids constitute the major bellows of the calf muscle pump and do not constrict with exercise.

Venous dilatation is seen in response to barbiturates, reserpine, guanethidine, nitroglycerin, nitroprusside, phenoxybenzamine, phentolamine, and many anesthetic agents.[16] In the volume-depleted patient, this may lead to sudden intraoperative hypotension during induction of anesthesia.

PATHOPHYSIOLOGY

Venous pathology is usually due either to obstruction of flow or venous valvular insufficiency.[9,20] Other clinical conditions involving the venous system are trauma and tumors. Management of traumatic venous injuries is complicated and beyond the scope of discussion here. However, one thing that is very clear about traumatic injuries is that venous repair is vitally important in extremity replantation following traumatic amputation. Tumors may involve the venous system either by extrinsic compression or by intramural spread. Primary tumors of the venous system are infrequently encountered and will not be discussed here.

Venous Obstruction

The clinical manifestations of venous obstruction, including venous distention and edema, are due to venous hypertension. Most commonly this occurs because of formation of thrombus within the deep venous system. Clinical sequelae and the development of venous hypertension are related to the degree, location, length, and chronicity of obstruction. Nonocclusive thrombi in the major deep veins cause very little changes in venous resistance and remain clinically silent until they embolize into the pulmonary artery, resulting in a pulmonary embolus.[21-23] More distal DVT typically presents with leg swelling, dilated superficial veins, and calf and thigh tenderness.

The physiologic consequences of venous obstruction in the leg are due to venous hypertension, secondary to increased venous resistance. Because of abundant collateral channels, chronic and isolated venous obstruction seldom alters venous resistance appreciably. Superficial venous thrombosis usually presents with local signs such as erythema, induration, and tenderness, and most calf vein thrombi are asymptomatic. Acute, extensive DVT often increases venous resistance significantly. For this reason, acute ileofemoral vein thrombosis, which blocks venous drainage not only from the profunda femoris and femoral veins but also from the greater saphenous vein, has a much more dramatic clinical presentation. In the supine patient, venous pressures are 8-18 mm Hg when clots are confined to the below-knee veins, 20-51 mm Hg when the femoral vein is involved, and 32-83 mm Hg in cases with ileofemoral vein thrombosis.[24] Occasionally, the rapid increase in venous pressure may obstruct arterial flow, leading to gangrene. This entity, known as phlegmasia cerulea dolens, is both a limb- and life-threatening condition.[13]

The musculovenous pump increases venous return to the heart during exercise. The emptying of the deep venous system and prevention of retrograde flow during relaxation by competent valves maintains low venous pressure and a high flow system. Venous pressure at the ankle, typically 80-90 mm Hg, is rapidly decreased to 20 mm Hg or less by walking as few as five steps[11] (Fig. 2-7).

The usual exercise-induced fall in venous pressure is absent in the setting of an acute DVT.[25] Chronic venous hypertension may result from associated valvular incompetence and venous insufficiency. Engorged collateral veins may occasionally be visible. Swelling also results from edema formation as fluid leaks from the high-pressure capillaries into the interstitial spaces.

With the increasing use of invasive hemodynamic monitoring, total parenteral nutrition (TPN), and hemodialysis access catheters, upper-extremity DVT is being encountered more commonly, although less frequently than lower-extremity DVT.[4-6] Other predisposing factors that may cause upper-extremity DVT are the presence of a cervical rib or muscular band that causes venous compression, or effort thrombosis. Although upper-extremity DVT is only occasionally associated with pulmonary embolization,[26] it does lead to a high incidence of late sequelae of arm swelling and discomfort with exercise.[6]

Venous Valvular Insufficiency

During calf muscle contraction, blood flows toward the heart in the deep as well as the superficial system. However, when the muscles relax, blood flows retrograde in the superficial system and enters the deep venous system through perforators. Flow of blood in the reverse direction does not occur when the venous valves are competent.

In patients with valvular incompetence and CVI, blood pools in the superficial as well as the deep venous systems. The postexercise reduction in venous pressures does not occur, and most of the changes related to valvular incompetence are due to the associated venous hypertension.

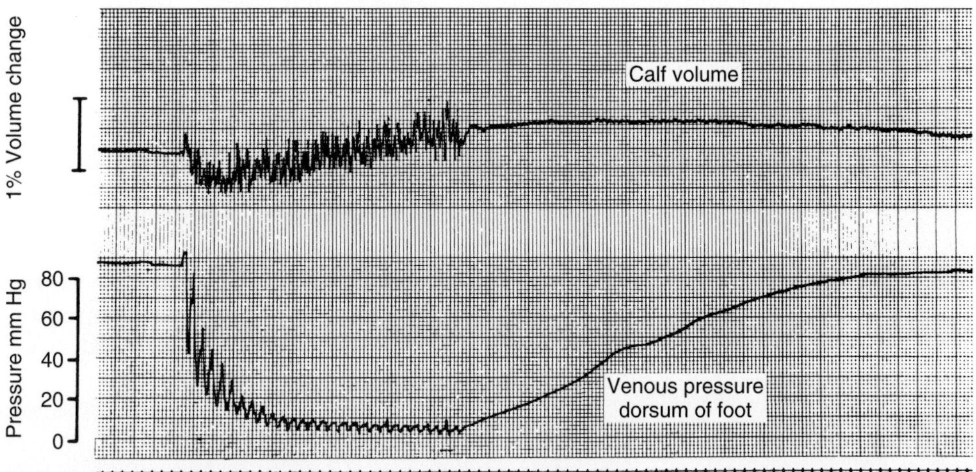

FIG. 2–7. The musculovenous pump mechanism is responsible for the normal decrease in venous pressure associated with exercise. (From Strandness DE Jr, Sumner DS: *Hemodynamics for surgeons,* New York, 1975, Grune & Stratton.)

Resolution of thrombosis with recanalization of the venous lumen occurring in the vast majority of cases[16,27] of DVT renders the valves of the perforators and deep veins permanently incompetent. The unidirectional flow pattern across these valves is usually irreversibly destroyed by the inflammatory reaction of the thrombotic process[13,16] (Fig. 2-8). This process is further exaggerated by a variable element of associated venous obstruction due to the presence of residual bands and webs within the lumen. Because of the obstruction and valvular incompetence of the deep venous system and perforators, blood flows into the superficial system from the deep venous system as a means to provide collateral venous drainage. This results in the formation of varicosities. As pressure in the superficial veins increases, they begin to dilate and this causes the valves within them to become incompetent, making the whole process worse.

Patients with primary varicose veins have incompetent valves of the deep and superficial systems in the absence of previous episodes of DVT. Primary valvular reflux is the most common cause of CVI and the primary cause of varicose vein development. These varicosities usually involve the greater saphenous system but approximately 12 percent of the time involve the lesser saphenous vein.

Primary valvular insufficiency may be due to congenital absence of the valves in the common femoral vein and external iliac vein.[12] This causes increased venous hydrostatic pressure cephalad to the most proximal saphenous valve, resulting in venous dilatation with loss of coaptation of the valve leaflets, resulting in reflux.[2] Other authors have implicated an abnormally distensible vein wall that results in abnormal valvular function.[16] Hormonal as well as mechanical factors may increase venous pressure and distention that result in the venous valvular incompetence and varicosities associated with pregnancy.[13]

Continuous columns of blood extending from the ankles to the heart in the superficial and deep systems result in massive increase in venous pressure. This increased venous pressure is transmitted to the capillaries in the subcutaneous tissues, which results in exudation of plasma and red cells into the interstitium. With time, the protein organizes, the red cells degenerate, and the tissues become hyperpigmented. Such thickened, pigmented, usually hot red and tender skin is referred to as lipodermatosclerosis. Dermal tissue fibrosis in patients with CVI is associated with increased transforming growth factor-β1 gene expression and protein production.[28] These changes are most commonly seen just proximal to the ankle where the venous hypertension is the greatest. Minor trauma results in the formation of venous ulcers, typically seen proximal to the medial malleolus, overlying the ankle perforators.

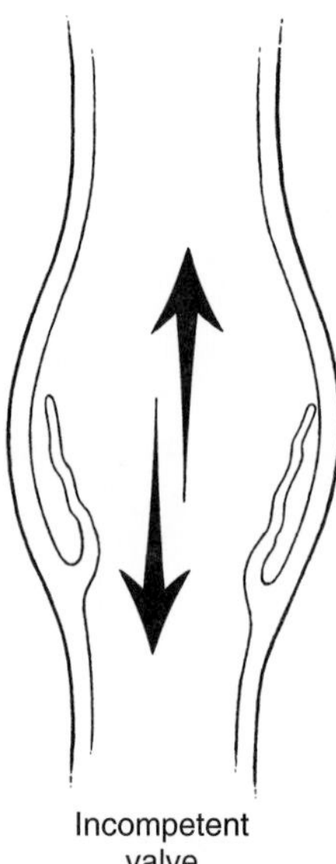

FIG. 2–8. An incompetent valve is unable to prevent retrograde flow of blood.

Patients with primary valvular insufficiency and postphlebitic veins fail to show the characteristic exercise-induced emptying of the deep veins and the associated pressure drop. High venous pressures and massive increases in venous volume in the presence of obstructed venous flow and venous valvular incompetence may occasionally present with a severe bursting kind of calf pain often referred to as venous claudication.[29]

REFERENCES

1. Strandness DE: Applied venous physiology in normal subjects and venous insufficiency. In Bergan JJ, Yao JST, eds: *Venous problems*, Chicago, 1976, Year Book, pp 25-45.
2. Crane C: The surgery of varicose veins, *Surg Clin North Am* 59:737-748, 1979.
3. Wolfe WG, Sabiston DC Jr: *Pulmonary embolism*, Philadelphia, 1980, WB Saunders.
4. Hoffman MJ, Greenfield LJ: Central venous septic thrombosis managed by superior vena cava Greenfield filter and venous thrombectomy: a case report, *J Vasc Surg* 4:606-611, 1986.
5. Warden GD, McDouglas WM, Pruitt BA: Central venous thrombosis: a hazard of medical progress, *J Trauma* 13:620-626, 1973.
6. Tilney NA, Griffith MD, Edwards EA: The natural history of major venous thrombosis of the upper extremity, *Arch Surg* 101:792-796, 1970.
7. Gloviczki P, Kazmier FJ, Hollier LH: Axillary-subclavian venous occlusion: the morbidity of a nonlethal disease, *J Vasc Surg* 4:333-337, 1986.
8. Shimokawa H, Takeshita A: Endothelium-dependent regulation of the cardiovascular system, *Intern Med* 34:939-946, 1995.
9. Hallet JW Jr, Brewster DC, Darling RC: *Manual of patient care in vascular surgery,* Boston, 1982, Little, Brown & Co.
10. Ludbrook J: Applied physiology of the veins. In Dodd H, Cockett FB, eds: *The pathology and surgery of the veins of the lower limb,* Edinburgh, 1976, Churchill Livingstone, pp 50-55.
11. McCarthy WJ, Fahey VA, Bergan JJ et al: The veins and venous disease. In Corry RJ, Perry JF (eds): *Principles of basic surgical practice,* Philadelphia, 1987, Hanley & Belfus, pp 453-466.
12. Basmajian JV: Distribution of valves in femoral, external iliac and common iliac veins and their relationship to varicose veins, *Surg Gynecol Obstet* 95:537-542, 1952.
13. Sumner DS: Venous anatomy and pathophysiology. In Hershey FB, Barnes RW, Sumner DS, eds: *Noninvasive diagnosis of vascular disease,* Pasadena, 1984, Appleton Davis, Inc, pp 88-102.
14. Dodd H, Cockett FB: The surgical anatomy of the veins of the lower limb. In Dodd H, Cockett FB, eds: *The pathology and surgery of the veins of the lower limb,* Edinburgh, 1976, Churchill Livingstone, pp 18-49.
15. Giordana JM, Trout HH III: Anomalies of the inferior vena cava, *J Vasc Surg* 3:924-928, 1986.
16. Sumner DS: Hemodynamics and pathophysiology of venous disease. In Rutherford RB, ed: *Vascular surgery*, ed 4, Philadelphia, 1995, WB Saunders, pp 1673-1698.
17. Ludbrook J: The musculovenous pumps of the human lower limb, *Am Heart J* 71:635-641, 1966.
18. Moneta GL, Bedford G, Beach K et al: Duplex ultrasound assessment of venous diameters, peak velocities, and flow patterns, *J Vasc Surg* 8:286-291, 1988.
19. Shepard JT: Reflex control of the venous system. In Bergan JJ, Yao JST, eds: *Venous problems,* Chicago, 1976, Year Book, pp 5-23.
20. Kistner RL: Diagnosis of venous insufficiency, *J Vasc Surg* 3:185-188, 1986.
21. Wheeler HB, Rohrer MJ: Diagnosing and preventing venous thromboembolism, *J Respir Dis* 9:25-40, 1988.
22. Haeger K: Problems of acute venous thrombosis: 1. The interpretation of signs and symptoms, *Angiology* 20:219-223, 1969.
23. Heijbuer H, Ten Cate JW, Buller HR: Diagnosis of venous thrombosis, *Semin Thromb Hemost* 17(suppl 3):259-268, 1991.
24. De Weese JA, Rogoff SM: Phlebographic patterns of acute deep venous thrombosis of the leg, *Surgery* 53:99-108, 1963.
25. Husni EA, Ximenes JOC, Goyette EM: Elastic support of the lower limbs in hospitalized patients: a critical study, *JAMA* 214:1456-1462, 1970.
26. Campbell CB, Chandler JG, Tegtmeyer CJ et al: Axillary, subclavian, and brachiocephalic venous obstruction, *Surgery* 82:816-826, 1977.
27. Killewich LA, Bedford GR, Beach KW et al: Spontaneous lysis of deep venous thrombi: rate and outcome, *J Vasc Surg* 9:89-97, 1989.
28. Pappas PJ, You R, Rameshwar P et al: Dermal tissue fibrosis in patients with chronic venous insufficiency is associated with increased transforming growth, *J Vasc Surg* 30(6):1129 -1145, 1999.
29. Killewich LA, Martin R, Cramer M et al: Pathophysiology of venous claudication, *J Vasc Surg* 1:507-511, 1984.

3

Lymphedema

CINDY L. FELTY □ THOM W. ROOKE

Lymphedema, which affects more than 1 percent of the U.S. population and over 150 million people worldwide, is the swelling of a body part (often an extremity) caused by an abnormal accumulation of protein-rich fluid in the interstitial spaces. It occurs secondary to an anatomic or functional obstruction in the lymphatics or the lymph nodes.[1] Lymphedema can be a difficult and frustrating condition to treat. Because most patients cannot be helped by surgery, therapy is focused around education about the disease, elastic compression, physical therapy, drugs, hygiene, and other conservative measures. Treatment is important; without it, the condition typically worsens, leading to repeated infections, enlargement of the limb, thickening of the skin, disfigurement, and potential disability. Because of lack of understanding of the theoretical and practical aspects of lymphedema treatments by many health care professionals, suboptimal therapy is received by these patients.

ANATOMY AND PHYSIOLOGY

The lymph system is a complex network composed of fine lymphatic vessels and lymph nodes, along with other specialized structures such as spleen, thymus, and tonsils. It helps maintain water and protein balance in the tissues and assists the immune system.

Lymph is a clear, colorless fluid formed by the transudation of plasma into the tissue spaces. The composition of lymph varies depending upon its location, but it generally includes proteins and lymphocytes and may contain certain foreign substances such as bacteria. Interstitial protein is collected in lymph fluid and returned to the plasma. The lymphocyte, a white blood cell present in the lymph fluid, helps fight infection. Lymph fluid may also contain foreign substances such as bacteria or chemicals that have been removed from the tissues; these are broken down or removed by the lymph nodes located in places such as the neck, axilla, and groin.

Lymph is continually removed from the tissues in order to maintain the body's balance of fluid and protein. As edema develops, tissue pressure builds and tends to push fluid from the interstitial space into the lymph vessels. Valves located within the lymphatics ensure that the lymph flows in only one direction.[2] Small lymphatics join to form larger ones, and the biggest lymph channels eventually combine into two separate lymph ducts through which lymph fluid ultimately returns to the blood. Lymph from the upper left side and lower part of the body flows primarily into the thoracic duct, while lymph from the right side of the head, neck, chest, and right arm empties into the right lymphatic duct located in the right side of the chest. The rate of lymph flow can be increased by skeletal muscle contraction, increased heart rate, and passive movements from other body parts. The velocity of lymph flow may increase by tenfold over resting values during exercise.

PATHOPHYSIOLOGY

Lymphedema develops when the lymphatic load exceeds the transport capacity of the lymphatic system. When this occurs, the tissue becomes inundated with protein-rich edema fluid. Without treatment, the protein-rich interstitial fluid is eventually replaced by fibrous

TABLE 3–1 Stages of Lymphedema

Stage I	Stage II	Stage III
Skin pits on pressure	Nonpitting on pressure	Overproduction of connective tissue
Reduces with elevation	Not reduced by elevation alone	Hardening of the skin
None or slight fibrosis	Moderate to severe fibrosis	Elephantiasis

tissue and collagen, which can lead to progressive fibrosis and, in later stages, irreversible tissue enlargement.

Lymphedema is often described by stages (Table 3-1). The first stage, also called the reversible stage, is manifested by edema of a pitting nature. The edema is soft, and the swelling typically resolves overnight with simple elevation of the affected limb. If the lymphedema remains untreated, it produces a progressive hardening of the tissues, which occurs secondary to scarring and the proliferation of connective and/or adipose tissue. This stage of lymphedema, known as irreversible or stage II lymphedema, is manifested by edema that does not resolve with overnight elevation. At this point, the skin loses its pitting character and begins to thicken. Stage III (or lymphostatic elephantiasis) is manifested by a tremendous increase in the volume of the affected limb. The hardening of the dermal tissues and papillomas that subsequently develop can give the patient the appearance of having elephant skin (Fig. 3-1).

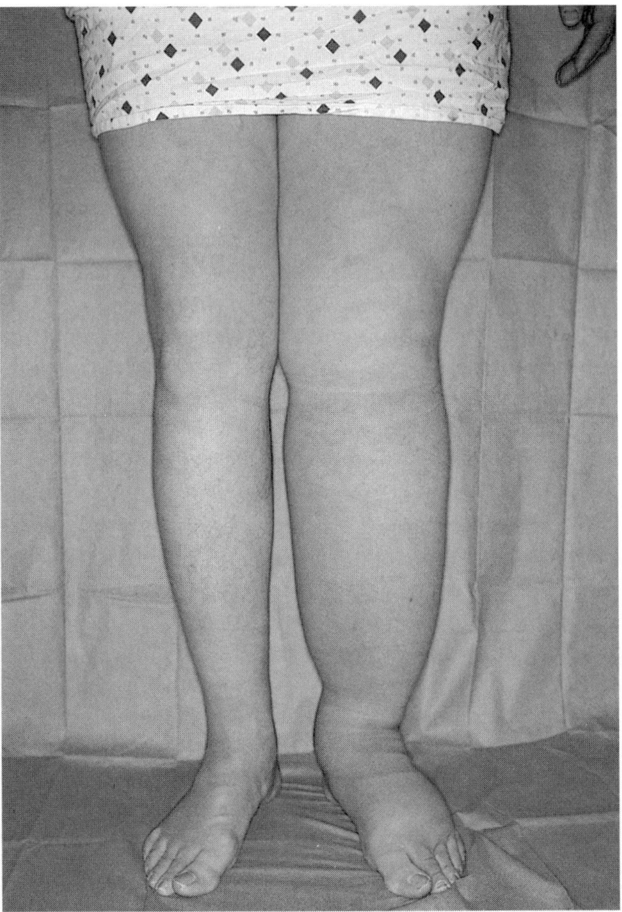

FIG. 3–1. Primary lymphedema—painless swelling of the leg and foot. The toes are involved and may appear squared when viewed on end. Stage II lymphedema does not resolve with overnight elevation of the extremity.

CLASSIFICATION

Lymphedema can be characterized as primary or secondary. Primary lymphedema occurs in the absence of any obvious cause. It is more common in females and usually occurs in the lower extremity. Primary lymphedema is thought to arise from an inborn defect in the development of lymphatic vessels. Primary lymphedema can be present at birth or may occur before the age of 1, in which case it is classified as congenital lymphedema. Lymphedema occurring between the ages of 1 and 35 is referred to as lymphedema praecox.[3] Lymphedema tarda is generally the name given to primary lymphedema occurring after the age of 35.[4] Congenital lymphedema, which occurs in a familial pattern, is referred to as Milroy's disease.[3]

Secondary lymphedema is caused by injury, scarring, or excision of the lymph nodes. It may occur as a result of surgery in which the lymph nodes are removed, or it may develop as a side effect of radiation therapy. Secondary lymphedema is occasionally caused by trauma or by chronic infections of the lymph system. Infections of the lymph system are generally bacterial in nature, with streptococci being the most common pathogen. In some parts of the world, especially in the tropics, secondary lymphedema is usually caused by parasitic infections.

EVALUATION AND DIAGNOSIS

Before treatment is initiated, the cause of the edema should be determined. The diagnosis of lymphedema can frequently be made by obtaining an accurate history and performing a good physical examination. Patients with primary lymphedema will give a history in which swelling occurs spontaneously; this may develop at birth or in association with puberty, childbirth, or a minor injury. There may also be a familial history of limb swelling. Patients exhibiting secondary lymphedema can usually describe the precipitating event such as surgery, radiation therapy, or infection.

The physical examination will typically reveal swelling with an appearance and distribution consistent with lymphedema. The patient may present with swelling of the extremity; this often starts at the ankle and may progress to involve the entire limb. It is usually painless. Examination of the extremity may reveal a square appearance to the toes, and the skin may be thick and/or the edema hard and nonpitting.[5] In addition, the skin may have a red discoloration due to recurrent episodes of lymphangitis and cellulitis. Other changes of the skin such as verrucae and small vesicles (containing clear lymph) may also be present. Ulcerations of the skin may be present in advanced cases.

There are other conditions that may mimic lymphedema or may be present in addition to lymphedema. These include congestive heart failure, venous disease, infective cellulitis, drug-induced swelling, reflex sympathetic dystrophy, tumor, lipedema, renal disease, and a host of others. The physical examination will frequently differentiate lymphedema from other entities, but occasionally the presentation is atypical enough to warrant specific testing. It is important to identify and treat the nonlymphedematous components of the limb swelling as well.[5]

For patients over 40 years of age with new-onset lymphedema, malignancy must be excluded.[5] Cancer (with or without surgery or radiation) is responsible for 94 percent of upper-extremity and 52 percent of lower-extremity secondary lymphedema.[6]

Lymphangiography has long been recognized as the gold standard test for diagnosing lymphedema. It is performed by cannulating a small lymph channel on the dorsum of the hand or foot and injecting a lipid-soluble contrast material. Unfortunately, it is possible for acute lymphangitis to result from this invasive procedure, and it should therefore be avoided whenever possible.

Lymphoscintigraphy provides a safe and simple alternative to demonstrate whether edema is of lymphatic origin. Technetium-99m labeled colloid is injected into the web spaces of the foot or hand.[7] Images are subsequently obtained as the colloid progresses along the limb (imaging is typically performed at 30 minute, 1 hour, 3 hour, and 6-hour intervals). Candidates for microvascular anastomosis may sometimes be identified using this technique.[8]

Magnetic resonance imaging (MRI) and computerized tomography (CT) can be used to distinguish some of the features of lymphedema and to evaluate possible lymphatic obstruction. MRI and CT can evaluate the subcutaneous tissue; the presence of multiple branching, nonenhancing tubular structures in an enlarged subcutaneous tissue compartment is suggestive of lymphedema.[9] The presence of mild-to-moderate skin thickening may also be helpful in the diagnosis.[10]

After the diagnosis is confirmed with a reasonable degree of certainty, the underlying cause of the lymphedema should be readdressed. One question that must be answered is whether or not lymphatic flow can be improved. Are the lymphatics obstructed by an infection or neoplastic process that might respond to antibiotics or chemotherapy? Are antiparasitic drugs indicated? Can lymphatic reconstructive surgery be performed? Unfortunately, most types of lymphedema do not have causes that are amenable to definitive therapy.

MEDICAL THERAPY

The goals of medical therapy are (1) to prevent lymphedema from occurring, or if it occurs, to treat the disease in its early stages, (2) to remove excess fluid and dissolved substances (protein) from the lymphedematous area, (3) to prevent fluid reaccumulation, (4) to maintain the limb at its smallest size possible by using the simplest methods available, (5) to avoid factors that can aggravate or worsen the edema, (6) to provide adequate information and motivation for the patient to become an active participant in the care of the lymphedematous limb, and (7) to determine the intensity of the treatment so that it matches the severity of the disease in a way that not only meets the needs and expectations of the practitioner and the patient, but also ensures that the patient will comply with the recommendations (Table 3-2).

A lymphedematous limb may be reduced using a number of methods, alone or in combination.

Bed Rest/Leg Elevation

The patient is instructed to elevate the limb to 45°, using either a foam wedge or a lymphedema sling (Fig. 3-2). Although leg elevation should ideally be maintained until the leg is fully reduced, it is unrealistic to do this in the outpatient setting. Elevation is, therefore, typically performed during the night, and during the day when possible. Leg elevation uses gravity to drain fluid from the edematous limb; the higher the limb, the greater the benefit. The limb should be wrapped whenever it is dependent in order to maintain reduction between sessions of elevation. Several days of this treatment will usually reduce all but the most resistant cases of lymphedema.

Vasopneumatic Pumps

Vasopneumatic compression pumps are an integral part of many treatment programs in the United States. The goal is to move fluid along the limb in a distal-to-proximal direction. Most pumping sessions last about 1 hour and are performed one to three times daily. Pumps can be used in either the inpatient or outpatient setting. Between sessions, the limb is wrapped to prevent reaccumulation of edema. Pumping is continued until maximum reduction of fluid is achieved, at which time maintenance therapy is initiated.

Single-Chamber

These pumps have an inflatable single-chamber sleeve, which encases the limb. During inflation, the limb is compressed at pressures of 50-100 mm Hg for 1-2 minutes. The uniform pressure forces fluid out of the limb through the remaining lymphatics.

Multichamber

These pumps use multiple-chamber sleeves, which sequentially inflate the chambers in the sleeve, causing fluid to be "milked out" of the swollen limb. These pumps may be more effective than the single-chamber pumps but are also more expensive (Fig. 3-3).

TABLE 3–2 Findings and Therapy for the Stages of Lymphedema

	Stage I	Stage II	Stage III
SKIN OF AFFECTED LIMB	Taut, stretched, warmer temperature, normal texture, pitting	Minimal changes, color, some redness, dry, flaky pitting or nonpitting	Shiny, brawny, may leak fluid from lymph, nonpitting, coarse texture, chronic redness
POTENTIAL COMPLICATIONS	Cellulitis	Recurrent cellulitis	Angiosarcoma (rare), chronic cellulitis
THERAPY			
Elevation of limb	Helpful	Helpful	Helpful
Compression pumps	Helpful but not essential	Often helpful	Usually helpful
Manual lymphatic drainage	Helpful but not essential	Often helpful	Usually helpful, may benefit from returning for additional sessions in 6 months
Compression wrap	Elastic	Nonelastic, multilayered	Nonelastic, multilayered
Compression garment	Ready-made, class I for upper extremity, class II for lower extremity	Ready-made class II-III	Custom-made, class III or 50-60 mm Hg
Exercise	Strengthening/range of motion	Increased range of motion/increased range of strengthening	Motion/flexibility
Diet	Maintain goal weight or achieve goal	Maintain or achieve goal weight	Reduce to goal weight, involve dietitian
Support	Support group, education, offer resources	Support group, education, offer resources	Support group, education, offer resources

Cardiac-Gated

These pumps use single-chamber sleeves, which inflate during a specific portion of the cardiac cycle, then deflate during the rest of the cardiac cycle. The pressure exerted by these sleeves is typically 50-100 mm Hg. The cardiac-gated pumps are effective at treating lymphedema but usually require a trained person to operate them. They may cost $10,000 or more to purchase.

Complex Decongestive Therapy

Although massage has been used for centuries to force fluid from swollen limbs, a variation of massage-based therapy known as manual lymphatic drainage has more recently been developed. Manual lymphatic drainage was developed in the early 1930s by Dr. Emil Vodder and has become one of the more popular methods for massaging swollen limbs.

Manual lymphatic drainage refers to a light massage technique that is usually initiated by massaging the chest or abdomen in order to empty the central lymphatic vessels and prepare them to receive peripheral lymph fluid from the limb (Fig. 3-4). The therapist then massages distally to proximally along the affected limb. Light massage is used to stimulate lymphatic flow and gently coax fluid through the obstructed vessels. Two sessions (lasting 1 hour or more) are usually performed each day. The limb is wrapped between sessions to enhance reduction and prevent reaccumulation of fluid. It typically requires about 2 weeks of therapy to maximally reduce the limb. Between massage sessions, exercise is performed (while the

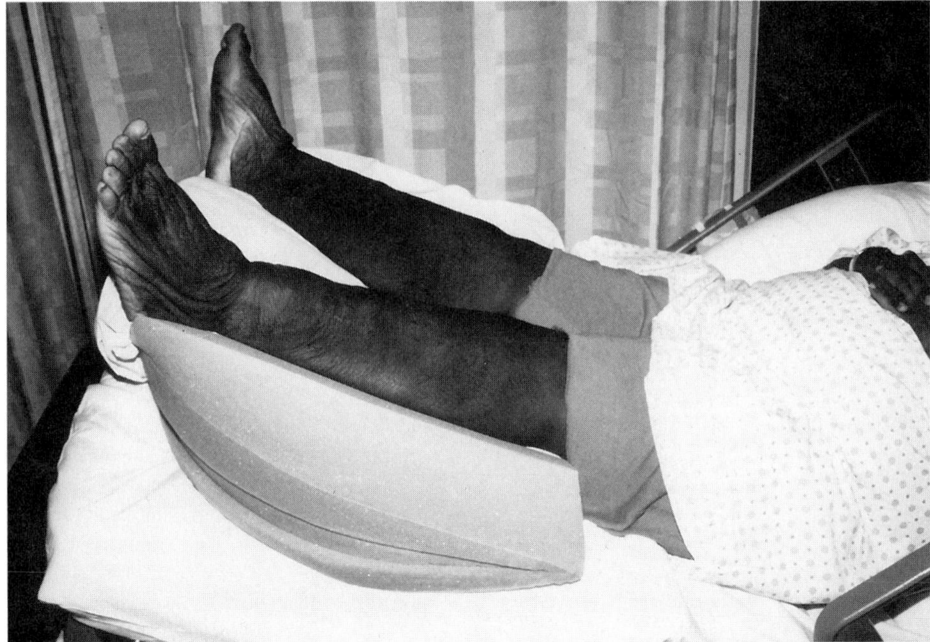

FIG. 3–2. Elevation of the limb to at least 45° using a foam wedge can help reduce limb edema.

limb is wrapped) to enhance reduction of the limb. Although it is possible for patients to do the massage themselves, they are usually advised to have a "significant other" learn and perform the technique.

Dr. Földi[11] later described a combination of lymphatic massage and other therapies, named complex decongestive therapy (CDT). CDT combines (1) the use of massage to reduce the limb with (2) a well-defined program of exercise, compressive bandaging of the extremity, lymphedema extremity exercises, education (especially about the importance of meticulous skin care), and, ultimately, the use of compression garments. As a result of the pioneer work of

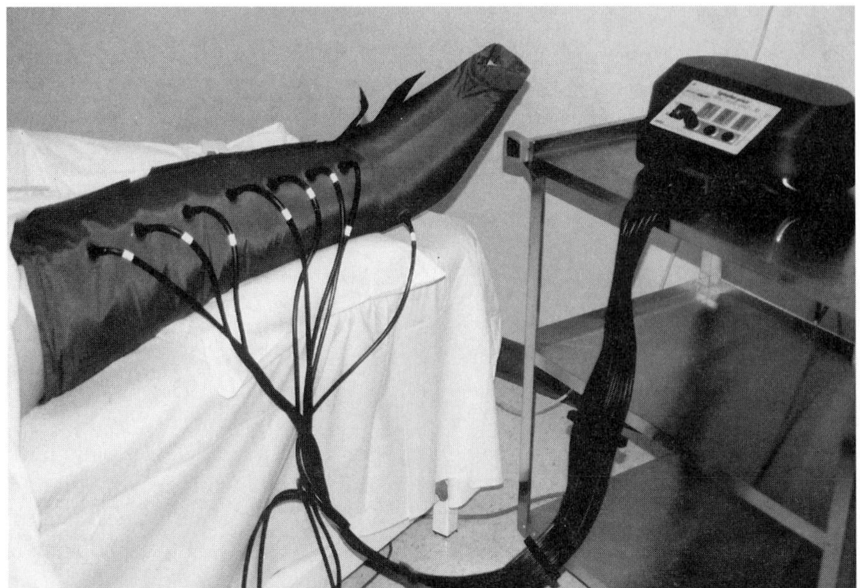

FIG. 3–3. Lymphapress (Myovatec Surgical Systems Ltd., New Delhi, India). Multiple chamber pump that sequentially inflates in a distal-to-proximal direction, moving fluid from the foot toward the trunk. Vasopneumatic pumping can be used at home.

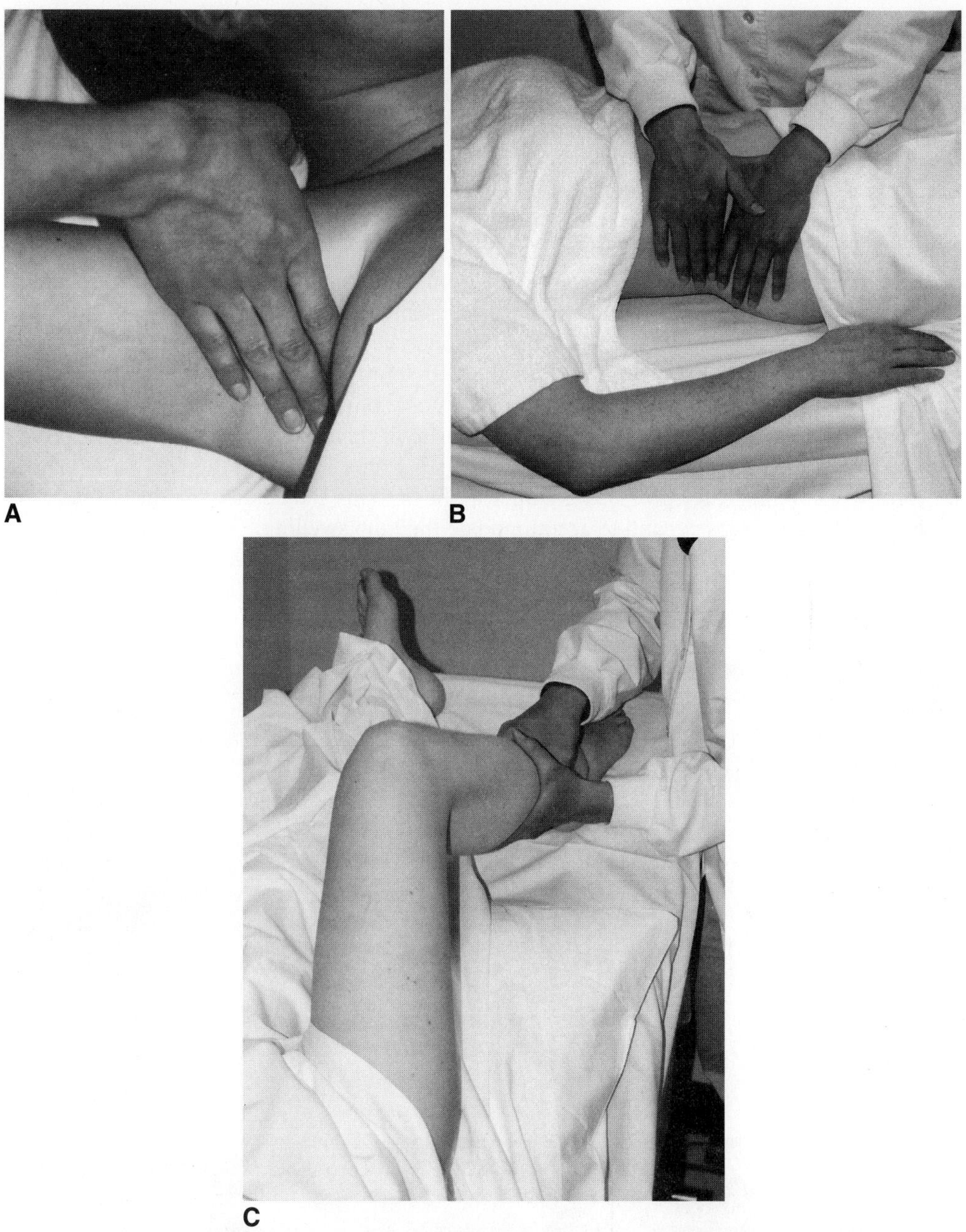

FIG. 3–4. Manual lymphatic drainage is performed by a physical therapist on a patient with lower-extremity lymphedema. **A,** Manual lymphatic drainage is started in the axillary regions to prepare and clear lymph nodes around the thorax. **B,** Therapy is used to stimulate and empty nodes in the trunk area. **C,** The leg is massaged, moving fluid proximally while the therapist progresses along the limb.

Földi,[11] these techniques are quite popular in Europe and Australia and are becoming widely available in the United States and Canada.

CDT is very effective in reducing the affected limb; however, data are limited when comparing its efficacy with other limb-reducing modalities. Boris et al[12] reported in 1994 on complex lymphedema therapy (a technique of manual lymph drainage, compressive bandaging, and exercises), which was used to treat 38 patients for a period of 1 month. Eighteen of these patients had unilateral lower-extremity lymphedema; 16 were females with arm lymphedema secondary to breast surgery; and 4 had bilateral leg disease. Reduction of edema averaged 73% in patients with arm disease and 88% in patients with leg edema.

Bandaging

Compression bandaging should be performed immediately after each session of elevation, vasopneumatic compression, or massage (Fig. 3-5). Bandaging of the extremity not only keeps fluid from reaccumulating in the limb, but also increases venous and lymphatic drainage. Elastic or nonelastic compression can be used. With lymphedema that is nonpitting, nonelastic compression with special foam pads fitted into areas of significant fibrotic tissue tends to be effective at enhancing limb reduction. During active edema reduction therapy, the bandages may be worn at night, as well as during the day. During maintenance therapy, bandages may be worn only at night or not at all in conjunction with elastic compression stockings during the day. Some situations might warrant the use of elastic bandages in lieu of compression stockings.

Bandage wraps come in a variety of types. The most commonly used are either long stretch (Ace®, Conco®, DuPey®, and Setopress™) or short stretch (Komprex, Comprilan) wraps. Long stretch wraps (as their name implies) stretch 100% or more because of their elastic component, whereas short stretch wraps do not have elastic in their material and, therefore, stretch 70% or less of their length. Because the short stretch wraps are stiffer, they may provide better control of swelling (they provide resistance to the limb instead of allowing the limb to grow as the long stretch wraps expand to accommodate the limb swelling). They tend to cost more than long stretch wraps, but long stretch wraps need to be replaced every 4-8 weeks whereas short stretch wraps may last 6 months before needing to be replaced. Short stretch wraps may

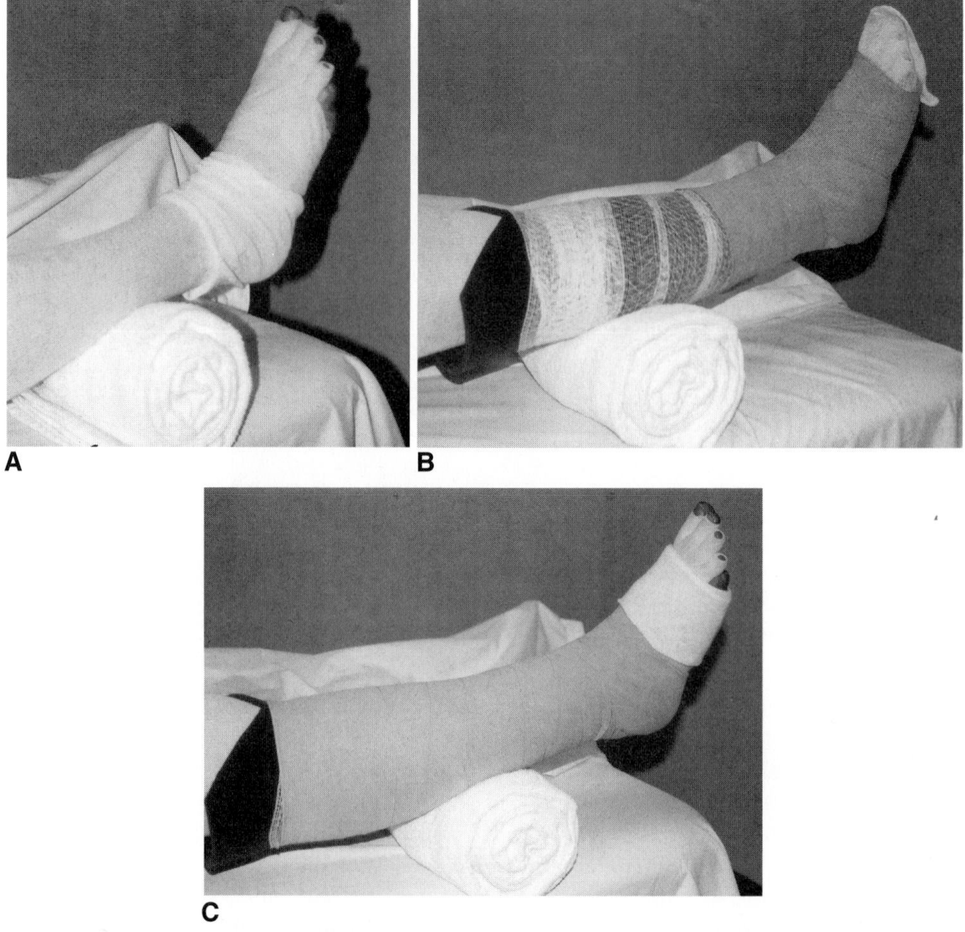

FIG. 3–5. Compression bandaging maintains the limb reduction during the interval between manual lymphatic drainage or pump sessions. A cotton stockinette is applied first **(A)**, followed by a circumferential foam pad (to keep the compressive forces uniform over the affected areas) **(B)**, and short stretch wraps, such as Comprilan (BSN-Jobst, Charlotte, North Carolina), are applied over the foam to provide limb compression **(C)**.

be used in conjunction with soft foam or cotton batting to make a composite wrap system that is comfortable, nonelastic, and remains in place throughout much of the day (see Fig. 3-5).

There are several methods for applying wraps. The most common are the spiral and figure-of-eight technique. The degree of compression is determined by (1) how much the wrap is stretched as it is applied and (2) the degree of overlap that occurs each time the limb is encircled. Rewrapping needs to be performed two to three times a day because as elasticity is lost, the effectiveness of the bandage is reduced.

The limb is usually measured after every treatment session. When the measurements do not reduce any further after two sessions, the limb is considered maximally reduced. The limb is usually measured early the following morning for compression garments, and the patient continues the treatment program until the stocking is available. The compression garment is applied for the first time in the morning, when the limb should be at its smallest.

Exercise

Exercise generally involves a light remedial program designed to increase venous and lymphatic drainage. Specific exercises are typically performed while the patient is wearing compressive bandaging to enhance the reduction process. Leduc, Peeters, and Bourgeois[13] have demonstrated that repeated muscle contraction of the hand with the limb bandaged results in increased reabsorption of protein and enhanced lymphatic flow.

Maintaining Limb Reduction

After the limb has been maximally reduced, elastic compression in the form of graduated elastic compression stockings is recommended. The use of compression garments remains the key to maintaining limb size for most patients (Fig. 3-6). It should be remembered that compression stockings are meant only to maintain the size of the reduced limb, not reduce the edema. Compression sleeves or stockings provide circumferential, graduated pressure

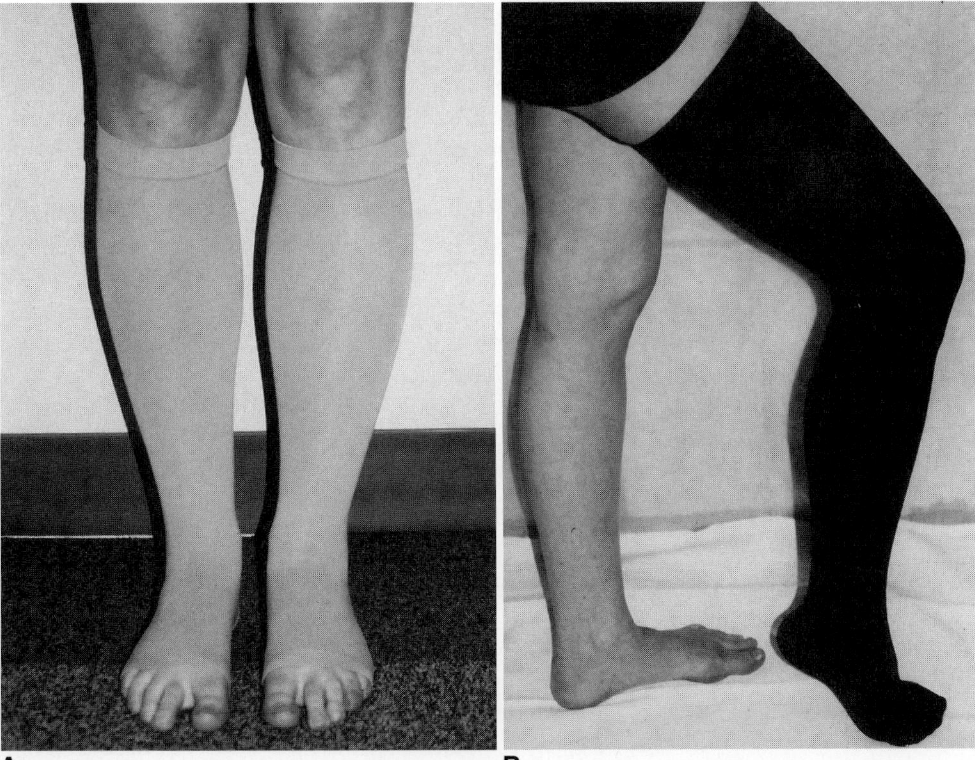

FIG. 3–6. After the limb is maximally reduced, graduated compression stockings are worn to maintain limb size. **A,** Knee high with open toes. **B,** Thigh high closed-toe with silicone band.

along the length of the limb and are characterized according to the amount of pressure at the distal end of the garment.

Compression garments usually require a prescription and can be purchased ready-made in medical supply stores (Table 3-3). Custom-made garments can be designed to accommodate larger limbs or an unusually shaped limb and are frequently required for patients with lymphedema in order to obtain an optimal fit. The garment should ideally be long enough to cover all swollen portions of the limb. It is important that the fit be correct for the limb size. Compression garments come in many different styles and colors. One pair of ready-made stockings will last about 4-6 months. Custom-made garments may last about 4 months. Patients should be remeasured every year or more if the patient experiences a 15-pound weight gain or loss, to ensure a near-perfect fit.

In order to maintain a reduced limb, the compression garment must be applied shortly after getting up in the morning, to avoid refilling of edema of the limb. When swelling is difficult to control, some patients may need to reapply nonelastic bandages at night, in addition to compression garments during the day. Some patients may have a tendency to accumulate edema while showering or in a warm bathtub and are usually advised to shower at night just before retiring.

Other devices that may be used for long-term edema maintenance include devices such as the CircAid (Fig. 3-7) (CircAid Medical Products Inc., San Diego, California), which is made of a nonelastic fabric that encircles the limb and uses a Velcro closure system to accommodate individual variations in limb circumference.

The key to successful maintenance therapy is to correctly match the intensity of the treatment to the severity of the disease. Maintenance therapy is a lifelong program; if a program is too aggressive, the patient may find it difficult to be fully compliant, yet an inadequate program will lead to swelling. The program must be aggressive enough to maintain the correct limb size, but reasonably easy to comply with. Involving the patient in the treatment plan and keeping the patient's lifestyle in mind will ensure greater success in maintaining the reduction achieved.

Diet

Another component of therapy is weight control. Patients should achieve or maintain their ideal weight and avoid excessive weight gain in order to better control swelling in the affected limb. Excessive weight tends to worsen lymphedema (the excess adipose tissue tends to make the limb more susceptible to lymphedema formation). Generalized obesity may also contribute to swelling by impairing venous return, or by interfering with exercise, pneumatic pumping, limb elevation, and other edema-reducing activities that are dependent upon limb mobility.

Another important consideration is to avoid unnecessary salt intake. Too much salt can lead to an increase in total body fluid, which may aggravate the lymphedema as well.

Drug Therapy

There are some pharmacologic therapies that have been shown to be effective in treatment of lymphedema. The most commonly used class of medications is antibiotics for cellulitis and lymphangitis, especially in the treatment of acute infection. Patients with lymphedema who have had recurrent episodes of cellulitis and lymphangitis are frequently instructed to take

TABLE 3–3 Amount of Compression Generally Worn to Maintain Limb Reduction According to Classification of Lymphedema

Class	Pressure Delivered	Amount of Edema
I	20-30 mm Hg	Mild upper-extremity edema
II	30-40 mm Hg	Mild to moderate edema
III	40-50 mm Hg	Severe lymphedema
–	50-60 mm Hg	Severe resistant lymphedema

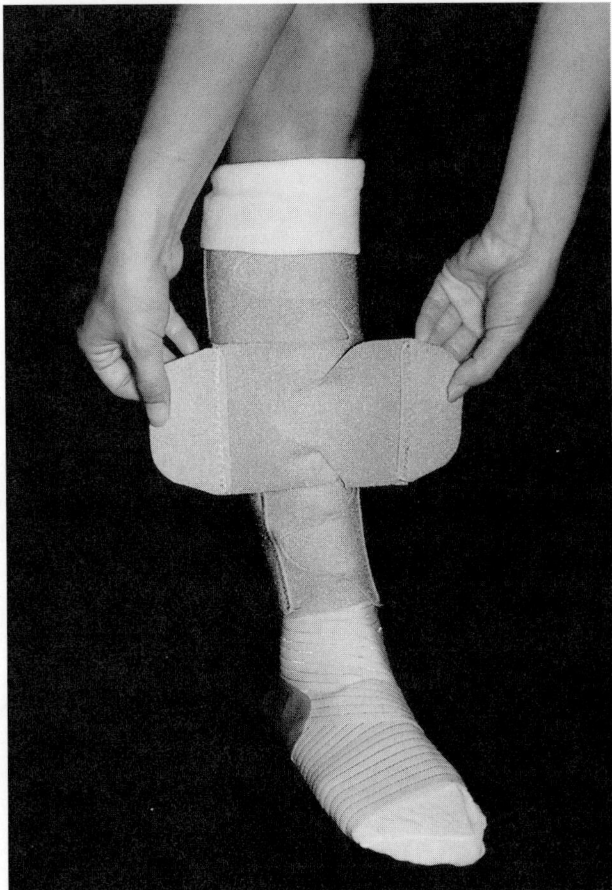

FIG. 3–7. The CircAid® (CircAid Medical Products, Inc., San Diego, Calif.) device can enhance graduated compression. It can also be used as a nonelastic wrap for patients who do not tolerate compression stockings.

antibiotics at the first sign of infection and immediately contact their primary care provider. Some patients (especially those who have had four to six infections in a year) may be instructed to take a week of antibiotics prophylactically each month to prevent repeated bouts of infection. Fungal infections, a complication of lymphedema, should be treated with antimycotic drugs. Topical antifungal agents may also be prescribed for prophylactic therapy as well. Filariasis is often treated with ivermectin or diethylcarbamazine.

Diuretic agents may occasionally be helpful during the early phases of lymphedema. Use of diuretics long-term is discouraged, as this is only marginally beneficial. Lymphedema in advanced stages will produce tissue that is fibrotic and hard, and diuretics seem to have little effect on these changes.

Many drugs can cause fluid retention and aggravate lymphedema; they should be avoided if possible. Nonsteroidal anti-inflammatory drugs, calcium channel blockers, steroids, and estrogens are the drugs most commonly known for enhancing fluid retention.

Oral benzopyrones, which initially were in Europe and Australia, have recently been pulled off the market in those countries as well as Canada and the United States. Early reports by Casley-Smith, Piller, and Morgan[14] suggested that oral benzopyrones were beneficial in expediting the reduction of lymphedema tissue; however, this benefit has not been substantiated by later reports, and a significant incidence of liver toxicity has been reported.[15] Information regarding the use of topical powders or creams containing benzopyrones has not been studied as closely.

Immunologic therapy attempts to boost immunity by the intraarterial injection of lymphocytes; however, this therapy is still in experimental stages.

Skin Care

It is important to prevent breaks in the skin that can lead to infection. Patients are encouraged to moisturize dry skin using a lanolin-based lotion or similar agent. Antifungal creams or powders are prescribed as indicated. Instruction should be given on proper care of toenails. If toenails are thick, nail care should be provided by a podiatrist. If the affected limb is injured, patients are instructed to aggressively care for the wound, sometimes with topical antibiotic ointments, limb elevation, and additional compression over the injured area to enhance healing and reduce the likelihood of infection.

PATIENT EDUCATION

The educational needs of the patient with lymphedema are numerous. A program is unlikely to be successful if the patient is not motivated to learn about the disease or to improve the edema. Lymphedema is a chronic, usually incurable disease, and therapy will be lifelong; however, early recognition, acceptance, and motivation will help the patient avoid long-term complications. The focus of education with the patient generally involves addressing the following:

- The meaning of lymphedema.
- Specific instructions regarding individual therapy program in the active phase of therapy and in the maintenance phase.
- Instruction on use of pneumatic pump or how to perform manual lymphatic drainage. Patients should be encouraged to consider comfort, ease of operation, and cost when purchasing a pump.
- Signs and symptoms of infection or worsening lymphedema that should be reported to primary caregiver.
- Proper skin care.
- Application and care of compression garments.
- How to measure limb to assess changes in limb size.
- Contingency plan for reducing limb when stocking becomes ineffective.
- Exercise program instructions.
- Dietary considerations.
- Special instructions when traveling.

Support

One of the most important things that caregivers can provide to patients is a source of support. Patients should be encouraged to return for follow-up care and reevaluation as needed to ensure a successful program. The nurses or therapists in the clinic should routinely call patients within a few weeks after dismissal to assess the effectiveness of the program. This is often the time when many questions arise regarding maintenance therapy in the home environment. It provides a good opportunity for nurses (1) to emphasize the importance of continued therapy, (b) to assist in devising creative treatment alternatives, and (c) to help patients recognize when they should seek professional help.

Although most patients adapt reasonably well to the challenges of lymphedema, not all do. Counseling may be a valuable component of medical and physical therapy. This may be seen more often in adolescents with new onset of the disease, where body image, physical appearance, and issues of self-esteem are especially important.

Assessment of Physical Limitations and Home Setting

Careful assessment of the patient's home situation allows the caregiver to help the patient establish a routine and perform the necessary treatments over the course of the day with a minimum alteration in the patient's lifestyle. It also provides an opportunity to assess the patient's ability to perform the prescribed program. Allowing the patient to demonstrate the wrapping technique, stocking-donning technique, and massage or pump application also helps to ensure that the patient will remain compliant with the program. The degree of patient involvement in the program, and the patient's knowledge about the disease process, will also help determine success. Patients should be encouraged to ask questions, learn as much as they can about the disease, actively participate in their care, and take personal responsibility for their own well-being.

SURGICAL THERAPY

There have been a number of surgical procedures suggested as a means to treat lymphedema. Unfortunately, less than 10 percent of patients with lymphedema are candidates for surgical repair.[16] The types of operations that are generally recommended are (1) reduction operations, which remove excess tissue and decrease the volume of the extremity, or (2) operations to improve lymphatic drainage of the extremity. Two classic procedures are the Homans' and Charles' operations, both of which reduce the volume of the extremity. The Homans' operation involves resection of a portion of the edematous and underlying tissues; with closure of the wound, the size of the limb is reduced. The Charles' operation involves complete excision of the skin, subcutaneous tissue, and fascia.[17] The muscle is then covered with a split thickness skin graft that is taken from healthy skin. Upper-extremity procedures have been reported to be more successful than lower-extremity procedures. These surgeries are generally undertaken only when extensive lymphedema has not been manageable by aggressive medical means, or occasionally when there have been repeated unrelenting episodes of lymphangitis.

Liposuction with controlled compression therapy is another surgical procedure that has received attention. Brorson[18,19] has reported the use of liposuction with upper-extremity lymphedema, where hypertrophied adipose tissue is removed with a resultant reduction in limb volume. The mechanism behind the hypertrophy of adipose tissue may be that macrophages and adipose cells take up lipids from the lymph, but the lipids cannot be transported further because of the interrupted lymph flow. The subcutaneous adipose tissue thickens, and chronic swelling ensues.[20,21] Later, an ingrowth of fibrosis is seen in the subcutaneous adipose tissue, which makes the condition more difficult to treat. Fibrosis may occur because fibroblasts are stimulated by the high protein concentration in the lymph.[19] Following liposuction, Brorson[18] reported that skin blood flow was maintained, lymph transport was not further compromised, a reduced incidence of cellulitis was observed, and there was a decrease in volume of 50% as compared with a group who received controlled compression therapy alone.

Procedures to surgically restore lymphatic flow include lymphatic-to-venous anastomosis,[17,22-24] lympho-lympho anastomosis,[23] lymph vessel autotransplantation, and cross-femoral lymph vessel transposition.[25] Lymphatic-to-venous anastomosis is made between lymphatic vessels and nearby small veins; lymph is allowed to flow from the obstructed area directly into the venous system. Lymph-to-venous operations at Mayo Clinic show an initial 50% patency rate.[22] Although lymph-venous and lymph-nodal venous shunts are promising, these procedures require confirmation of long-term patency (e.g., imaging by lymphoscintigraphy) and demonstration of improved lymphatic tracer transport (objective measurements of long-term efficacy). Clinical experience with these procedures over the last 20 years suggests that results are better and more lasting if surgery is performed early in the course of lymphedema before irreversible fibrosclerosis occurs.

Lymphatic autotransplantation, in which lymphatic vessels are removed from one portion of the body and used to bypass the blockage in another part of the body,[17,25] requires the presence of large donor lymphatic vessels. Long-term patency following these microsurgical operations has been unpredictable.

Potential complications of surgical procedures include poor healing of incision sites, infection, prolonged hospital stays, poor cosmetic results, and failure to provide significant relief of swelling. In addition, most patients must still wear a compression garment after surgery.

Lymphedema is a challenging medical problem. Success of therapy correlates with the amount of support provided to the patient while in the program and the enthusiasm of the patient to participate proactively as well.

The knowledge of the nurse and the support and involvement in patients' therapy can be substantial and have many positive long-lasting benefits in assisting patients to achieve their goals.

REFERENCES

1. Browse NL, Stuart G: Lymphedema: pathophysiology and classification, *J Cardiovasc Surg* 26:91-106, 1985.
2. Edwards JM, Kinmonth JB: Lymphovenous shunts in man, *Br Med J* 4:579-581, 1969.
3. Allen EV: Lymphedema of the extremities, *Arch Intern Med* 54:606, 1934.
4. Kinmonth JB, Taylor GW, Tracy GD et al: Primary lymphoedema: clinical and lymphangiographic studies of a series of 107 patients in which the lower limbs were affected, *Br J Surg* 45:1-10, 1957.
5. Spittell JA, Schirger A: Edema, peripheral. In Taylor RB, ed: *Difficult diagnosis,* Philadelphia, 1985, WB Saunders, pp 130-137.
6. Gloviczki P, Calcagno D, Schirger A et al: Non-invasive evaluation of the swollen extremity: experiences with 190 lymphoscintigraphic examinations, *J Vasc Surg* 9:683-690, 1989.
7. Stewart G, Gaunt JL, Croft D, Browse NL et al: The value of lymphoscintigraphy in the investigation of lymphedema, *Immunol Haematol Res Monogr 2,* 1982:209-213.
8. Cambria RA, Gloviczki P, Naessens JM et al: Non-invasive evaluation of the lymphatic system with lymphoscintigraphy: a prospective, semi-quantitative analysis in 386 extremities, *J Vasc Surg* 18:773-782, 1993.
9. Huang A, Fruauff A, DiCarmine F et al: Case report 861: primary lymphedema of the lower extremity, *Skeletal Radiol* 23(6):483-485, 1994.
10. Hadjis NS, Carr DH, Banks L et al: The role of CT in the diagnosis of primary lymphedema of the lower limb, *AJR Am J Roentgenol* 144(2):361-364, 1984.
11. Földi M: Physiology and pathophysiology of lymph flow. In Clodius L, ed: *Lymphedema,* Stuttgart, 1977, Georg Thieme, pp 1-11.
12. Boris M, Weindorf S, Lasinski B et al: Lymphedema reduction by noninvasive complex lymphedema therapy, *Oncology (Huntingt)* 8(9):109-110, 1994.
13. Leduc O, Peeters A, Bourgeois P: Bandages. Scintigraphic demonstration of its efficacy on colloidal protein reabsorption during muscle activity. In Nishi et al, editors: Progress in lymphology XII, *Excerpta Med,* Amsterdam, 1990, Elsevier, pp. 421-425.
14. Casley-Smith J, Piller N, Morgan RG: Behandlung Chronischer Lymphödeme der Arme and Beine mit 5,6-Benzo-(alpha)-pyron: placebokontrollierte Doppelblind-cross-over-Studie über die Dauer von einem Jahr, *Therapiewoche* 12:1068-1076, 1986.
15. Loprinzi CL et al: Lack of effect of Coumarin in women with lymphedema after treatment for breast cancer, *New Engl J Med* 340:346-350, 1999.
16. Gloviczki P: Treatment of acquired lymphedema—medical and surgical. In Ernst CB, Stanley JC, eds: *Current therapy in vascular surgery-II,* Philadelphia, 1991, BC Decker, pp 1030-1036.
17. Savage RC: The surgical management of lymphedema, *Surg Gynecol Obstet* 159:501, 1984.
18. Brorson H: Liposuction gives complete reduction of chronic large arm lymphedema after breast cancer, *Acta Oncol* 39(3):407-420, 2000.
19. Brorson H, Svensson H, Norrgren K et al: Liposuction reduces arm lymphedema without significantly altering the already impaired lymph transport, *Lymphology* 31(4):156-172, 1998.
20. Ryan TJ, Curri SB: Blood vessels and lymphatics, *Clin Dermatol* 7:25, 1989.
21. Ryan TJ: Lymphatics and adipose tissue, *Clin Dermatol* 13:493, 1995.
22. Gloviczki P, Fisher J, Hollier LH et al: Microsurgical lymphovenous anastomosis for treatment of lymphedema: a critical review, *J Vasc Surg* 7:647-652, 1988.
23. Campisi C, Boccardo F, Tacchella M: Reconstructive microsurgery of lymph vessels; the personal method of lymphatic-venous-lymphatic (LVL) interpositioned grafted shunt, *Microsurgery* 16(3):161-166, 1995.
24. Campisi C, Boccardo F, Alitta P et al: Derivative lymphatic microsurgery: indications, techniques, and results, *Microsurgery* 16(7):463-468, 1995.
25. Baumeister RG, Siuda S, Bhomert H et al: A microsurgical method for reconstruction of interrupted pathways; autologous lymph-vessel transplantation for treatment of lymphedemas, *Scand J Plast Reconstr Surg* 20:141-146, 1986.

PART TWO

Perioperative Evaluation and Management

4

Clinical Assessment of the Vascular System

VICTORA A. FAHEY

Despite new developments in noninvasive and invasive testing, the basic foundation for diagnosis in vascular disease remains a good history and physical examination. The assessment should also include regular health habits and risk factors. On the basis of the information obtained, appropriate interventions can be planned toward achieving optimal patient health. Such an assessment is one of the primary responsibilities of professional nursing.

The goal of nursing intervention is to help the patient achieve the highest quality of life compatible with the illness. In addition to the physical examination, the patient's level of knowledge and attitude about the disease and readiness to learn should be assessed. Nursing assessment should also focus on the patient's and family's perceived needs, including physical, psychosocial, spiritual, financial, and safety issues. It is important to evaluate these responses, which vary greatly, because psychosocial factors strongly influence a patient's adaptation to vascular disease.[1]

The history and physical examination provide an opportunity to establish a positive nurse-patient relationship. Achieving a good rapport may help increase the accuracy of the history and improve and maintain the patient's health state.

This chapter will focus on the skills and techniques required to obtain an accurate history and perform a physical examination of the peripheral vascular system. It is beyond the scope of this chapter to discuss every symptom and sign that may be present, but the significant features of arterial and venous disease are emphasized. More specific signs and symptoms and special examinations will be discussed in the appropriate chapters in this text. Clinical assessment of lymphedema is discussed in Chapter 3. Because signs and symptoms of arterial and venous disease have specific characteristics, this chapter is divided into assessment of the arterial system and the venous system and further subdivided into body regions.

PREPARATION FOR HISTORY AND PHYSICAL EXAMINATION

Prior to the assessment, an explanation of the history and physical examination should enhance the patient's willingness and ability to contribute pertinent information. Conditions that are essential to performing a good physical examination include good lighting in a warm, comfortable room and full exposure of all extremities while preserving privacy. In addition to standard equipment, a portable Doppler ultrasound, stethoscope, and sphygmomanometer should be easily accessible to enhance efficiency of the examination. Gloves should be used when examining the patient.

A systematic order of assessment should be established. After a complete health history including the chief complaint is obtained, the physical assessment of the patient is then performed, including inspection, palpation, and auscultation. Assessment should be performed bilaterally, always comparing one extremity or side with the contralateral one. Nonverbal communication exhibited by the patient can also reveal important information.

ASSESSMENT OF THE ARTERIAL SYSTEM

Atherosclerosis is a systemic process, and persons with peripheral arterial disease may also have significant cerebrovascular or coronary artery disease. Because of this, the initial patient evaluation should include an examination of the entire arterial system. Although the patient's cardiac status is significant, evaluation of this aspect of the cardiovascular system is not included in this chapter.

Patient History

Obtaining a comprehensive history is key to performing an accurate assessment. Components of a complete health history are included in Box 4-1. The disease may often be localized by history alone. The chief complaint is the reason the patient is seeking medical attention. Chief complaints will be discussed under each body region. It is important to listen and ask specific questions about these complaints.

Nurses play an important role in primary and secondary prevention of vascular disease. Obtaining risk factor information is an essential part of the history in order to plan appropriate intervention. Patients who smoke heavily have a more rapid progression of disease and worse prognosis.[2] Atherosclerotic disease is often accelerated in patients with diabetes.

Additional information to be gathered from the patient's history includes recent weight gain or loss, generalized weakness, problems with eating, gastrointestinal disturbances, and musculoskeletal problems. If significant malnutrition is suspected, a complete nutritional assessment should be performed. Protein-calorie malnutrition increases the risk of sepsis, delayed wound healing, pulmonary complications, and fluid and electrolyte imbalances.[3] Sepsis and delayed wound healing pose a serious threat of morbidity and mortality in vascular patients, especially when synthetic graft material has been used. Risk factors for the development of malnutrition are included in Box 4-2. Preoperative and postoperative nutritional supplements and correction of electrolyte imbalances will help decrease perioperative complications.

Head and Neck

Chief Complaint

The patient may present with an asymptomatic bruit identified on physical examination. Clinical symptoms of cerebrovascular insufficiency may vary from a minor transient neurologic event to a catastrophic stroke with paralysis and coma.[4] Symptomatic patients exhibit either carotid manifestations (hemispheric) affecting the anterior circulation or vertebrobasilar manifestations (nonhemispheric) affecting the posterior circulation (Table 4-1). Other nonspecific symptoms such as headache, seizures, or altered states of consciousness or cognition may occur. The symptomatology of cerebrovascular disease often mimics that of other neurologic entities. Classification of neurologic deficits is discussed in Chapter 14.

Inspection

A baseline neurologic assessment should be performed, including the following:

- Orientation with respect to person, place, and time
- Pupil size
- Reaction to light
- Grasp strength and equality
- Movement of all extremities
- Facial symmetry
- Tongue deviation
- The ability to communicate (speech) and swallow

Inspect the carotid arteries for pulsation. Normally, carotid pulsation is not visible, although it may be visible at the base of the right neck with longstanding hypertension, with a tortuous carotid artery, and possibly with a carotid artery aneurysm or carotid body tumor.[5]

BOX 4–1

Components of a Complete Health History

CHIEF COMPLAINT/HISTORY OF PRESENT ILLNESS
Location
Character (severity of symptoms)
Date of onset
Precipitating factors (stress, activity, medication)
Relief methods
Frequency of symptoms
Duration of symptoms
Progression of symptoms

SIGNIFICANT MEDICAL-SURGICAL HISTORY
Cardiac history (angina, arrhythmias, myocardial infarction)
Claudication
Hypertension—if yes, age at onset, severity, medications
Neurologic events or disorders: cerebrovascular or peripheral (loss of motor or sensory function, speech deficit, visual disturbances, dizziness, syncope, epilepsy, Parkinson's, multiple sclerosis)
Past injuries/spinal cord injury
Past surgeries and endovascular interventions
Infections
Renal artery disease/renal function
Malignancy
Diabetes
Collagen vascular disease
Clotting abnormalities (see Chapter 9)
Venous thromboembolism
Allergic reactions
Pregnancies
Present/past medications—Certain drugs can mimic or actually cause arterial occlusion. Inderal may increase patient's symptoms by decreasing cardiac output and systemic blood pressure. Ergot preparations for headache may cause arterial occlusion (see Chapter 1).

FAMILY HISTORY
Arterial disease (cerebral, coronary, and peripheral or aneurysm disease)
Venous disease
Cholesterolemia
Clotting abnormalities

PSYCHOSOCIAL HISTORY
Occupational history: current and past—use of vibratory tools; standing all day; professional athlete
Tobacco use
Drug abuse
Current activity level
Stress level
Dietary intake/obesity/weight loss
Alcohol intake
Emotional state
Activities of daily living/exercise program
Hygiene habits/foot care

If the patient has experienced amaurosis fugax, an ophthalmoscopic examination should be performed. Bright, reflective spots may be seen in the retinal arteries. These are known as Hollenhorst plaques and represent cholesterol emboli from ulcerated plaque in the carotid or innominate arteries.[5] The fundi may also reveal evidence of severe hypertension, diabetes mellitus, or extensive atherosclerosis.[6]

BOX 4–2

Risk Factors for the Development of Malnutrition

Oral or gastrointestinal disturbances	Cancer
Inadequate nutritional intake	Radiation therapy
Sepsis	Chemotherapy
Multiple surgical procedures	End-stage cardiac disease
Severe pulmonary disease	Excessive alcohol intake

Palpation

The common carotid pulse is palpated in the middle or lower neck between the trachea and the anterior border of the sternocleidomastoid muscle (Fig. 4-1). To palpate the carotid artery, feel the trachea and roll fingers laterally into the groove between it and the sternocleidomastoid muscle, which lies below and medial to the angle of the jaw. Each carotid artery should be palpated separately; massage or compression of the artery should be avoided to prevent reflex bradycardia or syncope related to carotid sinus manipulation. A palpable carotid pulse is not a significant finding, because in the presence of a totally occluded internal carotid artery, a carotid pulse may be palpable if the external carotid artery is patent. The superficial temporal artery, a branch of the external carotid artery, can be palpated just anterior to the tragus of the ear. This suggests a patent external carotid artery.

The base of the neck and the supraclavicular fossa should be palpated for a pulsatile mass indicating an aneurysm or a carotid body tumor. The vertebral arteries are not readily accessible to palpation because they lie deep at the posterior base of the neck and are surrounded by cervical bone for most of their course.[5]

TABLE 4–1 Differentiation Between Carotid/Hemispheric Manifestations (Anterior Circulation) and Vertebrobasilar/Nonhemispheric Manifestations (Posterior Circulation)

Carotid/Hemispheric	Vertebrobasilar/Nonhemispheric
Amaurosis fugax (fleeting monocular blindness)	Bilateral visual defects
Diplopia: no	Diplopia: yes
Contralateral motor and sensory deficits: weakness, tingling, numbness of extremity	Bilateral motor and sensory deficits: vertigo, syncope, dizziness, ataxia, dysphagia
Dysphasias (if dominant hemisphere is involved)	Drop attack/headache, confusion/memory loss

Auscultation

A bruit, the French word for noise, is an audible sound associated with turbulent blood flow created by a change in the diameter of the arterial lumen. While having the patient hold his or her breath, auscultate the carotid artery with the bell of the stethoscope from the base of the neck to the angle of the jaw. You are listening for a bruit, which usually signifies arterial stenosis at or proximal to the site of auscultation. Carotid bruits are usually loudest in the upper third of the neck in the area of the carotid bifurcation. If a bruit is heard, move the stethoscope toward the clavicle. If the sound intensifies, the bruit probably originates in the heart (aortic stenosis) or the subclavian artery; a diminished sound usually signifies the bruit originates in the carotid artery.[7]

A totally or near-totally occluded artery, as well as an artery with a hemodynamically insignificant stenosis but an ulcerating plaque, may not produce a bruit. Thus, the absence of a bruit does not rule out a significant carotid lesion. If a carotid bruit was auscultated and then disappears at a later time, the carotid artery may have occluded during the interim. The severity of the stenosis cannot be determined by the loudness of the bruit because a tight carotid stenosis may have minimal flow and a faint bruit.[5] To evaluate the hemodynamic

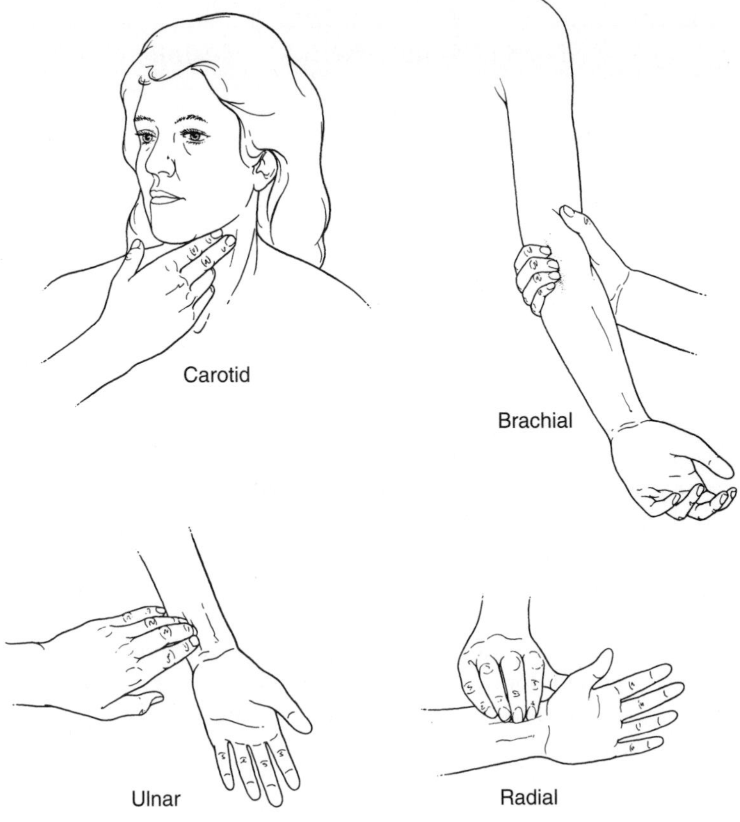

FIG. 4–1. Palpation of the carotid, brachial, radial, and ulnar arterial pulses.

significance of a carotid bruit, a carotid duplex scan is performed (see Chapter 5). A vertebral artery bruit may be faint and is best heard over the tip of the shoulder.[7] The significance of carotid bruits is discussed in Chapter 14.

Upper Extremities

Chief Complaint

The most common symptoms exhibited with upper-extremity arterial insufficiency are acute onset of pain, chronic exertional muscle fatigue of the upper arm, and Raynaud's phenomenon (cold sensitivity). Acute arterial ischemia, characterized by severe pain, pallor, pulselessness, poikilothermia, and later paresthesias and paralysis (the six *P*s of acute arterial occlusion) (Box 4-3), is usually the result of embolism, proximal thrombosis, or occasionally a subclavian artery aneurysm or an iatrogenic arterial injury. Muscle fatigue and discomfort occurring after prolonged use of the arm is similar to intermittent claudication of the lower extremity. The fatigue may be due to a proximal subclavian or axillary stenosis or occlusion. Thoracic outlet syndrome can also produce fatigue, paresthesias, and numbness in the arm with activity. The symptoms are usually initiated by elevation or hyperabduction of the arm and result from neurovascular compression (see Chapter 15).

Intermittent hand coolness, pain, and numbness may suggest Raynaud's phenomenon. It is characterized by episodic digital vasospasm associated with skin color changes precipitated by exposure to environmental cold, occupational exposure to specific types of vibratory equipment, and/or emotional stress.[5,8] Triphasic color changes of the digits occur; fingertips turn pale (white), then cyanotic (blue), then hyperemic (red). This most often occurs in the hands and fingers but can also occur in the toes and feet. Skin ulceration may be seen in the presence of collagen vascular disease (scleroderma).

BOX 4–3

Six *Ps* of Acute Arterial Occlusion

Pain	Poikilothermia
Pulselessness	Paresthesias
Pallor	Paralysis

Inspection

Examine the color of the extremity and fingertips. Check capillary refill. Note the time it takes to return to normal color; color should return within 3 seconds or less. With diminished blood flow, the return to normal color is delayed. Superficial skin lesions, ulceration, and gangrene of the digits may be present secondary to an occlusive or embolic source.

Inspect the size of the upper extremities, noting muscle atrophy, hematoma, edema, fingertip lesions along the nail edge, skin ulceration, or gangrene (Fig. 4-2). Note the presence of needle tracks. If Raynaud's is suspected, inspect the fingers for tapering, a waxy appearance, joint mobility, and skin tautness or signs of scleroderma including shiny, atrophic skin. Observe for ulnar deviation of the hand, indicating possible rheumatoid arthritis.

Examine motor and sensory function of the hands and fingers, which may be diminished in the acutely ischemic limb. Have the patient flex and extend the fingers. Test sensory function with a dull object or light touch with a feather. A neuromotor examination of the upper extremity should be performed and documented prior to and after any invasive diagnostic or therapeutic intervention.

Palpation

Pulses should be palpated for their presence, rate, equality, regularity, and strength. For simplicity, pulses can be graded from 0 to 2 as absent (0), diminished (1), or normal (2). An especially prominent pulse should raise suspicion of an aneurysm.[9]

The presence or absence of peripheral pulses provides important information regarding the condition of the arteries and the level of disease. A diminished or absent pulse indicates the presence of an arterial stenosis or occlusion proximal to the site of examination. An

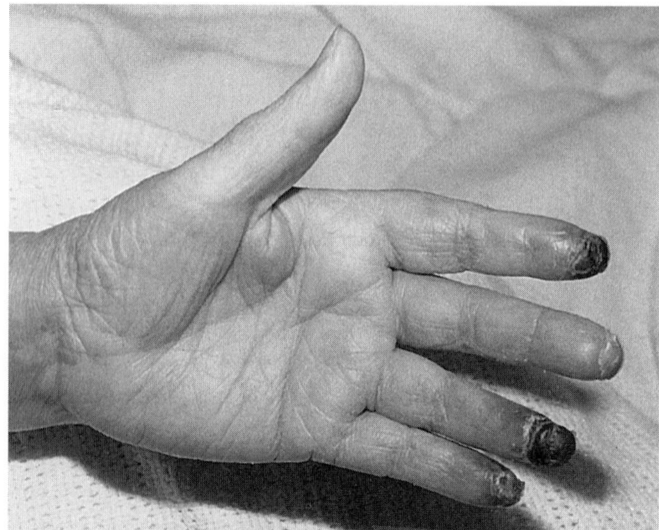

FIG. 4–2. Ulceration and gangrene of the digits.

abnormally strong pulse may suggest occlusion distal to the examination site or the presence of an aneurysm.

In the upper extremity, palpation of the axillary, brachial, radial, and ulnar artery pulses should be performed (see Fig. 4-1). The axillary artery is in the upper medial arm in the groove between the triceps and biceps muscle; the brachial artery is located medial to the biceps muscle at the antecubital fossa above the elbow; the radial artery is located at the lateral wrist over the distal radius; and the ulnar artery may be palpated at the medial wrist over the distal ulna. Because of its anatomic location, the ulnar artery may be difficult to palpate. Doppler ultrasound may be used to assess arterial signals when pulses are not palpable. Postural changes may cause alterations in the pulse; therefore, monitoring of the radial pulse in the various thoracic outlet maneuvers (see Chapters 5 and 15) should be performed.

The supraclavicular and infraclavicular regions should be palpated for a pulsatile mass suggestive of a subclavian aneurysm or a bony mass suggestive of a cervical rib. The ulnar artery should be palpated for the presence of an aneurysm even in the palm. Skin temperature of the upper extremities can be palpated using the back of the hand. The temperature of the extremity becomes cool just distal to the arterial occlusion.

The radial and ulnar arteries are interconnected by two arches within the hand, which protects blood supply to the hands and fingers. Arterial patency of the palmar arch can be determined by performing the Allen test (Fig. 4-3), as follows: The patient holds the hand to be tested with the palm facing up. The radial artery of one wrist is compressed by the fingers of the examiner. The patient is asked to open and close the hand rapidly for 1 minute to squeeze the blood out of the hand, and then asked to extend the fingers quickly. When the hand is opened, the palm is mottled and pale. The radial artery is released, and the hand is inspected for return of color and capillary refill. The response is normal if recovery of normal color is complete within a short period of time (less than 6 seconds). If pallor remains,

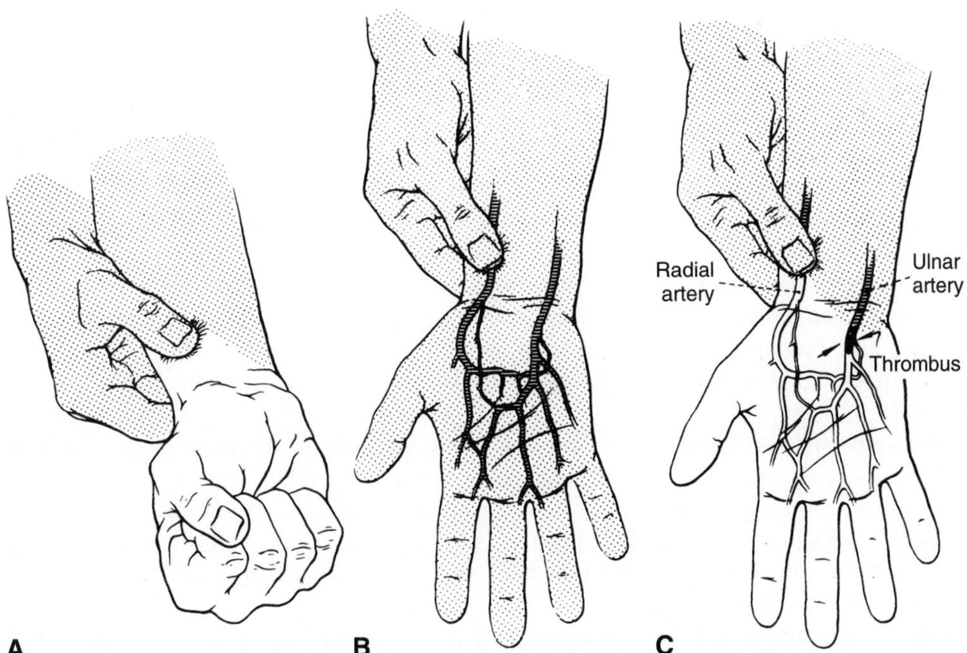

FIG. 4–3. Allen test for patency of the palmar arch: **A,** Pallor induced by the clenched fist with radial artery compression. **B,** Return of the palm perfusion on relaxation of the hand with patent ulnar artery. **C,** Continued pallor of the hand due to ulnar artery occlusion. (From Fairbairn JF: Approach to the patient with peripheral vascular disease. In Fairbairn JF, Juergens JL, Spittel JA, eds: *Peripheral vascular disease,* ed 4, Philadelphia, 1972, WB Saunders, p 27.)

incomplete continuity of the palmar arch is indicated, as well as occlusion of the radial artery; the hand is dependent on the ulnar artery for blood flow. This test should then be repeated with extended compression of the ulnar artery.[10] A positive Allen test is found in hypothenar hammer syndrome, in which repetitive trauma to the hand by either blunt or vibratory mechanisms can result from use of the palm of the hand in activities that involve pushing, pounding, or twisting.[11]

Auscultation

Auscultation of the upper extremity includes measurement of brachial blood pressure bilaterally using a stethoscope or Doppler transducer. If more than 20 mm Hg difference exists between arm pressures, it may indicate a stenosis in the innominate, subclavian, or axillary artery on the side of lower pressure. The left subclavian artery is more often affected by atherosclerosis than the right subclavian artery. If such asymmetry of upper-extremity blood pressures is detected, it is important to inform the patient of this finding and document it in the medical record. This is significant not only from a vascular standpoint, but also because blood pressure medication may be given based on an inaccurate blood pressure if pressures are not checked bilaterally.

A palpable distal pulse is usually only possible with a pressure of 70 mm Hg or greater. When pulses are not palpable, the Doppler can be used to assess arterial signals. The Doppler is so sensitive it can pick up an arterial flow signal in a vessel that has only 20 mm Hg pressure. However, a tone obtained using a Doppler does not equal a palpable pulse.[12]

The supraclavicular fossa should be auscultated for the presence of a subclavian or innominate bruit, which may signify arterial pathology of the proximal artery. An innominate artery stenosis may produce a bruit in both the subclavian and carotid arteries; this should be differentiated from a bruit caused by aortic stenosis, which decreases in intensity on ascending the carotid artery. Auscultation of the subclavian artery should be performed in a neutral position and in thoracic outlet maneuvers (see Chapter 15).

The Abdomen

Chief Complaint

With an abdominal aortic aneurysm (AAA), the patient may present with no symptoms but a pulsatile abdominal mass is found on physical examination. Some patients with an AAA feel as though they have a "second" heartbeat. Turbulent blood flow within the aneurysm may cause distal embolization, in which the patient presents with a blue or painful toe (Fig. 4-4). Although unusual, a large aneurysm may cause duodenal compression with weight loss and indigestion or iliac vein compression resulting in lower-extremity edema.

A patient with a symptomatic aneurysm (leaking or ruptured) may present with abdominal pain radiating toward the back or groin, scrotal pain, syncope, shock, or hypotension. Tenderness of the abdomen may exist in the presence of an inflammatory aneurysm. Discoloration of the abdomen, flank, or scrotum may occur due to extravasation of blood.

With aortoiliac occlusive disease, the chief complaint will be discussed under the lower-extremity section. In males, sexual impotence characterized by inability to maintain an erection is a complaint associated with aortoiliac occlusive disease (see Chapter 11). Impotence can also be a result of medications, psychologic factors, or diabetes.

With chronic mesenteric ischemia, intestinal angina may occur 15 to 30 minutes after eating, also known as postprandial pain. The relationship between pain and food ingestion leads to food fear. Because a person avoids eating to prevent this discomfort, significant weight loss can result. Acute intestinal ischemia may present as severe abdominal pain out of proportion to physical examination, followed by vomiting and/or diarrhea and an elevated white blood count (see Chapter 17).

Uncontrollable hypertension and new onset of renal failure may be indicative of renovascular hypertension (see Chapter 16).

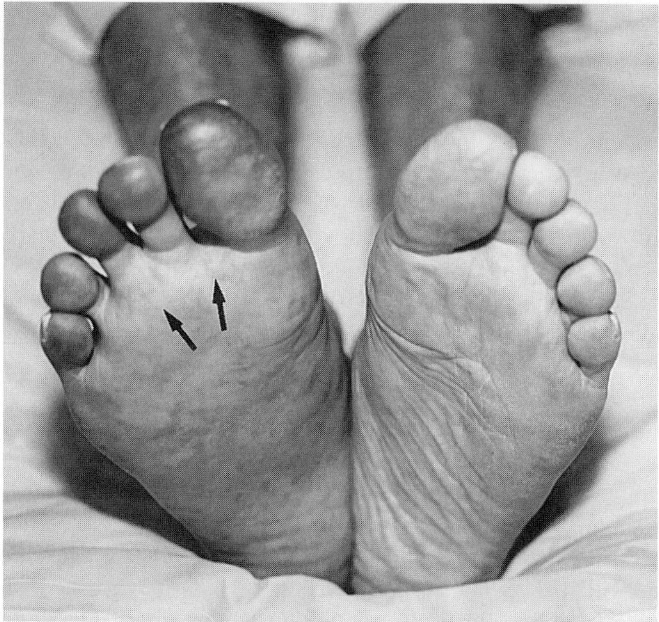

FIG. 4–4. Blue toes *(arrows)* secondary to distal embolization.

Inspection

The retroperitoneal position of the abdominal aorta and its branches limits the amount of information that can be obtained from the physical examination. Inspect the patient in a supine position, noting the contour of the abdomen and the presence of pulsations, obesity, ascites, distention, or discoloration. Note incisions from previous surgery. Blue toe syndrome may be present secondary to an embolic source in the aorta.

Palpation

The aorta bifurcates at the level of the umbilicus, and the aortic pulse may be palpated just above this in the nonobese patient. The normal size of the aorta approximates the width of a patient's thumb. To palpate, press fingers firmly deep into the abdomen to identify the aortic pulsation. If the pulse is prominent or feels wide, place the thumb along one side of the aorta and the fingers along the other side. An abdominal aortic aneurysm should be suspected if the width feels larger than 4-5 cm.[5] If the mass appears to extend to the xiphoid and costal margins, suspect a suprarenal or thoracoabdominal aneurysm. While palpating the abdomen, note any abdominal tenderness or referred pain; this may indicate aneurysm rupture, leak, or inflammation. Iliac artery aneurysms of significant size may be palpable on rectal exam.

Auscultation

A bruit may be heard when significant occlusive disease of the aorta and its branches is present. Aortoiliac disease may cause a bruit in the middle and lower abdomen. Renal artery bruits may be faint and localized in the upper abdominal quarter just lateral to the midline. Mesenteric artery stenoses are associated with epigastric bruits.[5] Although bruits may be detected, their significance is variable. Further diagnostic tests, including ultrasound, computed tomography (CT) scan, and/or arteriogram, are required to obtain the necessary information.

Lower Extremities

Chief Complaint

Although patients may be asymptomatic, a pulse deficit, a bruit, an abnormal pulsation, or an aneurysm may be found on routine physical examination. Symptoms may be disguised in patients whose activity levels are limited because of other health problems such as cardiac disease.

The most common presenting symptom in lower-extremity arterial disease is pain. The degree of pain depends on whether the problem has an acute or chronic onset, the severity of the disease (the extent of blood flow reduction), and the adequacy of collateral blood supply.

Chronic arterial insufficiency of the lower extremity causes two characteristic types of pain: intermittent claudication and ischemic rest pain. Claudication, derived from the Latin infinitive "to limp" *(claudicare)*, is defined as cramping muscle pain brought on by walking a predictable distance and relieved by brief periods of rest.[13] The pain may vary from a slight ache to a severe, cramp-like pain. The patient may describe weakness or tiredness with exercise.[14] Claudication, similar to angina, indicates inadequate arterial blood supply to contracting muscles.

The location of muscle pain indicates the level of arterial occlusion (Fig. 4-5). The muscle groups affected will generally be one joint below the occlusive lesion. With aortoiliac occlusive disease, the chief complaint is buttock and thigh claudication. Cramping calf pain usually results from a superficial femoral or popliteal artery stenosis or occlusion.

Pain in the legs brought on by exercise is a common complaint and not always due to arterial occlusive disease.[14] Patients with neurospinal compression or musculoskeletal disease may also present with pain while walking[15] (Fig. 4-6). Other causes of leg pain may be peripheral neuritis in diabetics, arthritis, sciatica, and reflex sympathetic dystrophy or minor causalgia, which is a burning pain in nature. The differential diagnosis of claudication is listed in Table 4-2.

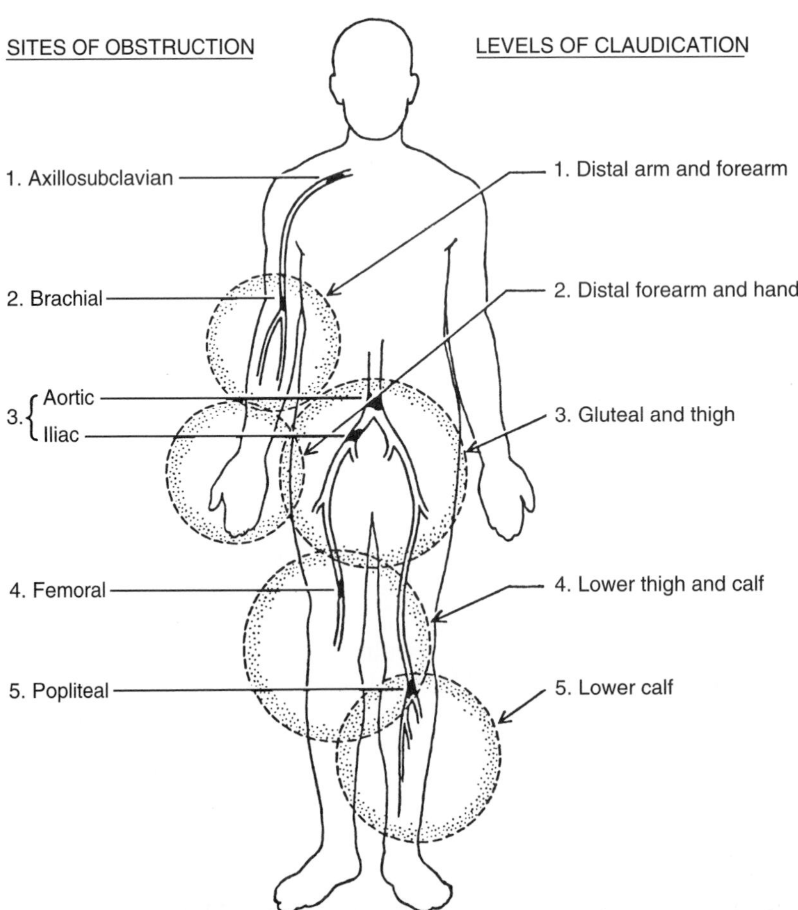

FIG. 4–5. Sites of obstruction and corresponding levels of claudication.

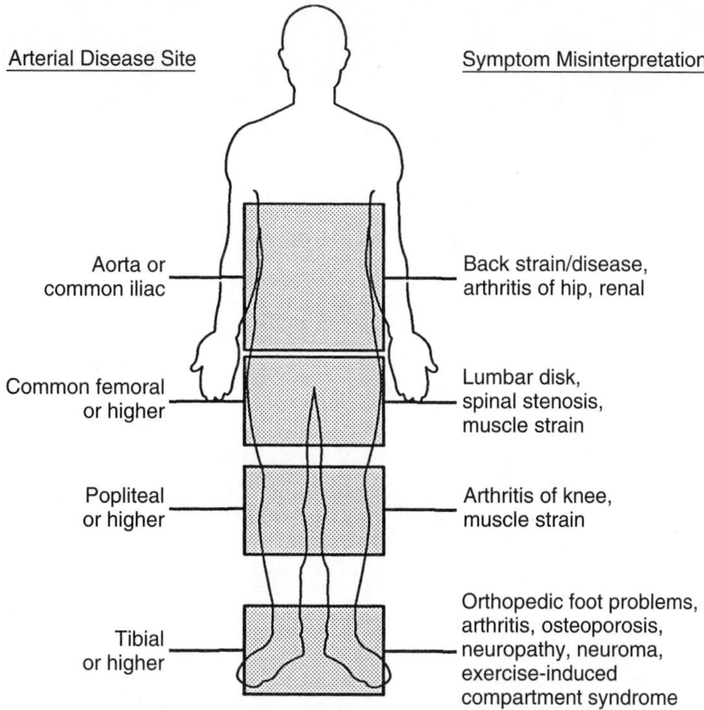

FIG. 4–6. Common misinterpretations of lower-extremity claudication, which often mimics neurologic or musculoskeletal disorders. Assessment of onset, precipitating factors, and relief methods is important for an accurate diagnosis.

Vascular intermittent claudication can be differentiated from neurogenic claudication if the following criteria are met:

1. The pain must start as a muscle cramp in the thigh, buttocks, or calf after walking a predictable distance.
2. The pain must be relieved by rest in a standing position after a predictable period of time.
3. The patient must then be able to walk a similar distance again, and again experience pain and then obtain relief after stopping for the same period as before.[16]

Calf cramps should not be confused with those that occur at night in older patients, some of whom may even have pulse deficits or other signs of arterial disease. Nocturnal muscle cramps have no known vascular basis; instead, they are thought to result from exaggerated neuromuscular response to stretching.[14]

Rest pain, which occurs with advanced arterial occlusive disease, is described as pain in the toes or metatarsal head area when the extremity is resting in a supine position. Rest pain initially occurs at night and interferes with the patient's sleep. Relief is obtained when the foot is placed in a dependent position, such as dangling it over the side of the bed. Pain may be relieved by strong analgesics or opiates.

Ischemic ulceration is caused by inadequate blood supply. The ulcer usually occurs at the tips of the toes, over pressure areas where local pressure causes further decrease in arterial perfusion (Fig. 4-7), the heels, and occasionally between the toes (Fig. 4-8). Neurotrophic ulcers (Fig. 4-9) or interdigital ulcers in diabetics must not be confused with those due to severe ischemia (Table 4-3).

Tissue loss such as gangrene of the toes (Fig. 4-10) or forefoot in conjunction with rest pain represents the most severe form of ischemia. Superficial skin gangrene resulting from microembolization must not be confused with ischemic gangrene. In blue toe syndrome secondary to atherosclerotic debris, microemboli, or aneurysms, the digits are typically cold and

TABLE 4–2 Differential Diagnosis of Intermittent Claudication

Condition	Location of Pain or Discomfort	Characteristic Discomfort	Onset Relative to Exercise	Effect of Rest	Effect of Body Position	Other Characteristics
Intermittent claudication (calf)	*Calf muscles*	*Cramping pain*	*After same degree of exercise*	*Quickly relieved*	*None*	*Reproducible*
Chronic compartment syndrome	Calf muscles	Tight, bursting pain	After much exercise (e.g., jogging)	Subsides very slowly	Relief speeded by elevation	Typically heavily muscled athletes
Venous claudication	Entire leg, but usually worse in thigh and groin	Tight, bursting pain	After walking	Subsides slowly	Relief speeded by elevation	History of iliofemoral DVT, signs of venous congestion, edema
Nerve root compression (e.g., herniated disc)	Radiates down leg, usually posteriorly	Sharp lancinating pain	Soon, if not immediately after onset	Not quickly relieved (also often present at rest)	Relief may be aided by adjusting back position	History of back problems
Symptomatic Baker's cyst	Behind knee, down calf	Swelling, soreness, tenderness	With exercise	Present at rest	None	Not intermittent
Intermittent claudication (hip, thigh, buttocks)	*Hip, thigh, buttocks*	*Aching discomfort, weakness*	*After same degree of exercise*	*Quickly relieved*	*None*	*Reproducible*
Hip arthritis	Hip, thigh, buttocks	Aching discomfort	After variable degree of exercise	Not quickly relieved (and may be present at rest)	More comfortable sitting, weight taken off legs	Variable, may relate to activity level, weather changes
Spinal cord compression	Hip, thigh, buttocks (follows dermatome)	Weakness more than pain	After walking or standing for same length of time	Relieved by stopping only if position changed	Relief by lumbar spine flexion (sitting or stooping forward) pressure	Frequent history of back problems, provoked by increased intra-abdominal pressure
Intermittent claudication (foot)	*Foot, arch*	*Severe deep pain and numbness*	*After same degree of exercise*	*Quickly relieved*	*None*	*Reproducible*
Arthritic, inflammatory processes	Foot, arch	Aching pain	After variable degree of exercise	Not quickly relieved (and may be present at rest)	May be relieved by not bearing weight	Variable, may relate to activity level

From Rutherford RB: Initial patient evaluation: the vascular consultation. In Rutherford RB, ed: *Vascular surgery,* ed 5, Philadelphia, 2000, WB Saunders, pp 1-13. Reprinted with permission.

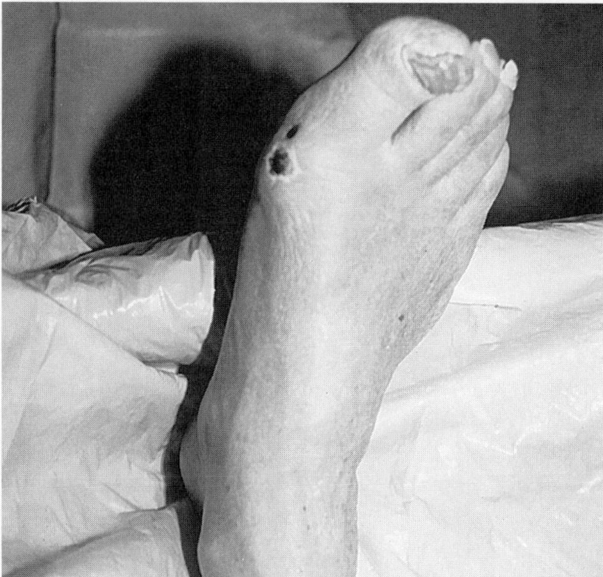

FIG. 4–7. Ulceration over bony prominence.

painful (see Fig. 4-4). Gangrene of the toes may also be present in diabetics with palpable pedal pulses.

Acute arterial occlusion of the lower extremities, the sudden decrease in limb perfusion, is characterized by the six *P*s: sudden onset of pain, pallor, pulselessness, and poikilothermia (coolness) in the affected extremity; paresthesias and paralysis occur in later stages (see Box 4-3). These signs and symptoms may not be present in all patients.[13] With an acute aortic occlusion, patients may experience sudden onset of bilateral leg pain and coolness.

Inspection

The lower extremities should always be inspected bilaterally. Color of the extremities should be examined with the patient in different positions. Elevate the patient's legs 30°-45°. If arterial

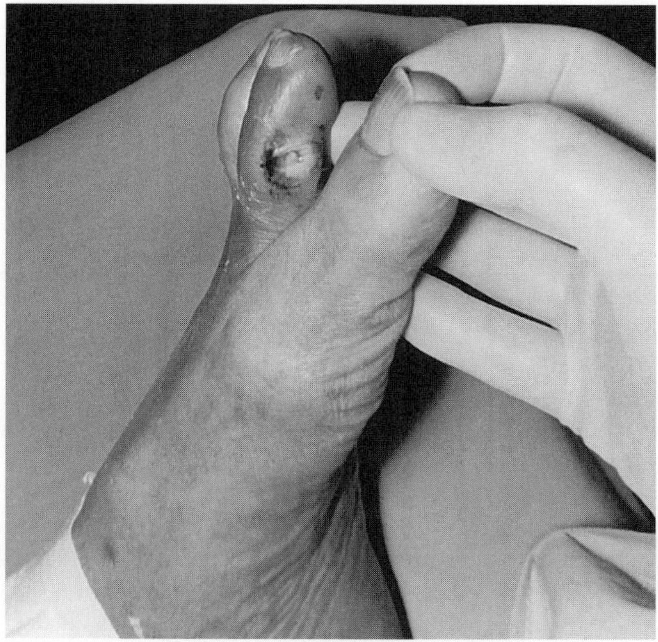

FIG. 4–8. Ulcer between the toes.

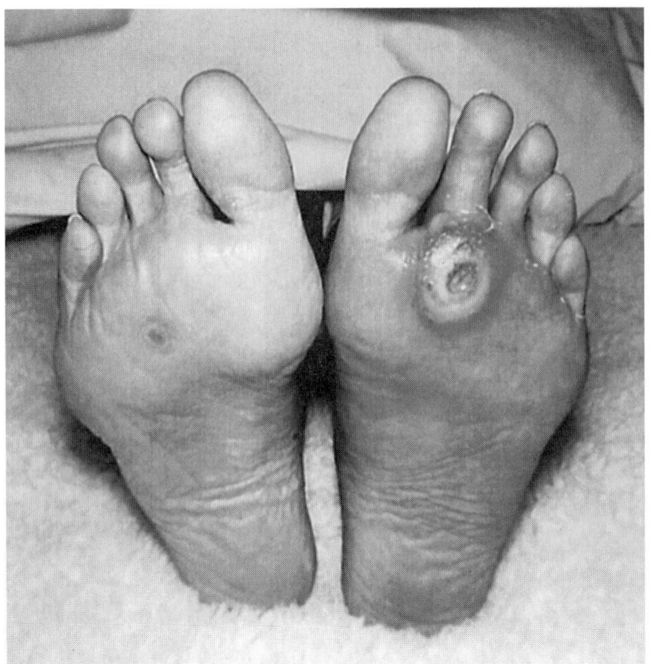

FIG. 4–9. Neurotrophic ulcer.

TABLE 4–3 Characteristics of Common Lower-Extremity Lesions

Characteristic	Ischemic Ulcer	Venous Stasis Ulcer	Neurotrophic Ulcer
Onset	Traumatic or spontaneous	Traumatic or spontaneous	Spontaneous
Location	Toe, heel, dorsum of foot	Medial distal third of leg	Sole of foot under calluses or pressure points
Pain	Severe at night; relieved by dependency	Mild pain when infected; aching with dependency; relieved with elevation	None
Skin around ulcer	Atrophic; may be inflamed	Stasis dermatitis; pigmentation changes	Callous
Ulcer edge	Definitive	Uneven	Definitive
Ulcer base	Pale, eschar	Healthy	Healthy or pale
Pulses	Decreased or none	Normal	Normal
Associated signs	Trophic changes Gangrene may be present	Edema No gangrene Decreased sensation Diabetes	Neuropathy No gangrene

Data from Pousti TJ, Wilson SE, Williams RA: The clinical examination of the vascular system. In Veith FJ, Hobson RW, Williams RA et al, eds: *Vascular surgery principles and practice,* New York, 1994, McGraw-Hill, pp 74-89.

disease is significant, the legs become pale, a phenomenon known as "pallor with elevation"; the arterial system cannot pump adequate blood into the capillary system against gravity through the arterial blockages.

The patient should then hang his or her legs over the side of the bed. The legs should remain a healthy pink color. With arterial disease, a deep red color (dependent rubor) occurs as a result of blood pooling in the arterioles. The color changes reflect increased oxygen saturation and blood flow in the capillary venous plexus of the skin that occurs because of loss of the sympathetic reflex vasoconstriction normally found in dependency.[6] Capillary refill time, the time taken for a blanched area to "pink up," is a crude indication of blood flow. It

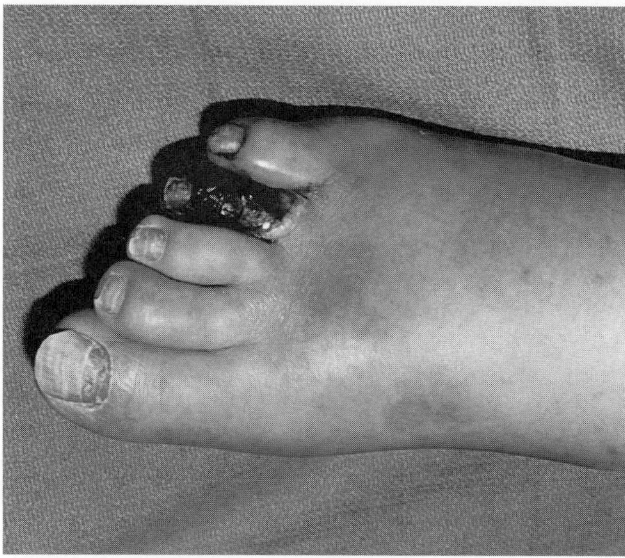

FIG. 4–10. Gangrene of toe with cellulitis.

can be checked by pressing on the tip of the toes or sole of the foot with a finger and then releasing pressure.

Inspect the extremities for trophic changes secondary to tissue malnutrition from arterial compromise. Trophic changes include the following:

- Hair loss on the affected extremity
- Thin, smooth, shiny skin
- Thick, brittle nails with or without fungal infection (Fig. 4-11)
- Tapering of toes or fingers
- Any skin breakdown (possibly traumatic), ulceration, or gangrene

Ischemic ulcerations are usually located over pressure points, i.e., heels, toes, and bony prominences, and on the dorsum of the foot and over metatarsal heads, especially I and V. Note the size and depth of the ulcer, color of the base (usually pale), and the presence and/or odor of drainage. Gangrene may be dry, mummified, blue-black eschar on toes, forefoot, or heel, or it may be moist (wet gangrene). Areas of discoloration on the toes or foot from microembolization (blue toe syndrome) should be noted.

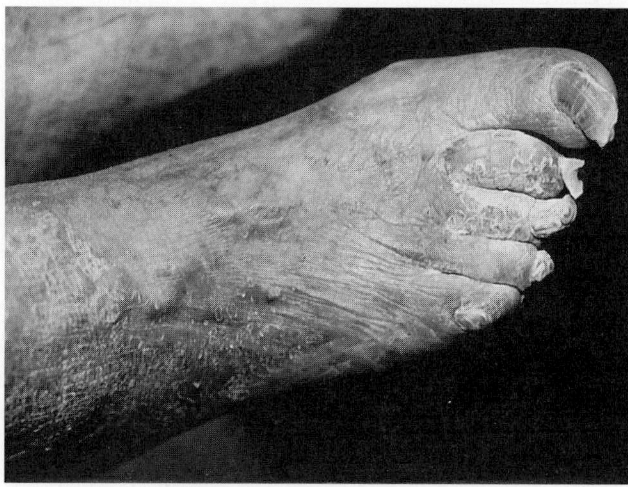

FIG. 4-11. Thick, deformed nails.

Inspect the extremities for size and symmetry, muscle atrophy, or edema that may be present secondary to the leg being in a dependent position or a potential compartment syndrome. Also note the absence of a limb or digit or any scarring on the extremities from previous surgery or injury. Diabetes can lead to bone abnormalities and foot deformities.

Acute ischemia reduces blood supply to distal nerve fibers and muscles; therefore, motor and sensory function of the extremities may be diminished or absent. The three findings that separate a threatened from a viable extremity are the presence of persistent pain, sensory loss, and muscle weakness.[9]

Sensory function can be assessed by touch, pressure, or nailbed compression. Ask the patient to tell which toe is being touched while using a blunt-edged instrument such as a hemostat or paper clip. Invasive instruments such as safety pins should be avoided to prevent a break in the skin. Diabetic neuropathy as well as previous surgery can contribute to impaired sensation.

Motor function is evaluated by eliciting movement of muscle groups whose blood supply is derived from arteries distal to the occlusion. Instruct the patient to perform digital flexion and extension as well as to move the extremity.[14] Drop foot may be present with advanced ischemia.[9] Muscle rigor, tenderness, or pain with passive movement are late signs of advanced ischemia and probable tissue loss.

Palpation

One can determine the location of disease with examination of the pulses. Examination of the lower-extremity pulses includes palpation of the femoral, popliteal, posterior tibial, and dorsalis pedis arteries (Fig. 4-12). While palpating the pulses, note aneurysmal dilation. With the patient supine, the common femoral pulse can be palpated just distal to the inguinal ligament, midgroin, between the pubic bone and the anterior superior iliac spine. It is difficult to palpate in an obese person. The examiner should stand on the side being examined and press deeply. The popliteal pulse is located deeply on the posterior medial aspect of the knee joint. With the patient's knee slightly flexed and calf muscles relaxed, cup both hands and press fingertips behind the knee against the flat surface of the tibia. If the pulse cannot be palpated in this position, have the patient lie on his or her abdomen and flex the knee 45°; then palpate again. If the popliteal pulse is easily palpated, a popliteal aneurysm should be suspected. The posterior tibial artery is found in the groove behind the medial malleolus of the ankle, one-third the distance from the malleolar prominence to the edge of the tendon. To palpate the left pulse, stand on the left side, with right fingertips curved behind the medial malleolus. The dorsalis pedis pulse, a continuation of the anterior tibial artery, is found on the dorsal midportion of the foot between the first and second metatarsals. Standing at the foot of the bed using the hand on the same side as that of the foot being palpated, place three fingers on the dorsum of the foot on an imaginary line drawn between the midpoint between the malleoli and the first web space. Because of anatomic variations, the posterior tibial and dorsalis pedis pulses may be absent in about 10 percent of the population.[14] If the dorsalis pedis pulse is not palpable, the lateral tarsal artery, the terminal branch of the peroneal artery located laterally and in the midportion of the foot, should be palpated. Because the peroneal artery lies medial to the fibula behind the lateral malleolus, it is not usually palpable.

Patients with intermittent claudication may have superficial femoral artery disease and therefore have femoral pulses but absent distal pulses. Diabetics commonly have infrapopliteal disease and thus have palpable femoral and popliteal pulses but absent distal pulses. Intermittent claudication may occur in the presence of palpable pedal pulses; however, the pulse may disappear after exercise.[9] The "disappearing pulse phenomenon," described by DeWeese,[17] can be demonstrated by repeat palpation of pedal pulses after exercise. The patient can rise up on the toes repeatedly or walk on a treadmill until claudication develops. Pulses disappear because of the marked decrease in vascular resistance that occurs in exercising muscle distal to an obstruction and because of the increased distribution of flow to muscle beds proximal to the obstruction.[7] The presence of normal pulses after exercise

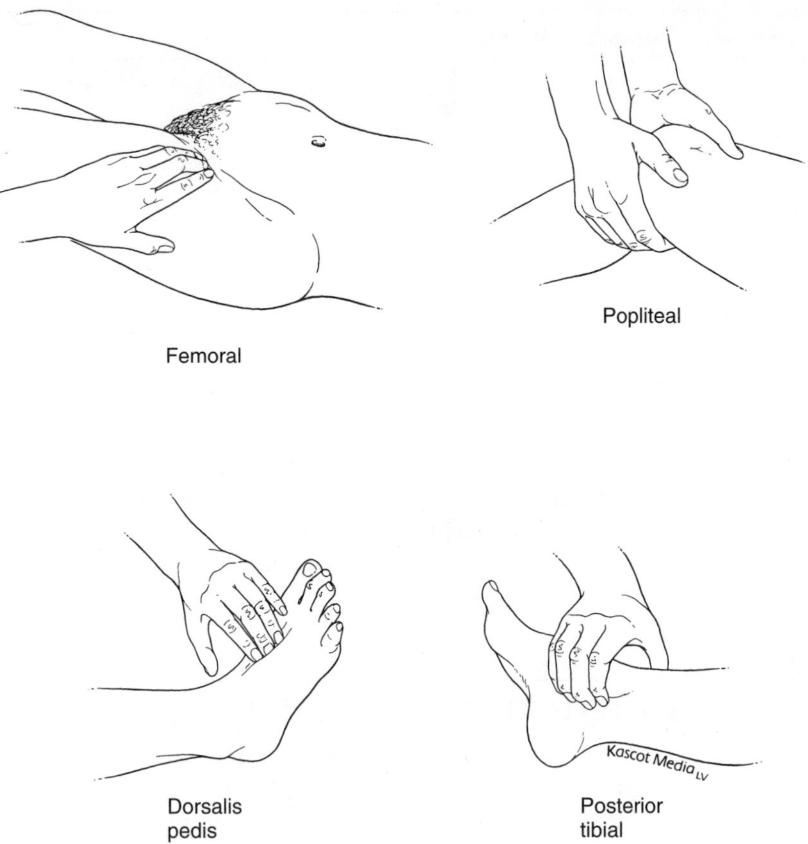

FIG. 4–12. Palpation of the femoral, popliteal, posterior tibial, and dorsalis pedis arterial pulses.

strongly suggests a nonarterial cause.[2] If a young person has a history of claudication with palpable pedal pulses, pulses should be rechecked during active plantar flexion or passive dorsiflexion. Popliteal artery entrapment syndrome may be present. Pedal pulses may be normal in the presence of microemboli.[9]

After completing the pulse evaluation, use the back of the hand to assess the skin temperature of the lower extremities. In addition to absent pulses, a temperature demarcation can be felt one skeletal segment below the site of arterial occlusion. Symmetric coolness usually indicates peripheral vasoconstriction; asymmetric coolness may represent arterial insufficiency. If infection is suspected in the foot, it should be palpated for tenderness and fluctuation.

Auscultation

The femoral artery may be auscultated for a bruit. The bruit occlusion test may help localize the stenosis, differentiating between iliac and superficial femoral artery disease. If the initial auscultation reveals a bruit, the examiner compresses the superficial femoral artery distal to the site of the stethoscope. If the bruit disappears or decreases in intensity, a stenosis in the superficial femoral artery is likely. Conversely, if no change or an increase in intensity occurs, the profunda femoris artery or another branch artery may be stenotic. By repeating this maneuver with the stethoscope placed above the inguinal ligament, the examiner may detect a stenotic lesion in the iliac artery.[6] Also, auscultation is important to confirm a suspected arteriovenous fistula, which is characterized by a continuous to-and-fro bruit.

By auscultating blood pressure measurements over the arteries in the leg, the examiner can determine the level and severity of disease. Normally, the systolic blood pressure at the ankle level is equal to or slightly higher than the brachial systolic pressure. To determine the

TABLE 4–4 Ankle-Brachial Index

No symptoms	= .7-1.0 or greater
Claudication	= .5-.7
Rest pain, ulcer, gangrene	= .3 or less

Data from Benjamin ME, Dean RH: Examination of the patient with vascular disease. In Dean RH, Yao JST, Brewster DC, eds: *Current diagnosis and treatment in vascular surgery*, Norwalk, Conn, 1995, Appleton & Lange, pp 1-4

percentage of blood supply to the extremity, the ankle pressure is divided by the highest brachial pressure.

$$\frac{\text{Ankle Pressure}}{\text{Brachinal Pressure (Highest)}} = \text{Ankle-Brachinal Index (ABI)}$$

Any decrease in pressure indicates arterial stenosis (Table 4-4). This is further discussed in Chapter 5. Calcification of the arterial wall, which occurs in diabetics and patients with renal failure, can result in a falsely elevated ankle pressure because the vessel is incompressible. When a prosthetic graft is tunneled through soft tissue, the graft is not compressible, also resulting in an invalid pressure measurement.

ASSESSMENT OF THE VENOUS SYSTEM

Venous disease, unlike arterial occlusive disease, is usually localized to one anatomic area and occurs most commonly in the lower extremities, although the upper extremities can be affected, especially with the increased use of central venous lines. Physical assessment of the venous system is less precise than the arterial system.

Head and Neck

Dilated jugular veins may indicate an arteriovenous fistula, congestive heart failure, or venous occlusion proximal to the dilated veins. If both sides of the neck and both arms have dilated veins, a superior vena cava syndrome is suspected.[6]

Upper Extremities

When venous disease involves the upper extremity, acute or chronic obstruction of the axillary or subclavian vein is the most likely cause.[18] Acute deep vein thrombosis (DVT) usually results from central venous cannulation for parenteral nutrition or intravenous therapy, thoracic outlet syndrome, or shoulder injury. Acute thrombosis following vigorous exercise, work, or lifting may be referred to as effort thrombosis.[19]

In contrast to ileofemoral venous thrombosis, most subclavian-axillary thromboses are asymptomatic because of good collateral circulation and because the upper extremity is less susceptible than the lower extremity to gravitational forces.

Chronic venous obstruction may be a result of venous thrombosis or external compression of the vein by thoracic outlet syndrome or lymphatic obstruction. Lymphatic obstruction is usually associated with a history of a radical mastectomy, infection, or irradiation involving axillary lymph nodes (see Chapter 3).

Intermittent Subclavian Vein Obstruction

Intermittent swelling of the upper extremity may indicate intermittent subclavian venous obstruction. Discomfort and tightness in the arm and abnormally prominent superficial veins may also be present. These symptoms may be aggravated when the arm is raised above the head or when a patient's posture is unusually erect. The patient should be evaluated with his or her shoulders braced in the military position or with the arms hyperabducted and externally rotated at the shoulder.[19, 20]

Superficial Thrombophlebitis

With superficial thrombophlebitis, the main complaint is localized tenderness or pain (dolor) along the course of the affected vein. Inspect the affected vein for erythema and swelling. A cord may be palpable along the affected vein with increased skin temperature.

Inspect the arm for any break in the skin, which is a potential source of cellulitis. Purulent drainage and fever may indicate suppurative thrombophlebitis.

Deep Vein Thrombosis

Acute unilateral arm swelling is the chief complaint with a DVT and may be accompanied by an aching pain. Inspect the extremities for symmetry in size. Dilated superficial veins around the shoulder may be present (Fig. 4-13). Venous distention is not diminished when the arm is raised above the level of the heart.

Venous sounds are not usually audible with a stethoscope.[5] Patterns of abnormal venous flow in arms have not been as clearly defined as in the Doppler exam of the legs.[21] However, venous examination with Doppler ultrasound and duplex scanning is well recognized and discussed in Chapter 5.

Phlegmasia Cerulea Dolens

Severe venous obstruction can result in phlegmasia cerulea dolens, which is associated with intense upper-extremity swelling, pain, and bluish discoloration. It is usually seen in patients with advanced malignancy being treated with chemotherapy via a central line.[19] Venous gangrene of the upper extremity is rare.

Pulmonary Embolus

Signs and symptoms of pulmonary embolus (PE) are included in Box 4-4. Massive PE may also be accompanied by acute cor pulmonale and syncope. Neck veins may be distended. With a PE, pulmonic second heart sound is often accentuated. A friction rub may be present.[22]

Trauma

A penetrating injury or surgery of the arm may cause an arteriovenous fistula. Auscultate over the affected area to detect the presence of a bruit.

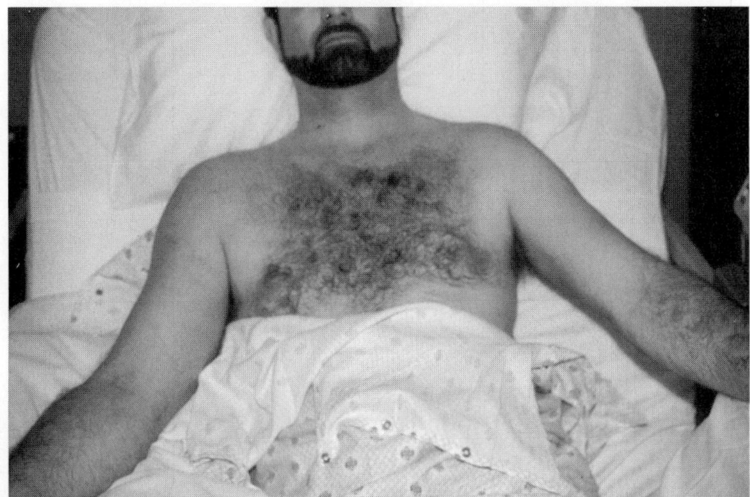

FIG. 4–13. Upper extremity venous thrombosis of the right upper extremity. Note unilateral right arm swelling and dilated superficial veins close to the surface of the skin.

BOX 4–4

Signs of Pulmonary Embolus

Chest pain	Dyspnea
Respiratory distress	Tachycardia
Sudden hypotension	Sweating

Lower Extremities

Superficial Thrombophlebitis

Symptoms of superficial thrombophlebitis in the lower extremity include localized pain or aching and possible swelling and warmth over the affected vein. There is usually redness over a firm mass or cord with surrounding induration along the course of the affected vein (Fig. 4-14).

Deep Vein Thrombosis

The most common symptom is sudden onset of unilateral edema or feeling of heaviness in the leg. Iliofemoral DVT may result in intense pain and swelling of the thigh and leg. Calf vein DVT may cause unilateral leg swelling below the knee. If the vena cava is involved, signs and symptoms are usually bilateral.

However, signs and symptoms may be absent or minimal depending on the size and location of the thrombus, the degree of obstruction, the phase of thrombus formation, and the adequacy of collateral circulation.[19] Thrombi in the leg veins are responsible for the majority of PEs but are recognizable prior to death in less than 55 percent of patients with fatal PE.[20]

Inspect the lower extremities for unilateral edema in the calf, ankle, or thigh. The lower-extremity circumference should be measured to establish a baseline and evaluate the effectiveness of therapy. For the most reliable comparison, measure at the same level each time by marking the areas. Inspect for dilation of superficial veins in the legs or pelvis, and note the color of the extremity. Palpate the pelvic and femoral areas for a mass that may cause external venous compression.

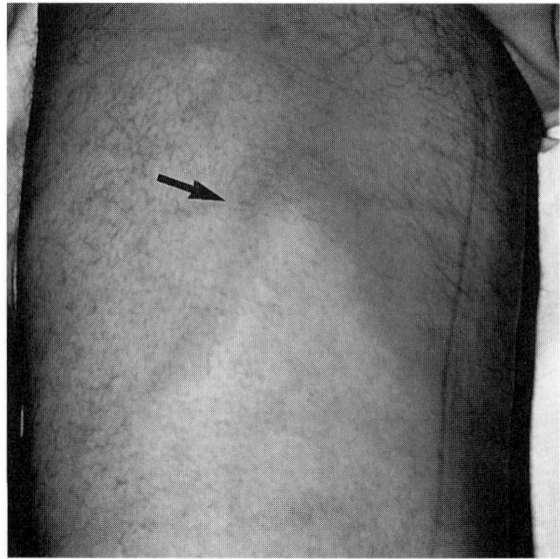

FIG. 4–14. Superficial phlebitis of the lower extremity.

Phlegmasia

Iliac vein thrombosis may cause the entire lower extremity to swell and become pale and painful, known as phlegmasia alba dolens. With extensive iliofemoral thrombosis, known as phlegmasia cerulea dolens, the leg is severely edematous, cyanotic, and painful, which can lead to venous gangrene.[5]

Varicose Veins

Patients with varicose veins (Fig. 4-15) complain of cosmetic disfigurement, unsightly veins with or without aching, cramping discomfort in their legs with prolonged standing, swelling in the evening, heaviness, and possibly night cramps. Discomfort is usually relieved with leg elevation. The pain may increase in severity prior to the menstrual period or during pregnancy.[20] Spider veins may be present, and the overlying skin color is purple or bright red. Reticular varices may render the skin a dark blue color.[19]

Patients being examined for varicose veins should stand to allow the long and short saphenous veins to fill. Inspect each leg for dilated, tortuous veins, usually located as tributaries to the greater saphenous vein. Note the location of the varicosities; any dilated suprapubic veins could be evidence of past iliofemoral or vena cava thrombosis.

Certain tourniquet tests may be performed to diagnose valvular competence in the veins. Incompetent valves in superficial and perforating veins can be detected by Trendelenburg's test. Patency of the deep veins can be determined by the Perthes test.[19, 22]

Varicose veins may be present with congenital vascular malformations.[21] A rare congenital pattern of varicose veins, called Klippel-Trénaunay syndrome, includes capillary malformations (port wine stains), atypical varicosities, and bony or soft tissue hypertrophy. These patients may have persistent lateral embryologic veins and an absent or abnormal deep venous system.[5]

Chronic Venous Insufficiency

Patients with chronic venous insufficiency complain of chronic swelling and aching discomfort in the legs when standing that is relieved by elevation of the legs above the heart.

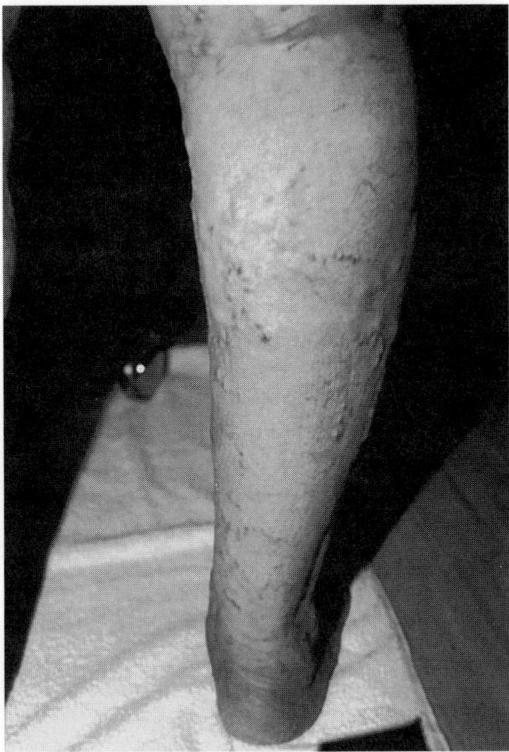

FIG. 4–15. Varicose veins.

Swelling secondary to high venous pressure can be venous (postphlebitic) or cardiac in origin, with right-sided heart failure or tricuspid valvular insufficiency. Night cramps may be common but are unrelated. Ulceration may be present. Although related pain is uncommon, patients may complain of bursting pain in the calf after walking about 100-200 yards, which is slowly relieved by rest and elevation. This condition, known as venous claudication, is secondary to venous outflow obstruction. This may occur after ileofemoral venous thrombosis, when recanalization and collateral development are poor. Exercising muscles significantly increase arterial inflow, and, in turn, venous outflow. As a result, venous pressures increase and the patient experiences a tight, almost bursting discomfort in the leg.[9]

Inspect the patient's lower extremities for edema, cellulitis, and hyperpigmentation of the skin around ankle ulceration, resulting from breakdown of red blood cells into deposits of hemosiderin that stain the tissue a characteristic brownish color. Also note eczema, stasis dermatitis (dry scaling), induration and scarring from previous ulceration, and the color of the legs when dependent. Note the presence and location of ulcers, their color, size, shape, and depth, and the presence of drainage or odor (see Table 4-3) (see Chapter 19).

The examiner may palpate a fascial defect along the course of the affected vein, representing the site of an incompetent perforator vein.[5] Palpation does not provide much useful information in the assessment of the postphlebitic leg. As in the upper extremities, auscultation with a stethoscope is not beneficial except in case of injury.

SUMMARY

The mainstay of diagnosis of vascular disease remains a good history and physical examination. Assessment of the vascular system is one of the fundamental activities of nursing practice. Its importance is paramount in providing quality nursing care as well as in initiating the nurse-patient relationship. In addition, the assessment provides the foundation of the nursing process: assessment, diagnosis, planning, implementation, and evaluation. See Chapter 3 for assessment for lymphedema.

REFERENCES

1. Ekers M: Psychosocial considerations in peripheral vascular disease. In Beaver BM, Wagner MW, eds: *Nursing clinics of North America: peripheral vascular dysfunction,* Philadelphia, 1986, WB Saunders, pp 255-263.
2. Benjamin ME, Dean RH: Examination of the patient with vascular disease. In Dean RH, Yao JST, Brewster DC, eds: *Current diagnosis and treatment in vascular surgery,* Norwalk, Conn, 1995, Appleton & Lange, pp 1-4.
3. Casey J, Flinn WR, Yao JST et al: Correlation of immune and nutritional status with wound complications in patients undergoing vascular operations, *Surgery* 93:822-827, 1983.
4. Imparato AM: Carotid endarterectomy: indications and techniques for carotid surgery. In Haimovici H, ed: *Vascular surgery: principles and techniques*, ed 4, Cambridge, 1996, Blackwell Science, pp 913-937.
5. Hallett JW, Brewster DC, Rasmussen TE: *Handbook of patient care in vascular diseases*, ed 4, Philadelphia, 2001, Lippincott, Williams & Wilkins.
6. Young JR: Physical examination. In Young JR, Graor RA, Olin JW et al: *Peripheral vascular diseases,* St Louis, 1996, Mosby, pp 18-32.
7. Pousti TJ, Wilson SE, Williams RA: The clinical examination of the vascular system. In Veith FJ, Hobson RW, Williams RA et al, eds: *Vascular surgery principles and practice,* New York, 1994, McGraw-Hill, pp 74-89.
8. Porter JM, Edwards JM: Occlusive and vasospastic diseases involving distal upper extremity arteries—Raynaud's syndrome. In Rutherford RB, ed: *Vascular surgery*, ed 5, Philadelphia, 2000, WB Saunders, pp 1170-1183.
9. Transatlantic Intersociety Consensus (TASC): Management of peripheral arterial disease (PAD), *J Vasc Surg* 31(1 Pt 2): 556-574, 2000.
10. Allen EV: Thromboangitis obliterans: method of diagnosis of chronic occlusive arterial lesions distal to the wrist with illustrative cases, *Am J Med Sci* 178:237-244, 1929.
11. Conn J, Bergan JJ, Bell JL: Hypothenar hammer syndrome: posttraumatic digital ischemia, *Surgery* 68:1122-1127, 1970.

12. Meacham PW, Dean RH, Smith BM: *Vascular physical diagnosis: the arterial system,* Nashville, 1985, Vanderbilt University School of Medicine.
13. Fairbairn JF: Clinical manifestations of peripheral vascular disease. In Juergens JL, Spittell JA, Fairbairn JF, eds: *Peripheral vascular diseases*, ed 2, Philadelphia, 1980, WB Saunders, pp 3-49.
14. Rutherford RB: Initial patient evaluation: the vascular consultation. In Rutherford RB, ed: *Vascular surgery*, ed 5, Philadelphia, 2000, WB Saunders, pp 1-13.
15. Callow AD: Clinical assessment of the peripheral circulation. In Callow AD, Ernst CB, eds: *Vascular surgery: theory and practice,* Norwalk, Conn, 1995, Appleton & Lange, pp 81-199.
16. Warren R: Two kinds of intermittent claudication, *Arch Surg* 111:739, 1976.
17. DeWeese JA: Pedal pulses disappearing with exercise, *N Engl J Med* 262:1214-1217, 1960.
18. Gloviczki P, Kaymier FJ, Hollier LH: Axillary-subcutaneous venous occlusion: the morbidity of a nonlethal disease, *J Vasc Surg* 4:333-337, 1986.
19. Bradbury A, Ruckley CV. Clinical assessment of patients with venous disease. In Gloviczki P, Yao JST, eds: *Handbook of venous disorders: guidelines of the American Venous Forum,* London, 2001, Arnold, pp 71-83.
20. DeWeese JA: Clinical examination of patients with venous disease. In Gloviczki P, Yao JST, eds: *Handbook of venous disorders,* London, 1996, Chapman & Hall, pp 63-80.
21. Yao JST: Non-invasive investigation of vascular disease, *Curr Pract Surg* 1:244-252, 1989.
22. Cho J, Gloviczki P: Venous diseases. In Corson JD, Williamson RCN, eds: *Surgery,* London, 2001, Mosby, Section 4, pp 1-16.

5

Noninvasive Vascular Testing

DONNA R. BLACKBURN □ LINDA PETERSON-KENNEDY

The past several decades have seen the emergence of noninvasive testing as a standard of care for the vascular patient. These techniques were designed to aid the clinician in the diagnosis and follow-up of peripheral vascular disease. Although certainly not all-inclusive, the information provided in this chapter will familiarize the vascular nurse with the fundamentals of noninvasive testing.

INSTRUMENTATION

Instrumentation currently available in the vascular laboratory provides both hemodynamic and anatomic information about the peripheral vascular system. The method employed is primarily diagnostic ultrasonography, including duplex imaging.

Ultrasound

Sound travels in waves that, when they strike an interface, are reflected back. In the 1800s, Christian Doppler[1] noted that there is a change in sound frequency in relation to a moving source. This change can be noted in the whistle of a moving train as it approaches and passes.

Sound is the result of vibration. One complete vibration is known as a cycle or Hertz (Hz), and the number of cycles per second is called frequency (also expressed in Hertz). One Hertz is one cycle per second. Ultrasound has a frequency greater than that detected by the human ear (greater than 20,000 Hz). Most ultrasonographic instruments used in the vascular laboratory employ ranges of 2-10 MHz (million cycles per second).

When the transmitted ultrasound waves strike moving red blood cells and other tissue interfaces, sound is reflected back to the transducer. Ultrasound reflected from moving red blood cells is shifted in frequency in an amount proportional to the velocity of the moving blood. Flow moving toward the transducer reflects sound at a higher frequency than that of the transmitted frequency. Conversely, the signal from receding flow has lower frequencies than the transmitted frequency.[2] Directional Doppler instruments have the capability of sensing flow direction by detecting these frequency changes.

Continuous-Wave Doppler Transducer

The continuous-wave Doppler is the one that is most frequently used to monitor ankle or arm pressures at the bedside. The continuous-wave Doppler transducer contains both a transmitting and a receiving crystal, which operate continuously. Flow at any point in the path of the sound beam will be detected with this device (Fig. 5-1). In handheld devices, direction cannot be detected.

Pulsed Doppler Transducer

One crystal acts as both a transmitter and a receiver in the pulsed Doppler transducer. Short pulses of sound are transmitted at regular intervals. The returning signal is received at specific times between transmissions (Fig. 5-2). The number of pulse repetitions per second can be

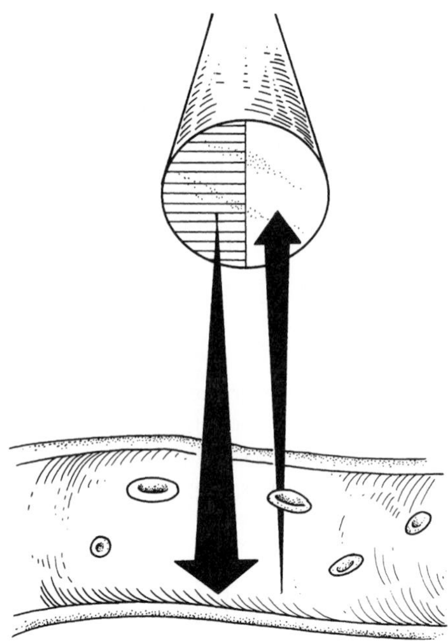

FIG. 5–1. Schematic illustration of a continuous-wave Doppler transducer. One crystal continuously emits an ultrasound beam; the other crystal continuously receives the backscattered signal. (From Pomajzl JM: *Real-time ultrasound imaging and pulsed/gated Doppler instructional manual,* Indianapolis, 1984, Biosound, Inc., p 35.)

varied with this system to allow sampling at a specific depth and site. This is the transducer used in duplex imaging; vessels are visualized, and the flow in them can be precisely evaluated.

The received Doppler data can be evaluated in several ways. Each returning echo can be displayed as a dot on the screen, creating a real-time image of the tissue beneath the transducer. The audible velocity of the blood within a vessel is processed through a spectral

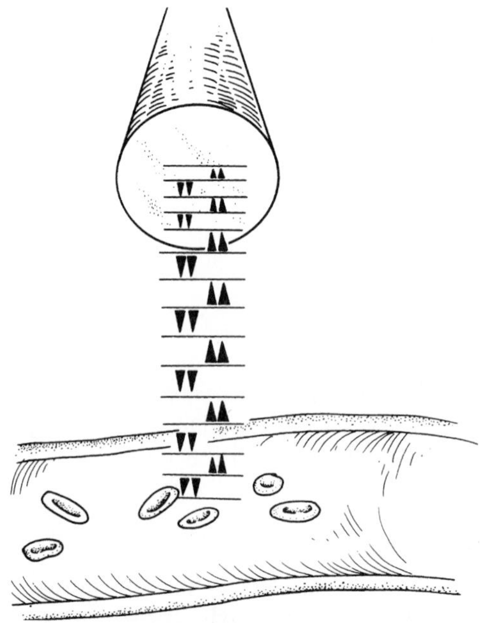

FIG. 5–2. Schematic illustration of a pulsed Doppler transducer. The same crystal acts intermittently as both a transmitter and a receiver. (From Pomajzl JM: *Real-time ultrasound imaging and pulsed/gated Doppler instructional manual,* Indianapolis, 1984, Biosound, Inc., p 35.)

analyzer to display exact velocities. Averaged velocities can be displayed through a zero crossing detector (the Doppler waveforms seen on an arterial Doppler exam).

Duplex Ultrasonography

Duplex imaging is a combination of visualizing the tissue in gray scale and listening to the Doppler information. Each tissue beneath the transducer changes or shifts the ultrasound beam in a characteristic manner. Ultrasound echoes reflected from tissue interfaces are displayed in shades of gray; the higher the density, the brighter the echoes. Because blood is a poor reflector of ultrasound, a blood vessel appears as an area of poor reflection surrounded by its walls, which are good reflectors.[3] Duplex imaging produces anatomic information in the image and physiologic information by analyzing the velocity information in the Doppler signal.

Color imaging is a method of displaying Doppler-shifted frequencies superimposed on the gray scale image to display simultaneous anatomic and hemodynamic information. Echoes reflected from moving red blood cells are displayed with colors that correspond to direction of flow.[2] Commonly, flow towards the transducer is displayed in red and flow away from the transducer is displayed in blue. The color scale on the side of the image guides the examiner for determining both flow direction and velocities (as velocity increases, the color will change according to the scale). Areas of stenosis cause the velocity to increase and the color to change. Poststenotic turbulence is represented by a mosaic pattern of all colors.

Plethysmography

Plethysmographs are used to directly or indirectly record volume changes in the limbs. The various plethysmographic devices available for use in the vascular laboratory differ in the type of transducer employed for assessing dimensional changes. Forms of plethysmography commonly used for limb volume measurement include air plethysmography and photoplethysmography (PPG).

Air Plethysmography

Air plethysmography is used to obtain volume pulse recordings. Pneumatic cuffs are applied at several locations on the extremity and inflated to a relatively low pressure to ensure skin contact. Volume changes within the limb result in pressure changes within the air-filled cuff and are displayed as waveforms.

Photoplethysmography

The PPG transducer contains an infrared light-emitting diode and a phototransistor that detects back-scattered light. Changes in cutaneous blood content in the skin alter the quantity of reflected light recorded by the photocell. This is used to detect pulses in the toes and fingers and also to detect venous refilling.

VENOUS TESTING: ACUTE VENOUS DISEASE

Duplex imaging is used to detect obstruction in the venous system of both the upper and lower extremities. Venous imaging has shown excellent correlation with venography in the diagnosis of deep venous thrombosis and has replaced it as the gold standard in all but the most complicated cases. The duplex image provides the ability to visualize and localize thrombus and, in many cases, to determine the age of the thrombus. In addition, physiologic information obtained in the Doppler signal may be processed and measured.

The patient exhibiting acute unilateral extremity pain or edema is a candidate for venous testing.[4] Testing is also indicated if pulmonary embolus is suspected. Venous testing is routinely performed in patients at high risk for development of deep venous thrombosis such as patients undergoing orthopedic or neurosurgical procedures or those on prolonged bed rest.

The lower-extremity examination is performed with the patient in a supine position. The transducer is placed in a transverse orientation over the common femoral vein. Light probe pressure is applied to determine if the walls of the vein compress against each other. The transducer is moved slowly down the common femoral, greater saphenous, superficial femoral, and popliteal veins, assessing for vessel compressibility every 1 or 2 cm.[5,6] If calf swelling is present, the posterior tibial, gastrocnemius, and peroneal veins are also assessed. Doppler flow characteristics are evaluated at the common femoral, superficial femoral, and popliteal veins.

Although deep venous thrombosis in the upper extremity is uncommon, routine use of central venous catheters has led to an increased incidence of upper-extremity venous thrombosis. Upper-extremity venous scanning is indicated in patients with edema of the arm or neck. The brachial, axillary, subclavian, and jugular veins are examined when thrombosis is suspected. Many peripherally inserted central catheters (PICC lines) are inserted into the basilic vein, so this vein is frequently studied.

The patient is placed in a supine position with the head of the bed flat. The internal jugular, innominate, subclavian, axillary, and brachial veins are sequentially scanned. Doppler flow patterns are evaluated at all levels. Compression maneuvers are performed over all segments not lying beneath a bony prominence.

Interpretation

Characteristics evaluated include vessel size, compressibility, flow patterns, presence of thrombus, and valve function. The normal vein has thinner walls and is slightly larger than the corresponding artery. Vein diameter fluctuates with the respiratory cycle, and the vessel size is augmented by a Valsalva maneuver. Normal veins compress with light pressure with the transducer (Fig. 5-3). In acute deep venous thrombosis, the vein usually appears dilated, soft echoes may be seen within the lumen of the vein, and the vein will not compress (Fig. 5-4). In the presence of very fresh thrombosis or obstruction in a proximal vein, the vein may appear black (normal), but the vein will not compress. In patients with chronic disease, the

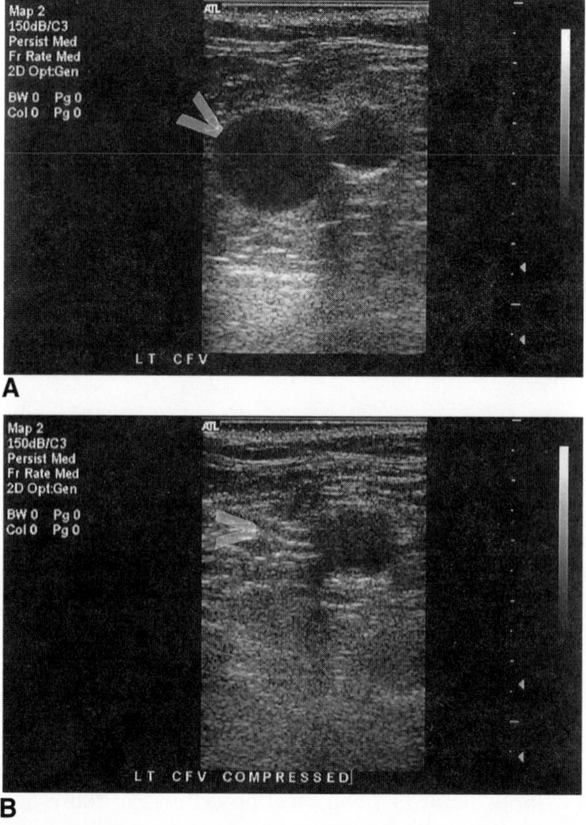

FIG. 5-3. Normal duplex exam at the common femoral level. **A,** Without probe pressure *(arrow)*. **B,** With light probe pressure *(arrow)*, the venous walls coapt, indicating thrombus-free lumen.

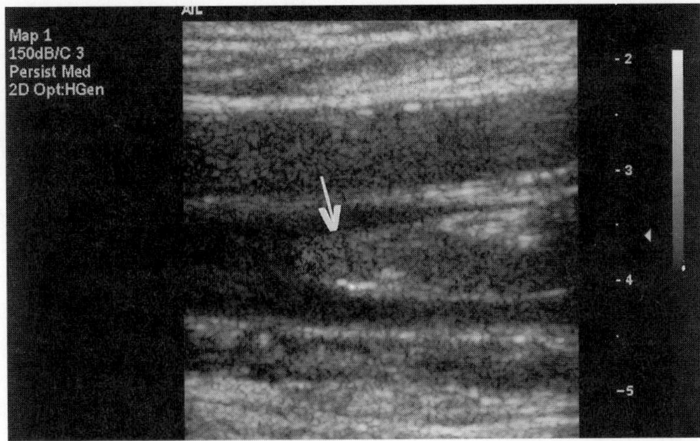

FIG. 5–4. Venous duplex demonstrating nonocclusive thrombus *(arrow)* within the lumen of the vein.

vein does not appear dilated and bright echoes can be seen along the walls of the vein. The vein is partially compressible, and respiratory variation is present.

The normal venous signal is spontaneous and phasic with respiration. Changes in intraabdominal pressure caused by respiratory movement of the diaphragm create phasic variations of the venous signal in the extremity. In the presence of deep venous thrombosis, flow signals are continuous or absent. Pulsatility of the leg veins is an abnormal finding most commonly seen in patients with congestive heart failure or fluid overload. The Doppler signals in the internal jugular, innominate, and subclavian veins are normally pulsatile due to their proximity to the heart (Table 5-1).

Limitations

Limitations include the following considerations: scanning may be difficult in obese or extremely muscular patients, and the small calf veins may not be easily visualized. Venous access may be limited in patients with dressings, contractures, intravenous catheters, central lines, or traction.

VENOUS TESTING: CHRONIC VENOUS DISEASE

Veins are equipped with one-way valves that open to permit the flow of venous blood toward the heart. If the valves become damaged or the veins stretched, the valves may no longer close adequately and reflux flow will occur.

Photoplethysmographic techniques indirectly assess venous valve function by detecting changes in cutaneous blood volume. Venous refilling time after exercise normally occurs as a result of arterial inflow across the capillary bed and is thus lengthy. Reflux flow through incompetent valves results in rapid postexercise refilling times. Duplex imaging allows assessment of the deep and superficial systems. The Doppler signal is evaluated to determine the presence and degree of venous reflux.

TABLE 5–1 Diagnostic Criteria for Venous Thrombosis

	Image Characteristics	Doppler Characteristics
Acute	Dilated Noncompressible Filled with soft echoes	Absent or continuous
Chronic	Nondilated Partially compressible Partially filled with bright echoes	Normal respiratory variation Reflux may be present

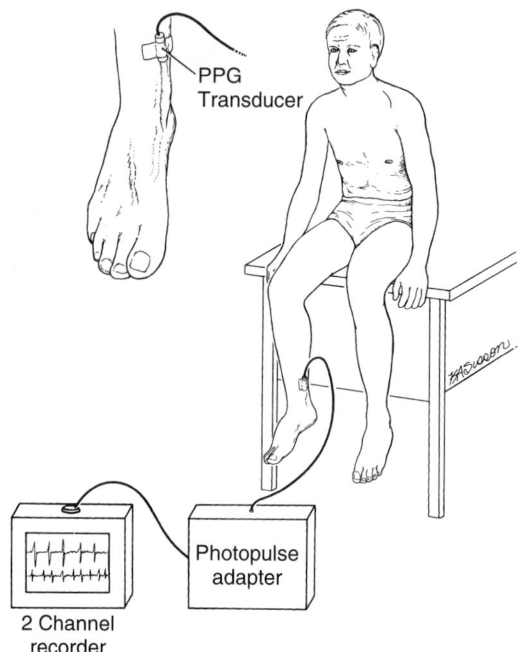

FIG. 5–5. The photoplethysmography examination is performed with the patient's legs dangling and the transducer applied to the medial aspect of the ankle.

Testing for venous valve function is indicated in the patient with stasis changes on the skin of the lower leg, varicose veins, nonhealing venous ulcers, or chronic lower-extremity edema after documented deep venous thrombosis.

Photoplethysmography

The patient is seated with the legs in a dependent, non–weight-bearing position. A PPG photocell is attached with double-faced tape to the skin just above the medial malleolus (Fig. 5-5). The patient is instructed to dorsiflex and plantar flex the feet five times and then to relax the limbs completely. If the patient is unable to exercise adequately, manual calf compression can be performed by the examiner. The superficial venous system may be occluded by application of a cuff or tourniquet at thigh or calf level, and the procedure repeated.

Recovery time is defined as the number of seconds required for the postexercise recovery curve to achieve a stable baseline (Fig. 5-6). A recovery time of 25 seconds or more is normal. Superficial incompetence is demonstrated by a recovery time of less than 20 seconds that normalizes after cuff application. A recovery time of less than 20 seconds both before and after tourniquet application indicates venous valve incompetence in the deep or perforating systems.[7]

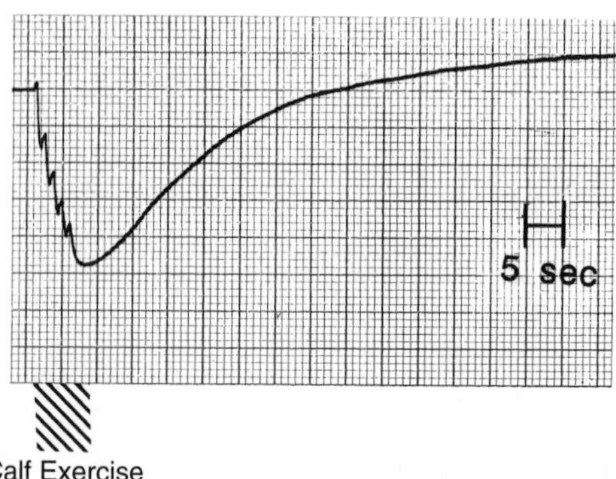

FIG. 5–6. Normal photoplethysmography curve. After exercise, there is a gradual refilling of the venous bed.

PPG is limited by the fact that probe placement may have to be altered in the patient with a stasis ulcer in the malleolar area.

Duplex Imaging

Patients are examined in a reverse Trendelenburg's position or standing. The Doppler signals are recorded over various sites in the deep and superficial systems with the patient breathing deeply or performing the Valsalva maneuver. Reversed flow (reflux) in the vein is timed, and reflux for greater than 1 second is considered abnormal.[8] The advantage of this procedure is that each venous segment is specifically interrogated.

ARTERIAL TESTING: LOWER EXTREMITY

Noninvasive techniques have been developed to evaluate the presence, severity, and location of arterial disease in the upper and lower extremities. Indications for arterial testing include screening patients for disease, defining disease severity, and postsurgical follow-up. Patients being medically treated or those placed on an exercise regimen also require periodic evaluation.

Segmental Waveforms

By examining the arterial system at various sites using a continuous-wave directional Doppler transducer, the diseased segment can be located. The vessels assessed are the common femoral, popliteal, dorsalis pedis, and posterior tibial arteries. Waveforms are obtained at each site for documentation in the permanent record.

The normal arterial signal has a sharp systolic component and one or more diastolic components (Fig. 5-7, *A*). This waveform implies relatively normal flow in an elastic, unobstructed artery. Minor degrees of stenosis do not usually significantly alter this waveform.

As the vessel becomes narrowed, the diastolic components are absent and the systolic component becomes wider (Fig. 5-7, *B*). In the occluded vessel, the systolic component of the waveform becomes blunted and there are no diastolic components (Fig. 5-7, *C*). An abnormal signal indicates disease proximal to the site at which that signal was obtained. In the patient with iliac disease, waveforms and signals will be abnormal at all levels (Fig. 5-8). With a superficial femoral artery occlusion, the common femoral artery will be normal and the popliteal and distal sites will be abnormal. The degree of abnormality will depend on the collateral flow and the state of the distal vessels. When multilevel disease is present, there will be a change in the waveform from one level to the next.

Sequential Volume Plethysmography

Pneumatic cuffs are placed at various levels on the extremity. A standardized quantity of air is used to slightly inflate the cuff. Volume changes that occur beneath the cuff are detectable and are converted to pulsatile pressure changes. These changes are recorded for analysis.

Strandness[9] described the changes that occur in the volume pulse recordings with occlusive disease (Fig. 5-9):

1. Normal—sharp systolic peak; prominent dicrotic wave
2. Mildly abnormal—sharp systolic peak; absent dicrotic wave; downslope bowed away from baseline

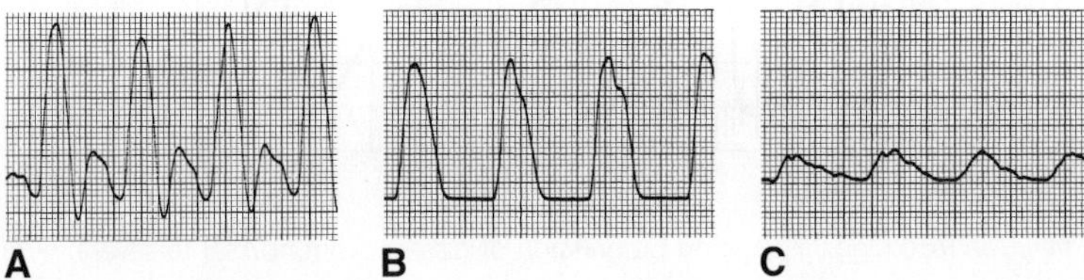

FIG. 5–7. Analog recordings obtained over normal **(A)**, stenotic **(B)**, and occluded **(C)** vessels.

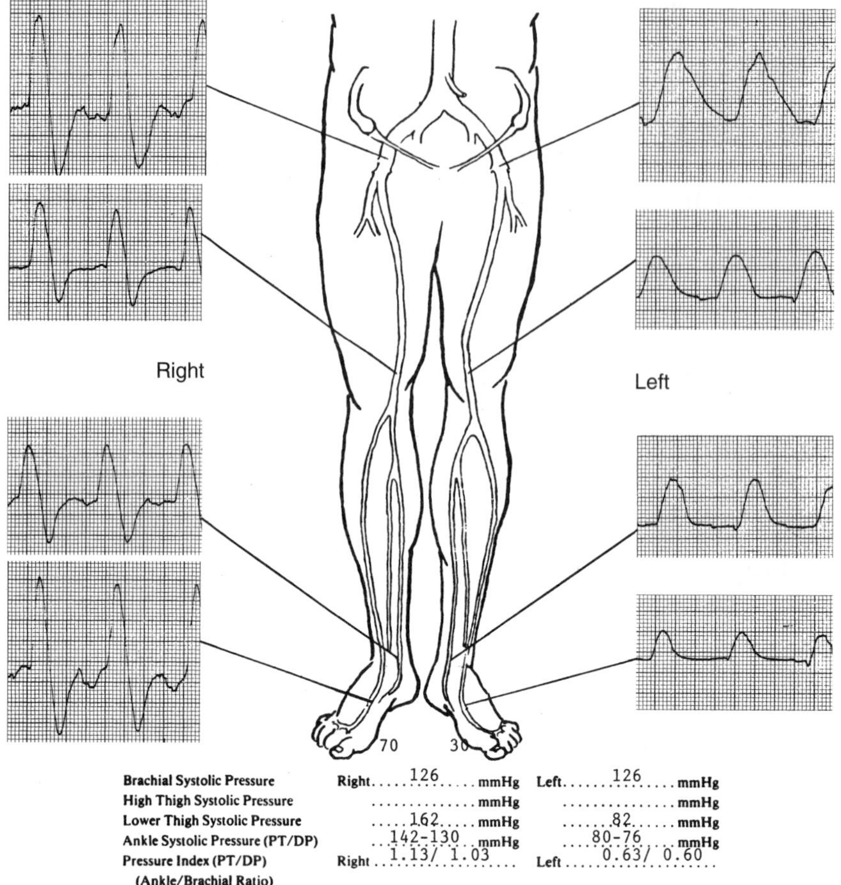

FIG. 5–8. Analog tracings and systolic pressures obtained in a patient with a left iliac occlusion. The right side is normal.

3. Moderately abnormal—flattened systolic peak; upslope and downslope nearly equal; dicrotic wave invariably absent
4. Severely abnormal—pulse wave of very low amplitude or entirely absent; if present, equal upslope and downslope time

Analysis of the volume pulse recordings from the different levels can determine the location of the diseased arterial segment and provide an estimate of the severity of the disease.

Segmental Pressures

Segmental pressures obtained with a Doppler are the most frequently used means of quantifying arterial flow.[10] Coupled with Doppler analog waveform analysis or volume plethysmography,

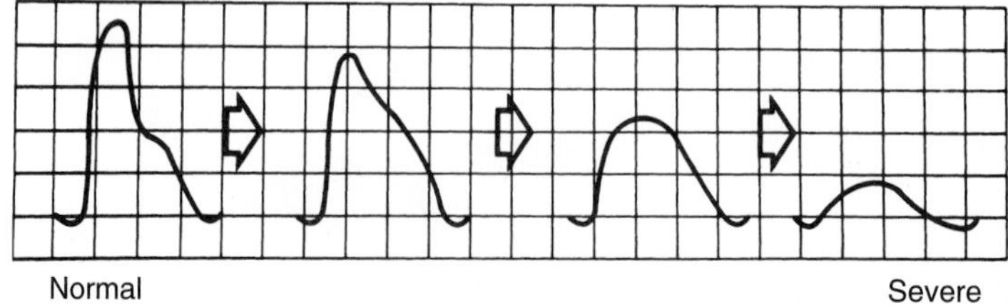

FIG. 5–9. Volume pulse recordings illustrating progression of disease from normal to severe. (From Kempczinski RF, Yao JST, eds: *Practical noninvasive vascular diagnosis,* Chicago, 1987, Year Book, p 141.)

TABLE 5–2 Ankle-Brachial Ratio: An Index of Disease Severity

Normal	1.00-0.95
Mildly abnormal	0.95-0.80
Claudicant	0.75-0.40
Ischemic	<0.40

they provide a thorough, concise examination in the vascular laboratory. Ankle-brachial indices are part of the standard vascular physical exam as recommended by the TransAtlantic Inter-Society Consensus.[11] In addition, they provide valuable information on limb perfusion in the postoperative period.

A standard arm cuff is placed immediately above the ankle to procure systolic pressure measurements at the dorsalis pedis and posterior tibial arteries. A standard thigh cuff is placed above the knee to obtain a low thigh pressure. Bilateral brachial pressures are taken, and the higher of the two is used to calculate an ankle-brachial index.

Normally, the systolic pressure in the leg is equal to or slightly higher than the systolic arm pressure. This is due to the highly resistant vascular bed in the lower extremity. With occlusive disease, the systolic pressure drops proportionately to the severity of disease. The ratio of the segmental pressure to the systolic arm pressure provides a method of quantifying the severity of disease.[12] This can be applied to all pressures; however, most frequently used is the ankle-brachial ratio index. In addition, this ratio is necessary for comparison with the previous studies, because the systemic pressures will vary from one examination to another. This ratio is proportional to the degree of ischemia present (Table 5-2).

Ratio changes within a 0.15 range are considered within normal limits because of changes in absolute pressure and intraexaminer variability. A change in ratio greater than 0.15 indicates a significant improvement or deterioration. Importantly, ankle pressures obtained postoperatively that do not increase by at least 0.15 indicate no improvement in arterial perfusion.[12]

A difference of more than 30 mm Hg between segments indicates disease. The popliteal pressure is especially useful in predicting healing in patients undergoing amputation. If the thigh pressure exceeds 60 mm Hg, the probability is high that a below-the-knee amputation site will heal.[13]

Calcification of the arterial wall prevents accurate pressure measurements. Pressures can be falsely elevated (frequently to above 300 mm Hg) because of an incompressible vessel. This condition is most frequently seen in patients with diabetes and chronic renal failure. A prosthetic distal graft, if tunneled through soft tissue, will be incompressible. Pressure measurements in these patients are invalid, and diagnosis must be based on waveform/signal analysis.

Toe Pressure Measurements

Great toe measurements are frequently performed to assess distal arterial flow. This is especially useful in diabetics in whom calcification of the larger vessels is present. A 2.5 × 9 cm cuff is placed proximally on the toe. The distal arterial signal is obtained with a Doppler transducer or a PPG. A systolic pressure is then obtained.

The normal toe pressure is 60 mm Hg.[14-16] The toe pressure is useful in predicting healing of toe and forefoot wounds and toe amputation sites. If the toe pressure exceeds 30 mm Hg, chances are high that a forefoot wound or amputation site will heal (Table 5-3).

TABLE 5–3 Toe Pressures

Normal	≥60 mm Hg
Reduced	>30, <60 mm Hg
Ischemic	<30 mm Hg

Stress Testing

Stress testing is indicated when resting flows are not grossly abnormal, when symptoms do not correlate with the resting flows, and in cases of back disturbances that may simulate claudication (neurogenic claudication).[17] Exercise testing provides objective documentation in the evaluation of the effectiveness of medical or exercise treatment regimes. The optimal method of stress testing involves performance of the activity associated with the patient's symptoms (i.e., walking). Because of the high percentage of concomitant cardiac disease, cardiac monitoring during exercise is strongly recommended.[18,19]

Exercise Testing

Following a resting study, the patient is asked to walk at a standardized speed and grade (1.5 mph at a 10 percent grade) until disabling claudication occurs. A maximum walking time of 5 minutes is standard. After exercise, the ankle pressure (dorsalis pedis or posterior tibial artery) is recorded in each limb at 1-minute intervals until pre-exercise levels are reached. Measurements are terminated if resting levels are not reached in 10 minutes.

Normally, flow increases with exercise. In the diseased state, flow and pressure decrease distal to a stenosis. This pressure drop is proportional to the severity of the disease and will be most abnormal with multilevel disease.[20]

Peripheral Arterial Scanning

Images generated from the duplex scanner provide anatomic as well as hemodynamic information and can precisely locate diseased segments.[21] Duplex imaging is most commonly used as a guide in localizing and grading the severity of stenosis in patients with known peripheral arterial disease. The technique should be used in conjunction with standard analog waveforms and segmental pressures.

A 7-4 MHz linear transducer is used to evaluate the upper and lower extremities. A low-frequency abdominal probe is required for examination of the aortoiliac segment and in obese patients. Each vessel is interrogated along its entire length. Doppler velocity samples are recorded prestenosis, at the stenosis, and poststenosis.

A greater than 100 percent increase in velocity between the proximal and stenotic segments or a peak systolic velocity of more than 100 cm/sec is consistent with a 50-99 percent reduction in diameter.

Arterial Trauma

Arterial catheterization for diagnostic and therapeutic procedures can result in complications such as pseudoaneurysms (Fig. 5-10), arteriovenous fistula, vessel dissection, or intimal flaps. Duplex studies are useful in determining the presence of arterial injury. The most common postcatheterization injury, pseudoaneurysm, is now being treated with ultrasound-guided thrombin injection immediately following diagnosis.[22-24]

The ultrasound transducer is positioned over the aneurysm, a spinal needle with an echogenic tip is inserted into the center of the aneurysm, and 0.5 to 1.0 ml of a 1000-U/ml thrombin solution is slowly injected, resulting in instantaneous thrombosis of the aneurysm. This procedure is quick and relatively pain free in comparison to either manual compression of the aneurysm or surgical repair. The patient is able to ambulate immediately following treatment. Preprocedure and postprocedure ankle-brachial indices are performed to ensure that arterial patency has been unaffected. Patients are rescanned in 3-4 days to document complete thrombosis of the aneurysm.

Arterial Graft Assessment

Duplex imaging provides a means for determining the patency and evaluating the hemodynamics of arterial bypass grafts. Graft surveillance for the first 2 years has been recommended by the TransAtlantic Inter-Society Consensus.[11] Protocol can vary between institutions; however, a baseline scan after suture removal, at 3 and 6 months postoperatively, and then annually is a typical surveillance program. Imaging is also indicated if there

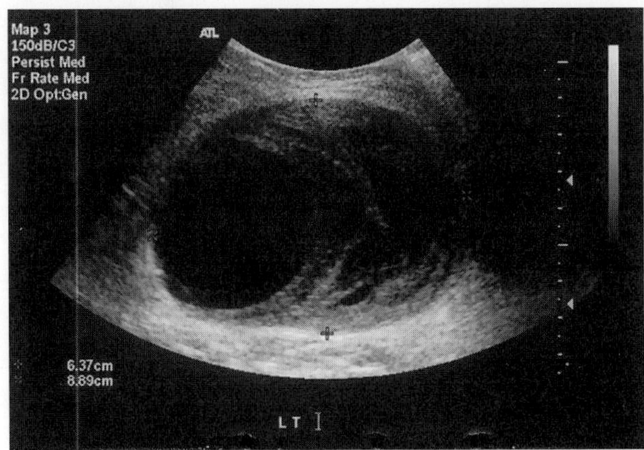

FIG. 5–10. Duplex image of a pseudoaneurysm arising from the common femoral artery.

is a drop in ankle-brachial indices, new claudication has developed, or a bruit or thrill is noted over the graft.

The graft is examined from the proximal to the distal anastomosis. Doppler velocity recordings and vessel diameter measurements are made throughout the length of the graft and in both the inflow and outflow vessels.

With all grafts, careful assessment of the proximal and distal anastomotic sites is mandatory, because these areas are the most common site of graft stenosis. In addition, focal stenosis (Fig. 5-11) within a vein graft may occur as a result of injury to the vein wall, incomplete

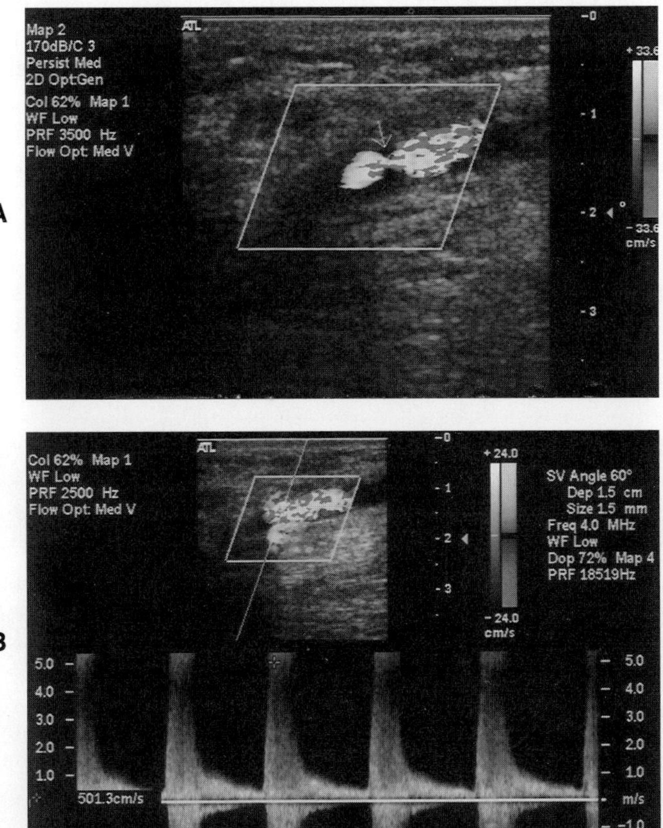

FIG. 5–11. Duplex images showing narrowing within an in situ graft *(arrow)* **(A)** and the associated turbulent, stenotic Doppler spectral waveform **(B)**.

valve lysis, or torsion of the graft. Care should be taken in the assessment of in situ grafts for retained valves (Fig. 5-12) and residual arteriovenous fistulae. If found, these sites are usually marked for the surgeon to repair. Synthetic grafts are not amenable to scanning in the first week postoperatively due to air within the graft walls, which prevents ultrasound penetration. Later in the postoperative period, these grafts can be visualized and followed as any other graft.

ARTERIAL TESTING: UPPER EXTREMITY

The same principles and techniques used for assessing the lower extremity may be applied to the upper extremity. Indications for upper-extremity evaluation include decreased or absent pulses, a pressure gradient of more than 20 mm Hg between arms, frank ischemic changes (coolness, pallor, cyanosis, pregangrenous or gangrenous changes), and nonhealing wounds.

Doppler waveforms are recorded at the axillary, brachial, radial, and ulnar arteries. Pressures are taken over the brachial, radial, and ulnar arteries. There should be no more than 30 mm Hg difference between segments of the same arm or between segments of one arm and like segments of the opposite arm. Normal and abnormal waveforms are analyzed in a manner similar to that used in the lower extremity.

The palmar arch is assessed by means of a modified Allen's test. The Doppler probe is placed in the flexion crease of the palm to locate the signal over the palmar arch. Alternate radial and ulnar artery compressions are then performed.

Normally, the palmar arch is supplied by both the ulnar and radial arteries. With compression of one artery, a signal remains in the palmar arch. If the arch is totally dependent on one vessel, the signal in the palmar arch will obliterate with compression. An incomplete arch (supplied by only one vessel) is present in 20 percent of normal subjects[25]; it is an important finding. Thus, arterial punctures of the dominant artery should never be performed. This being an important finding, the patient should be notified in case an arterial puncture is required in the future.

Digital pressures are indicated in patients exhibiting ischemic changes in the hands and fingers. A digital cuff is placed proximally on the finger, and the distal arterial signal is obtained with a Doppler device or PPG. Systolic pressures are recorded in this manner on each digit.

The digital pressure should be equal to the proximal adjacent arterial pressure. There should be less than 20 mm Hg difference between the digital pressures and pressures taken at the wrist level. There should be no difference in pressure from one digit to the next. When proximal disease is present, all digits will have an equally reduced pressure.

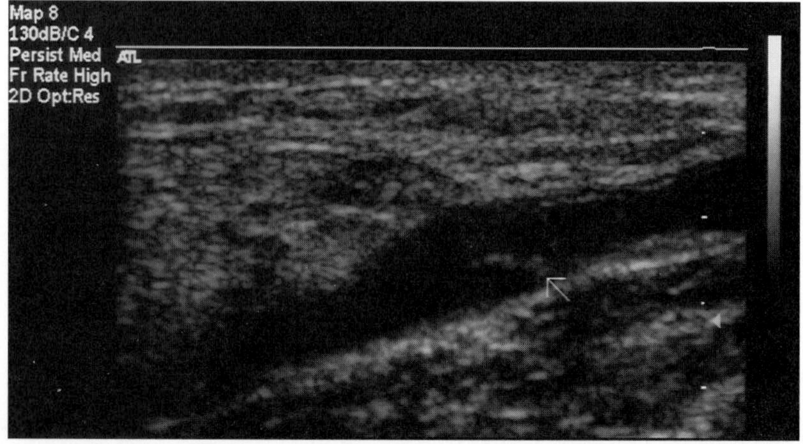

FIG. 5–12. Duplex image of a retained valve cusp *(arrow)* in an in situ graft.

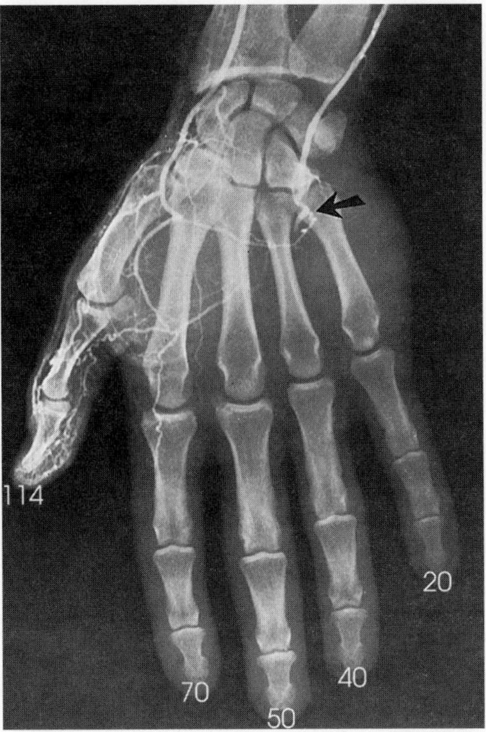

FIG. 5–13. Upper-extremity arteriogram demonstrates distal ulnar artery occlusion *(arrow)*. No digital arteries are visualized in the fingers, and all finger pressures are abnormal.

Only the affected digits will have lower pressures when digital artery occlusion is present (Fig. 5-13).

Cold Sensitivity

Cold-sensitivity testing may be added to the upper-extremity examination in those patients whose presenting symptom is hypersensitivity to cold. A standard upper-extremity examination, including digital pressures, should be performed to exclude an organic cause of these symptoms. If the standard examination is normal, testing for Raynaud's disease is indicated.

A thermistor sensor is attached to the distal portion of each finger, and baseline temperatures are recorded. The hands are then submerged in ice water for 20 seconds. Temperatures are taken immediately after the ice bath and every 5 minutes for 30 minutes or until temperatures return to preimmersion levels.

Normal digits will rewarm in 20 minutes or less. In the patient with Raynaud's disease, digital temperatures in all fingers will remain below pre–ice bath levels for more than 20 minutes (Fig. 5-14). In patients with digital artery occlusion, only the affected digits will have a prolonged recovery time.[26]

Thoracic Outlet Evaluation

Patients with complaints of pain and paresthesia in the neck, shoulder, and upper extremity are candidates for thoracic outlet testing. In addition, young patients with ischemia of the hand should be evaluated for the presence of thoracic outlet syndrome. An aneurysm of the subclavian artery may occur as a result of intermittent arterial compression at the thoracic outlet. Distal embolization can result from such an aneurysm.

The patient is studied in a sitting position with the hands resting on the lap. A photoplethysmograph is placed on one finger of each hand, and a tracing of the arterial pulse is made. The arms are then moved to a 90° horizontal position, directly over the head (180°), and an exaggerated military position is adopted, with the arms bent at the elbow and the

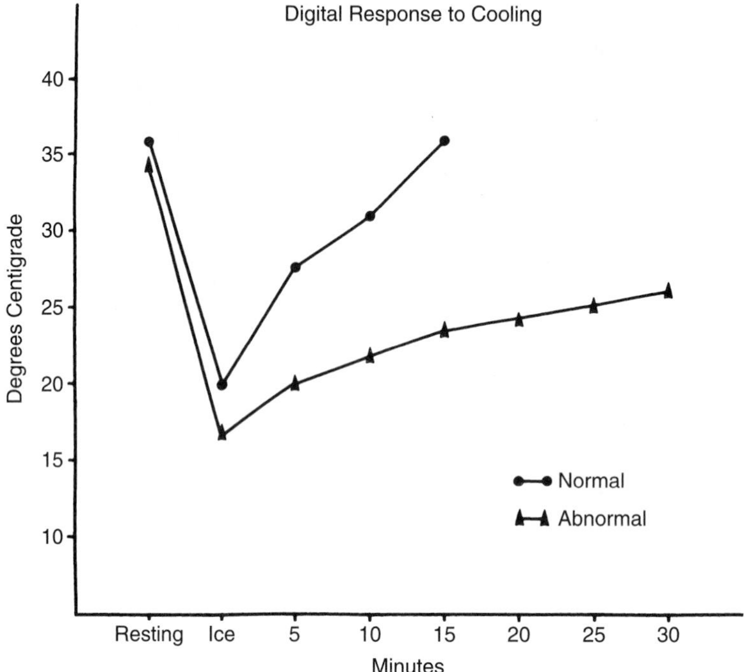

FIG. 5–14. Digital temperature recovery times in normal subjects and in those with cold sensitivity. (From Bartel P, Blackburn DR, Peterson LK, et al: The value of noninvasive tests in occupational trauma of the hands and fingers, *Bruit* 8:15-18, 1984.)

shoulders thrust back. The Adson maneuver is performed by having the patient extend the neck, turn his or her head to the side, and take a deep breath. Tracings are obtained and recorded in each position.

Obliteration of the arterial pulse in any position indicates compression of the artery and is considered positive. Compression may occur between the rib and clavicle and also from abnormal muscle insertion or muscle hypertrophy. Diminution of the arterial pulse is not considered a positive finding. If the PPG findings are abnormal, duplex scanning may be performed over the axillary and subclavian arteries to determine the presence of an aneurysm and to localize the area of obstruction. This procedure evaluates only the presence or absence of arterial compression at the thoracic outlet. Symptoms may be caused by compression of the vein or nerve that also pass through the thoracic outlet.

CAVERNOSAL DUPLEX IMAGING: TESTING FOR IMPOTENCE

Duplex imaging is used to directly image and assess flow characteristics in the cavernosal arteries to determine the cause of impotence. Erectile dysfunction can be caused by arterial insufficiency, venous leak, nerve dysfunction, psychogenic causes, or a combination of these factors.

A color duplex system with a high-frequency transducer is used to obtain diameter measurements and flow velocities both before and after an intracavernosal injection of 30 mg of papaverine or 10 μg of prostaglandin E_1.

Normally, vessel diameter will increase after injection by 50 percent, peak systolic velocities will increase 100 percent and are greater than 25 cm/sec, and the end-diastolic velocities are below 5 cm/sec.

Arterial insufficiency is demonstrated by the fact that the diameter does not increase by 50 percent and the peak systolic velocity does not increase by 100 percent and does not reach 25 cm/sec. A venous leak is indicated when the vessel diameter increases by 50 percent, the peak systolic velocity increases by 100 percent and is above 25 cm/sec, but the end-diastolic velocity is greater than 5 cm/sec.[27,28]

ABDOMINAL DUPLEX IMAGING

Mesenteric Arterial Duplex

Indications for mesenteric scanning include postprandial abdominal pain (intestinal angina), unexplained weight loss, or an abdominal bruit.[29] Patients should receive nothing by mouth at least 8 hours before examination. It is preferable for patients to have these studies done early in the morning after an overnight fast. A low-frequency transducer, usually 3 MHz, is required to examine the deep abdominal vessels. With the patient in the supine position, the scan head is placed just below the xyphoid process; the supraceliac aorta is identified, and Doppler velocity signals are recorded. The celiac trunk is the first visceral branch of the aorta. The celiac branches into the hepatic and splenic arteries. On the duplex image, this bifurcation looks like "gull wings." The superior mesenteric artery (SMA) arises anteriorly from the aorta just distal to the celiac trunk (Fig. 5-15). The inferior mesenteric (IMA) arises from the anterior aorta, distal to the renal arteries. The IMA may be difficult to image because it is lower down in the abdomen and bowel gas may obscure the origin of the artery. These vessels are interrogated, and Doppler velocity samples are obtained. After the fasting examination, stress testing may be performed on patients with equivocal studies. A high-calorie liquid meal (8 oz Ensure Plus or an equivalent product) is ingested by the patient. The celiac trunk and the SMA are restudied 30-40 minutes postprandially.

The normal celiac signal demonstrates forward flow throughout diastole with a window below the spectral wave. Both systolic and diastolic flow velocities will normally increase after a test meal. A peak systolic velocity of more than 200 cm/sec is indicative of a stenosis of 70 percent or greater.

The normal SMA signal in a fasting patient is biphasic or triphasic. Postprandially, both systolic and diastolic flow velocities will increase and the signal will convert to a lower resistance pattern because of peripheral vasodilation in the gut. A peak systolic velocity of more than 275 cm/sec in a fasting patient and an SMA-aortic ratio of equal to or greater than 3.5 indicates a stenosis of the SMA of at least 70%.[30] Studies may be inadequate because of obesity, excessive bowel gas, and/or recent abdominal surgery.

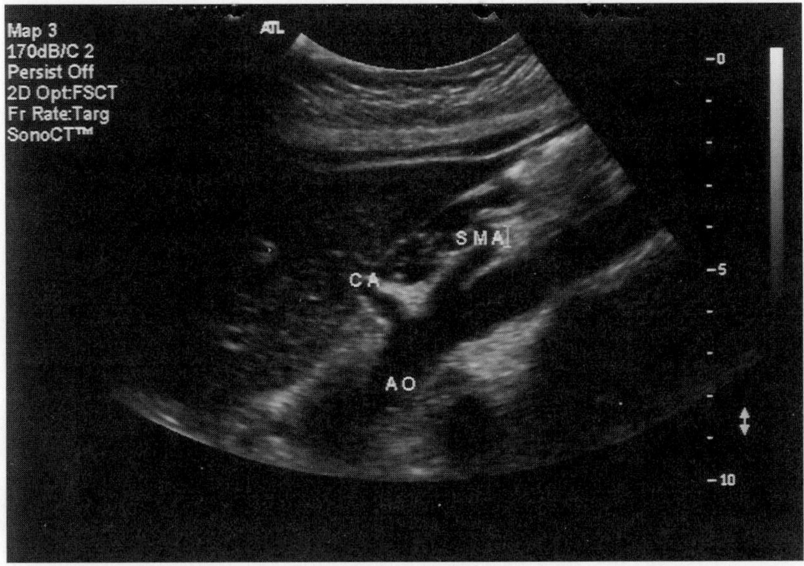

FIG. 5–15. Image of the abdominal aorta *(AO)*, celiac axis *(CA)*, and superior mesenteric artery *(SMA)*.

Renal Arterial Duplex

Renal artery imaging is indicated in patients in whom renovascular hypertension is suspected. This would include patients with hypertension that is difficult to control medically, young patients with a new onset of hypertension, and patients with severe atherosclerotic or aneurysmal disease with hypertension. It is also a useful tool in the follow-up of patients undergoing renal artery bypass or stent procedures.

Patients should maintain at least an 8-hour fast before examination. The procedure is performed with a low-frequency transducer while the patient is in the supine position. The SMA is identified in long axis and aortic velocities recorded in this area. The transducer is rotated into a transverse plane, and the left renal vein is observed crossing between the aorta and the SMA. The right renal artery usually arises first. It arises from the anterior/lateral aorta around 11 o'clock and travels beneath the inferior vena cava to the right kidney. The left renal artery arises just distal to the right from about the 4-5 o'clock position (Fig. 5-16). Flow velocities from the proximal, mid, and distal renal arteries are obtained at a 60° angle whenever possible. The patient is rotated onto each side and the kidneys interrogated via this flank approach. The kidney size is noted as well as flow in the upper, mid, and lower poles of the kidney. The renal veins are assessed for patency.

The renal artery Doppler signal normally demonstrates continuous flow throughout diastole like that seen in the internal carotid artery. Vessel stenosis causes an increase in flow velocity. A ratio of the peak systolic velocity in the renal artery and the aorta is calculated.

$$\frac{\text{PSV renal artery}}{\text{PSV aorta}} = \text{Rental-aortic ratio}$$

A ratio greater than 3.5 indicates a greater than 60 percent renal artery stenosis.[31]

Most renal artery stenoses occur at the origin of the vessel, and this ratio applies. However, in patients with fibromuscular dyplasia, the narrowing in the vessel frequently occurs in the mid to distal renal artery. In those cases, a doubling of the velocities from the proximal renal artery indicates a significant stenosis.

The resistive index of flow within the kidney is calculated by averaging measurements from the upper, middle, and lower poles of the kidney. A resistive index of 80 or greater is indicative of renal parenchymal disease. Patients who have renal artery stenosis and a resistive

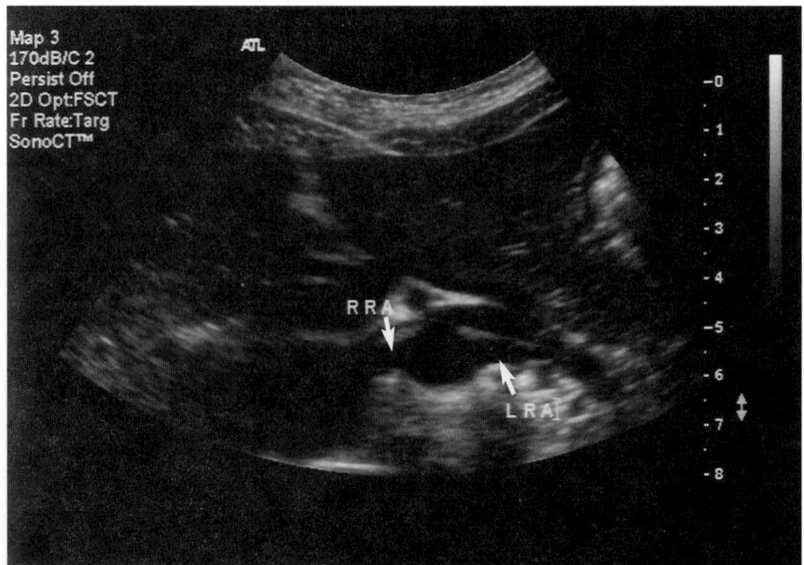

FIG. 5–16. Transverse image of the aorta and the origin of the bilateral renal arteries *(arrows)*.

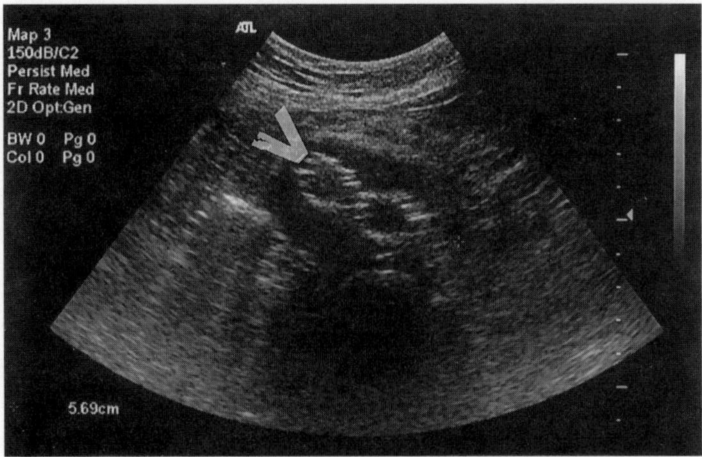

FIG. 5–17. Duplex image of an aortic bifurcated endograft *(arrow)*.

index of 80 or greater do not improve following intervention, and in fact, the intervention frequently makes them worse.[32]

Aortic Duplex

Duplex imaging is useful in detecting patients with aortic aneurysms. The size and location of the aneurysm can be determined. In addition, duplex scanning has been used in assessing patients after endovascular repair of abdominal aneurysms.[33] Flow in the endograft is assessed (Fig. 5-17). The aneurysm sac is measured and should shrink over time after graft placement. Leaks from the endograft into the lumen of the aneurysm can be detected; a leak should be considered if the aneurysm enlarges.

CEREBROVASCULAR TESTING

Noninvasive studies that examine the extracranial carotid artery are divided into two groups: those that examine the carotid artery directly and those that assess flow through the carotid artery indirectly by examination of its distal branches. By far the most common diagnostic study is duplex imaging. Today indirect testing is rarely used (see previous editions for discussion of indirect modalities). The most accurate way to detect disease in the extracranial carotid and vertebral arteries is by direct assessment of the vessels.[33]

Carotid testing is indicated in patients with hemispheric symptoms of stroke; transient ischemic attacks; amaurosis fugax; nonhemispheric symptoms, including dizziness, loss of memory, drop attacks, and blurred vision; and in patients with an asymptomatic bruit. Carotid duplex scanning is used to detect operable lesions, to evaluate disease progression in medically treated patients, and to follow patients post carotid endarterectomy or post carotid stent placement (Fig. 5-18).

Cerebrovascular Duplex

Most ultrasound machines used today perform three functions: direct visualization of the vessels with B-mode imaging and assessment of flow characteristics with both Doppler spectral waveforms and color flow imaging. The images themselves provide anatomic information. High resolution images allow for definition of plaque morphology. Soft versus calcified plaque can be defined, and smooth plaque can be differentiated from irregular plaque and ulcerative lesions. Aberrant anatomy and vessel tortuosity can be defined. Because both vessel wall and residual lumen can be visualized, the percentage of diameter reduction can be accurately measured.

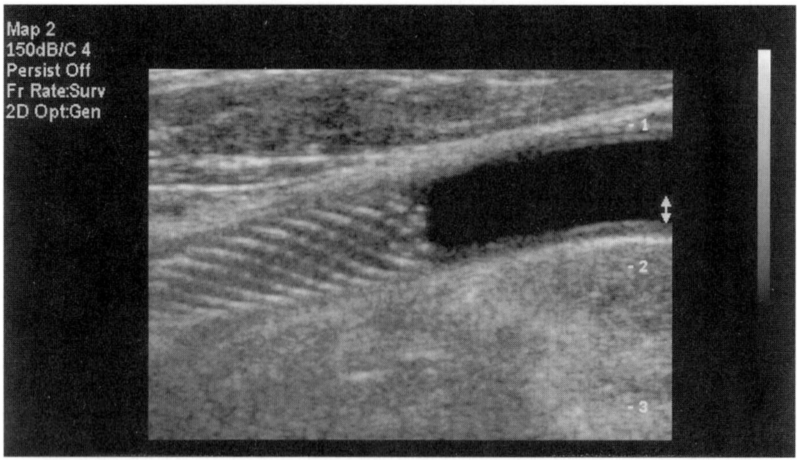

FIG. 5–18. Image of a carotid stent.

The examination is performed while the patient is in a supine position with the neck extended. The Doppler transducer is placed as low on the neck as possible, and a signal from the common carotid artery (CCA) is located. The probe is slowly advanced up the neck to the carotid bifurcation (approximately at the level of the thyroid cartilage). The signals from the internal carotid artery (ICA) and the external carotid artery (ECA) are located and recorded. These vessels should be imaged from the base of the neck to the level of the jaw in both the longitudinal and transverse plane. Following examination of the carotid vessels, the vertebral artery is evaluated by moving the transducer laterally from the CCA until the vertebral bodies are visualized. Flow signals are taken in the vertebral artery between the vertebral bodies. The vessel should be examined from the upper neck to its origin at the subclavian. A Doppler signal is then taken in the subclavian artery.

Interpretation

Normally, the intima is visualized throughout the common, internal, and external carotid arteries (Fig. 5-19). In diseased states, plaque is identified and classified, diameter reduction is measured, and flow signals are evaluated (Fig. 5-20).

Flow in a normal artery is laminar. In the presence of stenosis, flow velocities will increase as blood passes through the area of narrowing. In addition, just distal to the area of narrowing, flow becomes turbulent as the red blood cells bounce off the walls of the artery. This creates flow in many directions. These changes are reflected in the spectral waveform. Flow velocities and turbulence increase in proportion to the degree of stenosis. In total occlusions, no signal can be obtained in the vessel.

Flow direction, velocity, and turbulence can also be displayed using color. Flow towards the Doppler probe is displayed in one color while flow in the opposite direction is displayed in another color. As flow velocities increase, the color will change from a deep tone to a lighter and brighter color, for instance from red to orange to yellow. Turbulence is noted by a mosaic of colors corresponding to flow going in numerous directions at numerous velocities.

The ICA, ECA, and CCA all have individual normal flow characteristics. The ICA supplies a low-resistance vascular bed (the brain). The signals from the ICA, therefore, show constant flow, even in diastole (see Fig. 5-19, *B*). The ECA supplies a high-resistance bed (the scalp, face, and skin). Therefore, the flow signal in the ECA sounds very much like that of a peripheral artery, where there is reversal of flow in diastole. The CCA has a combination of the ICA and ECA flow characteristics. The criteria for interpreting flow signals obtained in the ICA with a 5-MHz pulsed Doppler instrument is shown in Table 5-4.[34]

Direct testing is able to detect disease only below the angle of the jaw. If the bifurcation is high in the neck, the ICA and ECA may not be adequately evaluated.

Normal vertebral flow is toward the brain with flow signals similar to the ICA.

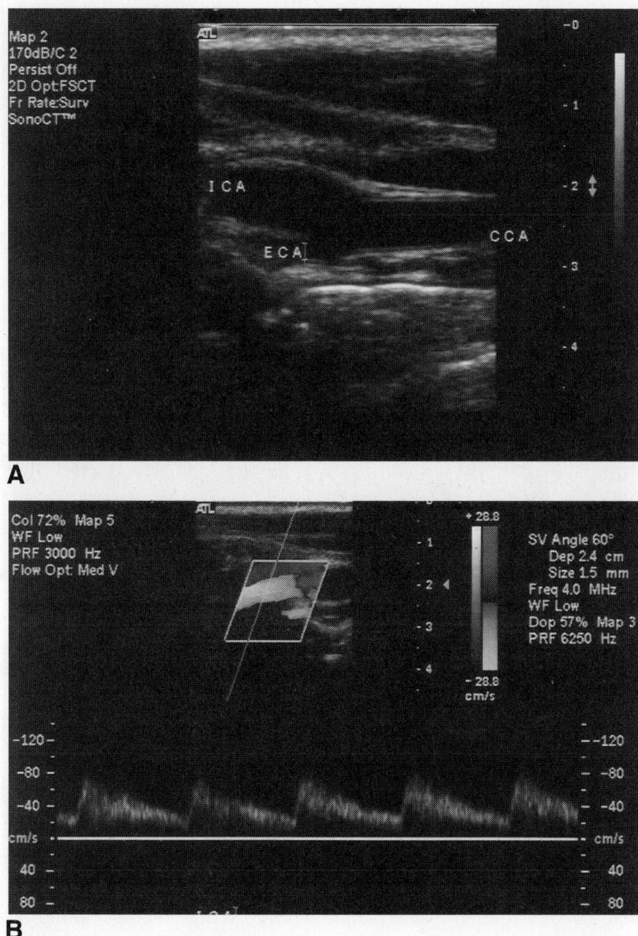

FIG. 5–19. Duplex image of a normal carotid bifurcation **(A)** and normal Doppler spectral waveforms **(B)**.

Transcranial Doppler

The transcranial Doppler examination uses a low-frequency (2 MHz) pulsed Doppler transducer to assess the intracranial arteries and the circle of Willis.[35] The exam may be performed with a pulsed Doppler or duplex imaging.

Transcranial Doppler examination is used to assess flow in patients suspected of having intracranial stenosis, to assess collateral circulation in patients with ICA occlusions, to assess patients with vertebrobasilar insufficiency, and to measure cerebral vasospasm after subarachnoid hemorrhage.

Ultrasound does not penetrate bone very well, so several acoustic "windows" are used where the skull is thin (Fig. 5-21). The transtemporal window is used to assess the middle cerebral artery, the anterior cerebral artery, and the posterior cerebral artery. The orbital window is used to evaluate the ophthalmic artery and the carotid siphon. The foramen magnum is used to evaluate the distal vertebral arteries and the basilar artery.

Interpretation

Normal values and flow direction for the transcranial examination are seen in Table 5-5.

QUALITY CONTROL

The noninvasive modalities discussed in this chapter have been extensively used in the clinical setting. Most examinations are subjective and rely on the expertise of the examiner.

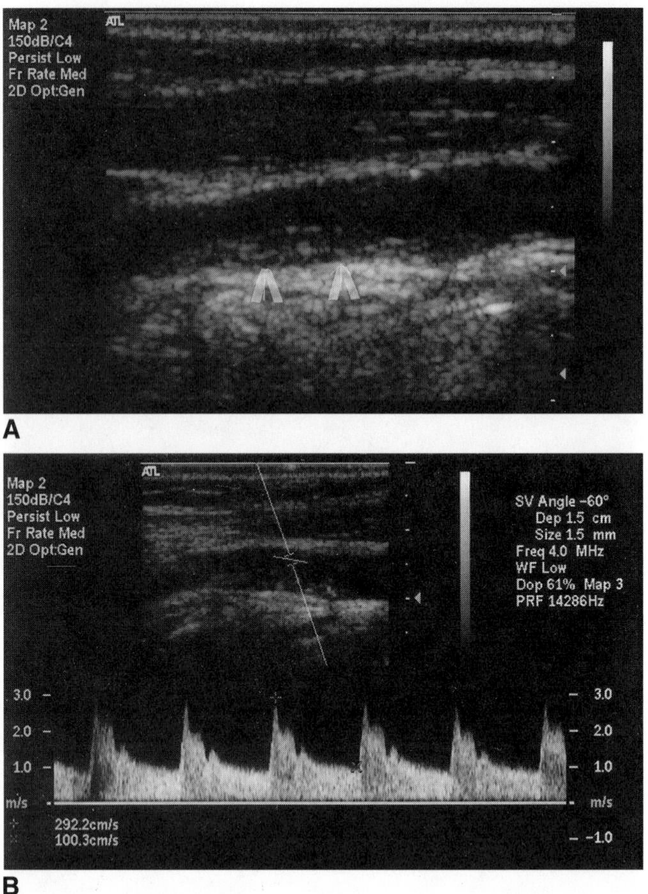

FIG. 5–20. Duplex image demonstrating mixed plaque *(arrows)* in the internal carotid artery **(A)** and spectral waveforms **(B)** within the area of stenosis. Diagnostic criteria would indicate a 60-80 percent diameter reduction.

Regular conferences in which laboratory results are compared with the "gold standard" are mandatory. Accuracy rates in each laboratory for each procedure should be assessed; if these rates vary from the reported literature, reexamination of technique or interpretation must be made. Vascular laboratory accreditation helps ensure that quality standards are in place. In

TABLE 5–4 Criteria for the Classification of Internal Carotid Stenosis by Duplex

Degree of ICA Stenosis	Peak Systolic Velocity	End-Diastolic Velocity	Spectral Waveform Characteristics	Image Characteristics
None	<2 × CCA PSV		No spectral broadening	Walls free of plaque
<60%	<260 cm/sec	<80 cm/sec	Spectral broadening	Plaque visualized
60-79%	>290 cm/sec	>80 cm/sec <140 cm/sec	Turbulent	Plaque visualized
80-99%	>290 cm/sec	>140 cm/sec	Turbulent	Plaque present
Total occlusion			No flow signal in ICA/ decreased diastolic flow in CCA	Lumen filled with plaque/thrombus

ICA, internal carotid artery; *CCA*, common carotid artery; *PSV*, peak systolic velocity.

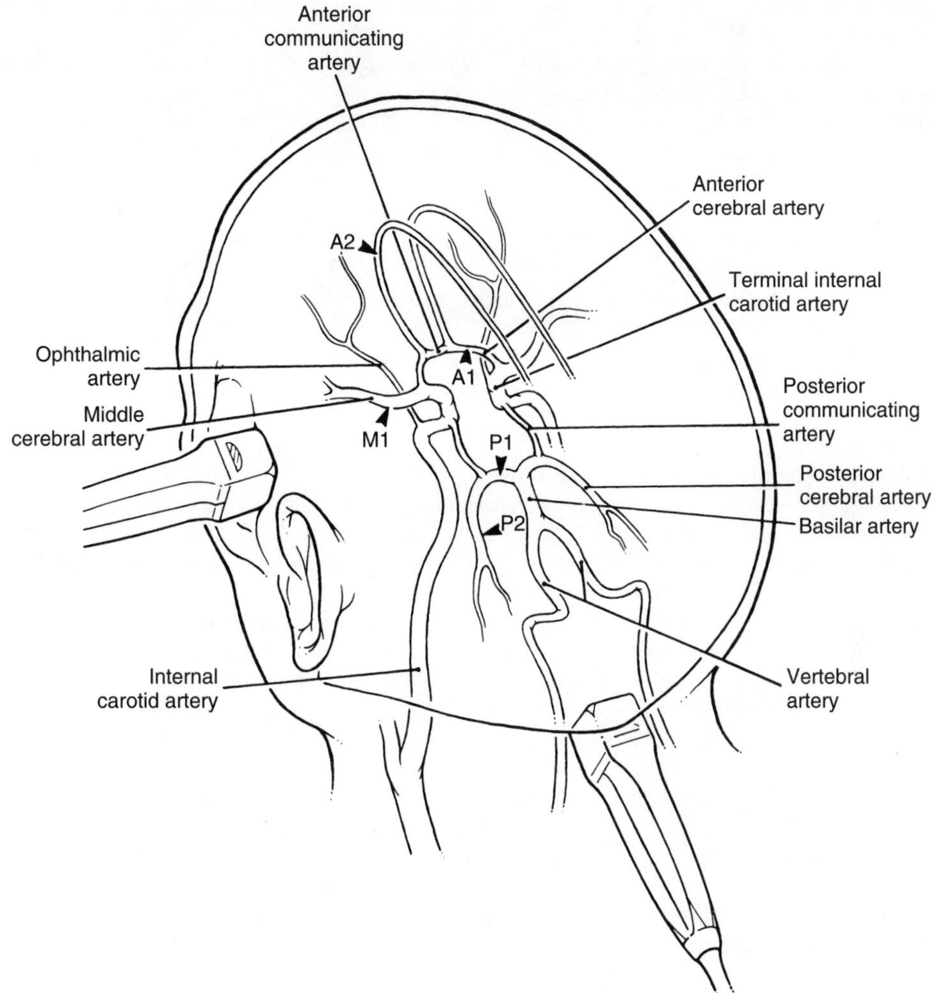

FIG. 5–21. Diagram of the normal circle of Willis and the window used in transcranial examination. (From Advanced Technology Laboratories: *Vascular scanning protocols,* Bothell, Wash, 1992.)

many states, Medicare will only reimburse for those studies performed in an accredited laboratory or by a registered vascular technologist.

TABLE 5–5 Normal Values and Flow Direction for Transcranial Examination

Vessel	Mean Velocity (cm/sec)	Depth From Probe	Flow Direction
MCA (M1)	62 ± 12	40-60 mm	Towards
ACA (A1)	50 ± 12	65-75 mm	Away
ICA	Varies	65 mm	Towards
PCA (P1), (P2)	42 ± 10	65-75 mm	Towards/Away
Vertebral	36 ± 10	60-85 mm	Away
Basilar	39 ± 10	>85 mm	Away

From Advanced Technology Labs: *Advanced Scanning Protocols,* Bothell, Wash, 1992.
MCA, middle cerebral artery; *ACA,* anterior cerebral artery; *ICA,* internal carotid artery; *PCA,* posterior cerebral artery.

REFERENCES

1. Doppler C: *Abh K Bohm Ges Wiss* 2:465, 1842.
2. Kremkau FW: *Diagnostic ultrasound: principles and instruments,* Philadelphia, 1998, WB Saunders.

3. Pomajzl MJ: *Real-time ultrasound imaging and pulsed/gated Doppler instructional manual*, Indianapolis, 1984, Biosound Inc.
4. Fowl RJ, Strothman GB, Blebea J et al: Inappropriate use of venous duplex scans: an analysis of indications and results, *J Vasc Surg* 23:5, 881-885, 1996.
5. Talbot SR: B-mode evaluation of peripheral veins, *Semin Ultrasound CT MR* 9:295-319, 1988.
6. Zwiebel WJ, ed: *Introduction to vascular ultrasonography*, Philadelphia, 2000, WB Saunders, pp 329-343.
7. Abramowitz HB, Queral LA, Finn WR et al: The use of photoplethysmography in the assessment of venous insufficiency: a comparison to venous pressure measurements, *Surgery* 86:434-441, 1979.
8. Bundens WP, Bergan JJ. In Zwiebel WJ, ed: *Introduction to vascular ultrasonography,* Philadelphia, 2000, WB Saunders, pp 347-368.
9. Strandness DE: *Peripheral arterial disease: a physiologic approach,* Boston, 1969, Little, Brown & Co.
10. Aburahma AF, Khan S, Robinson PA: Selective use of segmental Doppler pressures and color duplex imaging in the localization of arterial occlusive disease of the lower extremity, *Surgery* 118(3):496-503, 1995.
11. Dormandy JA, Rutherford RB: Management of peripheral arterial disease (PAD). TASC Working Group. TransAtlantic Inter-Society Consensus (TASC), *J Vasc Surg* 31(1 Pt 2):S1-296, 2000.
12. Lijmer JG, Hununk MG, van den Dungen JJ et al: ROC analysis of noninvasive tests for peripheral arterial disease, *Ultrasound Med Biol* 22(4):391-398, 1996.
13. Yao JST, O'Mara CS, Flinn WR et al: Postoperative evaluation of graft failure. In Bernhard VM, Towne JB, eds: *Complications in vascular surgery,* Orlando, 1980, Grune & Stratton, pp 1-19.
14. Dean RH, Yao JST, Thompson RG et al: Predictive value of ultrasonically derived arterial pressure in determination of amputation level, *Am Surg* 41:731-737, 1975.
15. Ramsey DE, Manke DA, Sumner DS: Toe blood pressure: a valuable adjunct to ankle pressure measurement for assessing peripheral arterial disease, *J Cardiovasc Surg* 24:43-48, 1983.
16. Bone GE, Pomajzl MJ: Toe blood pressure by photoplethysmography: an index of healing in forefoot amputation, *Surgery* 89:569-574, 1981.
17. Goodreau JJ, Creasey JK, Flanigan DP et al: Rational approach to the differentiation of vascular and neurogenic claudication, *Surgery* 84:749-757, 1978.
18. Cardullo PA: ECG monitored arterial exercise tests, *Bruit* 7-9, 1983.
19. Carroll RM, Rose HB, Vyden J et al: Cardiac arrhythmias associated with treadmill claudication testing, *Surgery* 83:284-287, 1978.
20. Strandness DE, Bell JW: An evaluation of the hemodynamic response of the claudicating extremity to exercise, *Surg Gynecol* Obstet 119:1237-1242, 1964.
21. Kohler T, Andros G, Porter J et al: Can duplex scanning replace arteriography for lower extremity arterial disease? *Ann Vasc Surg* 4:280-287, 1990.
22. Kang S: Technique and results of ultrasound guided thrombin injection for pseudoaneurysms. In Pearce, Yao JST, eds: *Advances in vascular surgery*, Chicago, 2002, Precept Press, pp 333-339.
23. Lenox A, Griffin M, Nicolaides A et al: Percutaneous ultrasound guided thrombin injection: a new method for treating postcatheterization femoral aneurysms, *J Vasc Surg* 28:1120-1121, 1998.
24. Hessel SJ, Adams DF, Abrams HL: Complications of angiography, *Radiology* 132(2):273-281, 1981.
25. Coleman SS, Anson BJ: Arterial patterns in the hand based upon a study of 650 specimens, *Surg Gynecol Obstet* 113:409-424, 1961.
26. Porter JM, Snider KL, Bardana EJ et al: The diagnosis and treatment of Raynaud's phenomenon, *Surgery* 77:11-14, 1975.
27. Lue TF, Hricak H, Marich KW et al: Vasculogenic impotence evaluation by high-resolution ultrasonography and pulsed Doppler spectrum analysis, *Radiology* 155:777-781, 1985.
28. Kadioglu A, Erdigru T, Karoidag K et al: Evaluation of penile arterial system with color Doppler ultrasonography in nondiabetic and diabetic males, *Eur Urol* 27(4):311-314, 1995.
29. Flinn WR, Rizzo RJ, Park JS et al: Duplex scanning for assessment of mesenteric ischemia, *Surg Clin North Am* 70:99-107, 1990.
30. Moneta G, Yeager RA, Dalman R et al: Duplex ultrasound criteria for diagnosis of splanchic artery stenosis or occlusion, *J Vasc Surg* 14:511-520, 1991.
31. Olin JW, Piedmonte MR, Young JR et al: The utility of duplex ultrasound scanning of renal arteries for diagnosing significant renal artery stenosis, *Ann Intern Med* 122:833-838, 1995.
32. Redemacher J, Chavan A, Bleck J et al: Use of Doppler ultrasonography to predict the outcome of therapy for renal artery stenosis, *N Engl J Med* 344(6):410-417, 1002.
33. Matsumura JS, Ryn RK, Ouriel K: Identification and implications of transgraft microleaks after endovascular repair of aortic aneurysm, *J Vasc Surg* 34(2):190-197, 2001.
34. Moneta GL, Edwards IM, Papanicolaou G et al: Screening for asymptomatic internal carotid artery stenosis: duplex criteria for discriminating 60-99% stenosis, *J Vasc Surg* 21:989-994, 1995.

35. Aaslid R, Nornes H: Non-invasive transcranial Doppler ultrasound recording of flow velocity in basal cerebral arteries, *J Neurosurg* 57:769-774, 1982.

ADDITIONAL READING

Kremkau FW: *Diagnostic ultrasound, principles and instruments,* Philadelphia, 2002, WB Saunders.
Strandness DE: *Duplex scanning in vascular disorders,* Philadelphia, 1993, Raven Press.
Talbot SR, Oliver M: *Techniques in venous imaging,* Pasadena, 1992, Appleton Davis.
Zwiebel WL, ed: *Introduction to vascular ultrasound,* Philadelphia, 2000, WB Saunders.

6

Percutaneous Endovascular Intervention and Imaging Techniques

ROBERT L. VOGELZANG

The imaging and percutaneous treatment of vascular disease has undergone explosive change in the last 5 years. After a long period of development, testing, and introduction of new devices such as stents and thrombectomy devices and further improvements in older devices such as angioplasty balloons, endovascular therapy has now become widely accepted as the standard method to treat many forms of vascular disease that were previously exclusively treated by open surgery. It was in the early 1970s that angioplasty and other techniques, which are now widely used, began to be taught and applied. These methods included angioplasty, transcatheter infusion for vascular thrombosis, and embolization for treatment of hemorrhage and control of tumor growth. Simultaneous with the development of these innovative percutaneous methods, imaging techniques such as computed tomography (CT), magnetic resonance imaging (MRI), and high-resolution digital subtraction angiography (DSA) were invented and disseminated. These advances enabled the interventional radiologist to see anatomic structures with immensely more clarity than had previously been possible. They also permitted complex interventions to be undertaken with far more confidence and assurance.

All these developments, however, essentially set the stage for the introduction of the metallic endoluminal stent, which has revolutionized the field of vascular therapy in the 10 or so years since its approval for use in humans. The stent has markedly expanded the range of vascular beds that can be effectively treated with percutaneous techniques, including the carotid artery, that were strictly off-limits prior to this development. The addition of coverings to stents to make stent-grafts has had an even greater impact so that aortic aneurysms are now treated without open surgery (endografts). Stents have also been shown to produce better short- and long-term results and as a result have, in many situations, supplanted angioplasty as the method of choice for percutaneous treatment of vascular occlusive processes.

Drug therapy associated with the procedures has also changed considerably; new generations of anticoagulants such as enoxaparin (Lovenox) and antiplatelet agents such as clopidogrel also have radically changed the outcome of these treatments.

The widespread use of these new methods demands that appropriate indications be understood so that tests and treatments are not duplicated. With newer transcatheter intervention, different complications occur, sometimes with greater frequency than with conventional arteriography. This chapter will attempt to address the indications, techniques, complications, and results of these procedures and to emphasize the role of nursing in preprocedural assessment, periprocedural care, and postprocedural management.

OVERVIEW OF INTERVENTIONAL RADIOLOGY AND ENDOVASCULAR NURSING

As more complex procedures are performed on larger numbers of patients (many of whom are critically ill) and as other specialties in addition to interventional radiology such as cardiology and vascular surgery have become more and more involved in the performance of endovascular procedures, the need for skilled, dedicated periprocedural nursing care has grown. As a result, a new nursing discipline has emerged: those skilled and knowledgeable in endovascular, percutaneous therapy. The nurse has a number of responsibilities, some of which are new to the field and others that continue to involve the essential skills of nursing practice directed towards the particular needs of the endovascular patient. On a personal level, nurses working in an interventional endovascular procedural area have a responsibility to understand and practice radiation safety. The basic requirements involve wearing film monitoring badges and protective lead aprons but also include knowledge of the effects of excessive exposure to ionizing radiation on themselves and their patients. Of course, the basic nursing responsibilities of comfort, reassurance, support, and preservation of patient dignity must remain foremost in the nurse's role. The presence of "high tech" machinery and waiting periods in an unfamiliar, busy department may create an apparently hostile environment to which the nurse must orient the patient.

The nurse should discuss the procedure with the patient and help allay any anxieties he or she may have. In addition, specific nursing needs such as the presence of urinary catheters, surgical dressings, or central venous lines should be noted; patients may require special attention for a variety of reasons including recent surgery, chronic disabilities, and/or medical conditions, all of which affect the conduct of the procedure.

During the procedure, nursing needs are intensive and include such activities as starting intravenous lines, preparing and directing the puncture site, and most importantly monitoring the physiologic status of the patient. Basic monitoring includes electrocardiographic recording of rate and rhythm, measurement of blood pressure and respiration at regular intervals (every 5 to 10 minutes), and continuous monitoring of oxygen saturation via fingertip pulse oximetry. In many vascular procedural areas, nurses are responsible for administering intravenous sedatives and narcotics to supply a pain-free, comfortable condition for the patient. The use of fentanyl and midazolam is now standard care for intraprocedural medication. These drugs also provide the added benefit of production of retrograde amnesia about the procedure. Safe induction of conscious sedation must be accompanied by accurate documentation of level of consciousness, vital signs, and oxygen therapy periprocedurally.

After the procedure, the nurse will assess the patient's suitability for transfer to the nursing floor/intensive care unit and provide a written nursing summary on the chart. Prior to transfer, an oral report to the patient's nurses from the interventional nursing team is extremely beneficial. This exchange will ensure that any specific conditions requiring special attention are highlighted. This may include issues as diverse as the insertion of a urinary catheter during the procedure, a notation about a stable hematoma, the presence and status of a catheter or sheath in a peripheral artery, or details about an ischemic limb undergoing therapy, which may need monitoring by careful and regular Doppler and physical examination of the peripheral pulses.

ARTERIOGRAPHY

Indications

The indications for arteriography have narrowed since the 1950s and 1960s, when arteriography was used not only for the detection of vascular disease but for identification and characterization of many tumors throughout the body. The introduction of CT, ultrasound, and MRI/ magnetic resonance angiography (MRA) has markedly reduced the use of arteriography in tumor detection and in most cases eliminated it altogether. In the 1990s, arteriography was mainly used for the identification of abnormalities confined to the vessel itself or for intravascular therapy. In the past 5 years, MRA has had a dramatic effect on the use of diagnostic arteriography, in many situations largely eliminating it altogether or reducing its use to highly selected or special circumstances. Current indications for arteriography include the following.

Vascular Disease

The most common indication for the performance of arteriography is the presence of occlusive arterial disease in the extremities, extracranial or intracranial circulation, or visceral arteries for renovascular hypertension or intestinal ischemia. Patients with aneurysms of the aorta or extremities also may undergo arteriography.[1,2]

Arteriography is not a screening technique; a patient with symptoms of peripheral or cerebral arterial disease should first have a thorough physical examination, including palpation of pulses and arterial auscultation as well as a detailed clinical history. In addition, these patients require appropriate screening with noninvasive techniques such as Doppler and real-time ultrasound imaging of the affected vessels. As indicated earlier, MRA has largely replaced routine peripheral arteriography, including carotid arteriography. At Northwestern Memorial Hospital, for example, the incidence of routine lower-extremity runoff arteriography has been reduced by 90% in the past 3 years, largely as a result of MRA.

If arterial disease of sufficient severity is detected on clinical examination and noninvasive testing, arteriography may be obtained in patients who are candidates for surgery or endovascular intervention. Other candidates for arteriography include postoperative patients with suspected graft occlusion or pseudoaneurysm formation.

Tumor Detection

Arteriography has been used extensively in the past for the detection of tumors in solid organs such as the liver or kidney. In order to identify these tumors, catheterization and injection of the vessel supplying the organ is performed, and the radiologist searches for changes produced by the tumor. These changes include displacement of vessels, the presence of abnormal tumor vessels, or vascular occlusions, which may allow differentiation between benign and malignant masses. In general, however, arteriography is only used to define the vessels supplying the tumor before surgery.

Access for Transcatheter Therapy

The most common transcatheter therapies now performed for vascular disease are percutaneous transluminal angioplasty (PTA) and stenting. The optimal use of these newer endovascular therapies requires careful patient selection to determine which lesions can and should be treated because long-term results vary depending on the lesion characteristics and location.

Transcatheter therapy may also be used to lyse clot within a vessel or graft due to embolus or thrombosis.[3] Transcatheter thrombolysis is usually most effective when performed early after the occluding episode, but chronic thrombosis within a graft or (more commonly) within a native artery may also be lysed. Thrombolysis should be used cautiously and in the correct patient because the complication rate is higher than the rate for other endovascular procedures.

Catheter-based therapy may also be used to occlude vessels as well as to open them. Therapeutic transcatheter embolization involves injection of occluding materials such as surgical gelatin, particulate matter, liquids, or steel coils to occlude the vascular supply to a selected region. The technique may be performed to control hemorrhage in a patient who cannot undergo surgery or whose bleeding site is obscure or not readily located surgically.[4] Embolization may also be used to primarily control congenital arteriovenous malformations by selectively catheterizing feeding vessels and injecting particles or liquids that occlude the central vascular mass. In endovascular graft placement, embolization is frequently used to treat endoleaks or side branches that may potentially be a source for endoleaks.

Technique

Virtually all arteriography and interventional radiologic procedures are performed using the so-called Seldinger technique, which was invented by Sven Ivar Seldinger[5] in 1953. The method, elegant in its simplicity, involves needle puncture of the artery followed by placement of a wire through the needle into the lumen of the vessel. Over this wire, a catheter may be safely placed within the vessel, with the wire acting as a "guide" to the catheter (hence the designation of the wire as a guidewire). The guidewire is then withdrawn, and the catheter can be directed to a specific location and an injection made.[6] The guidewire technique also allows numerous and repetitive changes of a catheter to be performed without excessive trauma to the vessel wall. The technique is summarized graphically in Fig. 6-1.

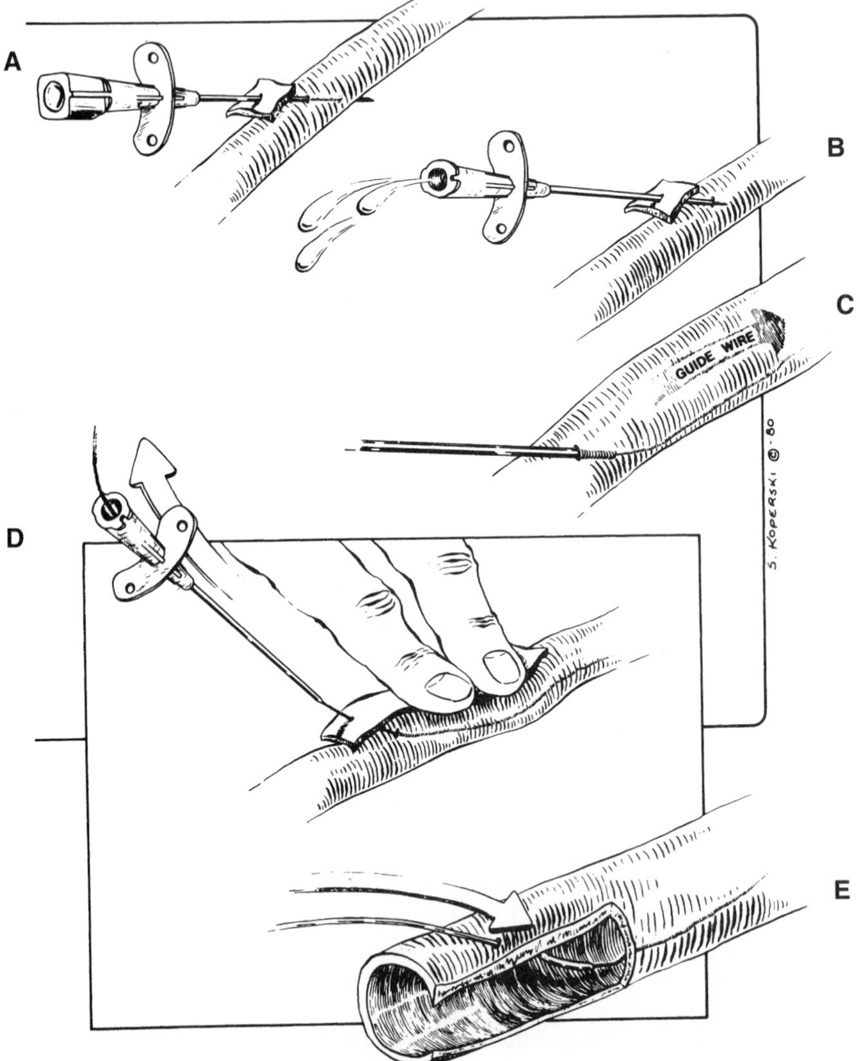

FIG. 6–1. Seldinger technique for arterial catheterization. **A,** The artery is percutaneously punctured. Note that the needle punctures both walls of the artery. **B,** The inner sharpened stylet is removed and the outer cannula withdrawn until the cannula lies within the arterial lumen and there is free return of blood. **C,** The guidewire is advanced into the artery through the cannula. **D,** After full advancement of the guidewire into the artery, the cannula is withdrawn and pressure is applied over the arterial puncture site to prevent bleeding. **E,** A catheter is threaded over the guidewire and advanced into the artery. (From Neiman HL: Techniques of angiography. In Neiman HL, Yao JST, eds: *Angiography of vascular disease*, New York, 1985, Churchill Livingstone, p 5. With permission.)

In order to be used to gain access to the arterial system, a vessel to be punctured must meet the following requirements: (1) it should be readily accessible, (2) it should be sufficiently large so that the catheter does not occlude the vessel, and (3) it should not be diseased. Three arteries that generally meet these qualifications are the common femoral artery, the axillary artery, and the brachial artery.[7,8]

The transfemoral approach is the most widely used, safest, and most effective route for arteriography (Fig. 6-2). If the femoral artery is not available for catheterization due to prior surgery, arterial stenosis, or occlusion, alternate routes for arteriography include the brachial approach, in which puncture is made in the brachial artery at or just above the antecubital fossa, and the axillary approach, in which the proximal brachial artery is punctured near the axilla. The choice of arterial access sites depends on many factors; each site has advantages and disadvantages and may be used in different circumstances. The brachial route is used in patients with aortoiliac occlusive disease and minimally palpable or nonpalpable femoral pulses or in those patients with previous femoral or aortic grafts, although graft puncture is not definitely contraindicated. If a patient has had a prior history of stroke, the brachial route may be contraindicated because the proximity of the catheter to the cerebral vessels increases the risk of stroke following the examination. The brachial approach also has specific complications associated with this approach, such as hematoma formation with brachial plexus compression that can result in long-term morbidity.

This complication occurs when small amounts of bleeding into the brachial sheath can cause compression and ischemic injury of the nerve plexus contained in the sheath. The clinical sequelae can range from small sensory deficits to major motor deficits. The angiographer's goal is to select the approach that provides the best diagnostic films with the least amount of risk to the patient.

Variously shaped catheters for specific purposes and vessels may be placed into the vascular system during a procedure. The most commonly used catheter in lower-extremity arterial disease is the "pigtail" catheter, which allows injection of a large amount of contrast material with a great deal of safety. These catheters are usually placed in the aorta, where contrast injection can be made with the blood flow carrying the material into the lower extremities for subsequent filming. Branches of the aorta and their subdivisions are selectively catheterized via the use of an appropriately shaped catheter designed to "seek" the vessel to be examined (Fig. 6-3).

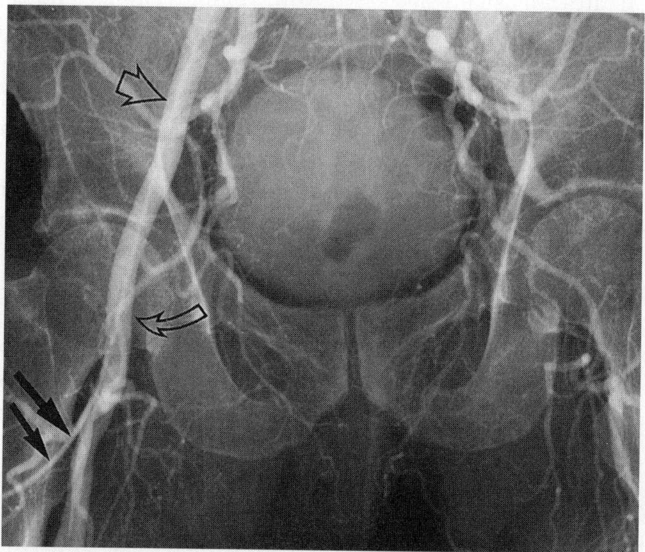

FIG. 6–2. Catheterization of the common femoral artery. Catheter *(arrows)* enters the right common femoral artery *(curved arrow)* and passes up the external iliac artery *(open arrow)*. The left femoral artery is occluded.

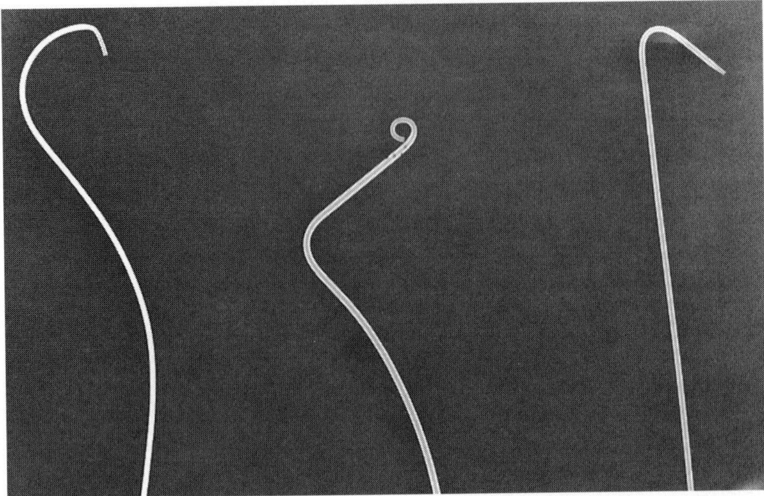

FIG. 6–3. Various catheter shapes designed for different purposes. A "cobra" shape (left) is used for injection into branches of the aorta. A catheter with a small "pigtail" at the tip *(middle)* is used for pulmonary arteriography. Its right-angle bend is designed to aid passage of the catheter through the right atrium and right ventricle. The catheter on the right is a simple bent catheter for entry into branches of the aorta.

Although many catheters exist, an angiographer generally will use only a small number of catheters with which he or she is familiar. Other highly specialized catheter shapes may be made by forming the catheters under steam in the angiographic laboratory. Guidewires also have specific functions and have different shapes for various requirements. They come in sizes ranging from 12 thousandths (.012) of an inch to 38 thousandths (.038) of an inch, with the majority in the .035- and .038-inch sizes. Catheter sizes usually change from 4 French to 7 French, although there is occasional need for catheters as small as 2 French and as large as 10 French. (One French equals one third of a millimeter.) Interventionalists now always use a vascular sheath that allows multiple catheter exchanges to be made with less arterial damage and less risk of bleeding.

After proper placement of the catheter, contrast material is injected using a pressure injector that is programmed for the appropriate flow rate and total volume to be given. For example, average flow rates and volumes for arteriography of the abdominal aorta (aortography) would be approximately 15-25 ml/sec, for a total of 30-50 ml of contrast material. In aortic branches, injection rates are usually decreased, with volumes adjusted for the capacity of the vessel in question. Renal artery injections average 6 ml/sec for a total of 9 ml, whereas injection into the superior mesenteric artery averages 8-10 ml/sec, for a total of 50-70 ml. Because of the renal toxicity of contrast agents, the total dose for an exam should not usually exceed 350 ml, although in extended procedures larger amounts can be used.

Due to the potentially thrombogenic nature of the catheter, heparinized flush solution is constantly used to keep the catheter free of clot. The guidewire has a heparin coating, and the catheter materials are designed to be of low resistance and have relatively little friction. In addition, the position of the catheter is critical, so that blood flow can occur around the catheter and not be occluded by it. The catheter and guidewire combination is never forced into a narrowed area or placed directly adjacent to an area of disease, unless a therapeutic intervention is being performed. Following the arteriogram, the catheter is withdrawn and manual compression of the artery that has been punctured is applied to prevent hematoma formation. After an appropriate period of time, usually 15-20 minutes, pressure is released; if no bleeding occurs, the patient is transferred back to the hospital room.

Complications

The interventional radiologist is concerned with the safe conduct of the examination. Complications of arteriography for which the patient is carefully monitored during and after the examination are discussed in Table 6-1.

TABLE 6–1 Complications of Arteriography

Complications	Findings	Symptoms	Information	Therapy
Puncture site hematoma	Stable or expanding swelling at puncture site and/or pulse loss	Pain, swelling, paresthesia, coolness of extremity, sensory and motor loss (in axillary or brachial artery punctures)	Pulse, blood pressure, pulse character, sensory and motor function, size and rate of expansion of hematoma	Direct pressure, cold pack, surgery
Pseudoaneurysm	Firm, pulsatile mass over puncture site	Pain, swelling, arterial compromise	Size and rate of expansion, vital signs, distal pulses	Ultrasound-guided compression, surgery
Local arterial occlusion (thrombosis)	Cool, pulseless extremity	Pain, sensory and motor loss	Vital signs, sensory and motor function, pulses	Heparinization, surgery, transcatheter fibrinolysis
Embolus	Loss of a distal pulse	Pain, coolness, sensory and motor loss	Vital signs, sensory and motor function, pulses	Heparinization, surgery, transcatheter fibrinolysis
Contrast-induced allergy and/or anaphylaxis	Urticaria, wheezing, dyspnea, cardiac arrhythmias, cardiac arrest (reactions may be immediate or delayed)	Itching, flushing, hives, nausea, shortness of breath, respiratory stridor	Vital signs, cardiac status, respiratory status	Intravenous fluids, intravenous epinephrine, respiratory support
Contrast-induced renal failure	Anuria/oliguria	Few	Urine output, creatinine	Fluid management, diuretics, dialysis
Neurologic complications	Aphasia, confusion, unconsciousness, hemiparesis	Blurred vision, speech deficit, motor or sensory deficits	Vital signs, neurologic status	Heparinization, CT or MRI scan, careful monitoring

CT, computed tomography; *MRI,* magnetic resonance imaging.

Nursing Management

Nursing care of the patient who undergoes diagnostic arteriography includes patient education, preangiographic preparation, and periprocedural and postangiographic monitoring. The nursing care process begins with accurate assessment of the patient's overall condition upon arrival in the department. Specific diagnoses relevant here are anxiety, deficient knowledge, pain, impaired gas exchange, risk for aspiration, risk for infection, risk for imbalanced fluid volume, ineffective tissue perfusion, and altered coagulation.

Routine orders and restrictions vary according to each institution and operator. Preprocedural preparation and orders usually include the following: (1) an accurate appraisal of renal function by blood urea nitrogen (BUN) and creatinine determinations; this is significant because contrast material is potentially nephrotoxic and postprocedure monitoring of the renal function requires a baseline test; (2) assessment of coagulation parameters by measurement of partial thromboplastin time (PTT), prothrombin time (PT), and platelet count; (3) adequate hydration with intravenous fluids and oral intake; good hydration is essential in order to prevent the occurrence of renal failure induced by contrast material;

(4) no solid foods after midnight; and (5) discontinuation of heparin or other anti-coagulation.

After the procedure, careful monitoring of distal pulses is vital, because a change in the pulse status may indicate a complication such as arterial thrombosis or embolus. Prompt detection of arterial occlusion is a high priority in preventing further complications. The nurse must monitor the patient for the development of a puncture-site hematoma (nonpulsatile mass), false aneurysm (pulsatile mass), contrast reactions, and contrast-induced renal failure. Some difficulties in postprocedural assessment may arise; for example, a hematoma at a puncture site may be confused with simple fullness or fleshiness. This sometimes-confusing distinction can often be made by comparison with the opposite groin and remembering that hematomas are generally firm and not soft. The findings and appropriate therapies for many of the complications of diagnostic and therapeutic arteriography are listed in Table 6-1.

Routine postprocedural orders include the following: (1) frequent checks of vital signs, neurologic function, and pulses in both extremities with particular attention to the extremity that has been catheterized (q 15 minutes × 4, and q 1 hour × 2); (2) assessment of the puncture site for hematoma and the appearance of the extremity distal to the puncture site; (3) bed rest for 6-8 hours, with the punctured extremity kept straight; (4) intravenous hydration continued for 6-8 hours; (5) BUN and creatinine levels assessed the next day; a complete blood count should be obtained if a translumbar approach has been used; and (6) resumption of preprocedural dietary and medication orders. If a patient has been on heparin, the drug is not resumed for a minimum of 4 hours.

VENOGRAPHY

Indications

Venography is used to demonstrate venous abnormalities in the lower and upper extremities, as well as in the vena cava and its branches such as the hepatic or renal veins.[9,10] It is usually performed to assess patency of the deep venous system and the presence of deep venous thrombosis; the test is indicated when noninvasive studies are indeterminate or negative in the face of a strong clinical suspicion of thrombotic occlusion. Venography allows differentiation between acute thrombosis and chronic venous occlusion and can accurately assess venous anatomy prior to surgical procedures. The test can also distinguish intrinsic thrombus formation from that secondary to venous compression and can evaluate congenital venous anomalies.

Technique

The technique for venography involves placement of the patient in a 45° upright position, with the leg to be examined in a non–weight-bearing position. Contrast material is injected into a distal foot vein to fill the entire venous system of the extremity. Fluoroscopy and filming then allows the detection of flow patterns and of venous occlusion. Thrombus is identified as a filling defect within the vein (Fig. 6-4). If visualization of larger veins such as the vena cava is required, puncture of a centrally located vein such as the femoral or antecubital vein may be performed with catheter placement into the appropriate location. Serial filming then takes place after rapid injection of contrast material.

Other techniques include transcatheter venous pressure monitoring, which is useful in obstructive diseases of the veins such as portal hypertension. Selective catheterization of veins such as the renal or hepatic veins can allow samples to be withdrawn for analysis of specific products, such as renin in the evaluation of renovascular hypertension. Selective venography may also be performed.

Complications

The main complication associated with venography is thrombophlebitis. Contrast material has been shown to injure venous endothelium and induce clot formation. As a preventive

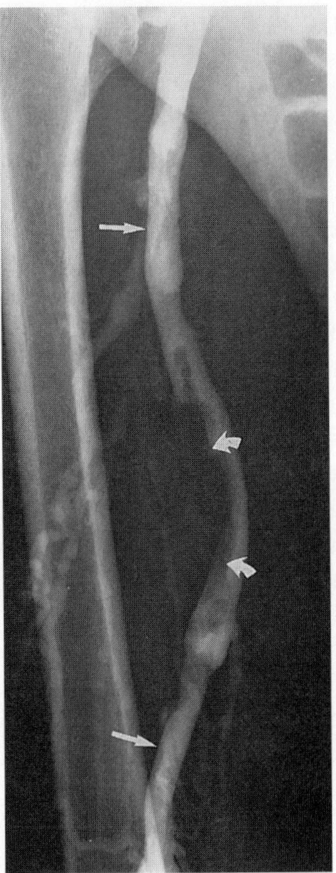

FIG. 6–4. Venogram of the femoral vein *(arrows)* demonstrates a "filling defect" *(curved arrows)* within the vein, diagnostic of thrombosis.

measure, all contrast material should be flushed from the venous system using heparinized saline. Despite these measures, however, postvenographic thrombosis can and does occur.

Extravasation of contrast at the injection site may cause inflammation and even lead to skin necrosis; this complication is fortunately quite rare and usually is only seen in patients with compromised blood flow in the area of extravasation. Hypersensitivity (allergic) reactions to contrast may also occur.

Nursing Management

Nursing care is directed toward patient education because the procedure may involve multiple attempts at finding and puncturing a vein, detection of complications at the injection site, monitoring for the presence of contrast-induced thrombophlebitis, and maintaining adequate hydration. The patient is usually on clear liquids for 3-4 hours prior to the procedure. The patient is to remain at bed rest for 2 hours after the procedure if the femoral vein in the groin is punctured.

BALLOON ANGIOPLASTY AND STENTING

Transluminal angioplasty has had a major impact on the treatment of vascular disease. Charles Dotter[11] of the University of Oregon invented the technique in 1964, and it was popularized in Europe. The original Dotter technique dilated vessels by the passage of progressively larger catheters through an area of arterial blockage or narrowing. Lower-extremity arteries, such as the iliac and femoral vessels, were amenable to this therapy, but branch arteries such as the renal or coronary vessels could not be dilated. In 1974, Andreas Gruntzig[12] devised a usable balloon-dilating catheter that provided increased safety and broader range of application. The technique has been successfully used in every major artery in the body, including lower-extremity, renal, coronary, and brachiocephalic vessels.[13-15]

Balloon angioplasty, however, has major limitations. Principal among the limitations is a relatively high rate of recurrence after angioplasty (as much as 50% recurrence or restenosis at 1 year).[15] Other problems included the failure of angioplasty to effectively treat long-segment arterial occlusions and/or occlusions and stenoses in the majority of patients with femoropopliteal disease. These drawbacks led many investigators to devise and use different methods and devices such as catheters that mechanically or via lasers removed plaque. In the 1980s a large number of these atherectomy and laser devices were invented and investigated, of which very few proved to show improved results over conventional balloon angioplasty.

The invention of vascular stents, however, radically changed the face of vascular intervention. These endoluminal metallic devices not only were rapidly proven to be useful but were considered a significant improvement over angioplasty in many vascular territories and became the preferred method of treating occlusive arterial lesions. Stents have also broadened the range of vessels and lesions treatable with these techniques[14,16,17] (Fig. 6-5).

From a nursing standpoint, all vascular recanalization procedures are quite similar in that the patients are essentially identical to those undergoing balloon angioplasty. Postprocedural nursing care will thus concentrate on assessment of the treated limb or organ and the puncture site. In this section, transluminal balloon angioplasty and stenting as a general model for this group of procedures will be discussed; later, differences between these newer therapies and balloon angioplasty from a nursing and technical (procedural) standpoint will be described.

Indications

In the lower extremities, transluminal angioplasty and stenting are indicated for treatment of arterial occlusive disease. In general, angioplasty is used in the treatment of segmental (less than 10 cm in length) stenoses and occlusions of the aortoiliac, femoropopliteal, and tibial arteries. Balloon dilatation of lesions more than 10 cm long has shown to be less durable, and

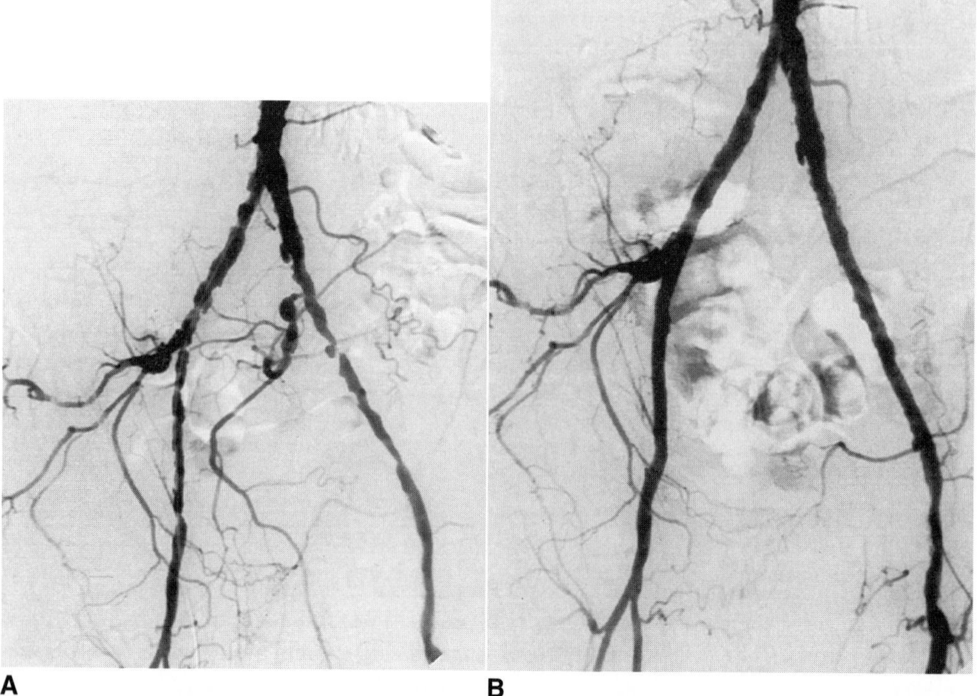

FIG. 6–5. Treatment of bilateral diffuse iliac artery disease with extensive stenting. **A,** Multifocal bilateral disease. **B,** After bilateral stenting with Wallstents.

in the iliac circulation stents are now quite routinely placed for long-segment occlusions and stenoses. In the femoropopliteal vessels, angioplasty of long lesions is still undertaken in patients with ischemia who are not operative candidates. Angioplasty of long areas of disease may allow limb salvage or convert a proximal amputation to a more distal one. In diabetic patients with ischemia and a nonhealing foot ulcer, angioplasty of less-than-ideal lesions may often permit adequate wound healing. Routine stenting of femoral and popliteal artery lesions is still controversial, and many interventionalists still reserve the use of stents for acute failures of angioplasty[17] (Fig. 6-6), although newer drug-eluting stents seem to offer considerable promise in reducing restenosis. The tibial arteries are very rarely treated with stents.

Angioplasty and stenting also frequently serve an adjunctive role to surgery. For example, a patient with an iliac stenosis proximal to a femoral artery occlusion may benefit from stenting of the iliac stenosis prior to femoral artery bypass surgery. Improved iliac artery inflow is a prerequisite to the femoral surgery and PTA/stenting may help to avoid a proximal surgical procedure.

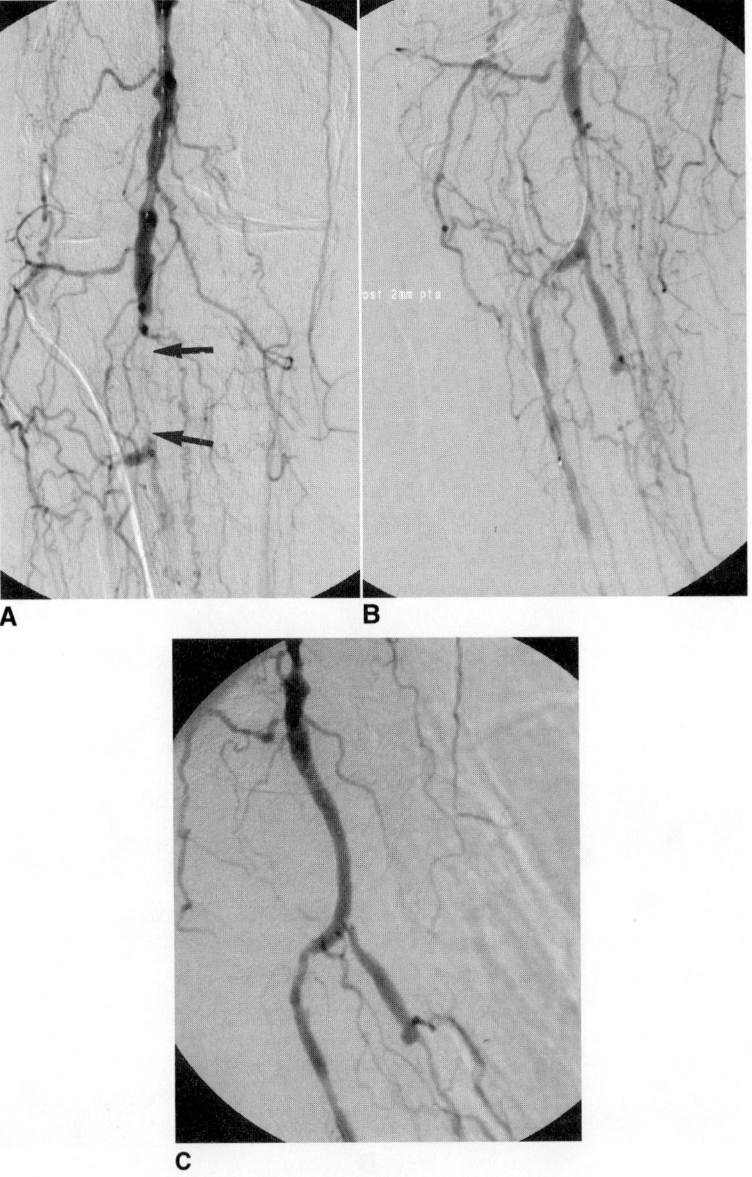

FIG. 6–6. Treatment of popliteal artery occlusion with stent. **A,** Initial popliteal artery occlusion *(arrows)* in a patient with severe ischemia. **B,** After angioplasty there is minimal improvement. **C,** After stenting.

Renal artery angioplasty and stenting is indicated for the nonoperative treatment of renovascular hypertension in those patients with amenable lesions, including (1) patients with fibromuscular dysplasia (Fig. 6-7) or atherosclerosis of the main renal artery (Fig. 6-8) (angioplasty is the generally the treatment of choice for fibromuscular dysplasia), (2) patients with segmental lesions of the proximal branches, and (3) patients with renal transplants who develop stenoses at the arterial anastomosis.[13]

Brachiocephalic artery angioplasty and/or stenting is indicated in specific lesions of the subclavian, innominate, vertebral, and/or carotid arteries such as fibromuscular disease of the common or internal carotid artery and atherosclerotic lesions of the proximal subclavian and/or innominate artery (Fig. 6-9). In the past 5 years, the use of stenting as a primary treatment of carotid artery atherosclerotic lesions has markedly accelerated based on very positive

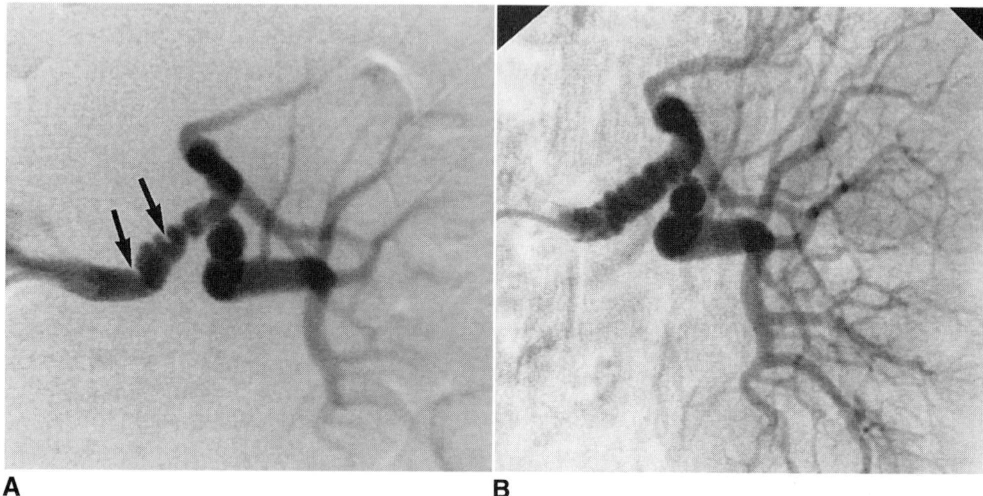

FIG. 6–7. Renal angioplasty for renal artery stenosis in a 42-year-old woman with severe refractory hypertension. **A,** Left renal arteriogram shows "string of beads" appearance of main renal artery *(arrows)* characteristic of dysplasia. **B,** After balloon angioplasty, considerable luminal widening is noted with elimination of stenoses. The patient had excellent clinical response and was normotensive off all medications following the procedure.

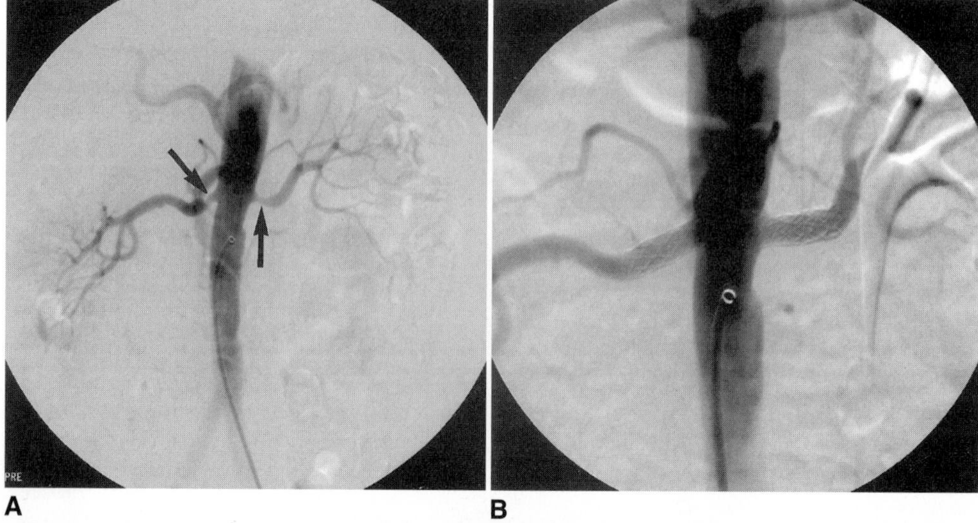

FIG. 6–8. Stenting for bilateral renal artery stenosis. **A,** Aortogram demonstrating bilateral high-grade renal artery lesions *(arrows)*. **B,** Aortogram following successful bilateral renal artery stenting.

clinical and research experiences with newer, low-profile devices. It appears quite likely that stenting of the carotid artery may become a preferred method of treatment for many carotid artery occlusive lesions.[18]

Many other vascular sites may be dilated or stented successfully. Some of the most common include hemodialysis access fistulae stenoses and stenoses of veins caused by trauma, malignancy, or old thrombosis (Fig. 6-10). Postoperative arterial anastomotic stenoses and bypass vein graft stenoses can also be dilated successfully.

Technique

The techniques for angioplasty and stenting are similar to those used for arteriography, with the exception that the catheter and guidewire are maneuvered across areas of narrowing or occlusion. Additionally, larger holes are made in the punctured artery by these larger devices

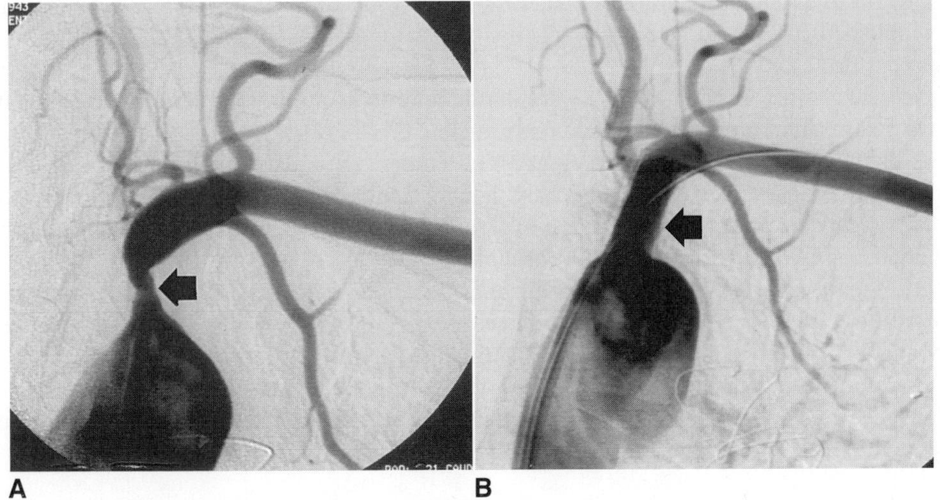

FIG. 6–9. Treatment of subclavian artery stenosis with stenting. **A,** Proximal left subclavian artery stenosis *(arrow)* was responsible for posterior fossa symptoms related to subclavian steal. **B,** After placement of Palmaz stent; good filling of the left vertebral artery *(arrow)*. Symptoms resolved.

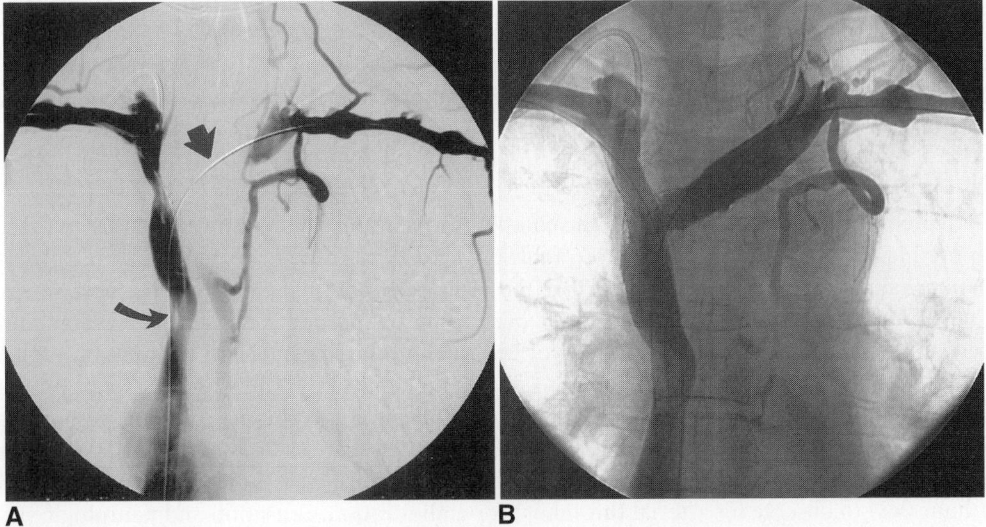

FIG. 6–10. Stenting for treatment of superior vena cava syndrome. **A,** Pretreatment with occlusion of left innominate vein *(arrow)* and high-grade vena cava stenosis *(curved arrow)*. **B,** After extensive stent reconstruction.

and the vascular sheaths needed to introduce them. After the blockage has been passed with a wire, an angioplasty catheter with an attached balloon of appropriate diameter is placed across the lesion. The dilating catheter is a double-lumen catheter that has an inflatable but nondistensible balloon at the tip. It has a distal end-hole that permits monitoring of pressure or infusion of contrast material or medication during the procedure. Typical balloon lengths are between 2 and 6 cm, with balloon diameters of 4 to 15 mm. Balloons of smaller and larger sizes may occasionally be used for specialized circumstances.

After positioning the catheter across the lesion, heparin is given to prevent thrombosis of the distal vessel while flow is temporarily occluded during balloon inflation. A vasodilator, such as nitroglycerin, is frequently administered intraarterially at a dose of 200 μg. The balloon is inflated in the diseased segment for 30 seconds; contrast material is used to inflate the balloon so that it may be seen fluoroscopically. Radiopaque metallic markers are also located at both ends of the balloon to allow precise localization in the stenotic area (Fig. 6-11). After dilatation, the catheter is placed proximal to the dilated segment and an angiogram is obtained to assess the success of the procedure. If an adequate result is not accomplished (persistent stenosis or residual pressure gradient), repeat dilatation or stenting is performed.

Arterial stenting is conducted in a similar manner to angioplasty except that the operator has two basic stent types and a number of available products from which to choose. The two types of stents are the self-expanding and the balloon expandable; the benefits and disadvantages of each are taken into account by the operating physician. For instance, renal arteries are usually recanalized with balloon-expandable stents whereas iliac and femoral arteries are often best treated with self-expanding stents.

After successful completion of the angioplasty or stenting, the catheter is withdrawn. Because heparin has generally been given, the vascular access sheath is not usually withdrawn until the effects of heparinization have been reversed by protamine or wear off on their own. In some patients undergoing small vessel or complicated stenting procedures, antiplatelet agents may be given, which increases the risk of puncture site hemorrhage.

Complications

Complications of angioplasty/stenting occur in 2-4 percent of patients, but most are minor and do not require intervention. Complications requiring surgical or radiologic intervention occur in about 1 percent. Complications that can occur include distal embolization of fragments from the treated site with resultant ischemia, arterial dissection or occlusion at the dilatation site from local trauma, arterial thrombosis and occlusion, and hematoma or false aneurysm formation at the catheter insertion site.[19] These complications can require surgical treatment with the exception of small- or moderate-sized hematomas at the puncture site. Most occur in the periprocedural period, which emphasizes the need for attentive nursing care.

Nursing Management

Both preprocedural nursing care and the complications from PTA/stenting are similar to those in routine diagnostic arteriography (see Table 6-1). Postprocedural care requires astute observational skills and aggressive nursing care, because these complications may be more severe than in routine arteriography. Puncture site hematoma and pseudoaneurysm is of greater concern in these patients because of the use of heparin and the larger size of the puncture hole. The degree of fullness at the puncture site should be noted upon the patient's arrival on the nursing unit and any changes carefully noted. If a hematoma is initially present, its borders should be marked on the skin to allow quantification of change. Peripheral pulses must be monitored at 15-minute intervals (×4) followed by checks at ½-hour intervals (×2) and 1 hour (×2) to observe for arterial thrombosis or embolization. Sensation and neurologic status of the limb should also be assessed. Aspirin and other antiplatelet agents are also administered after angioplasty.

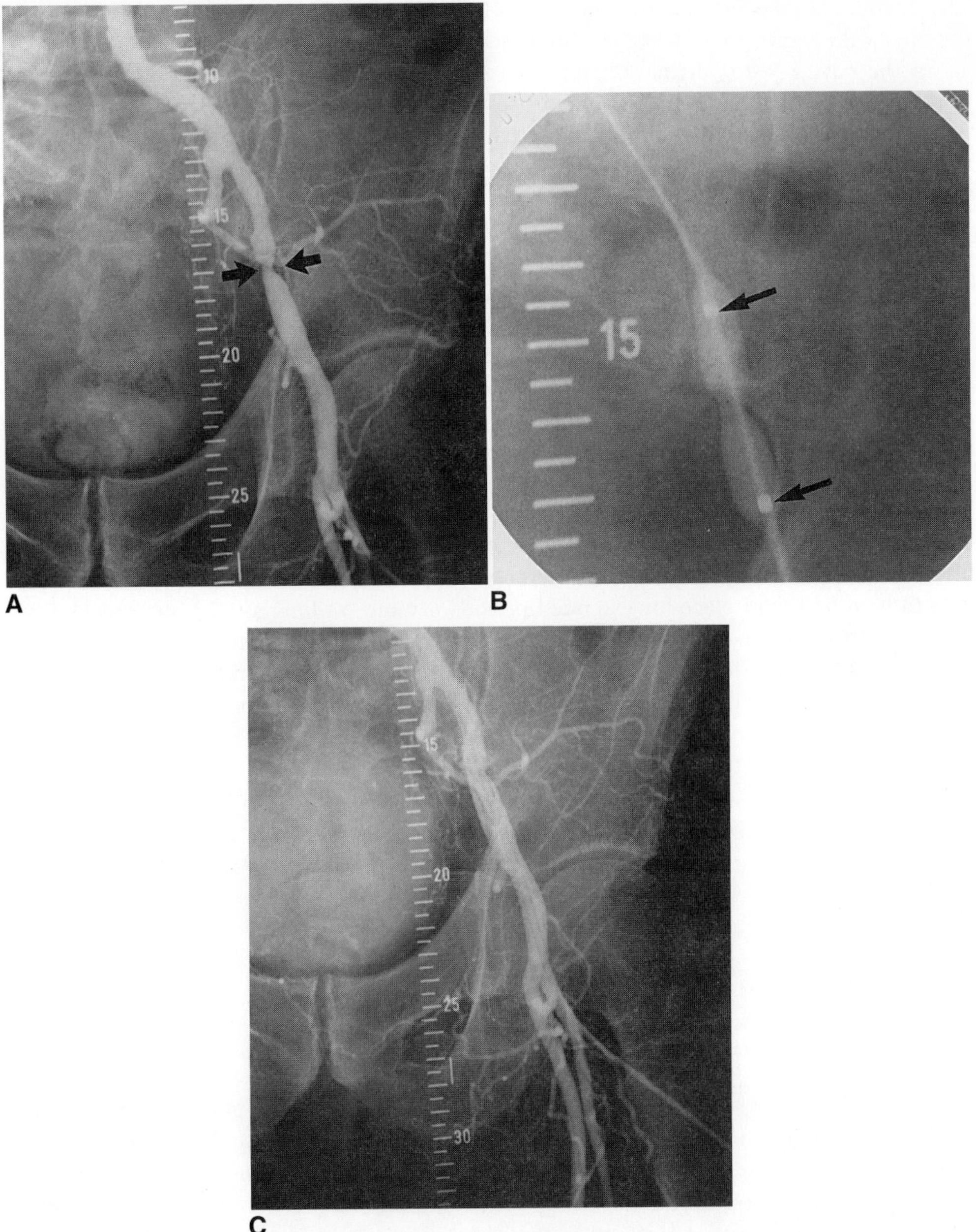

FIG. 6–11. Dilatation of an external iliac stenosis. **A,** Preangioplasty arteriogram performed via the femoral route shows a short left external iliac stenosis *(arrows)*. Radiopaque ruler allows localization of the stenosis at fluoroscopy. **B,** After insertion of balloon catheter across stenosis, the balloon is inflated with dilute contrast material. Notice narrowing of the balloon in the region of stenosis as the dilatation takes place. Small radiopaque markers *(arrows)* allow localization of the balloon prior to inflation. **C,** Postangioplasty arteriogram shows disappearance of stenosis.

TRANSCATHETER THROMBOLYSIS AND THROMBECTOMY

It has been known for many years that certain enzymes can accelerate the normal processes by which intravascular clot is lysed. These substances, mainly urokinase, have been administered systemically for the treatment of pulmonary emboli and coronary thrombosis, but clinical trials led to the conclusion that the complication rate was excessive. In an attempt to take advantage of these substances' lytic action against thrombosis but reduce their toxicity, lower doses of the enzymes were infused directly through a catheter into occluded vessels, with very encouraging results. Transcatheter dissolution of intravascular clot is now an accepted therapy in the treatment of vascular disease.

In the past 5 years, catheters and devices that mechanically macerate, pulverize, and remove clot have come into widespread use. These thrombectomy devices may be used in place of or along with thrombolysis in the patient with an occluded vessel.

Indications

Transcatheter fibrinolysis may be used as an alternative to surgical thrombectomy in patients with acute thrombosis of a bypass graft or native artery. Particular efficacy of fibrinolytic agents has been found in grafts and emboli to native arteries. Other indications for transcatheter fibrinolytic therapy include use when thrombotic or embolic complications occur during angioplasty. Iliac, femoral, popliteal, and subclavian deep venous thrombosis and pulmonary embolus have also been treated with local infusions[20,21] (Fig. 6-12). Contraindications to the use of these agents include recent surgery, hemorrhage, or trauma. Patients with a new stroke may also be at risk for the bleeding complications of this therapy.

Technique

Transcatheter thrombolysis is probably the most labor-and time-intensive procedure done by interventional radiology. It differs considerably from other procedures in that an arterial infusion catheter is left in place for extended periods of time (as long as 72 hours) as clot lysis progresses (Fig. 6-13). During this period of time, major demands are placed upon nursing personnel for monitoring of the drug infusion, catheter entry site, and the extremity under treatment. These added patient care requirements can only be met properly in an intensive care unit setting.

The technique of transcatheter thrombolysis involves insertion of a catheter directly into the thrombosis or embolus. In general, the catheter for lower-extremity occlusions is inserted

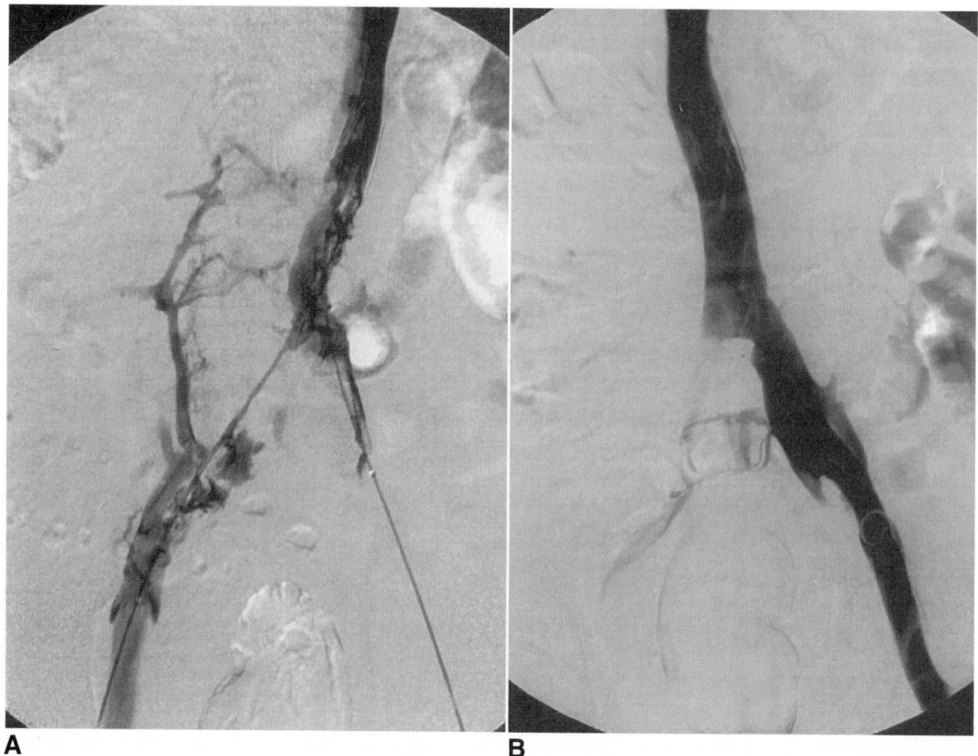

FIG. 6–12. Treatment of iliocaval thrombosis with local infusion of urokinase. Extensive iliocaval thrombosis **(A)** was treated with 72 hours of bilateral urokinase infusion with complete elimination of thrombus and disappearance of severe lower-extremity swelling and cyanosis **(B)**.

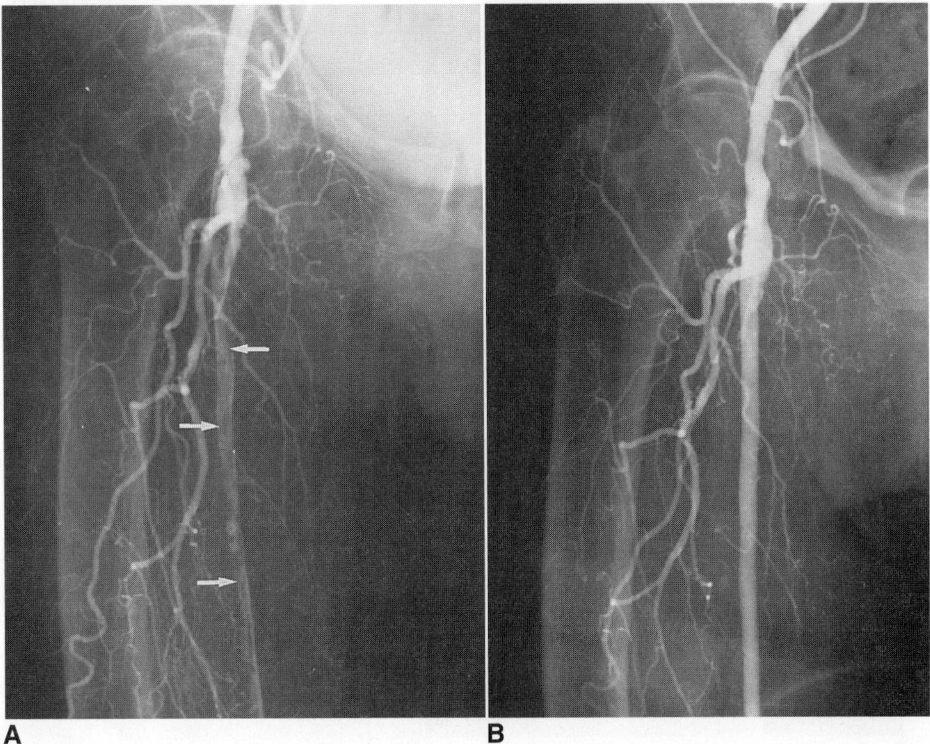

FIG. 6–13. Transcatheter lysis of thrombosed graft. **A,** Arteriogram prior to therapy shows multiple radiolucent filling defects within a previously placed femoropopliteal synthetic graft *(arrows)*. **B,** After 12 hours of transcatheter infusion of thrombolytic therapy, the graft was free of clot and distal pulses were restored.

in the opposite common femoral artery and passed around the aortic bifurcation, but other sites, including the femoral artery on the same side or the brachial artery, may be used. During the procedure, systemic anticoagulation with heparin is used to prevent thrombosis around the catheter or in the slowly flowing blood within the treated artery or graft. The procedure may also be combined with angioplasty if clot lysis uncovers a causative stenosis, or if there is a complication of angioplasty (Figs. 6-14 and 6-15). Some physicians will attempt to accelerate the clot lysis by forcefully injecting high doses of the thrombolytic drug into the clot.

Complications

The major complication rate of transcatheter thrombolytic therapy ranges between 2 and 10 percent. Most of the complications are hemorrhagic, with bleeding occurring at the catheter site or elsewhere. Other events that may occur include loosening of clot with distal embolization and formation of new clot around the indwelling catheter. Puncture site hematomas and pseudoaneurysms are also increased with this therapy.[20]

Nursing Management

As indicated above, thrombolytic therapy is the most nursing intensive vascular interventional procedure performed. Postprocedural orders reflect that complexity. A typical example of routine orders for thrombolysis is reproduced in Box 6-1. There are four major areas of nursing concern during this therapy.

Catheter Site Management

Catheter position is critical to this therapy; thus the catheter is carefully secured, and an adhesive dressing is placed. Despite these precautions, flexing of the thigh and other movements may dislodge the catheter; avoidance of such movements is thus mandated. Patients will, however, require shifting and movement for bed linen changes and use of a bedpan; these

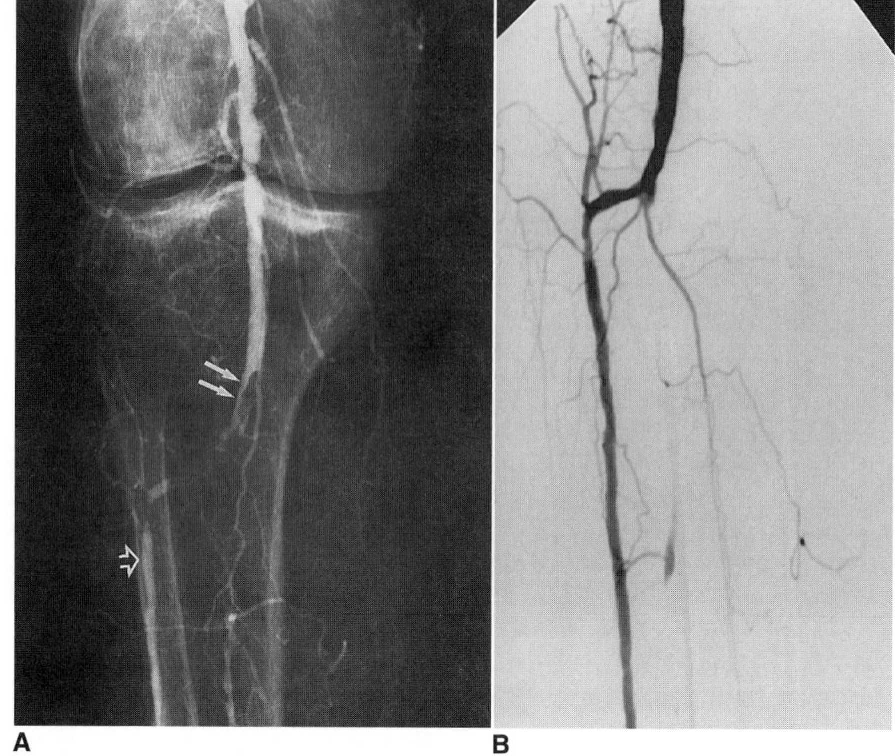

FIG. 6–14. Lysis of spontaneous arterial thrombosis. The patient was an 82-year-old woman suffering from acute onset of right lower-extremity rest pain. **A,** Initial angiogram showed occlusion of the distal popliteal artery by filling defect *(arrows)* with collaterals reconstituting the anterior tibial *(open arrow)*. **B,** Following overnight infusion of urokinase at the site of occlusion, there was complete opening of the popliteal and anterior tibial artery with excellent clinical results.

should be accomplished with assistance. The catheter insertion site must also be monitored for the development of bleeding or hematoma formation, complications that occur with increased frequency in light of the concurrent use of heparin. Minimal catheter site oozing is typically seen and generally is controlled by light pressure. Repeat angiography is also frequently performed. During the repeat visits to the radiology suite (when the concealing dressings are likely to be removed), careful checking of the catheter insertion site for hematoma should be made.

Drug Management

There are several agents available for thrombolytic therapy, including tissue plasminogen activator (TPA), and doses given are dependent on the drug used. For example, TPA doses usually are in the range of 0.2-1.0 mg/hr. Careful calculation of drug concentration and infusion flow rates, always administered by infusion pump, is thus critical to avoid potentially catastrophic dosing errors. In addition, anticoagulation with intravenous heparin is frequently used and must be monitored by maintaining the PTT at $1\frac{1}{2}$ to 2 times control value.

Hematologic Monitoring

Thrombolytic therapy can and does cause major alterations in systemic coagulation and hemostasis. Careful observation of the patient for signs and symptoms of local or remote hemorrhage, including gastrointestinal or intracranial bleeding, is thus mandated. Oozing from intravenous puncture sites may be seen; unnecessary punctures should be avoided because of the patient's altered clotting parameters. Also, laboratory values such as fibrinogen, platelets, PT, and PTT must be monitored at 4- to 6-hour intervals. The fibrinogen level should not fall below a value of 100 mg/100 ml.

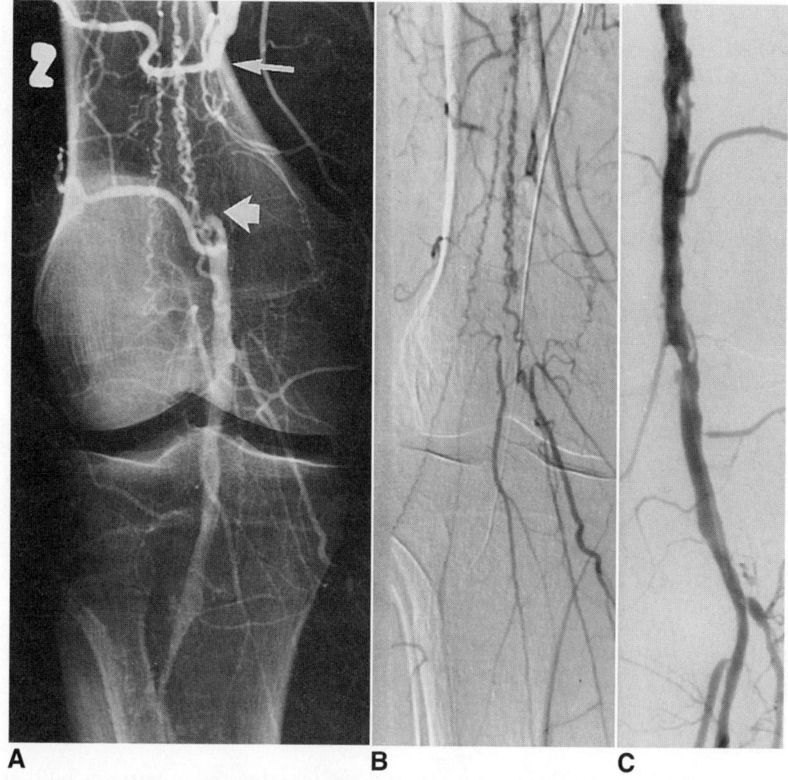

FIG. 6–15. Use of thrombolysis to treat a thrombotic complication of transluminal angioplasty. The patient was a 56-year-old man with right lower-extremity claudication. **A,** The original arteriogram demonstrated a short-segment occlusion of the popliteal artery *(arrows)*. **B,** Following dilatation, complete thrombosis of the femoral popliteal artery was observed. **C,** Urokinase was infused overnight with restoration of patency.

BOX 6–1

Thrombolytic Infusion

1. Monitor vital signs, distal pulses, affected limb temperature, sensory and motor function and puncture sites ______________ q 15′ × ________; q 30′ × ________.
2. Monitor closely for signs of hemorrhage from any area of the body.
3. No arterial punctures/avoid unnecessary venipunctures.
4. Strict bed rest with ________ hip extended/arm rest.
5. Patient may be logrolled side to side.
6. Head of bed elevated ________°.
7. Ensure that dressings are intact; do not manipulate catheter.
8. Follow-up angiogram scheduled on: ________
9. Notify SERVICE and INTERVENTIONAL RADIOLOGY FELLOW (include phone numbers) for:
   - Fibrinogen level <100 mg/100 ml.
   - Change in vital signs; decreased or absent pulses; urine output <200 ml/8 hrs; change in color, temperature, or sensation in either lower/upper extremity; bleeding or hematoma at puncture site (apply pressure to site); presence of pain in any area of the body. Do not apply sandbags over puncture site at any time.
10. Time TPA infusion started: ____________ hours on (date) ____________.
    - Rate started at ____________ units/min.
    - Infuse above rate for ____________ hours.
    - Then infuse at ____________ units/min for ____________ hours.
11. Start heparin infusion at ____________ units/hours.
12. PT, PTT, fibrinogen, FDP at ____________ and at every ____________ hour(s).

TPA, tissue plasminogen activator; *PT,* prothrombin time; *PTT,* partial thromboplastin time; *FDP,* fibrin degradation products.

Monitoring of the Limb under Treatment

Thrombolytic therapy is generally used for ischemic conditions of the extremity. As lytic therapy progresses, changes in the perfusion of the limb can be expected to occur. Certainly, if therapy is successful, return or strengthening of distal pulses may be auscultated or palpated. Color and temperature of the extremity can be expected to improve as well. These changes may occur gradually or rather suddenly depending on the nature of the occlusion and the efficacy of therapy.

During thrombolytic therapy, an acute worsening of the extremity manifested by pain and/or loss of pulses can result from "showering" of distal embolization of fragmented clot distally. Although this may be initially alarming, the sudden development of ischemic signs and symptoms should be correctly identified as progress and therapy continued because the signs and symptoms will generally improve with continued infusion. Side effects of the fibrinolytic agent may include generalized body shaking, anxiety, impaired gaseous exchange, fever, and hypertension. The reaction is generally short-term, and the patient is usually continued on the drug.

TRANSCATHETER EMBOLIZATION

Arteriography can be used to diagnose areas of hemorrhage and to identify tumors. The same catheter used to diagnose can also be used to occlude the blood supply to tumors and site of hemorrhage by injecting materials that block the blood supply to those areas.

Indications

Transcatheter occlusion of vessels is indicated as definitive therapy in patients who are not candidates for surgery or in certain conditions such as arteriovenous malformations. Transcatheter occlusion can also be a useful adjunct to surgery. In these patients, preoperative embolic occlusion of the vascular supply to neoplasms may reduce surgical blood loss considerably. Additionally, malignant liver tumors not amenable to surgery are also now being effectively treated. When performed appropriately, these catheter techniques may be lifesaving and provide levels of occlusion not obtainable surgically. This is most dramatically seen in the treatment of arteriovenous malformations, which may be difficult to excise or control surgically. Transcatheter therapy may obliterate these lesions without surgery (Fig. 6-16); however, multiple procedures

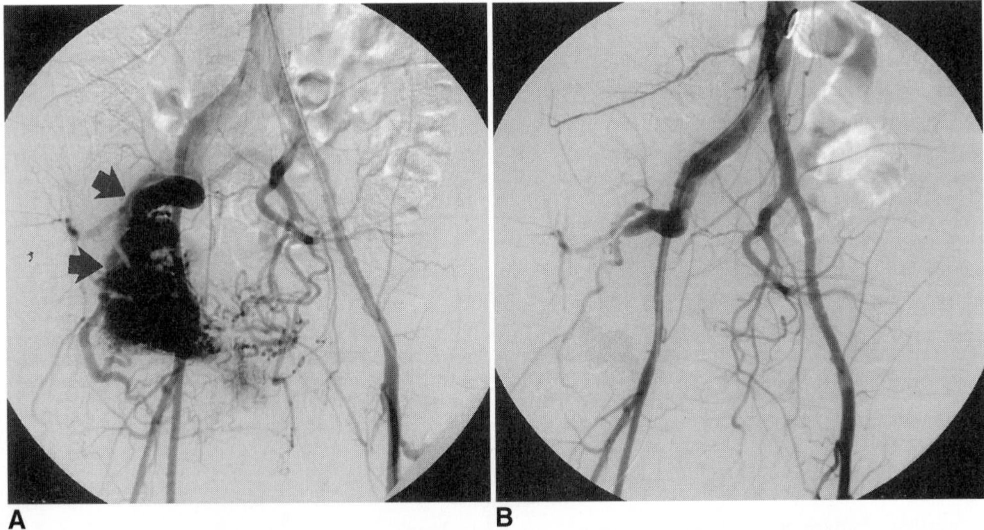

FIG. 6–16. Transcatheter cure of pelvic arteriovenous malformation. **A,** Pretreatment with large shunting hypervascular arteriovenous malformation on right side of pelvis *(arrows)*. **B,** One year after final treatment with disappearance of arteriovenous malformation.

may be required to progressively occlude the malformation. Control of gastrointestinal, postsurgical, or posttraumatic hemorrhage is also possible (Fig. 6-17).[22-24]

Technique

In this technique, the catheter is positioned in the vessel to be occluded. Once catheter position is obtained, the vessel may be occluded with a variety of substances, including particles such as pieces of surgical gelatin (Gelfoam) or small plastic bits. Other substances used include liquids such as alcohol or tissue adhesive (bucrylate); devices for large vessel occlusion include steel coils and inflatable detachable balloons.

Complications and Nursing Management

The main complications associated with transcatheter embolization therapy are local catheter entry site problems and, most important, inadvertent occlusion of vessels outside the target area. Pain may also be commonly seen after an embolization; this is related to ischemia produced in the intended area of embolization and should not be seen as a complication. In general, good medication management can eliminate this problem, which is seen most intensely in the first 24 hours. Postoperative care also requires careful assessment of distal pulses, as well as constant monitoring of the patient for signs of infarction of other organs or tissues depending on the location of embolization.

PERCUTANEOUS INFERIOR VENA CAVA FILTER PLACEMENT

Introduction

Vena cava filters have been in wide use for about the last 20 years, primarily in the form known as the Greenfield vena cava filter, which was implanted operatively through a venotomy. Recently, however, a new generation of smaller filters that have proven to be as effective and as safe as the Greenfield filter have been introduced; these devices are now placed percutaneously.[25,26]

Indications

Pulmonary embolism (PE) is a life-threatening complication of deep venous thrombosis. It is estimated that about 30 percent of patients will die of the disease if it is left untreated.

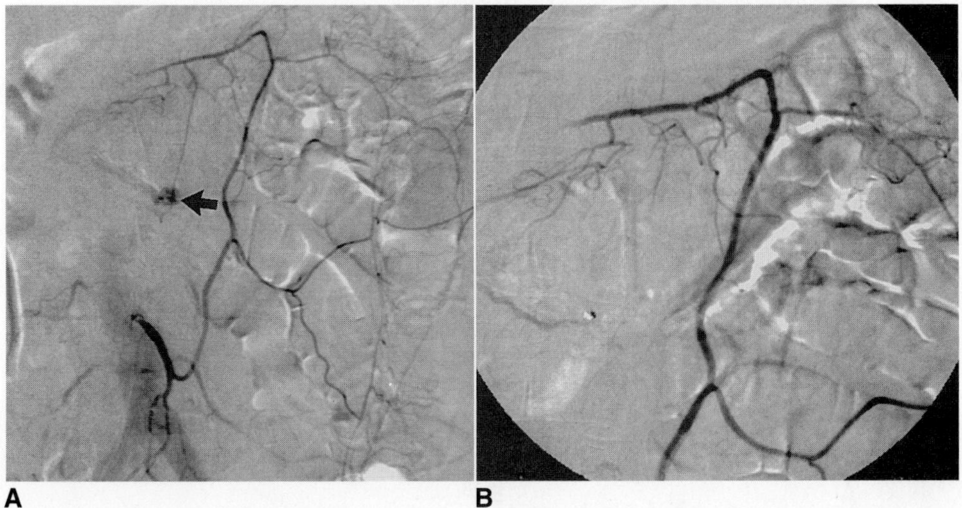

FIG. 6–17. Embolization of gastrointestinal bleeding. **A,** Postoperative lower gastrointestinal bleeding was documented by contrast extravasation on inferior mesenteric arteriography *(arrow)*. **B,** After embolization with microcoils and surgical gelatin pledgets, bleeding and contrast extravasation are no longer evident.

Treatment usually consists of anticoagulation therapy with heparin and coumadin, which reduces the mortality of PE considerably, to less than 5 percent. There are, however, a number of patients in whom anticoagulation therapy cannot be used, usually because of a bleeding tendency, anticipated surgery, or a history of recurrent PE on adequate anticoagulation. Other patients may not be able to tolerate any further episodes of PE because of reduced cardiac or pulmonary capacity, or they may be at risk for massive embolus from a large clot in the vena cava or iliac veins. These selected individuals are candidates for placement of a vena cava filter in order to prevent PE.

Technique

Vena cava filters are placed through the right internal jugular or the right femoral venous approach. The procedure itself is simple and straightforward in that catheterization of the vena cava is performed under local anesthesia. A venacavogram is first done to identify any abnormalities and to ensure that no clots are present in the cava. If this exam appears unremarkable, the filter is deployed in the infrarenal cava below the renal veins through a sheath that ranges in size from 6 French to 12 French in diameter depending on the device that is used (Fig. 6-18). Following filter deployment, the catheter is withdrawn, hemostasis achieved, and the patient is returned to his or her room.

Complications

Complications of vena cava filter insertion can be either immediate or delayed. Immediately, improper deployment or positioning of the filter may reduce filtering efficiency. Perforation of the vena cava with retroperitoneal bleeding has also been very rarely described. Late complications of vena cava filter placement include movement or migration of the filter with

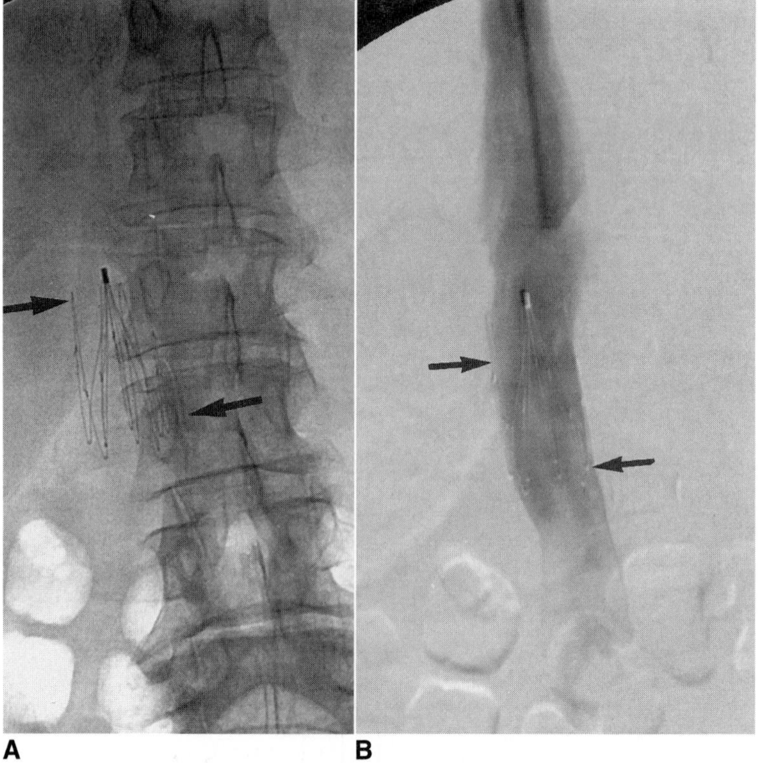

FIG. 6–18. Vena cava filter. **A,** Plain film of the abdomen showing VenaTech LP filter in position *(arrows)*. This is an updated version of the VenaTech filter. **B,** Venocavogram performed after filter insertion. Notice the well-centered position of the filter.

some filters rarely migrating to the heart or pulmonary artery. Occlusion of the vena cava can also occur because a large embolus has been trapped.[26]

Nursing Management

Nursing management for insertion of vena cava filters involves several areas. Frequently, these patients are quite ill and may have a number of other coexisting medical conditions that require nursing management. Deep venous thrombosis with attendant leg swelling may often be present, or there may be a recent episode of PE that produces cardiovascular or pulmonary instability. The filter insertion is relatively straightforward and not painful; however, post-procedural management will concentrate mainly on observation for hematoma or venous thrombosis at the site of insertion and any signs or symptoms of filter migration. Follow-up with plain abdominal x-ray is usually obtained 1-2 days after a filter insertion to ensure that the filter is sufficient. In rare circumstances, the patient may be continued on anticoagulation. In these cases, the anticoagulation should not be begun for at least 4 hours after the insertion of the filter and withdrawal of the deployment sheath.

TRANSJUGULAR INTRAHEPATIC PORTOSYSTEMIC SHUNTS

Introduction and Indications

Portal hypertension, usually caused by parenchymal liver disease relating to viral or alcoholic hepatitis, is a major cause of morbidity and mortality in the United States. Portal hypertension, defined as increased pressure in the portal vein, results from progressive scarring and fibrosis within the liver parenchyma. As a result of this scarring, increased resistance to portal flow develops and a large number of portal venous collateral channels are formed, including collateral veins around the stomach and gastroesophageal junction. These veins can bleed massively and are the cause of many of the problems caused by portal hypertension. Therapeutic options in the past have included endoscopic sclerotherapy, in which injection of sclerosing liquids into the varices prevents bleeding, or surgical shunting of the obstructed portal vein into the vena cava by the use of a portocaval shunt. Unfortunately, surgical mortality is very high in the patients who are actively bleeding and who have the poorest liver function. Surgical mortality in this group (Child's class C) may be greater than 50 percent.

Technique

Transjugular intrahepatic portosystemic shunt (TIPS) is an interventional radiologic therapy that is now widely used and largely supplants traditional surgical shunts. It allows nonsurgical placement of a large-caliber shunt between the portal vein and the hepatic vein (the outflow vein of the liver). The procedure is generally performed under general anesthesia but may be done using intravenous sedation. A large steerable needle is placed through the right internal jugular vein into the hepatic vein and a passage made between the hepatic vein and the portal vein that lies a short distance (2-4 cm) away from the hepatic vein. After entry of the portal vein, a guidewire is passed and the tract through the liver dilated. The tract is then held open by placement of a metallic vascular stent (Fig. 6-19). The procedure provides a large decompressive shunt that reduces flow in the varices and stops bleeding.[27]

Complications and Nursing Management

Patients with cirrhosis and portal hypertension present complex nursing management difficulties. These patients may be actively bleeding with many associated hemodynamic problems. The patient is usually in the intensive care unit and generally requires nursing management during the entire procedure, such as fluid management, cardiovascular and respiratory management, and appropriate sedation. Following the procedure, careful observation of the patient for continued bleeding and/or complications of the procedure such as hepatic encephalopathy or high output cardiac failure is necessary.

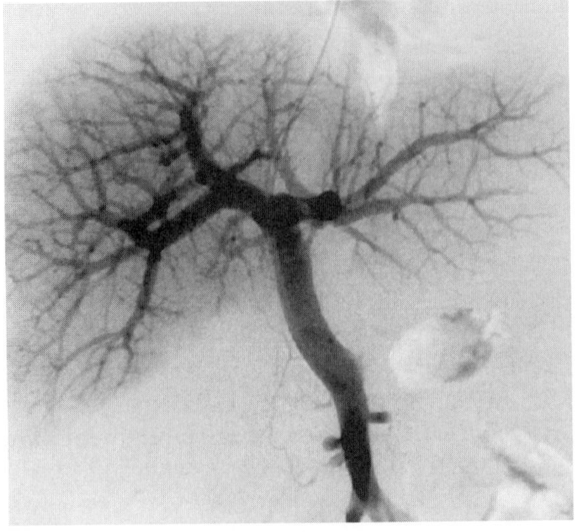

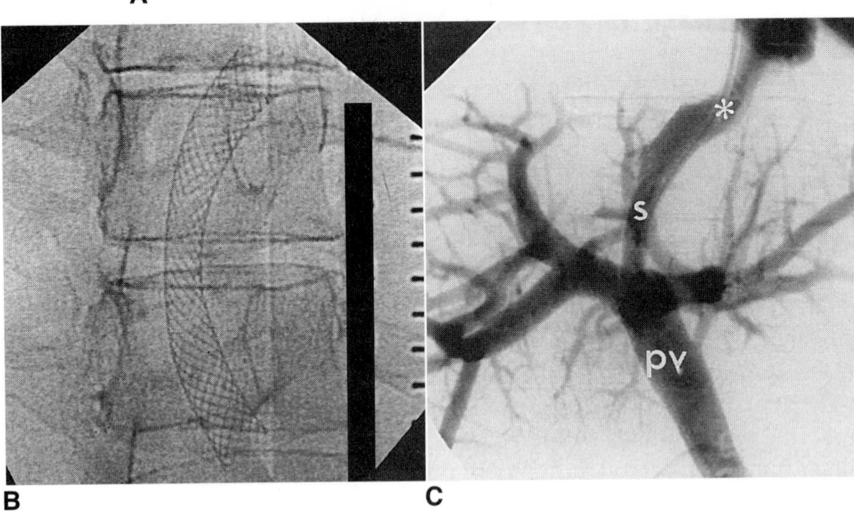

FIG. 6–19. Transjugular intrahepatic portosystemic shunt (TIPS). A patient with progressive portal hypertension and variceal bleeding underwent the transjugular procedure. **A,** After placement of a catheter from the hepatic vein through the hepatic parenchyma into the portal vein, a portal venogram was performed. **B,** After balloon dilatation of the tract, a metallic shunt was placed, which causes shunting of blood between the portal vein and hepatic vein. **C,** Portal venogram following the procedure shows contrast in portal vein *(pv)* with flow through shunt *(s)* directly into hepatic vein *(*)*.

DIAGNOSTIC ULTRASOUND

Indications

Ultrasound examination of the vascular system is widely used because it is accurate, inexpensive, and noninvasive. Indications include the evaluation of abnormalities of blood flow using Doppler and frequency analysis and direct depiction of anatomic abnormalities, such as aneurysm and plaque disease. Ultrasound is useful in screening for the presence of aneurysms of the aorta and of the femoral or popliteal arteries, as well as the detection and treatment of postcatheterization femoral artery pseudoaneurysms. It can readily differentiate hematoma from pseudoaneurysms. Ultrasound can also detect the presence of fluid, hematomas, seromas, and perivascular abnormalities. Detection of intraabdominal masses or fluid collections in the postoperative vascular patient is another important indication for diagnostic ultrasound.

Technique

The body part to be examined is scanned using a variety of transducers of various frequencies. In general, lower frequencies such as 3 MHz (3 million cycles/sec) are used for imaging of deeper structures such as the retroperitoneum and abdomen. Higher-frequency transducers, such as 7 MHz, provide more detail and are best used for superficial structures, such as the gallbladder. Ultrahigh-frequency transducers up to 10 MHz usually provide a small field of view and substantially reduced penetration (a few centimeters), but provide exceptional detail of small superficial structures such as the thyroid gland, as well as of superficially located vessels and grafts. Sound waves generated by the transducer penetrate the body part and are reflected, refracted, or absorbed. Those sound waves are reflected and refracted by the structures beneath the transducer and are detected by the same transducer that is sending the signals. These returning sound waves are then converted to images and displayed on a television monitor. In most cases, "real-time" ultrasound is used, which allows detection of motion as well as blood flow.

Ultrasound does have several limitations. In the abdomen, the image may be degraded or blocked by gas and/or fat, which cannot be penetrated by sound waves. Obese patients or patients with excessive bowel gas may not be candidates for complete ultrasound evaluation. Bowel gas can be eliminated by the ingestion of liquid by mouth or the introduction of a water enema for reduction of gas artifact from the colon. Bowel gas may also be shifted in the abdomen by having the patient assume different positions.

Ultrasound-guided compression of postcatheterization femoral artery pseudoaneurysms has been particularly useful. This technique, which was only recently described, has eliminated the need for surgical repair of 90-95 percent of catheter-related femoral artery pseudoaneurysms. The procedure is simple in that the same transducer that has been used to demonstrate flow within the pseudoaneurysm is used to directly compress the pseudoaneurysm at the point of communication with the underlying artery. Manual compression by the examiner takes place until flow ceases within the pseudoaneurysm and thrombosis occurs. Several cycles of compression of up to 10 minutes each may be necessary to accomplish thrombosis of the pseudoaneurysm unless there is an underlying coagulopathy or the pseudoaneurysm is chronic.

Complications and Nursing Management

Complications of diagnostic ultrasound are essentially nonexistent. Nursing care is directed toward patient education and preparation for the examination, which is relatively simple. For evaluation of the abdominal organs, the patient is usually on NPO (nothing by mouth) status 8 hours prior to testing to reduce gas and to maximally distend the gallbladder. Water may also be administered orally during the examination. Postexamination care is minimal, because contrast is not given.

Ultrasound-guided compression of pseudoaneurysms is generally very well tolerated. The patient may experience some pain during forceful compression of the pseudoaneurysm that might require sedation or injection of local anesthesia at the site of compression. After ultrasound-guided compression obliterates the pseudoaneurysm, careful monitoring of the site for the return of a pseudoaneurysm should be performed clinically, because occasionally these may recur. Typically, the patient is followed with a repeat ultrasound at 24 or 48 hours to ensure that no pseudoaneurysm remains. The limb under examination should be monitored during and after compression therapy to ensure that all the distal pulses are intact and that there has been no change in the perfusion of the extremity due to the forceful compression of the common femoral artery.

COMPUTED TOMOGRAPHY

Introduction and Indications

CT is a powerful imaging tool in vascular disease. CT scanning is routinely used for accurate staging of abdominal aortic aneurysms, as well as in complex postoperative problems such as graft infection, repetitive graft occlusion, hemorrhage, or abscess. In addition, CT can be used for guidance of biopsy procedures. All of these developments in CT have been made possible by the technical improvements in the machines available for clinical use. Initially, body scanning was performed with an 18-second scan time and a small number of x-ray detectors. Current scanners are capable of completing a scan in 2 seconds, which substantially reduces motion artifact. These machines also possess an increased number of x-ray detectors, which improves image quality and resolution. The major advantage of CT over other imaging modalities, including arteriography, is that CT allows direct depiction of the arterial wall and accurately defines processes and structures around the vessel wall that are indicators of disease (e.g., fluid, air, and hematoma).

Technique

CT produces axial slices of the body, so that anatomy is depicted in cross section. This sectioning of the body is performed by placing the patient in a circular gantry around which are arrayed an x-ray tube and multiple x-ray detectors. The tube moves around the body while emitting x-rays that are confined to a very narrow beam or slice. The rays pass through the body and are detected on the opposite side by the detectors. The information from the detectors is then processed by high-speed computer and an image is generated. Various sections are obtained by moving the patient through the gantry. The thickness of the slice taken can also be varied between 2 and 10 mm.

For the majority of cases, contrast is administered orally and intravenously. Oral contrast allows identification of bowel and avoids confusion with pathologic masses. Intravenous contrast administration causes enhancement of vessel lumens and allows them to be distinguished from processes such as thrombus in the peripheral portion of an aneurysm, vessel, or graft (Fig. 6-20). It also allows identification of whether a graft or vessel is occluded. Intravenous contrast administration also causes many parenchymal organs, such as the kidney, liver, and spleen, to enhance or become denser. This aids in the detection of benign and malignant masses, which usually do not enhance to the same degree as do normal parenchyma.

Biopsies and drainage procedures are also frequently performed under CT guidance, which allows precise localization of masses and fluid collections. A needle, catheter, or guidewire can be placed into collections or masses, using CT to avoid overlying structures. In this manner, postoperative abscesses are drained and deep masses are biopsied.

Complications and Nursing Management

Complications in CT are minimal because the technique is noninvasive. Patients may experience contrast-induced renal failure or reactions, so urine output and creatinine must be monitored and the patient should be observed for contrast reactions. Additionally, biopsy or drainage procedures performed under CT guidance may rarely have hemorrhagic or septic complications. Nursing care for CT thus revolves primarily upon adequate patient preparation, which includes the need for good hydration, because of the use of contrast.

MAGNETIC RESONANCE IMAGING AND ANGIOGRAPHY

Indications and Technique

MRI has now become an accepted imaging tool for vascular disease because of its ability to demonstrate vessels in multiple projection and because conventional intravenous contrast need not be used to demonstrate the vascular lumen. MRA has revolutionized the workup and evaluation of vascular disease and largely eliminated conventional arteriography of the lower extremities and carotid circulation (Fig. 6-21). CT continues to be used very commonly for evaluation of the thoracic and abdominal aorta; however, MRA is now the preferred technique of choice at many hospitals.

MRI is a simple examination in that no intravenous contrast is given, but not all patients are suitable for the examination. In particular, patients with pacemakers (particularly older

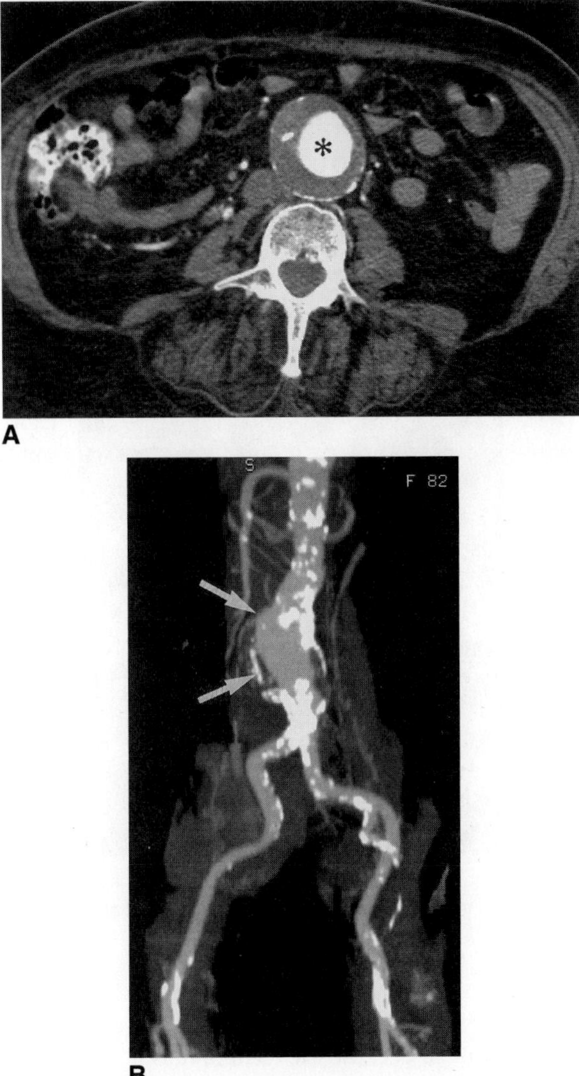

FIG. 6–20. Computed tomography of an abdominal aortic aneurysm. **A,** Axial image of enhanced scan showing opacified lumen *(*)* differentiating flowing blood from surrounding lower-density thrombus. **B,** Three-dimensional reconstruction of the abdominal aortic aneurysm shows exquisite detail achievable with modern imaging. Note aneurysm *(arrows)* and its relationship to the aortic bifurcation. White material on aorta represents calcium in wall.

varieties that have not been shielded from magnetic resonance frequencies) cannot be scanned due to inference with the pacemaker. Patients with implanted cardiac defibrillators also cannot have MRIs.

Metallic devices such as implanted surgical clips or vena cava filters, as well as joint replacements, can produce large artifacts that distort or obscure the image. Patients who have also had recent intracranial surgery with clips or aneurysm clipping should also not be scanned with MRI because of the possibility that clip movement may occur. Finally, critically ill patients who require extensive life support or respirators (which are made of metal) cannot be scanned using MRI because of the need for absence of any ferromagnetic objects in the room. The reason for their prohibition is simple: the extremely powerful magnet used in MRI can literally pull these devices into the magnet and cause bodily harm and, thus, they are prohibited from being placed anywhere in the scanning room. For these individuals, CT will continue to be the imaging technique of choice. MRI has also been used preliminarily as a guidance system for interventional procedures.

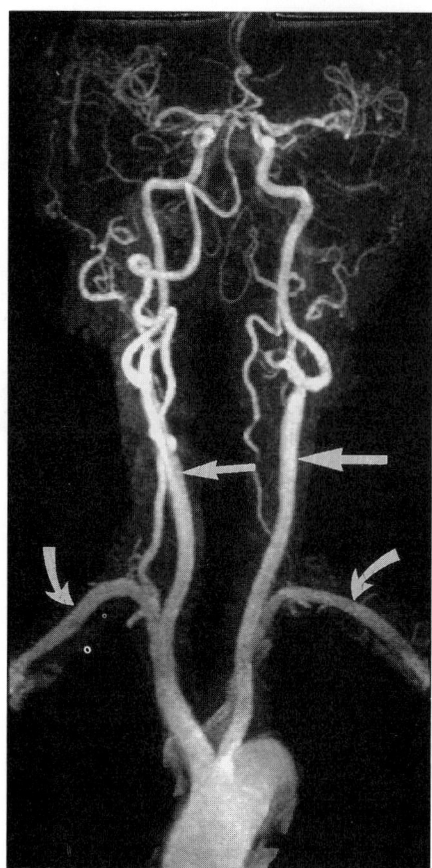

FIG. 6–21. Magnetic resonance angiography of aortic arch in a symptomatic patient. Note demonstration of carotid arteries *(arrows)* as well as the subclavian arteries bilaterally *(curved arrows)*.

Complications and Nursing Management

Complications in MRI are minimal because the technique is noninvasive. As indicated above, conventional intravenous contrast is not given and, therefore, the technique is ideal for patients with renal failure or those who are allergic to contrast. Magnetic resonance contrast is used; however, these agents have essentially no renal toxicity or allergic problems. The main issue surrounding nursing care of these patients is the fact that patients must lie relatively motionless during production of the scans, which generally take longer than CT (which usually takes 1-2 seconds per image). Ultrafast imaging is rapidly being developed, and these techniques make it much easier to obtain diagnostic information in most patients. For individuals who are not able to hold still or who are anxious, appropriate sedation is vital to enable production of good-quality diagnostic scans. Some patients may also become claustrophobic in the scanner because they must be placed in the gantry that completely surrounds their body. In these individuals, reassurance and/or sedation may alleviate the problem.

REFERENCES

1. Polak JF: Femoral arteriography. In Baum S, ed: *Abrams angiography*, ed 4, Boston, 1997, Little, Brown & Co, pp 1697-1742.
2. Hallisey MJ, Maranze SG: The abnormal abdominal aorta: arteriosclerosis and other diseases. In Baum S, ed: *Abrams Angiography*, ed 4, Boston, 1997, Little, Brown & Co, pp 1052-1072.
3. Ouriel K, Shortell CK, DeWeese JA et al: A comparison of thrombolytic therapy with operative revascularization in the treatment of acute peripheral arterial ischemia, *J Vasc Surg* 19:1021-1030, 1994.
4. Kadir S: Gastrointestinal bleeding: an overview. In Kadir S, ed: *Teaching atlas of interventional radiology*, New York, 1999, Thieme.

5. Seldinger SI: Catheter replacement of the needle in percutaneous arteriography: a new technique, *Acta Radiol* 39:368-371, 1953.
6. Braun MA, Nemcek AA Jr, Vogelzang RL, eds: *Interventional radiology procedure manual*, New York, 1997, Churchill Livingstone.
7. Kandarpa K, Aruny JE, eds: *Handbook of interventional radiologic procedures*, ed 2, Boston, 1996, Little, Brown & Co.
8. Crain MR, Mewissen MW: Abdominal aortography. In Baum S, ed: *Abrams angiography*, ed 4, Boston, 1997, Little, Brown & Co, pp 1013-1023.
9. Lea TM, Browse NL: Venography of the lower extremity. In Neiman HL, Yao JST, eds: *Angiography of vascular disease*, New York, 1984, Churchill Livingstone, pp 421-480.
10. Lea TM, McAllister V, Tonge K: The radiological appearance of deep venous thrombosis, *Clin Radiol* 22:295-305, 1971.
11. Dotter C, Judkins M: Transluminal treatment of arteriosclerotic obstructions: description of a new technique and a preliminary report of its applications, *Circulation* 30:654-670, 1964.
12. Gruntzig A, Kumpe DA: Technique of percutaneous transluminal angioplasty with the Gruntzig balloon catheter, *AJR Am J Roentgenol* 132:547-552, 1979.
13. Tegtmeyer CJ, Matsumoto AH, Johnson AM: Renal angioplasty. In Pentecost M, Baum S, eds: *Abrams angiography: interventional radiology*, Boston, 1997, Little, Brown & Co, pp 294-325.
14. Rholl KS: Percutaneous aortoiliac interventions in vascular disease. In Pentecost M, Baum S, eds: *Abrams angiography: interventional radiology*, Boston, 1997, Little, Brown & Co, pp 225-261.
15. Becker GJ, Katzen BT, Dake MD: Noncoronary angioplasty, *Radiology* 170:921-940, 1989.
16. Murphy TP: The role of stents in aortoiliac occlusive disease. In Perler BA, Becker GJ, eds: *Vascular intervention: a clinical approach*, New York, 1998, Thieme.
17. Henry M, Armor M, Ethevenot G et al: Palmaz stent placement in iliac and femoropopliteal arteries: primary and secondary patency in 410 patients with 2-4 year follow-up, *Radiology* 197:167-174, 1995.
18. Roubin GS, New G, Iyer SS et al: Immediate and late clinical outcomes of carotid artery stenting in patients with symptomatic and asymptomatic carotid artery stenosis: a 5-year prospective analysis, *Circulation* 103(4):532-537, 2001.
19. Levy JM, Hessel SJ: Complications of angiography and interventional radiology. In Baum S, ed: *Abrams angiography*, ed 4, Boston, 1997, Little, Brown & Co, pp 1024-1051.
20. Ouriel K: Thrombolytic therapy for occluded arteries and grafts: patient selection and results of disease. In Perler BA, Becker GJ, eds: *Vascular intervention: a clinical approach*, New York, 1998, Thieme.
21. Semba CP, Dake MD: Thrombolytic therapy for iliofemoral deep venous thrombosis: catheter-directed techniques disease. In Perler BA, Becker GJ, eds: *Vascular intervention: a clinical approach*, New York, 1998, Thieme.
22. Zuckerman DA, Bocchini TP, Birnbaum EH: Massive hemorrhage in the lower gastrointestinal tract in adults: diagnostic imaging and intervention, *AJR Am J Roentgenol* 161:703-711, 1993
23. Lang EK: Transcatheter embolization of pelvic vessels for control of intractable hemorrhage, *Radiology* 140:331-339, 1981.
24. Vogelzang RL, Yakes WF: Vascular malformations: effective treatment with absolute alcohol. In Pearce WH, Yao JST, eds: *Arterial surgery: management of challenging problems*, Philadelphia, 1996, Appleton & Lange, pp 553-550.
25. Webb MS, Dorfman GS: Vena cava filters. In Perler BA, Becker GJ, eds: *Vascular intervention: a clinical approach*, New York, 1998, Thieme.
26. Ferris EJ, McCowan TC, Carver DK et al: Percutaneous inferior vena caval filters: follow-up of seven designs in 320 patients, *Radiology* 181:851-856, 1993.
27. Haskal Z: Interventions in portal hypertension. In Pentecost M, Baum S, eds: *Abrams angiography: interventional radiology*, Boston, 1997, Little, Brown & Co, pp 525-546.

7

Intraoperative Nursing Care of the Vascular Patient

CAROL N. COX □ LYNN M. BORGINI

Beyond the "Surgery—No Admittance" sign is a technologically advanced world of highly skilled professionals who work in unison to provide care to a wide and varied surgical population. The team consists of two nurses (a circulating nurse and a scrub nurse), the surgeon and his or her assistants, an anesthesiologist, and ancillary personnel.

Health care workers and patients alike frequently perceive the operating room (OR) as a mysterious and threatening environment. Because of a lack of exposure to the OR during the formal education process, health care workers may be unfamiliar with OR protocols. They may also be intimidated by the many restrictions and strict adherence to technique that guide OR practice. The anticipation of surgery is a very stressful time for the patient and the family, resulting in high anxiety levels. Patients scheduled for surgery are sedated with drugs that have an antianxiety and amnesic effect. As a side effect of these drugs, the patient's recall of events during the perioperative phase is severely diminished or lost.

The information presented in this chapter is pertinent to the nurse who cares for the patient before and after surgical intervention as well as during the operative phase. The purpose of this chapter is to familiarize all nurses with the nursing process of assessment, planning, intervention, and evaluation and its application in the vascular OR suite. In addition, it will provide the novice vascular OR practitioner with the advanced knowledge and expertise necessary to aid the vascular patient through the operative phase.

The nurse plays a significant role in the vascular OR suite, thus needing a thorough knowledge of vascular anatomy and physiology as well as expertise in the technical component. It is an exciting role that continues to expand and challenge the vascular OR nurse.

The treatment for arterial disease has changed dramatically with endovascular surgery techniques. The current endovascular operating room suite functions as a fully equipped operating room as well as providing advanced digital imaging capabilities. Endovascular surgery procedures include diagnostic angiography, angioplasty and stent placement, and aortic endoluminal graft placement. The most commonly stented arteries are the iliac and femoral; the renal and mesenteric arteries are stented with less frequency. Stenting of the carotid artery is currently being evaluated with clinical trials. Combined endovascular and traditional arterial surgery may be performed such as an iliac artery balloon angioplasty and stenting performed in combination with a femoral to popliteal artery vein bypass.

INTRAOPERATIVE CARE

Collaboration

Intraoperatively, vascular patients require a multidisciplinary approach. Good communication skills are an essential priority within the specialty of perioperative nursing. The scrub and circulating nurses communicate throughout the operative phase. The circulating nurse works closely with the anesthesiologist, vascular nurse clinician, surgical intensive care unit, and ancillary departments. This collaborative effort among health team members is vital for a successful outcome.

Aseptic Technique

It is the dual responsibility of the scrub and circulating nurses to create, maintain, and monitor surgical asepsis to reduce the potential for infection. Throughout all phases of the operative procedure, a safe and aseptic environment is achieved through careful observance of the principles of asepsis. The principles of sterilization, disinfection, decontamination, and environmental monitoring are used in maintaining a surgically clean environment.

Equipment

To maintain an efficient, safe intraoperative environment, the scrub and circulating nurses must have a thorough working knowledge of all specialized equipment. They must coordinate and organize equipment and supplies on the basis of patient needs and type of surgical procedure. These items are selected in an organized, timely, and cost-effective manner. The nurse must make sure this equipment is in proper working order and readily available for the procedure. All supplies to be used on the operative field must be inspected for sterility. Package integrity and expiration date must be noted before placement on the sterile field (Fig. 7-1). The scrub nurse is responsible for the preparation and organization of all instruments and supplies on the sterile field and for the efficient handing of instruments to the surgeon and the surgeon's assistants throughout the procedure. The nurse anticipates the need for additional instruments and supplies due to unplanned changes in the surgical procedure. Both nurses count sponges, needles, blades, and instruments (according to hospital policy). The counts must be documented on the patient's operative record (Fig. 7-2). Counts are performed before the first incision and before closure of the incision sites.

Patient Care

The nurse's health assessment of the patient consists of the identification of physiologic, psychologic, and psychosocial data. Interpretation of this information assists the nurse in forming a plan of care and in identifying individual patient problems (Box 7-1). The nurse assesses the patient's coping mechanisms, expectations of care, and knowledge of the proposed

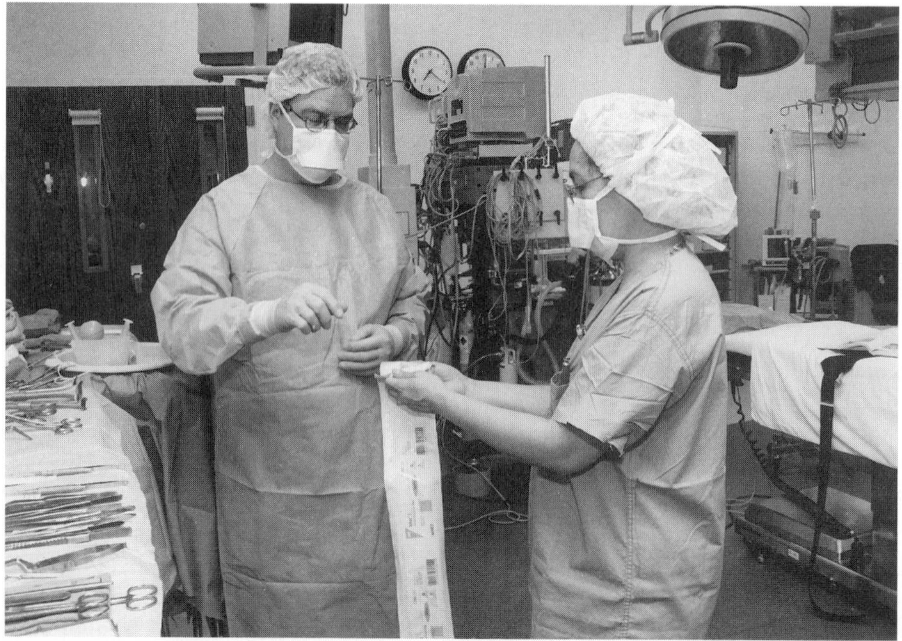

FIG. 7–1. Scrub and circulating nurses following aseptic technique when handling sterile items on the surgical field.

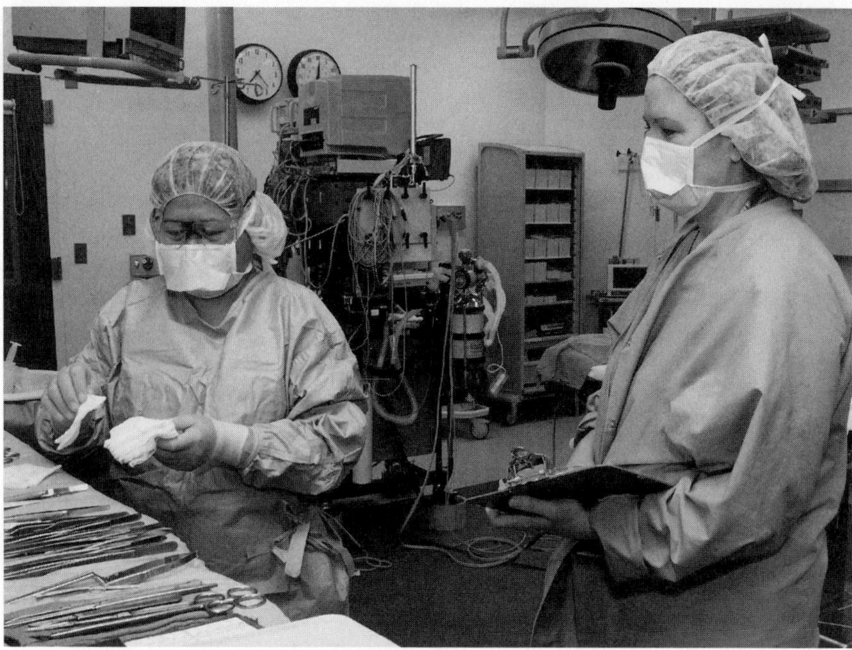

FIG. 7–2. Scrub and circulating nurses counting Raytec sponges before surgical procedure. The circulating nurse documents these counts on a separate count sheet and the operative record.

BOX 7–1

Nursing Diagnoses and Interventions

ANXIETY

Nursing Intervention

Assess patient's anxiety level.
Assess patient's knowledge and understanding of procedure.
Reinforce preoperative teaching.
Explain all procedures and preoperative preparation.
Discuss patient's questions and concerns in the preanesthetic area.
Provide comfort/security measures as needed (e.g., warm blankets, holding hand) during induction.
Introduce patient to personnel responsible for his or her care.
Maintain a quiet environment in the operating room suite.
Maintain patient dignity.
Maintain patient confidentiality.

IMPAIRMENT OF SKIN INTEGRITY

Nursing Intervention

Document presence of allergies.
Assess and document condition of patient's skin preoperatively, e.g., skin turgor, elasticity, rashes, bruises, or reddened areas.
Provide a preoperative clipping of body hair in the holding room to prevent breaks in patient's skin integrity.
Move patient slowly and gently onto the operating room bed.
Document type of skin preparation used for preoperative skin cleansing.
Provide adequate padding to all bony prominences, protecting nerve pathways.
Provide ongoing assessment of pressure points and relieve pressure as identified.
Place electrocautery dispersive pad on muscular body parts, avoiding bony prominences.
Document on the operative record all equipment and positioning devices.

Continued

BOX 7–1

Nursing Diagnoses and Interventions—cont'd

INFECTION

Nursing Intervention

Visibly inspect room for cleanliness prior to opening sterile supplies.
Provide sterile skin preparation to operative site.
Inspect sterile items for package integrity, expiration date, and sterilization process indicator.
Create effective barriers to transmission of microorganisms through proper gowning, gloving, and draping procedures.
Maintain aseptic technique throughout the procedure.
Initiate corrective action when break in technique occurs.
Limit traffic in the vascular suite during procedure.
Apply sterile dressings at end of procedure.
Administer antibiotics per physician's order.
Open prosthetic grafts as close to time of insertion as possible.

HYPOTHERMIA

Nursing Intervention

Assess patient's weight, height, and age.
Place warming blanket, and check correct temperature settings.
Increase room temperature before the patient enters vascular suite.
Place warm blankets on patient when entering vascular suite.
Limit exposure of patient during surgical preparation.
Provide warm intravenous fluids for anesthesia.
Provide warm fluids for irrigation of the surgical field.

SURGICAL INTERVENTION

Nursing Intervention

Assess and document preoperative level of consciousness.
Assess preoperative vital signs.
Assess preoperative laboratory values.
Anticipate potential blood loss.
Confirm and document availability of blood products for transfusion.
Implement use of blood salvage machine and/or rapid infusion when indicated.
Document amount of irrigation used on surgical field.

RETAINED FOREIGN BODY

Nursing Intervention

Follow established policy and procedures for sharp, sponge, and instrument count.
Confine and contain all discarded sponges, sharps, and instruments. Do not remove counted items or trash from the operating room suite after initiation of surgical count.
Notify attending surgeon when surgical counts are incorrect. Document corrective action and persons notified on incident form for risk management.
Document results of surgical counts on operative record.
Perform surgical count during change of shift, and document on surgical count sheet.

procedure and the specific operative site. The nurse reinforces what the surgeon has explained to the patient regarding the procedure, ensuring that the patient has a clear understanding of the operative event.

The circulating nurse has multiple responsibilities. The nurse must perform a thorough assessment of the patient in the preoperative holding area. After introducing himself or herself to the patient, the nurse verifies the patient's name and hospital number through analysis of the patient's addressograph plate and identification bracelet (Fig. 7-3). If blood products have been ordered, the patient's name and identification number on the blood band bracelet are confirmed with that on the blood products.

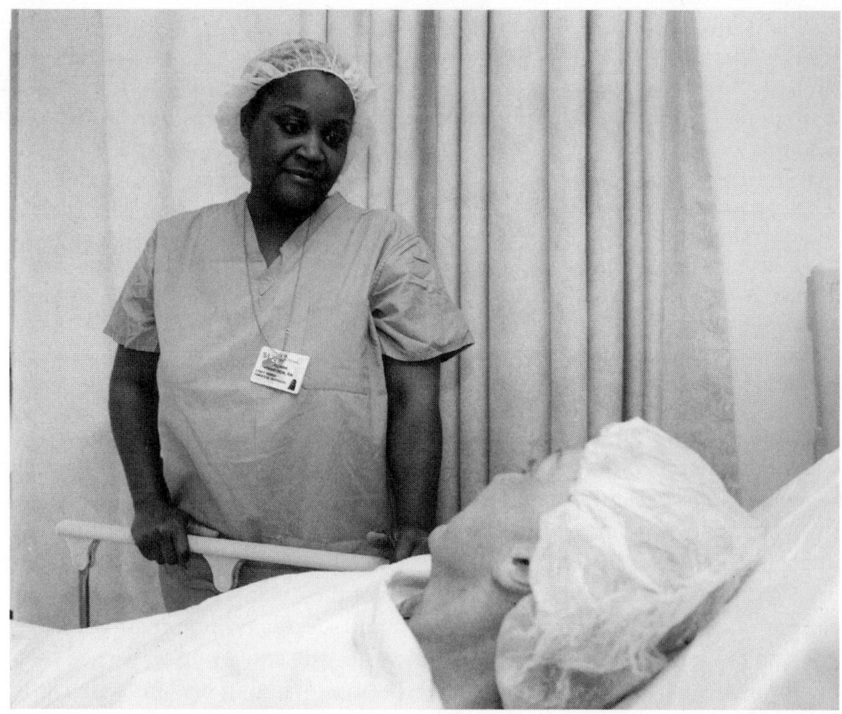

FIG. 7–3. Circulating nurse performing a preoperative assessment of the patient in the preoperative holding area.

Results of laboratory tests, coagulation profile, electrocardiogram, and chest radiograph are verified. Completed and signed operative and anesthesia consent forms, allergy and NPO (nothing by mouth) status are confirmed. The presence of any valuables such as dentures, eyeglasses, jewelry, or contact lenses should be documented and the valuables returned safely to the nursing unit or a family member.

In the preoperative holding area, the anesthesiologist interviews and assesses the patient. The various forms of anesthesia available, depending on age and concurrent medical conditions, are discussed. Intravenous and arterial lines are inserted; a Swan-Ganz catheter may be inserted in the OR suite if indicated.

In the OR suite, the circulating nurse and the anesthesiologist coordinate the safe transfer of the patient onto the OR bed. To ensure the patient's safety, a safety belt attached to the bed is applied above the knees. Monitoring equipment, a blood pressure cuff, a pulse oximeter, an arterial line, and electrocardiogram leads are applied.

This can be a very stressful time for the patient, who is surrounded by unfamiliar faces and equipment that can appear frightening. The circulating nurse continues to provide emotional support, comfort, and a quiet atmosphere. These measures can minimize stress during this time.

The temperature of the OR is quite cool, between 68° and 70° Fahrenheit. This cool temperature, as well as a low humidity setting, is used to prevent the growth of microorganisms. A warming blanket, warm intravenous fluids, and irrigation solutions are used throughout the procedure to prevent hypothermia.

The patient is anesthetized, and an indwelling Foley catheter is inserted into the bladder if the procedure dictates. An endotracheal tube and monitoring and infusion lines are secured and made easily accessible to the anesthesiologist. The circulating nurse places the dispersive pad for the electrocautery unit in a dry, well-padded area (usually the buttocks).

Positioning of the patient is a collaborative effort on the part of the surgeon, the circulating nurse, and the anesthesiologist. The circulating nurse obtains and arranges all equipment necessary for patient positioning before the patient is admitted to the OR. Positioning is performed slowly and carefully to provide maximal exposure of the surgical site without compromising respiratory, neurologic, and vascular function. All bony prominences and areas of potential circulatory compromise are padded.

Preparation of the operative site consists of a one-step prep consisting of iodophor (0.7 percent iodine) and 74 percent isopropyl alcohol. It provides rapid, long-lasting microbicidal action against a broad spectrum of microbes. The scrub nurse assists the surgical team in applying sterile drapes around the operative site. Equipment and supplies needed for the procedure (such as cautery, suction) are passed off the field by the scrub nurse. The circulating nurse connects the equipment to the appropriate unit and confirms any power settings with the surgeon.

CAROTID ENDARTERECTOMY

Carotid endarterectomy is performed for arteriosclerotic occlusive disease of the carotid artery. A carotid endarterectomy surgically removes the occluding atheroma and eliminates the source of emboli. Transient ischemic attacks (TIAs) and stroke are embolic or thrombotic in origin. As a result of potential atheromatous debris, emboli may arise from the carotid bifurcation and lodge in the ipsilateral cerebral hemisphere, or the internal carotid artery may occlude as a result of atheroma and/or thrombosis of the carotid artery (see Chapter 14).

Indications for carotid endarterectomy include severe asymptomatic stenosis of the carotid artery, a TIA, stroke, and recurrent carotid artery disease. A bruit, caused by turbulent blood flow through a narrowed artery, can often be auscultated in persons with carotid artery disease. This turbulence, which takes the form of vibrations, is transmitted to the skin surface. A TIA can cause motor and sensory deficits of the extremities on the contralateral side of the diseased carotid artery. Speech impairment may occur if the dominant hemisphere (speech center) is involved. Patients often ignore these symptoms because of rapid recovery. If these symptoms are ignored, a subsequent TIA can lead to a stroke.[1]

After the induction of anesthesia, the patient remains supine on the OR bed with a blanket roll under the shoulders. The patient's head is placed on a foam ring for support. This position allows for slight hyperextension of the neck for adequate surgical exposure of the carotid vessels.

A light touch is used during the surgical preparation to avoid dislodging atheromatous plaque in the carotid artery. A neck incision approximately 4 inches in length is made parallel to the sternocleidomastoid muscle. The incision begins medially and extends posteriorly under the lobe of the ear. Nerve injuries may result from inadvertent transection or surgical retractors. The cranial nerves must be identified and preserved. Injury to these nerves can result in deviation of the tongue to the operative side, with difficulty in speech and mastication.

The surgeon proceeds by dissecting down to the carotid sheath. The common facial vein that runs across the carotid artery is identified and divided. The carotid sheath is opened, and the common, internal, and external carotid arteries are identified and isolated with vessel loops. At this time the patient may experience bradycardia or hypotension as a result of manipulation of the carotid sinus. In this event, the surgeon injects 0.5-1.0 ml of local anesthetic (1 percent lidocaine) into the carotid sinus, which the scrub nurse has prepared on the surgical field.

The surgeon orders heparin to be administered intravenously by the anesthesiologist approximately 5 minutes before clamping of the arteries. Heparin is given to prevent thromboemboli while the carotid arteries are clamped.

Cerebral perfusion occurs via collaterals and the circle of Willis when the carotid artery is clamped. Internal carotid artery back pressure (stump pressure) is used to assess the adequacy of cerebral perfusion. Stump pressure is measured with a 21-gauge needle attached to a 4-foot pressure line. The needle is inserted into the common carotid artery. The opposite end of the line is passed to the anesthesiologist and attached to the arterial line. A pressure measurement is obtained before clamping of the common carotid artery. The common carotid artery is clamped with a vascular clamp, and a second pressure measurement is obtained. A stump pressure greater than 35 mm Hg (mean) is usually adequate for proper cerebral perfusion.

If the patient has bilateral carotid stenosis, a history of stroke, a stump pressure below 35 mm Hg, or recurrent carotid artery stenosis, an intraluminal shunt may be used to provide temporary cerebral perfusion. The shunt permits blood flow to the brain via the internal carotid artery. The shunt consists of silicone elastomer with stainless steel spring reinforcements to minimize kinking and occlusion of the cannula lumen. The ends of the shunt have cone-shaped bulbs to facilitate fixation of the shunt in the vessel (Fig. 7-4). These shunts come in different diameters to adapt to the patient's anatomy.

The distal end of the shunt is inserted into the common carotid artery; the proximal end of the shunt is inserted into the internal carotid artery. The previously placed vascular clamps are removed from the common and internal carotid arteries as each end of the shunt is inserted. A specialized clamp replaces each vascular clamp to secure the shunt.

Once the stump pressure has been measured, vascular clamps are placed on the common, external, and internal carotid arteries. The arteriotomy (surgical incision into the artery) is made with a No. 11 knife blade. The arteriotomy is extended with angled Potts vascular scissors.

The surgeon performs the endarterectomy around the shunt. The plaque is carefully peeled off the intima layer of the artery with a blunt instrument. The plaque is sent to the pathology department for examination and documentation. Before the artery is closed, the arteriotomy site is irrigated with heparin-saline solution to remove any small atheromatous debris left behind. Before complete closure of the arteriotomy, the three arteries are reclamped and the shunt is removed. The arteriotomy closure is completed with monofilament polypropylene suture material.

In some cases (such as with reoperative carotid endarterectomy and in patients with small arteries), a patch graft of autogenous vein or prosthetic material is used in reconstruction of the artery. Placement of such a patch, known as a patch graft angioplasty, prevents compromise in arterial diameter or blood flow. Before wound closure, hemostasis is achieved at the arteriotomy site and small bleeders are cauterized. Muscular, subcutaneous, and skin layers are closed, and a dressing is applied.

The patient is awakened in the OR to assess neurologic function. Assessment is performed by asking the patient to follow simple commands, such as moving the fingers and toes

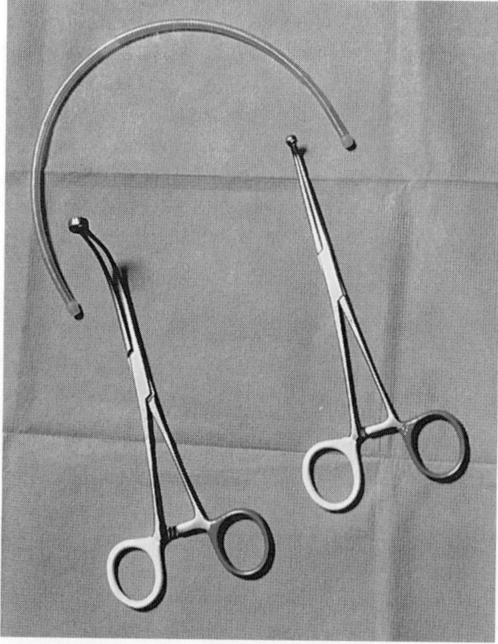

FIG. 7–4. Carotid shunt with cone-shaped bulbs to facilitate fixation of the shunt in the carotid artery. The shunt is held in place with specialized clamps.

contralateral to the affected carotid artery. Extremity strength is assessed by having the patient grasp the surgeon's hand. The patient is then discharged to the recovery room.

Postoperative complications include perioperative stroke, hypertension, hypotension, hematoma, cranial nerve injuries, and operative death. Neurologic deficit is caused by an intraoperative cerebral embolism or insufficient cerebral blood flow during carotid clamping. Factors contributing to hematoma formation include aspirin administered preoperatively, heparin given intraoperatively, coughing and straining during extubation, and technical factors. Hematomas should be treated aggressively because they can cause tracheal compression with airway compromise.

AORTIC SURGERY: ELECTIVE

Abdominal aortic aneurysm (AAA) and arterial occlusive disease are the major indications for surgery of the aorta. Risk factors for occlusive disease and aneurysm are similar: smoking, hypertension, age, diabetes mellitus, and genetics (see Chapters 11 and 12).

Arterial occlusive disease occurs as a result of atherosclerosis. Aneurysms are dilations of the arterial wall involving all layers of the artery. Recent clinical observations and research suggest that the pathogenesis of aneurysms may be more complex than initially believed and is probably multifactorial in origin.

The size of the AAA is a vital indicator in the decision for operative intervention. Symptoms of a leaking or ruptured aneurysm are the sudden onset of back and abdominal pain accompanied by hypotension. A computed tomography scan provides an accurate determination of the size and level of the aneurysm. An arteriogram delineates the renal, mesenteric, iliac, and lower-extremity arteries.

Elective treatment of an AAA involves resection of the aneurysm and replacement with a synthetic graft. Treatment of arterial occlusive disease involves replacement with a synthetic graft or occasionally an aortic endarterectomy. These synthetic grafts can be straight (tube) or bifurcated, extending to both iliac or femoral arteries. The disease process may dictate that one limb of the bifurcated graft extend to the iliac artery and the second limb to the femoral artery. Monitoring lines inserted preoperatively include an arterial line and, if indicated, a Swan-Ganz catheter. An epidural catheter may be placed preoperatively for postoperative pain management. General endotracheal anesthesia is induced, and a Foley catheter is inserted. The abdomen is prepared from the nipple line to the knees. A midline incision is made from the xyphoid to the symphysis pubis. The abdomen is explored for other pathologic conditions (i.e., malignant disease). If such conditions are found, the elective procedure may be cancelled so that these subsequent findings can be addressed. A table-mounted self-retaining retractor holds the abdomen open. A nasal gastric tube is inserted by the anesthesiologist, and its placement is checked by the surgeon. The bowels are lifted out of the abdominal cavity. Moist towels or lap sponges are placed over the bowels to eliminate exposure and provide protection.

Open Approach

Proximal control of the aorta is obtained by placement of a large vessel loop around the aorta. When required, the iliac and femoral arteries are also controlled with vessel loops. Before the vessels are clamped, heparin is given systemically by the anesthesiologist and allowed to circulate for 5 minutes. The iliac vessels are clamped first to prevent dislodgment of atheromatous debris into the legs. The proximal aorta is clamped, usually below the renal arteries in 90-95 percent of the cases. Clamping above the renal arteries for approximately 30-45 minutes is usually tolerated by the kidneys. An arteriotomy is made in the aorta with electric cautery and extended with scissors. In aneurysmal disease, the thrombus is evacuated and lumbar arteries are ligated within the aneurysm. Blood loss is suctioned into the cardiotomy reservoir of a blood salvage machine for reinfusion by the anesthesiologist (see section on "Blood Salvage").

The lumen of the aorta is assessed by the surgeon for proper size selection of a synthetic graft. The circulating and scrub nurses confirm graft size before placement on the surgical field. The end-to-end anastomosis between native aorta and graft is performed proximally. Prior to completion of the distal anastomosis, the graft is flushed with arterial blood to remove thrombus and debris that might otherwise embolize to the distal limbs. A straight tube graft is used if the iliac and femoral arteries are free of disease. If the iliac and/or the femoral arteries are diseased, a bifurcated graft is used.

The proximal clamp is slowly released to prevent hypotension. The rate of declamping is determined by continuous monitoring of the patient's blood pressure. If hypotension is detected, the aorta is temporarily reclamped and additional fluids are given by the anesthesiologist.

Hemostasis at the anastomotic suture lines is achieved to prevent postoperative hematoma formation. The old aneurysm wall is sutured over the synthetic graft. Closure of the retroperitoneum is essential to prevent erosion of the bowel into the synthetic graft and a resultant aortoduodenal fistula. At this time, the first sponge and needle count is performed by the scrub and circulating nurses.

The midline incision is closed with a heavy suture. A second sponge and needle count, as well as an instrument count, is performed. A final sponge and needle count is performed at the time of skin closure. The incisions are covered with sterile dressings, and the drapes are removed. The femoral and pedal pulses are assessed before the patient is extubated. Sterility of instrumentation is maintained by the scrub and circulating nurses until the patient leaves the OR. This is mandatory in the event of immediate reoperation.

Retroperitoneal Approach

Indications for a retroperitoneal approach to the aorta include pulmonary or cardiac insufficiency, multiple previous abdominal surgical procedures, and obesity. There are several advantages to retroperitoneal exposure of the aorta over the standard transperitoneal approach. The intestines are not exposed or manipulated with this approach. As a result, patients may resume oral intake sooner, body temperature is easier to maintain, and operative stress is decreased. A flank incision also causes less respiratory compromise than a midline abdominal incision. These are important factors in patients with significant heart disease and obstructive pulmonary disease. As a result of multiple abdominal procedures, adhesions form within the abdominal cavity. Adhesions require lysis with the standard midline abdominal incision; the retroperitoneal approach avoids these adhesions, which decreases incidence of bowel perforation.

Endovascular Approach

Endovascular surgery encompasses procedures ranging from simple percutaneous balloon dilatations to complex endoluminal graft placements.[2] Nursing care of the patient undergoing an endovascular graft placement presents a new and challenging role for the vascular nurse (Box 7-2). The endovascular graft is wound tightly in a catheter that is introduced through a skin incision into the femoral artery (Fig. 7-5). The catheter is then advanced to a level above the aortic aneurysm but below the renal arteries. The graft is then released from the catheter and attached into the aorta above the aneurysm with a series of hooks. A second type of stent graft that is released from the delivery catheter into the aorta expands to a preset size when it comes into contact with blood. The catheter is pulled back to a point below the aneurysm and attached in the same way. (see Chapter 12).

The vascular surgeon uses technology that involves fluoroscopic imaging, balloon catheter insertion, and guidewire manipulation. A dedicated endovascular suite in the OR combines the features of the traditional OR and the interventional radiology suite. A power injector, ceiling mounted C-arm, suspension monitors, and a fixed fluoroscopic table provide adequate digital imaging capability to perform these complex procedures safely and reliably (Figs. 7-6 and 7-7). This suite is also used by the vascular surgeon for diagnostic angiograms, balloon angioplasty, and stenting procedures. This allows the surgeon the ability to select the most appropriate operation.

BOX 7–2

Angiographic Catheters and Guidewires

DIAGNOSTIC ANGIOGRAPHY	ANGIOPLASTY/STENT
Puncture needle and J-wire	Preformed catheter
Introducer sheath	Guidewires (glide, angled, steerable)
Contrast media	Long introducer sheath
Multipurpose measurement catheter	Guiding catheter
Soft tip or J-guidewire	Balloons
Power injector	Inflation device
	Stents
	Contrast media
	Power injector

An arterial puncture is made in both femoral arteries with an 18-gauge needle followed by a guidewire and dilators. The femoral artery with the least amount of vessel tortuosity and atherosclerosis is used to deploy the graft. A femoral arteriotomy is required for the larger sheath that accommodates the endovascular graft. Further manipulations are made through the sheath and fluoroscopic guidewire.

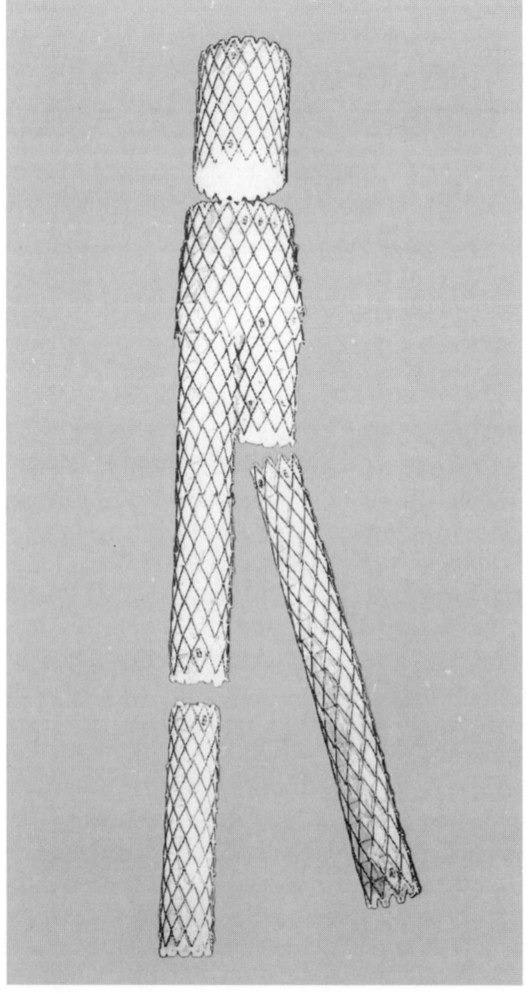

FIG. 7–5. Endovascular graft.

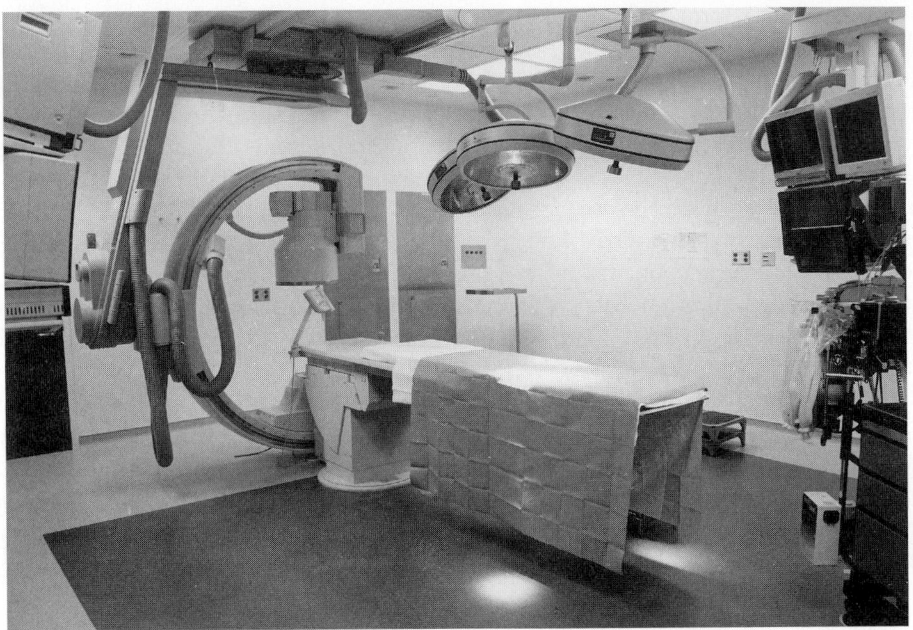

FIG. 7–6. Operating room endovascular suite.

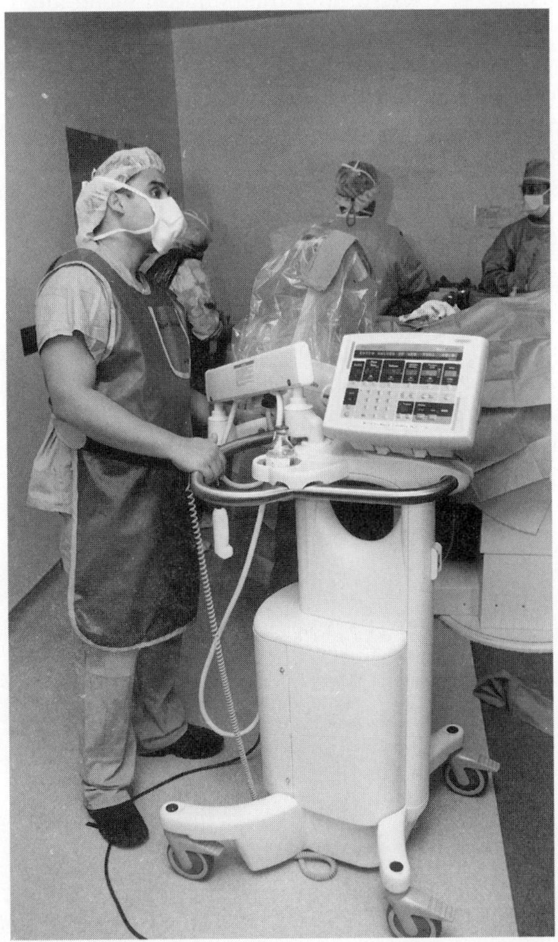

FIG. 7–7. A power injector is a pump for controlled injection of radiographic contrast material of specific volumes at specified rates.

To prevent clot formation in the femoral arteries, pressurized bags of 1000 ml 0.9% sodium chloride with 2,000 U of heparin are continuously infused. A large single basin with 1,000 ml sodium chloride and 5,000 U of heparin should be included in the set-up. The numerous guidewires and catheters can be coiled loosely and stored in this basin.

Following graft insertion, the surgeon repairs the arteriotomy site and achieves hemostasis. The femoral incision is closed in layers using a standard wound closure technique. A percutaneous approach may be used for the contralateral femoral artery. Closure of this artery can be performed using an 8- or 10-French percutaneous vascular surgical device. The device is composed of two components, a knot pusher and a sheath that contains two pairs of sutured needles as well as a needle guide and a rotating barrel that precisely controls the needles during deployment (Fig. 7-8). The knot pusher is used to advance surgical knots to the arteriotomy.

The complications of this procedure can include aneurysm rupture, peripheral embolization, and misdeployment of the graft, which all require emergency surgical intervention. Peripheral vascular instrumentation is used for the endovascular approach. In the event of a conversion to an open repair, abdominal vascular instrumentation should be readily available. Due to the urgency of conversion to an open procedure, time does not permit an instrument count; therefore, an x-ray should be performed prior to the patient leaving the OR.

AORTIC SURGERY: EMERGENT

An aortic rupture is usually characterized by the escape of blood into the space between the wall of the aorta and the periaortic sheath. The patient will experience a sudden onset of pain and a transient drop in blood pressure. This hematoma may be confined to the periaorta for a few hours or much longer. If the hematoma breaks through into the retroperitoneum and peritoneal cavity, hypovolemic shock occurs. It is crucial that these patients be transported to the OR and the aorta cross-clamped without delay.

Intraoperative nursing care of the patient undergoing elective repair of an AAA differs from that of the patient with a ruptured AAA. In the latter, time is of the essence to control aortic bleeding and save the patient's life. In this short span of time, multiple demands are placed on the OR nursing staff, and the knowledge and skills they bring to the task are of critical importance. It is essential that the scrub and circulating nurses be capable of prioritizing these responsibilities. An emergency abdominal vascular cart with instruments, supplies, and suture material should be available in the vascular OR suite at all times.

The OR nurses receive notification from the emergency room that a patient is being admitted directly to the OR. On arrival, the patient is taken directly to the OR suite, where

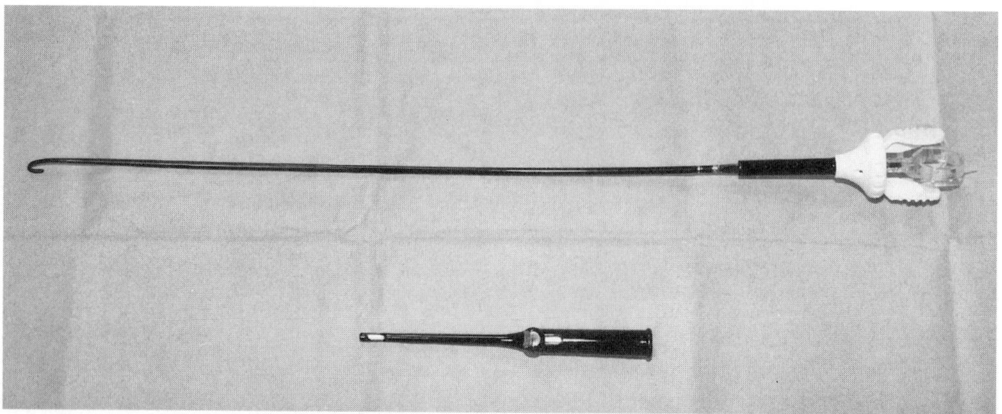

FIG. 7–8. Percutaneous vascular surgical device.

preparations to administer an anesthetic and to open the abdomen can proceed simultaneously. The circulating nurse opens the supplies while the scrub nurse gowns and gloves only. Time does not permit scrubbing the hands and arms before gowning and gloving. It is important for nurses and physicians to maintain sterility while circumventing some steps practiced in an elective procedure.

The circulating nurse is responsible for the availability of the blood salvage machine and all blood products. If personnel responsible for blood salvage are not readily available, the circulating nurse is responsible for the partial set-up of the blood salvage machine.

Blood Salvage

The patient's own red cells, which were previously lost to wall suction and discarded, can be salvaged with use of the blood salvage machine. This salvaged blood can be washed of coagulation factors (heparin, tissue, clots, and other debris) and returned to the patient in the form of packed red cells.

Autologous transfusion is not a new concept. Reinfusion of lost blood was employed as early as 1818 by James Blundell of Guy's Hospital in London. Preoperative blood donation was advocated by Bernard Fantus in 1937, the year he established the first blood bank in the United States. The primary stimulus for the rapid growth of autologous transfusion programs has been the fear of transfusion-transmitted disease, particularly acquired immunodeficiency syndrome (AIDS).[3] Increasing scarcity of banked blood and the risks of transfusion reactions and hepatitis are additional reasons.

The blood salvage machine is a fast, simple, and economical system. The hardware of the machine consists of a 2,200-ml cardiotomy reservoir with filter, a waste bag, a blood transfer pouch, and a 225-ml cone-shaped centrifuge bell. The hardware is interconnected by a tubing system to form a closed, sterile unit.

The blood loss from the surgical field is collected in the cardiotomy reservoir via sterile suction tubing. The fluid and blood are heparinized in the sterile suction tubing and cardiotomy reservoir by way of a heparinized drip solution. A roller pump transports the filtered, heparinized blood from the reservoir to the centrifuge bell. The cellular components are deposited onto the wall of the centrifuge bell at a rate of 5,650 rpm. When the erythrocyte sediment has reached the curved level of the bell, it is filled. In a second step, the erythrocyte sediment is rinsed with a normal saline solution until a clear rinse solution appears in the waste bag. The final step is the subsequent reversal of the roller pump, transporting the washed erythrocyte concentration into the blood transfer pouch. Once in the transfer pouch, the packed cells can be retransfused immediately to the patient.

A trained, dedicated team is essential for intraoperative blood salvage. Regulation and selection of cycling parameters, determination of the amount of anticoagulant, vacuum level adjustment, waste bag disposal, and documentation of the procedure are all responsibilities of the operator of the blood salvage machine. This team has 24-hour accountability for elective and emergency cases that require blood salvage (Fig. 7-9).

Before blood salvage became possible, numerous units of blood bank blood were required. Blood salvaging has decreased the number of units of blood bank blood required for the patient, thus reducing cost to the patient. However, the patient is charged for the use of the blood salvage machine. The cost includes the expense of the hardware and the operation of the machine. Each institution should decide on the use of banked blood versus blood salvage in terms of patient cost and patient safety.

Emergency Blood Salvage—Partial Set-Up

Supplies

- Blood salvage machine
- Cardiotomy reservoir
- 1 L 0.9 percent sodium chloride
- 40,000 U heparin
- 2 blood salvage suction tubings
- 1 standard suction tubing

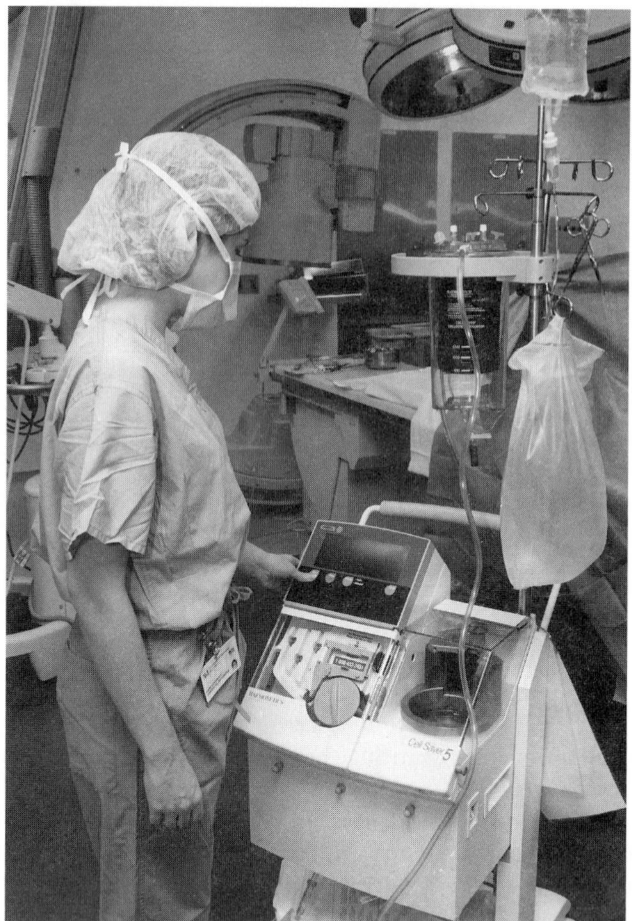

FIG. 7–9. Member of the blood salvage team reprocessing salvaged blood for reinfusion.

Instructions for Set-Up

- Open cardiotomy reservoir, and place into the ring on blood salvage machine.
- Hang 2 (1,000 ml) bags of 0.9 percent sodium chloride with 40,000 U heparin from the intravenous pole on the machine.
- Open two blood salvage suction tubings on the sterile field.
- Place one end of the standard suction tubing to the wall suction and the other end to the cardiotomy reservoir.
- The blood salvage suction tubing has one end consisting of an intravenous spike and suction port. This end is handed off the sterile field by the scrub nurse to the circulating nurse. The circulating nurse connects the spiked end to the liter of heparinized saline solution and the suction port to the cardiotomy reservoir.
- Allow 100 ml of heparinized solution to run into the cardiotomy reservoir, reducing flow to keep an open rate.

Partial set-up is complete.

Trained ancillary personnel may be needed to assist the circulating nurse in emergency care of the patient. They can access necessary blood products, notify emergency personnel, and provide additional support staff for nurses, the surgeon, and the anesthesiologist. This allows the circulating nurse to provide immediate, direct, intraoperative care to the patient.

Time does not permit an instrument or sharp count. However, lap sponges must be counted. It must be noted on the OR medical record that an instrument and sharp count was not performed due to an emergency. The surgeon must be notified and an incident report filed with risk management.

Before intubation by the anesthesiologist, the one-step prep is painted over the patient's abdomen from nipple line to knees. The surgeon gowns and gloves only. Sterile drapes are applied.

The instruments for elective and emergency AAA repair are essentially the same. Instrumentation will be specific to each institution. Initial, emergency instrumentation on the Mayo stand is listed in Box 7-3. For control of rupture, the aortic compressor is placed on the proximal end of the aorta, and the aorta is clamped proximally and distally with large DeBakey clamps (Fig. 7-10).

Hypothermia is most often a clinically important problem during prolonged operations that require a large surgical incision and large volumes of intravenous fluids. Heat loss is common in all patients during general anesthesia because anesthetics alter thermoregulation. An adverse effect of hypothermia is postoperative shivering. This is a risk, particularly in the elderly, because it increases the basal metabolic rate. Oxygen consumption increases, placing additional demands on the cardiac and pulmonary systems. In the elderly, if either of these systems cannot compensate, arterial hypoxemia may result.

All intravenous fluids should be kept warm by means of fluid warmers. A warmer supplied with saline irrigation and various intravenous fluids may be useful. The circulating nurse keeps these fluids readily available for when they are needed by the anesthesiologist and the scrub nurse. Warmth reduces blood viscosity and improves tissue blood flow. A warm OR at the outset of the procedure is beneficial until the patient is draped. Control of OR temperature throughout the procedure limits radiant heat loss from surgical incisions.

The patient will be discharged to the recovery room or directly to an intensive care unit. If the patient is to remain intubated and dependent on a ventilator, the circulating nurse receives ventilator settings from the anesthesiologist. The nurse then informs the intensive care nurse of the patient's direct admission, ventilator settings, and any other pertinent information. Additional responsibilities of the circulating nurse for patient transfer include availability of an Ambu bag, an oxygen tank, and an electrocardiogram monitor.

Improved operative techniques, better monitoring in the intensive care unit, and improved preoperative and postoperative management have reduced the risks associated with repair of

BOX 7–3

Mayo Stand Instrumentation for Abdominal Aortic Aneurysm

1 No. 10 knife blade
2 Hemostats
2 Boettcher hemostats (tonsil)
2 Vascular Mixters
2 Short DeBakey tissue forceps
2 Long DeBakey tissue forceps
1 9" Potts-Smith scissor (Richter)
2 Boettcher hemostats with 4-0 nonabsorbable suture pass points
1 Boettcher hemostat with 2-0 nonabsorbable suture pass points
1 2-0 nonabsorbable suture ligature to ligate lumbar arteries
2 Large DeBakey vascular clamps

In addition:

1 Self-retaining retractor (Grieshaber)
2 Blood salvage suction tubings
2 Wet radiopaque towels and lap sponges
1 Table-mounted retractor

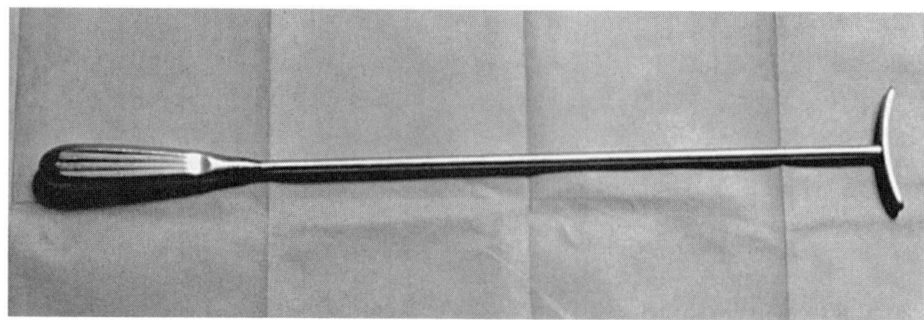

FIG. 7–10. The surgeon places the aortic compressor proximal to the point of aortic rupture to control hemorrhage.

the AAA. A successful outcome of this procedure depends on careful operative technique, close attention to anesthetic technique, and highly skilled perioperative nursing care.

FEMORAL ARTERY RECONSTRUCTION

Atherosclerosis is the most common cause of lower-extremity arterial occlusive disease. As the plaque enlarges within the artery, the lumen of the artery is reduced, resulting in decreased blood flow. When a patient has pain at rest, nonhealing lower-extremity ulcers, or gangrene of the toes or foot, arterial reconstructive surgery is indicated to increase blood flow to the lower extremity and prevent amputation.

Once the diagnosis of arterial insufficiency has been demonstrated by noninvasive testing, angiography may be performed. This is the most precise diagnostic tool for the assessment of arterial anatomy in the lower extremity, outlining the location and extent of arterial obstruction. Complete evaluation requires depiction of the aorta, iliac, femoral, popliteal, and tibial arterial segments. The common femoral artery is the most common site of angiographic access (see Chapter 13).

At the onset of the operation, the surgeon determines the proper bypass by selecting the best proximal site for inflow and the best distal site for outflow. Arterial bypass surgery may be done with a two-team approach. One team of surgeons makes the proximal incision on the upper thigh over the inguinal ligament where the femoral artery and saphenous vein are close together and can be easily dissected. The second team of surgeons makes an incision distally to expose the vessel of choice (i.e., popliteal, tibial, or peroneal artery).

Intraoperatively, an angiogram may be indicated prior to the bypass surgery when the tibial vessels are poorly visualized on the preoperative angiogram. The angiogram is performed after the femoral artery is first exposed through a groin incision. A 16-gauge angiocatheter or a 21-gauge butterfly is inserted into the femoral artery; the artery is then clamped proximal to the angiocatheter. The femoral artery is then injected with approximately 50 ml of contrast material. This enables the surgeon to visualize the tibial vessel with the least disease and best outflow to the foot. This vessel should be selected for the distal anastomosis.

The patient's own saphenous vein remains the graft of choice for arterial bypass surgery. The saphenous vein provides the best patency rate and can be reversed for use as an arterial bypass graft, allowing blood to flow unobstructed through the vein valves. The saphenous vein is removed from the leg, and the small end of the vein is anastomosed to the common femoral artery. The large end of the vein is anastomosed to the popliteal or tibial artery. The disadvantage of this technique is the size mismatch of the saphenous vein to the native vessel.

An alternative technique was developed to use the saphenous vein in its natural position without reversal. This technique is known as an in situ saphenous vein bypass. This procedure requires interruption of the valves within the saphenous vein. An advantage of the in situ bypass is the anastomotic size match of both ends of the saphenous vein to the native arteries. This technique may decrease ischemic damage to the vein graft wall because the saphenous vein is never entirely removed from the leg and therefore retains its adventitial blood supply.[4]

Preparation of the saphenous vein for use in situ entails exposure of the saphenous vein in the subcutaneous region of the affected leg. The proximal end of the saphenous vein is anastomosed to the common femoral artery. This produces arterial pressure within the vein graft and distends the vein to the most proximal vein valve. Side branches of the saphenous vein are dissected and ligated with ties of nonabsorbable suture material and stainless steel ligating clips. These venous branches are ligated to prevent arteriovenous fistulae when the vein is arterialized. The valve cusps are rendered incompetent through the use of a stainless steel valvulotome (Fig. 7-11). The valvulotome, which has a sharp blade, is placed into the vein through a venous side branch. The surgeon makes the valve incompetent by sharp division of each valve cusp, while preventing damage to the inner surface of the vein. The distal end of the saphenous vein is anastomosed to the distal vessel of choice (i.e., tibial or peroneal artery).[4]

If the saphenous vein has been removed for use in another operation or is not long enough or large enough, a synthetic graft is used. The synthetic graft most widely accepted is the polytetrafluoroethylene (PTFE) graft. Every effort should be made to use an autologous leg or arm vein for reconstruction, because PTFE anastomosed to the tibial vessels has a decreased patency rate.

On completion of the bypass, an intraoperative angiogram is performed to assess the technical competence of the arterial reconstruction, particularly the distal anastomosis and the distal runoff anatomy, which is valuable in future therapeutic decisions. If a technical error is detected, it can be corrected immediately. If the results of the angiogram are acceptable and adequate flow is confirmed, hemostasis is achieved at all incision sites. An absorbable suture material is used to close incision sites. The surgical drapes are removed, and dressings are applied.

As in all vascular procedures, it is important that the scrub and circulating nurses maintain the sterility of all instruments until the patient leaves the OR suite. Before the patient is awakened, the surgeon confirms the presence of dorsalis pedis and posterior tibial artery pulses with Doppler ultrasonography indicating adequate blood flow through the bypass graft. When the surgeon is satisfied with these pulses, the patient is awakened and transported to the recovery room.

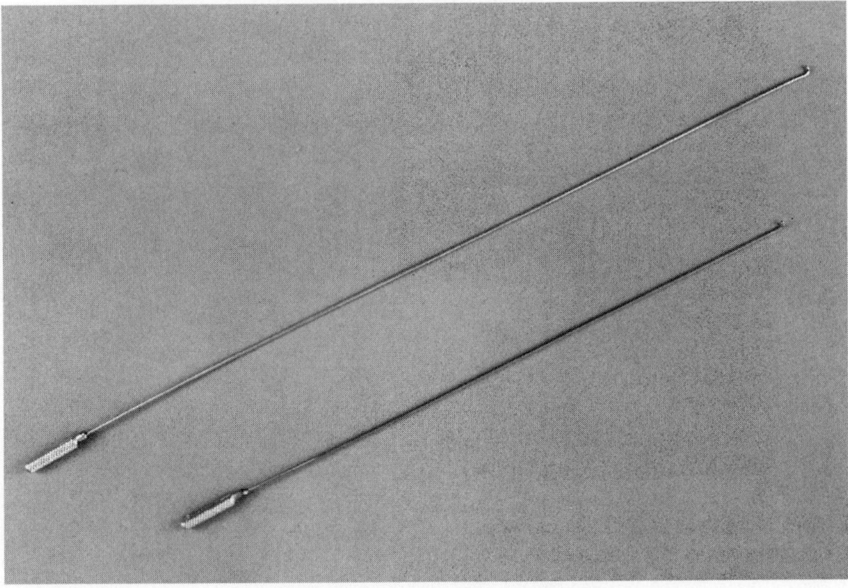

FIG. 7–11. Rigid stainless steel valvulotome.

Vascular Angioscopy

Angioscopy is a safe, accurate technique for intraoperative assessment and monitoring of lower-extremity arterial procedures. It provides the surgeon with a real-time, three-dimensional view of the reconstructed vessel. Angioscopy is used to identify previously unrecognized intraluminal defects, thus reducing the possibility of reocclusion; to visualize arterial plaque and/or thrombus within the native vessel or previous arterial bypass graft; to inspect anastomotic suture lines after bypass surgery; and to provide direct visualization of valve cutting in the in situ vein graft (Fig. 7-12, *A-D*). These findings ultimately may affect long-term patency of the graft, and clinical application of angioscopy may contribute to the understanding of graft failure.

The surgeon chooses an angioscope that is of the appropriate size for the bypass graft. The circulating nurse gives the sterilized angioscope and video camera to the scrub nurse. The video camera is sterilized with ethylene oxide for initial use. When subsequent use is required, a sterile plastic camera drape is employed.[5]

The vascular OR should have dedicated video equipment for angioscopy. This will ensure 24-hour availability of the equipment when requested by the surgeon. The OR nurses are responsible for the set-up and preparation of all angioscopy equipment. They should have a working knowledge of this equipment to facilitate an efficient and diagnostically accurate procedure. At the start of the procedure, the surgeon usually requests the angioscope. OR nurses trained in angioscopy can set up the equipment in 10 minutes; therefore, the occasional unexpected use of the angioscope does not present a problem.[5]

The circulating nurse prepares 1 L of 0.9 percent sodium chloride with 2,000 U heparin for use with the irrigation pump. This nurse is also responsible for assembling and priming the irrigation pump tubing. The scrub nurse hands the ends of the video camera cord and the light source cord off the sterile field to the circulating nurse, who then inserts the ends into

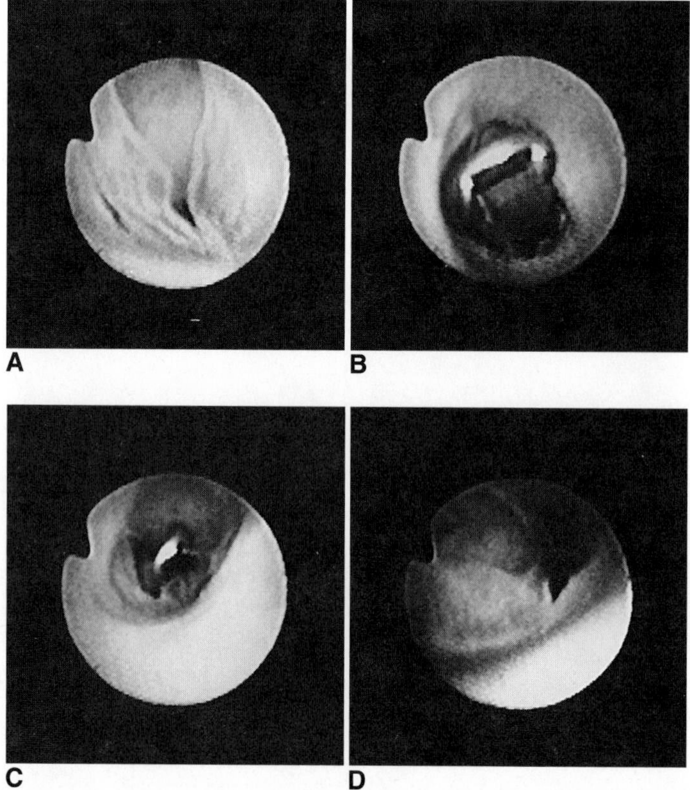

FIG. 7–12. View through an angioscope. **A,** Partially closed valve. **B,** Valvulotome above valve. **C,** Valve incision. **D,** Completed valvulotomy. (From Pearce WH, Baxter BT, Almgren CC, et al: The use of angioscopy in the saphenous vein bypass graft. In Yao JST, Pearce WH, eds: *Technologies in vascular surgery*, Philadelphia, 1992, WB Saunders, p 291.)

the camera unit and light source. One end of the irrigation pump tubing is passed off the sterile field to the circulating nurse, who connects it to the previously primed irrigation pump.[5]

The surgeon inserts the disposable angioscope into the vein bypass graft or synthetic bypass graft. The angioscope can also be inserted into the vein bypass graft through a side branch of the vein. The surgeon or the scrub nurse attaches the camera to the angioscope. The primed irrigation tubing is connected to the irrigation channel on the angioscope. A vascular clamp helps maintain occlusion of arterial inflow throughout the procedure.[5]

The irrigation pump is capable of delivering high- and low-volume flow rates. Typical rates are 50 ml/minute low and 150 ml/minute high. Surgeons using the irrigation pump should determine the standards of irrigation that best meet their visual needs (Fig. 7-13).[5]

The irrigation pump provides a continuous readout on total volume infused. Throughout the procedure, the circulating nurse informs the anesthesia staff regarding total fluid volume infused. This irrigation solution remains in the patient's vascular system and becomes part of the total fluid volume received by the patient intraoperatively.[5]

The irrigation pump is controlled by digital input and a bimodal foot pedal. One action of the foot pedal provides a high flow rate to initially clear the vessel of blood. The low flow rate is used to maintain clarity during the procedure. The key to successful angioscopy is the maintenance of a blood-free field. The smallest amount of blood flowing into the field significantly blurs the image on the monitor.[5]

The image from the angioscope is transferred directly to a high-resolution color monitor, which allows simultaneous viewing by the surgical team. The procedure can be recorded with the video cassette recorder. This information can be reviewed later for teaching and documentation.

The disposable angioscopes come in three sizes: a 1.5-mm, 100-cm; a 2.3-mm, 80-cm; and a 2.8-mm, 80-cm with irrigation channels (Fig. 7-14). Equipment required for angioscopy is listed in Box 7-4. Equipment used in vascular surgery organized by type of procedure is listed and pictured in Box 7-5.

The risks associated with angioscopy include the potential for endothelial trauma related to the mechanical passage of an angioscope through a graft and into the native artery, it is important that the smallest angioscope be used. Another risk is fluid overload due to the amount of irrigation fluid infused, usually 800 ml to 1000 ml. A significant amount of irrigation fluid is lost through the open distal vein.

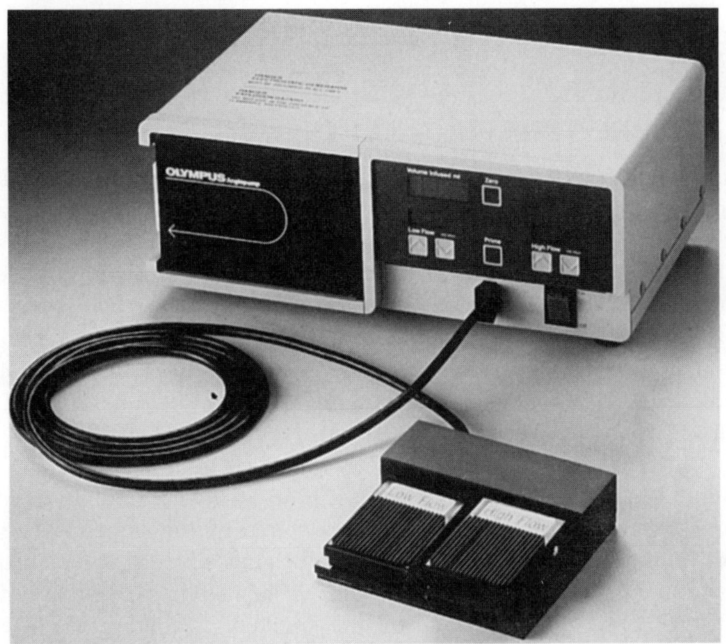

FIG. 7–13. The irrigation pump used in angioscopy. (Courtesy Olympus Corporation, Lake Success, NY.)

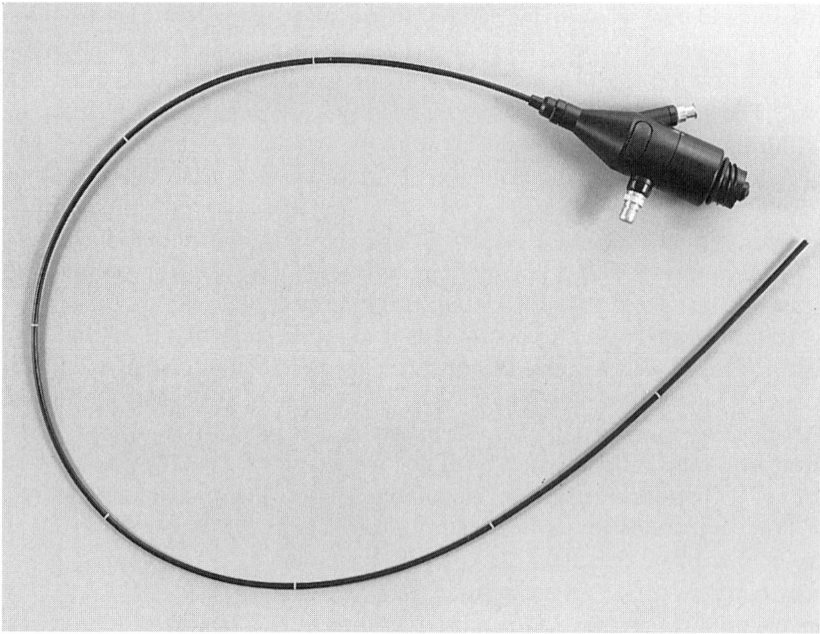

FIG. 7–14. 2.8-mm angioscope. (Printed with the permission of Baxter Healthcare Corporation, Vascular Systems Division.)

BOX 7–4

Equipment Required for Angioscopy

Video monitor
Combined video camera unit, light source
Videocassette recorder
Irrigation pump
Irrigation pump tubing
1000 ml of warm 0.9% sodium chloride containing 2000 U heparin for use with the irrigation pump

VASCULAR PROSTHETIC GRAFTS

To replace large-caliber arteries, the surgeon will select a polyethylene terephthalate (Dacron) or a PTFE prosthetic graft. Dacron grafts were among the earliest synthetic materials to be used. Dacron is a polymer made into fibers or threads that are then fabricated, with the use of textile technology, into a graft. There are three types of Dacron grafts: woven, knit, and knitted velour. Compared with knitted grafts, woven ones are more tightly constructed, less porous, and stiffer and, therefore, do not handle as well. However, most woven grafts have greater structural integrity than knitted grafts and are less likely to dilate after they are implanted in the patient. A Dacron graft can be lined with a microloop pile on the exterior or interior surface or on both surfaces. This is called a velour lining. Adding a velour to the construction of the graft increases the ease with which the graft is preclotted. The need for preclotting a graft can be eliminated if the graft is preclotted with albumin or collagen.[6]

Knitted and loosely woven grafts must be preclotted by the surgeon prior to systemic heparinization of the patient. The surgeon preclots the graft before it is implanted by soaking it in the patient's nonheparinized blood. The graft is then stretched several times to ensure that blood fills the fabric interstices and then is "milked" to remove excessive thrombus. Exposure of the blood-soaked graft to air activates the blood's clotting mechanism.[6]

BOX 7–5

Operating Room Trays for Vascular Procedures

PERIPHERAL VASCULAR BASIC TRAY (tray on left)

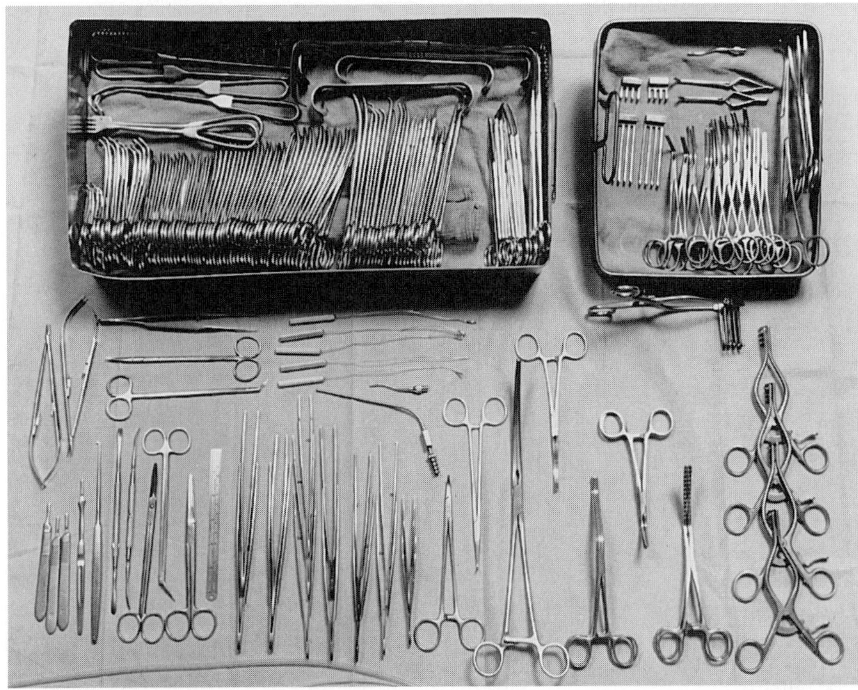

14 Towel clip
12 Mosquitoes, 5″ curved
6 Mosquitoes, 5″ straight
16 Hemostats, Kelly, curved
2 Allis, 6″
12 Péans, curved, 6″
2 Péans, curved, 8″
2 Sponge forceps, Foerster, 9 1/2″
2 Mixters, petit point
4 Mixters, Adson, curved
1 Mixter, regular, 7 3/4″
4 Boettchers, 7″ (tonsil hemostat)
3 Needle holders, Ryder, 7″ (regular)
4 Needle holders, Mayo-Hegar, 6 1/4″
2 Needle holders, Mayo-Hegar, 7″
2 Scissors, Potts-Smith, angled 60°
1 Scissor, Potts-Smith, 5 1/2″ (Richter)
3 Scissors, Potts-Smith, 7″ (Richter)
2 Scissors, Mayo, straight, 6 3/4″
4 Diamond tissue forceps, 7″
3 Gerald tissue forceps, 7 3/4″
4 DeBakey tissue forceps, 7 3/4″
2 Carmody tissue forceps, fine, 7 3/4″
2 Adson tissue forceps, 4 3/4″
1 Ruler, 6″

Continued

BOX 7–5

Operating Room Trays for Vascular Procedures—cont'd

PERIPHERAL VASCULAR BASIC TRAY (tray on left)—cont'd
2 Blunt hooks, Adson (nerve hook)
1 Suction tip, Frazier with stylet, No. 2 French size
1 Clamp, aortic, DeBakey, 19″ (for tunneling grafts)
2 Retractors, rake, 4-prong, sharp, 7¾″
2 Retractors, vein, straight, 10½″
2 Retractors, Cushing, 10½″
2 Retractors, ribbon, Sistrunk, small
2 Retractors, ribbon, large
2 Retractors, Richardson, double-ended, small
2 Retractors, Richardson, double-ended, large
2 Retractors, Army/Navy
2 Freer elevators
2 Knife handles, No. 3, 5½″
2 Knife handles, No. 7, 7″
4 Slings, Silastic, small
4 Slings, Silastic, large

PERIPHERAL VASCULAR CLAMP TRAY (tray on right, see p.147)
1 Edwards spring applicator (bulldog applier)
2 Henley clamps
2 Deep-angled Cooley clamps (patent ductus)
2 Straight Cooley clamps
7 Pediatric Cooley clamps

- 2 spoon-shaped jaws
- 2 60° angled
- 2 30° angled

2 Gregory bulldogs, angled, short
2 Baby "J" clamps (Dennis anastomosis clamps)
2 Profunda clamps
4 Weitlander retractors, medium
1 Henley retractor with:

- 2 short blades
- 2 medium blades
- 2 long blades

2 Webster cannulas, short

MICROVASCULAR TRAY

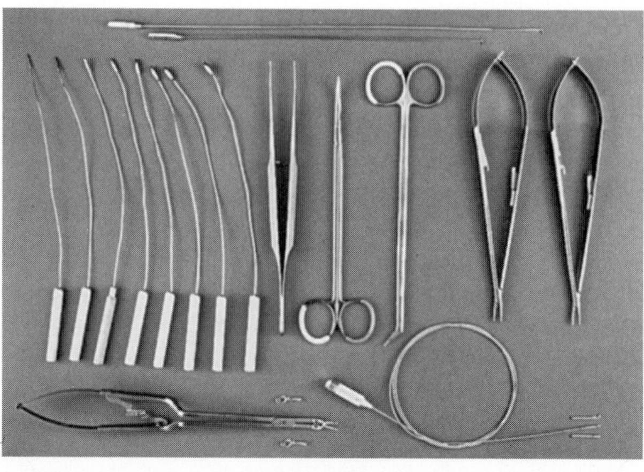

BOX 7–5

Operating Room Trays for Vascular Procedures—cont'd

MICROVASCULAR TRAY—cont'd
5 Castroviejo needle holders
1 Mills saphenous vein tissue forcep
1 Baby Potts scissor
1 Fine dissecting scissor
8 Coronary dilators, size 1 mm through 4.5 mm

ABDOMINAL VASCULAR BASIC TRAY (tray on left)

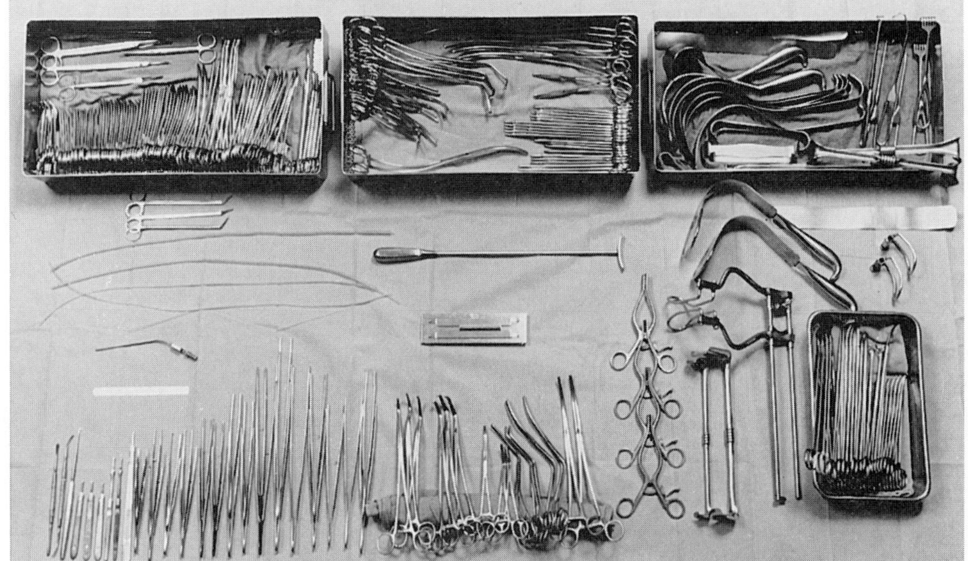

8 Towel clips, $5^{1}/_{2}''$
12 Mosquitoes, curved
6 Mosquitoes, straight
16 Hemostats, Kelly, curved
10 Kochers, $6^{1}/_{4}''$
12 Péans, 6″ curved
2 Péans, 8″ curved
4 Kochers, 8″
4 Sponge forceps, Foerster
2 Mixters, petit point
4 Mixters, Adson
2 Mixters, $7^{3}/_{4}''$
6 Boettchers, (tonsil hemostats)
2 Scissors, Potts-Smith, angled 60°
3 Scissors, Potts-Smith, 7″ (Richter)
2 Scissors, Potts-Smith, 9″ (Richter)
1 Scissor, Mayo, heavy, 9″ curved
1 Scissor, Mayo, $6^{3}/_{4}''$ curved
2 Scissors, Mayo, $6^{3}/_{4}''$ straight

Continued

BOX 7–5

Operating Room Trays for Vascular Procedures—cont'd

2 DeBakey tissue forceps, 12″
3 DeBakey tissue forceps, 9½″
4 DeBakey tissue forceps, 7¾″
3 Potts-Smith tissue forceps, 9″
2 Gerald tissue forceps, 7¾″
4 Diamond tissue forceps, 7″
1 Smooth tissue forcep, 12″
2 Potts-Smith tissue forceps, 10¼″
2 Tooth tissue forceps, short
2 Adson tissue forceps with teeth
2 Elevators, Freer
2 Knife handles, No. 3
2 Knife handles, No. 7
1 Knife handle, long No. 3
1 Ruler
2 Blunt hooks, Adson (nerve hook)
1 Suction tip, Frazier with stylet, No. 2

ABDOMINAL VASCULAR CLAMP TRAY (tray in middle, see p.149)

3 Mayo-Hegar needle holders, 8″
3 Mayo-Hegar needle holders, 7″
3 Mayo-Hegar needle holders, 6″
2 Sternal needle holders
6 Ryder needle holders, 9″
3 Ryder needle holders, 7″
1 Deep-angled Cooley clamp
2 Patent ductus clamps, straight
7 Pediatric Cooley clamps

  1 spoon
  2 curved jaws
  2 60° angle
  2 30° angle

2 Baby "J" clamps (Dennis anastomosis clamps)
2 Profunda clamps
2 DeBakey aortic clamps, "S" curved
3 DeBakey aortic clamps, large
2 DeBakey aortic clamps, small
1 DeBakey angled aortic clamp
4 Satinsky vena cava clamps
3 Harken clamps (No. 1, No. 2, No. 3)
2 Henley clamps
2 Wylie hypogastric clamps
2 Fogarty clamps, short
2 Fogarty clamps, long
1 Edwards spring applicator (bulldog applier)
1 Aortic compressor
2 2-ml glass syringes
2 Webster cannulas, short
4 Small slings, Silastic
4 Large slings, Silastic

BOX 7–5

Operating Room Trays for Vascular Procedures—cont'd

ABDOMINAL VASCULAR RETRACTOR TRAY (tray on right, see p.149)
2 Retractors, vein, straight
2 Retractors, Cushing
2 Retractors, Richardson-Eastman, large, double-ended
2 Retractors, Richardson-Eastman, medium, double-ended
2 Retractors, Deaver, wide
2 Retractors, Deaver, medium
2 Retractors, Deaver, narrow
1 Retractor, Mayo
2 Retractors, Glass
1 Retractor, Harrington
4 Retractors, Weitlaner, medium
2 Retractors, Parker, large
2 Retractors, Sistrunk
1 Retractor, malleable, 2″ curved
1 Retractor, malleable, 1½″ curved
1 Retractor, malleable, 1¼″
2 Retractors, rake, 6-prong, sharp
1 Retractor, extra-wide, Grieshaber with 2 long blades and 2 short blades

ABDOMINAL VASCULAR LONG INSTRUMENTS (front right tray, see p.149)
6 Boettchers, 7¼″
1 Scissor, Potts-Smith, 11″ (Richter)
2 Long Babcocks, 10½″
2 Needle holders, diamond jaw, 10¾″
2 Needle holders, Ryder, 10½″
2 Hemostats, deep bridge, curved, extra-long, 22¾″
2 Mixters, right angle, extra-long, 20¾″
2 Hemoclip appliers, large
2 Hemoclip appliers, medium
1 Base clip
1 Set table-mounted retractors (below)

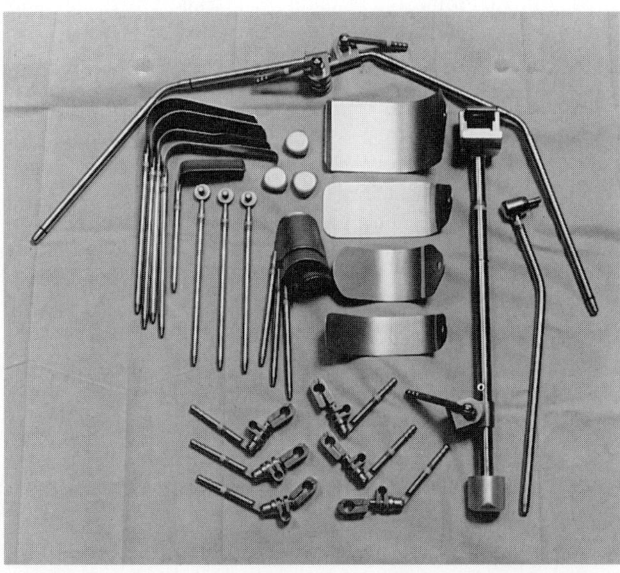

Low-porosity grafts are very stiff, having a porosity of 50 ml and they do not require preclotting. These grafts are used in procedures in which blood loss must be kept to an absolute minimum, such as repair of a thoracoabdominal aneurysm.

In 1976, expanded PTFE grafts were released for clinical use and became the preferred prosthetic conduit in femoropopliteal reconstructions. Surgeons prefer the PTFE graft because of its ease of handling and tight interstices that do not require preclotting. Accordingly, the use of Dacron for femoropopliteal reconstructions has declined. Dacron prosthetic grafts have been the standard for use in the abdomen. In 1980, however, PTFE grafts were released for use in the abdomen.[6]

THROMBOLYTIC AGENTS

Tissue plasminogen activator (TPA) is the thrombolytic agent used to treat acute arterial occlusion, arterial graft thrombosis, or distal embolization. TPA is usually infused via direct intraarterial infusion into a catheter through the femoral artery. Thrombolysis is designed to open up the arterial tree of occluding thrombus. Intraoperatively, 1 to 5 mg TPA may be injected into the affected vessel through a 16-gauge angiocatheter. This is injected intraarterially prior to the closure of the distal limb anastomosis (see Chapter 6).

Thrombolytic therapy is used to treat acute arterial occlusion, arterial graft thrombosis, or distal embolization. The thrombolytic agent is usually infused via direct intraarterial infusion into the femoral artery intraoperatively through a 16-gauge angiocatheter prior to the closure of the distal limb anastomosis (see Chapter 6).

CONCLUSION

The knowledge and skills required of the vascular OR nurse cover a broad spectrum, ranging from an endovascular procedure to a ruptured aortic aneurysm or an injury of a major blood vessel in a trauma patient. The nurse must continually strive to remain abreast of new technology. This knowledge allows for optimal intraoperative care of the patient.

ACKNOWLEDGMENTS

We thank Drs. James Yao, William Pearce, Jon Matsumura, Mark Morasch, and Mark Eskandari for their appreciation and recognition of our expertise in the perioperative care of their patients and our vascular nursing colleagues, Robert Johnson, Myrna Origenes, Maribeth DelaCruz, Peggy Schubrych, and Tess Reyes, for their contribution and knowledge in the care of the vascular patient.

REFERENCES

1. American Heart Association: Guidelines for carotid endarterectomy. a multidisciplinary consensus statement from the Ad Hoc Committee, *Circulation* 991:566-579, 1995.
2. Mansour MA: The new operating room environment: endovascular and minimally invasive vascular surgery, *Surg Clin North Am* 79(3):477-487, 1999.
3. Stehling L, ed: *Perioperative autologous transfusion: transcribed proceedings of a national conference*, Arlington, Va, 1991, American Association of Blood Banks, p xi.
4. Pearce WH, Baxter BT, Almgren CC et al: The use of angioscopy in the saphenous vein bypass graft. In Yao JST, Pearce WH, eds: *Technologies in vascular surgery*, Philadelphia, 1992, WB Saunders, pp 289-294.
5. Borgini L, Almgren CC: Peripheral vascular angioscopy: performance, equipment, technique, *AORN J* 52:543-550, 1990.
6. Pevec WC, Abbott WM: Femoropopliteal Dacron graft: five- to ten-year patency. In Yao JST, Pearce WH, eds: *Long-term results in vascular surgery*, Norwalk, Conn, 1993, Appleton & Lange, pp 273-277.

8

Medications Used in Vascular Patients

JANICE D. NUNNELEE □ MICHAEL A. FOTIS

There are many options for the medical management of vascular disorders. A thorough understanding of current medications, their purpose, actions, dosages, precautions, contraindications, and side effects is necessary to safely administer and assess medications and to properly educate patients.

This chapter discusses anticoagulants, thrombolytic agents, and antiplatelet agents.

ANTICOAGULANTS

Heparin

Heparin was first isolated and described as an anticoagulant while searching for procoagulants in 1916.[1] The compound was named heparin because of its abundance in the liver. Its use in prevention of thromboembolism in the postoperative period was not evident until Murray's research in 1937.[2] It was not until the mid-1960s that mini-dose heparin was introduced for prophylaxis against deep venous thrombosis (DVT). Heparin is now one of the most widely employed drugs used in vascular patients, and the indications are included in Box 8-1. Contraindications are seen in Box 8-2.

Heparin, found in the mast cell, is a complex heterogeneous polysaccharide (molecular weight 3000 to 30,000) with a strong negative charge.[6] Its physiologic function is unknown. Both unfractionated (high-molecular-weight heparin [HMWH]) and low-molecular-weight heparin (LMWH) convert antithrombin (heparin cofactor, previously known as antithrombin III) to a very active inhibitor of factor Xa. The majority of heparin's action is a result of a pentasaccharide sequence that has a high affinity for antithrombin.[6] Heparin, when properly dosed, prevents extension and embolization of thrombi. It does not dissolve thrombi but helps to prevent recurrence. Because of its large molecular size, it does not cross the placental barrier and this allows its use in pregnancy.[7] The chief disadvantage of heparin is the fact that it must be given parenterally.

Unfractionated (high-molecular-weight heparin) or low-molecular-weight heparin are often initiated alone in the presence of an active thrombotic process. In order to facilitate a safe transition to outpatient care, it is best to start warfarin as soon as a patient is able to take oral medications. Unfractionated or fractionated heparin must be given along with warfarin for 5 full days. Heparin should be stopped after 4-5 days of combined therapy and when the international normalized ratio (INR) (the INR is a measure of warfarin activity) is greater than 2.[8] Low-molecular-weight heparin may be given initially in the hospital and then in the outpatient setting, or may be administered solely on an outpatient basis.[9,10] In other cases, heparin is given until the cause of embolism is surgically treated and no outpatient anticoagulation is planned.

Unfractionated Heparin

Heparin must be measured according to a biologic standard of anticoagulant activity, expressed in international units (IU). This is due to the fact that each source of heparin produces different strengths if measured by weight or volume.

BOX 8–1

Indications for Heparin

- Preoperative and postoperative prophylaxis for deep venous thrombosis (DVT)
- Acute arterial and arterial graft occlusions
- Intraoperative use
- Postoperative prophylaxis for patients with synthetic grafts
- Flushing of various invasive lines
- Angiography
- DVT and pulmonary embolism (PE)
- Cerebrovascular embolic disorders
- Distal emboli (blue toe syndrome)
- Venous thrombotic events during pregnancy (warfarin is contraindicated in pregnancy)[3]

BOX 8–2

Contraindications/Precautions With Heparin

CONTRAINDICATIONS
Active or suspected bleeding (e.g., intracranial hemorrhage, decreasing hematocrit levels)
Known coagulation disorders (e.g., hemophilia, antithrombin III deficiencies)
During or following ophthalmic or neurosurgical procedures
Endocarditis
Threatened abortion
Heparin sensitivities
Heparin-induced thrombocytopenia

USE CAUTION IN THE PRESENCE OF:
Severe liver or kidney disease
Open wounds
Increased capillary permeability
Postoperative epidural catheter

Data from Fahey VA: Heparin-induced thrombocytopenia, *J Vasc Nurs* 13(4):112-116, 1995; Matula P: Management of patients undergoing vascular surgery who are receiving epidural analgesia, *J Vasc Nurs* 11(4):104-107, 1993.

Response to heparin varies among individuals and can also vary greatly in the same individual. Close monitoring is necessary to reduce avoidable complications. A laboratory test, the activated partial thromboplastin time (APTT), is available to measure the intensity of anticoagulation. An APTT of 2-2½ times control represents adequate anticoagulation.

If possible, a baseline APTT should be obtained prior to initiation of therapy. A prothrombin time is unnecessary.[11] The half-life of heparin is 60-90 minutes when administered in therapeutic doses by intravenous injection. When continuous intravenous therapy is given, the anticoagulant effect should be measured at 4-6 hours after initiation of the drug (three to four half-lives) and after every dose change. The APTT should be assessed at 4-6 hour intervals until two consecutive therapeutic APTTs are measured.[8] Daily measurement of the PTT is the minimum assessment of a patient who is stable on intravenous heparin. Variability in response to unfractionated heparin is secondary to the individual differences in plasma-binding proteins. In the first few days of therapy, the effect of heparin must be measured several times a day because doses may need altering. Later in therapy, particularly for DVT, the coagulation process will be slower and smaller amounts will be needed. Fewer measurements of the effect of heparin will be necessary.

Heparin is administered parenterally. There are three accepted means of heparin administration: continuous intravenous infusion, intermittent (pulse) intravenous injection, and subcutaneous injection in an aqueous solution. Because of erratic absorption and the risk of hematoma formation at the injection site, heparin should not be given intramuscularly. Continuous intravenous infusion of heparin diluted in a saline solution is the preferred route of administration for treatment of thromboembolic events. Prior to continuous infusion, a bolus injection may be given to introduce an immediate effect. Heparin is then delivered via an accurate infusion pump so that a known quantity is administered over a given time. Bolus amounts are determined by both the patient's weight and the extent of the clot. With large thrombi or pulmonary emboli, the bolus may be large, and up to 1800 units/hour may be given initially. The bolus dose is usually 80 units/kg of total body weight, followed by an infusion of 18 units/kg/hr.[8] Doses can vary according to patient characteristics. Continuous therapy offers the advantage of constant blood levels of heparin once the circulating volume is stabilized. Therefore, an APTT should be representative at any time that it is drawn. If the infusion is interrupted at any time in the hours before obtaining the APTT, the health care provider should be notified when the result is called. Disadvantages of constant infusion are the limitation of the patient's activity due to an intravenous line and potential for bleeding from the catheter insertion site. Other studies indicate that the cost of the hospital stay may not be justified.[6,9]

For intermittent (pulse) intravenous injection, heparin is given in an undiluted form via heparin lock, venipuncture, or a port in the intravenous tubing. Heparin is given at 4- to 6-hour intervals to maintain proper levels of circulating heparin. Dosage in this method is approximately 5000 units at each injection. Complications of this particular method of injection include infection and thrombophlebitis from constant venipuncture or invasion of an indwelling line. This type of therapy has been shown in some studies to create more frequent bleeding complications than other methods even with close monitoring.[12] PTTs are checked just prior to dose administration to assess the minimal heparin level for anticoagulant effectiveness. Although this method is rarely used today, it was often used in the past before accurate infusion pumps were readily available.

Subcutaneous heparin is rarely administered for DVT. It is often given for prophylaxis against DVT, especially in high-risk patients. Subcutaneous heparin given for venous thrombosis is administered at 4- to 12-hour intervals in doses of 5000-15,000 units. Absorption of the drug is erratic, and control is difficult during the treatment of any form of thrombosis. In the pregnant patient who receives intravenous heparin for treatment, the regimen for the duration of the pregnancy is administration of a dose sufficient to keep the PTT at 1.5-2.0 times normal. The dose may be administered every 8-12 hours. PTT is assessed 6 hours after injection.[7]

Subcutaneous heparin is administered for prophylaxis of DVT. Two hours prior to surgery 5000 units of heparin are given, and this is followed by doses every 8-12 hours until the patient is fully ambulatory. One problem frequently encountered with this method is pain and ecchymoses at the injection sites.

Low-Molecular-Weight Heparin

Low-molecular-weight heparins (LMWHs) were developed after the discovery that the antithrombotic effects of LMWH were the same as that of unfractionated heparin, but that LMWH was easier to use. LMWH is prepared by a chemical cracking process yielding fragments about one-third the size of heparin. The half-life is approximately two to four times that of unfractionated heparin.[11] The shorter LMWH strands do not have enough sites for binding both antithrombin and thrombin.[6,11] Because of this characteristic, LMWH primarily acts on factor Xa.

LMWH is dosed by patient weight, depending on the indication and the type of LMWH in use.[10] There are several LMWHs available, including dalteparin, enoxaparin, tinzaparin, and a pentasaccharide, fondaparinux. The anticoagulation action of LMWH is more predictable than that of unfractionated heparin because of its more reliable bioavailability.

Unfortunately, in contrast to unfractionated heparin, there is no readily available test to measure the intensity of anticoagulation with LMWH. It is very difficult to safely use LMWH in renal patients or patients weighing less than 50 kg or more than 100 kg. The incidence of severe bleeding is increased when LMWH is used in renal patients. The PTT does not accurately reflect the anticoagulant efficacy of the medication.

LMWH has been given with safety in the outpatient setting for DVT and has not resulted in increased mortality or morbidity.[3,6,9,12,13] A weight-based dose of LMWH has been found to be as effective as unfractionated heparin in treatment of DVT with or without pulmonary emboli. In addition, LMWH has the advantage of simplicity for home administration.[6,13]

Heparin Administration

Subcutaneous heparin must be injected into adipose tissue. The most common site is the abdomen, but the posterior arm, lateral thigh, and fat pad of the scapula may be used. Some centers have encountered problems with hematoma formation if injections are given within a few inches of an abdominal incision, so these areas should be avoided. The fat fold should be 1 inch when it is pinched between the thumb and the forefinger and should be free of induration or ecchymoses. A short needle (½-⅝ inch) should be inserted at a 45°-90° angle. Backflow should not be checked; a rotation chart should be made of injection sites. To avoid hematoma formation, the injection site should not be massaged.

Heparin Complications

The most frequent complication of heparin therapy is bleeding. Other uncommon complications are found in Box 8-3. Bony defects secondary to ascorbic acid deficiency can be enhanced by heparin; therefore, this deficiency is a relative contraindication to heparin treatment.

Heparin-induced thrombocytopenia with thrombosis (HITT) is an unusual yet extremely serious occurrence in heparin therapy, and its seriousness warrants further discussion. A modest decrease in platelet count during treatment with unfractionated heparin is common. Mild forms of thrombocytopenia generally are noted on the second to fifth day of heparin therapy, are often reversible, and usually are accompanied by few serious complications.[4] The platelet count rarely falls below 100,000 per microliter, and no treatment is necessary. The more severe form of HITT occurs in 1-3 percent of patients treated with unfractionated heparin for DVT. This syndrome is often accompanied by thrombosis and rarely hemorrhage[14,15] (Fig. 8-1). It appears to be less common with the use of LMWH, but it does occur. Thrombosis may include stroke, myocardial infarction, arterial graft occlusion, or DVT. The severe form may occur at any time during treatment but is most common between days 4 and 15. The platelet count drops precipitously below 100,000 per microliter. A drop from baseline of 40 percent or more in the platelet count is considered diagnostic of HITT.

The cause of HITT is believed to be an immune-mediated response.[4,16-18] Heparin-dependent antibodies bind to a heparin-platelet factor complex. These antibodies cause a secretion of adenosine diphosphate and thromboxane A, resulting in thrombocyte consumption (and

BOX 8–3

Uncommon Complications of Heparin Therapy

Hypersensitivity and anaphylaxis (rare)
Bronchoconstriction
Cutaneous necrosis
Urticaria
Alopecia
Osteoporosis (seen only with long-term therapy such as in pregnancy)
Pathologic features[3,12]

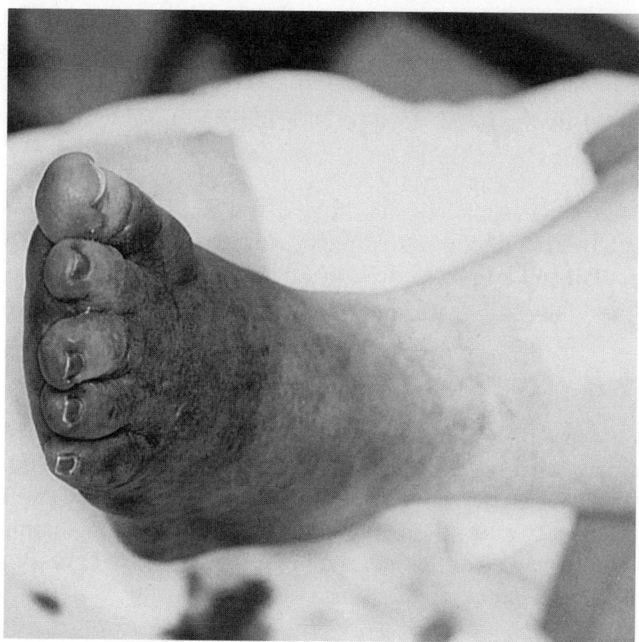

FIG. 8–1. Lower extremity arterial thrombosis secondary to heparin-induced thrombocytopenia.

bleeding) and/or activation of the coagulation cascade (and thrombosis). Both platelet counts and duration or amount of heparin therapy have been unrelated to the severity of either response. The etiology of this complication may be related to the biologic source of the heparin, as a higher incidence of HITT is associated with bovine preparations than porcine. Unfractionated heparin in any amount, and LMWH, are contraindicated in patients with a history of HITT.

Nursing Responsibility With Heparin

Nursing responsibility with any patient on heparin therapy begins with ensuring that the proper tests (PTT, platelet counts) are performed as ordered and results reported to the physician or vascular nurse. It is important to inform the responsible clinician if heparin therapy is interrupted at any time, because interruption would influence laboratory results. Appropriate dosing decisions are based not only on the most recent test result, but also should include the previous result, the present heparin dose, infusion time, and the previously adjusted dose. Additionally, it is the nurse's responsibility to ensure that unnecessary APTT tests are avoided if the patient is on LMWH.

Due to a short duration of action, simply holding the infusion for 1 hour and resuming the infusion at a decreased rate can often reverse heparin effects. When heparin activity is excessive, it can be reversed by slow intravenous infusion of protamine sulfate. An intravenous dose of 1-1.5 mg per 100 units of heparin remaining in the body will reverse the effect.[19] The action of protamine is thought to be due to its binding with heparin to prevent its reaction with antithrombin. If large amounts of heparin are being administered, a "heparin rebound" may occur, requiring additional protamine. Protamine is a protein derived from fish sperm. Serious allergic reactions to this protein include hypotension, bradycardia, dyspnea, and anaphylaxis. These effects can be reduced by slow injection. Research in a new protamine variant is being performed; this form holds promise for fewer side effects than with standard protamine.[20] Protamine can be used to reverse LMWH overdose, although this practice is clinically untested.

Nurses must observe for signs of bleeding and also educate the patient about these signs. Unusual ecchymoses, bleeding from mucous membranes, melena, hematemesis, hematuria, or cutaneous necrosis should be explained in lay terms and written instructions given to the patient. Menstruating women should report any radical changes in flow, and pregnant women should immediately report any vaginal bleeding or severe abdominal pain. However, it should be clear to the patient that failure to prevent further thrombosis is the most severe adverse event and that the benefits of anticoagulation far exceed the risk of side effects.

Instructions on the proper technique of self-administration, site rotation, and appropriate disposal of biohazardous waste are part of a complete discharge instruction plan. Reassurance to the patient and significant others regarding the ability to administer the medication is helpful. If alopecia occurs, the patient should be aware that this is temporary. Complications can best be avoided by strict attention to dosages, adequate determination of anticoagulation effects, and proper staff and patient education. In the patient with previous heparin therapy requiring hospitalization, the use of LMWH in the outpatient setting may require additional information and reassurance.

Oral Anticoagulants

Oral anticoagulants were identified in 1941 when the coagulation effects of spoiled sweet clover were noted. Since that time, warfarin drugs (warfarin, bishydroxycoumarin) have been synthesized and indanedione derivatives (diphenadione, phenindione) were made available. Warfarin is the drug of choice in the United States for oral anticoagulation. Indications are seen in Box 8-4. Long-term use of oral anticoagulants (with or without aspirin) after arterial reconstruction is dependent on individual patient characteristics.[21]

Except for pregnancy, contraindications to warfarin therapy are similar to those of heparin. Caution should be used in the presence of drainage tubes, malabsorption syndromes, dietary deficiencies, gastrointestinal ulcers, or impaired hepatic or renal function. Pregnancy is an absolute contraindication to the use of warfarin compounds. During pregnancy, warfarin compounds can cause teratogenic effects, especially if taken in the first trimester. Because these medications cross the placental barrier, the fetus may suffer from bleeding complications either before birth or during labor or delivery.[7]

Warfarin interferes with the interconversion of vitamin K. Vitamin K is a cofactor for the activation of coagulant proteins II, VII, IX, and X. The anticoagulant proteins C and S are inhibited by warfarin via the same mechanism.[22,23]

Warfarin has high bioavailability and is rapidly absorbed from the gastrointestinal tract. Warfarin (particularly the S-isomer) is eliminated through complex metabolism. The half-life of warfarin is about 36-42 hours. The half-life of anticoagulant protein C and of factor VII is about 6 hours. Factor IX and Factor II have half-lives of 24 and 96 hours, respectively. The antithrombotic effect of warfarin is dependent on the reduction of the activity of prothrombin (factor II).[22,23]

In the United States, the INR is the most commonly employed test to monitor warfarin therapy. The prothrombin time used earlier has been replaced by the more reliable INR. The INR

BOX 8–4

Indications for Oral Anticoagulants

Following heparin or thrombolytic therapy for:
- Deep venous thrombosis (DVT)
- Pulmonary embolism
- Arterial thrombosis
- Embolism
- Arterial or venous graft failures

Presence of a prosthetic valve
Valvular heart disease with subsequent embolism
Chronic or intermittent atrial fibrillation (to prevent embolism)
Inherited coagulation disorders
Cerebrovascular or extracranial carotid artery disease in patients who are poor surgical risks (controversial)

TABLE 8–1 Desirable International Normalized Ratio (INR) Values

2.0–3.0	2.5–3.5
Treatment of deep venous thrombosis (DVT)	Acute myocardial infarction
Prevention of DVT and pulmonary embolus	Valvular heart disease
Treatment after pulmonary embolism	Atrial fibrillation
Following select infrainguinal arterial bypass grafts	Recurrent systemic embolism
	Mechanical prosthetic valves

was devised in 1982 by the World Health Organization to provide a universal application to the monitoring of oral anticoagulation. It was not used extensively in the United States until the early 1990s. The INR is calculated by dividing the patient's prothrombin time by the mean prothrombin time, multiplied by the sensitivity index of the thromboplastin. The sensitivity index controls the variability of testing agents (thromboplastins) and is a comparison of the batch of thromboplastin to the international reference thromboplastin (value 1).[24] Desired levels of INR are seen in Table 8-1. The INR is the most accurate measure of anticoagulant control.

Warfarin therapy should be initiated with the average maintenance dose of 5 mg per day. Patients at risk for bleeding, those with liver disease or impaired nutrition, and the elderly should be started at reduced doses. A loading dose offers no advantage and may lead to adverse effects such as bleeding and/or thrombotic complications.[24] Successful patient management depends on a systematic process that includes careful assessment of the rate of change of the INR, as well as the absolute INR value, and an organized system of follow-up, patient communication, and education.[25] On the basis of the increase or decrease in test levels, the dosage is adjusted accordingly. Doses may vary from 1 mg daily in extremely sensitive patients to as high as 15-20 mg in a very few others. The physician, pharmacist, or vascular nurse monitoring the dosage will determine the frequency of blood tests. In some patients, the frequency may be every 2-4 weeks in long-term therapy, but in others more careful monitoring may be necessary.

More than 150 medications, nutritional agents, and herbals are reported to interfere with either the effects or the metabolism of warfarin.[23] During maintenance therapy, the INR may not reflect dose changes and/or the influence of interactive drugs until day 4 or longer. A partial list of drug interactions is seen in Table 8-2. For a complete list of information on a particular drug, a pharmacist or medication reference book should be consulted.

TABLE 8–2 Some Medications That Affect Warfarin (Coumadin)*

Decreases INR	Increases INR
Barbiturates	Aspirin
Rifampin	Heparin
Estrogens	Nonsteroidal anti-inflammatory drugs
Cholestyramine	High-dose penicillins
Griseofulvin	"Mycins"
Itraconazole (Sporanox)	Ticlopidine
Tamoxifen	Thyroxine
Quinidine	Cephalosporins
	Sulfa compounds
	Steroids
	Indomethacin
	Fluconazole
	Cimetidine

*Any medications that affect the cytochrome P-450 affect warfarin.
INR, International normalized ratio.

The advantage of warfarin drugs is their oral form, and their disadvantage is their prolonged action time. These medications should be discontinued 3-5 days prior to surgical procedures to ensure normal clotting. If surgery precludes the use of oral anticoagulants, interim coverage with heparin, LMWH, or mechanical interruption of the vena cava may be necessary (see Chapter 18).

There has been controversy regarding the initiation of warfarin therapy. It is generally best to begin at the same time as heparin therapy. Duration of therapy depends on the indication for therapy. Most physicians advise a 3- to 6-month course of therapy after initial heparin therapy.

Complications during warfarin therapy are similar to those during heparin treatment. Bleeding is the most common problem. Other side effects, which include gastrointestinal complaints and dermatitis, are infrequent.

A rare complication of warfarin therapy is skin necrosis. This has been reported to occur after one dose but is most common after 3-10 days of therapy. It occurs most frequently in females and in patients treated for a venous thrombosis rather than for cardiac or cerebrovascular disease.[26] The sites affected initially are commonly the breasts, thighs, buttocks, and legs.[26-31] Some studies link the presence of a carcinoma to the presence of skin necrosis.[31,32] Studies by several authors point to a connection between a protein C or S or antithrombin III deficiency and skin necrosis[33,34] (see Chapter 9).

The skin lesions that occur typically begin with intense pain, localized erythema, and petechiae. Swelling in the tissues follows, with color changes to a dark cyanotic appearance. Large blisters then develop over the area (Fig. 8-2). Necrosis may extend into subcutaneous or fat tissue. The tissue sloughs with resultant ulceration. The occurrence of skin necrosis is unrelated to dosage or elevated INR. The few pathology specimens from early changes point to a microvascular injury with fibrin deposition in small capillaries and veins.[26]

Treatment for this complication includes cessation of the drug, increase or reinstitution of heparin therapy, and comfort measures. Some early studies recommended the use of steroids, hypothermia, and administration of vitamins C and K. These measures have proven ineffective.[27,28,33] Surgical debridement, topical antibacterial ointments (especially sulfa compounds), and skin grafting may be necessary.

When an elevated INR occurs without hemorrhage, omitting a dose or several doses of the drug may correct the problem. The drug should then be restarted at a lower dose once the patient's INR is in the therapeutic range. If there is minor bleeding or the INR is exceptionally prolonged (between 5 and 9), once again warfarin should be held and resumed at a lower dose once the patient's INR is in the therapeutic range. Vitamin K, 1-2.5 mg given orally, is recommended if the patient is at increased risk for bleeding. These patients should be monitored more frequently in the future. If the INR is greater than 9, warfarin should be

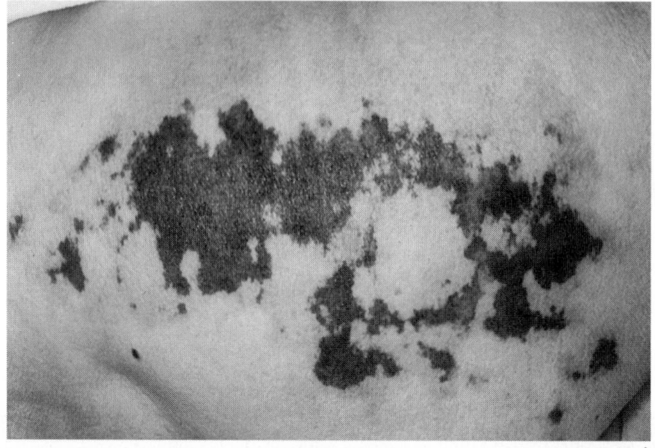

FIG. 8–2. Skin necrosis that occurred after 5 days of warfarin therapy. Note large dark blisters.

held and oral vitamin K, 2.5-5 mg, should be administered. The INR should be significantly reduced within 24-48 hours. The INR should be monitored more frequently and additional vitamin K administered as needed. Warfarin should be resumed at a lower dose once the patient's INR is in the therapeutic range. Patients may become refractory to warfarin after the use of vitamin K. With serious bleeding, vitamin K is administered by slow intravenous infusion and, depending on the severity, can be supplemented with fresh plasma or prothrombin complex. If anticoagulation is resumed at a later time, heparin may be used until the patient is once again sensitive to warfarin.[23]

Nursing responsibility at discharge begins with an assessment of the patient's level of comprehension. The patient and a significant other must be aware and capable of recalling the purpose, dose, side effects, precautions, and medical follow-up. The informed cooperation of the patient is essential to successful treatment. In addition, the nurse should assess the patient for a potential for falling, which might make oral anticoagulation dangerous outside of the hospital.

A flow sheet in simple form may assist the patient in recording and recalling warfarin doses and the times for INR determination. If the patient is incapable of traveling to a laboratory, arrangements should be made for home care to perform the test. Third-party payers generally cover regulation of anticoagulants and patient compliance for a period of time. If the patient has trouble determining the tablet strength, a single strength of 2-mg tablets (and no mixture of strengths) should be suggested to the physician. In addition, a daily dose packet may be made up by the discharge nurse and then the patient or family member. Simplicity of dosage may increase compliance.[34]

The patient should understand that the INR must be obtained as ordered. The patient should be instructed to call the clinician's office personally if no call is received with instructions following the test. The patient should be given an instructions sheet (Box 8-5). In addition to

BOX 8–5

Warfarin Discharge Instructions

Warfarin is used to reduce the blood's ability to clot. It prevents new clots from forming, or existing clots from becoming larger and causing more serious problems. It does not dissolve clots that already have formed. Warfarin is used as treatment for harmful clotting related to certain blood vessel, heart, and lung conditions.

A test called the INR shows how long it takes your blood to clot. When you first start taking warfarin, your INR will be checked often. Once the dose is set, the number of tests will be decreased. It will still be important to check your INR on a regular basis to help ensure the proper warfarin dose based on your needs. Too large a dose may cause bleeding. Too small a dose may allow blood clots to form.

MISSED DOSE

Take this medicine only as directed by your doctor or clinic. Do not take more or less of it, do not take it more often, and do not take it for a longer time than your doctor ordered. Take warfarin at the same time each day.

If you miss a dose, take it as soon as possible. Then go back to your regular schedule. If you do not remember until the next day, do not take the missed dose at all and do not double the next one. Call your clinic or doctor for instructions. Keep a record of each dose as you take it. Review this record with your clinic or doctor.

DIET

The effects of warfarin depend on the amount of vitamin K in your body. You should maintain your regular diet to promote consistent effects of your medicine. Any abrupt changes, such as crash diets, food fads, or nutrition supplements, may alter the normal amount of vitamin K in your body. Inform your clinic whenever you plan to change your diet.

Patients taking oral anticoagulants should avoid alcohol. Please talk with your clinic or doctor if you have questions about alcohol intake.

Continued

BOX 8–5

Warfarin Discharge Instructions—cont'd

DRUG INTERACTIONS

Many prescription medications can interfere with the action of warfarin. Tell all of your doctors (including dentist) that you are taking warfarin. Some over-the-counter (OTC) medicines and herbal remedies can also intensify or lessen the effect of warfarin. It is important to consult your doctor or pharmacist before you use any of these. You should consult your doctor or pharmacist before taking any vitamin supplements. It is not possible to have a complete list of drug interactions because of the large number of such medications.

SPECIAL INSTRUCTIONS

- If you cut yourself, apply pressure to the area for five minutes to make sure the bleeding has stopped.
- Do not begin taking this medicine during pregnancy, and do not become pregnant while taking it. This medicine can cause birth defects. Consult your doctor for added information.
- If you are to be away for any length of time, inform your doctor.
- It is important that you carry identification such as the Medic-Alert bracelet stating that you are taking this medicine so that proper treatment can be given in case of an emergency.
- Avoid activities and sports that may cause you to be injured. Report to your doctor any falls, blows to the body or head, or other injuries.
- Place a non-slip bath mat in the tub to prevent accidents.
- Be careful to avoid cutting yourself. This includes taking special care in brushing your teeth and in shaving. Use a soft toothbrush and use dental floss gently. Also, it is best to use an electric shaver rather than a razor blade.
- Keep all drugs out of the reach of children including discarded medication.
- Store away from heat and direct light.
- Do not store in the bathroom, near the kitchen sink, or in other damp places. Heat or moisture may cause the medicine to break down.
- Do not keep outdated medicine that is no longer needed.

NOTIFY YOUR DOCTOR IMMEDIATELY IF YOU NOTICE ANY OF THE FOLLOWING:

- Severe headache
- Prolonged bleeding, nosebleed, bloody gums, bloody sputum, blood in urine or stool
- Black stool (if not taking iron supplements)
- Unusual bruising or change in skin color, dizziness, or unusually heavy menstrual bleeding
- Unexplained swelling
- Shortness of breath, chest pain, pain in the joints or back, difficulty breathing or swallowing

From Fotis M, Patyk M, Fahey V: *Patient medication instructions—Warfarin*, Chicago, 1999, Northwestern Memorial Hospital.

the written sheet, verbal directions from the nurse, pharmacist, and community dietitian may assist in patient comprehension.

Documentation of instructions to the patient and the family is essential. Each piece of information given should be recorded in the hospital or home care record. Documentation of the assessment of level of understanding is crucial. Failure to document patient education carries significant medical-legal risks.

ANTIPLATELET AGENTS

Antiplatelet agents such as aspirin, dipyridamole (Persantine™), ticlopidine (Ticlid™), and clopidogrel (Plavix™) are used routinely to reduce the risk of platelet aggregation and thrombus formation.

Aspirin permanently inactivates the enzyme cyclooxygenase type-1 (COX-1) in the platelet, resulting in inhibition of the synthesis of thromboxane A2 (TXA_2). Platelets are unable to regenerate COX-1. TXA_2 induces platelet aggregation and vasoconstriction.[36] Once-daily administration of a low dose (80-160 mg/day) of aspirin results in almost complete inhibition of platelet TXA_2. Many times, higher doses of aspirin are needed to inhibit cyclooxygenase type-2 (COX-2), which is responsible for the analgesic and anti-inflammatory effects of aspirin. Low-dose aspirin acts as an effective antithrombotic with improved safety as gastrointestinal toxicity is dose related. Prostacyclin (PGI_2), generated via COX-2, acts to inhibit platelet aggregation and vasoconstriction. Low-dose aspirin is unable to sufficiently inhibit COX-2 and avoids promoting thrombosis via the COX-2 pathway. Aspirin has no direct effect on the coagulation cascade and is not used for treatment of active venous or arterial thrombosis.

The recommended antithrombotic dose of aspirin is 1 or 2 baby (80 mg) aspirin a day. Most studies indicate higher doses are not necessary and may in fact be harmful. Side effects are most frequently gastrointestinal (e.g., nausea, vomiting, epigastric distress, possible ulcers, gastrointestinal bleeding) and can be minimized somewhat if the drug is administered with a meal. Other possible effects are prolonged bleeding time, anemia, and dizziness. Aspirin in very high doses can cause confusion, neurologic disturbances, convulsions, acid-base disturbance, and tinnitus.

Dipyridamole has vasodilator and antiplatelet properties; however, its mechanism of action is unknown. The efficacy of dipyridamole both alone and with aspirin is suspect, as many trials find no benefit.[36] A single recent trial using a modified release form of dipyridamole with low-dose aspirin has shown modest benefit for the secondary prevention of stroke.[37] The Food and Drug Administration (FDA) recently approved this combination.

The related agents clopidogrel and ticlopidine are selective and irreversible inhibitors of ADP-induced platelet aggregation. Both clopidogrel and ticlopidine inhibit platelet aggregation and increase bleeding time. Like aspirin, the platelet effects of clopidogrel and ticlopidine are irreversible for the remainder of the platelet's life span. After discontinuation of therapy, platelet aggregation and bleeding time gradually return to baseline within 5 days.[36]

These medications are effective in the secondary prevention of atherosclerotic events (myocardial infarction, stroke, and vascular death) in patients with atherosclerosis documented by recent myocardial infarction, recent stroke, or established peripheral arterial disease.[38] They are considered alternatives to aspirin. It is not clear if any special patient population will get a better protection rate from clopidogrel than aspirin or ticlopidine. The side effects associated with clopidogrel therapy are similar to those reported with aspirin, but clopidogrel causes less neutropenia than ticlopidine.

Antiplatelet agents are indicated for the prevention of transient ischemic attacks, stroke, thromboembolic complications associated with artificial valves, myocardial infarction (post infarction and for primary prevention), graft occlusion in coronary or peripheral arterial bypass surgery, and following carotid endarterectomy. Aspirin has been studied for the prevention of DVT and has not proved effective.[36]

Contraindications to antiplatelet agents include known sensitivity to the drugs or active gastric ulcers. These agents should be discontinued 7 days prior to any elective surgical procedures where an antiplatelet effect is not desired. The use of high-dose aspirin should be avoided during pregnancy. Low-dose aspirin (80 mg/day) may be necessary in certain circumstances during the second and third trimester. Careful consideration should be given to the risks and benefits to both the mother and fetus before initiation of treatment.

Instructions to the patient should not be limited to information regarding side effects. It should be emphasized that the benefits of the medication outweigh the risk of adverse effects. Instruct the patient that the purpose of the medication is to prevent transient ischemic attacks and/or decrease the risk of thrombus formation. The patient must be informed in lay terms to watch for hematuria, melena, ecchymoses, hematemesis, abdominal pain, or dizziness. Alcohol should be consumed in moderation. Daily compliance should be emphasized.

ANTITHROMBOTIC AGENTS

Therapy for extensive venous or arterial thromboses was traditionally limited to anticoagulation, arterial thrombectomy, or embolectomy or arterial bypass surgery. Thrombolytic enzymes promote pharmacologic dissolution of blood clots by activating plasminogen. Plasmin (the active form of plasminogen) digests fibrinogen, leading to lysis. Thrombolytic agents help to reestablish patency more quickly than anticoagulants. These medications restore venous or arterial blood flow with minimal damage to the pulmonary vascular bed, venous valves, or graft material. It is believed that thrombolytic agents can reduce the risk of subsequent venous disease in the lower extremities or the risk of pulmonary hypertension.[39]

Urokinase (UK), streptokinase (SK), tissue plasminogen activator (t-PA), and reteplase are thrombolytic agents in current use. Thrombolytics may be indicated in a number of situations (Box 8-6). Strong medical contraindications to surgery and surgically inaccessible clots are also possible indications for thrombolytic therapy. Contraindications to therapy include those seen in Box 8-7. Caution should be used when patients have these relative contraindications. SK is antigenic and cannot be used repeatedly.[48] The costs of UK, reteplase, and t-PA are much greater than SK.

Urokinase is an enzyme that is produced from human neonatal kidney tissue cells. It acts directly to break the plasminogen molecule and yields plasmin. Streptokinase is a nonenzymatic protein produced by group C beta streptococci.[43,48] It works by reacting with plasminogen to produce an activator complex that converts plasminogen to the lytic enzyme plasmin. Alteplase is a naturally occurring enzyme that converts plasminogen to plasmin. The plasmin dissolves the clot by specifically working on the fibrin network. Reteplase is a genetically engineered version of alteplase.

Thrombolytic therapy works best in lesions of less than 7 days of age and in vessels that are not too small.[43,48] Massive thrombus requires a longer time to lyse than do smaller clots. If endogenous inhibitors are abnormally elevated, the fibrinolytic system may not activate adequately.

All agents are fast acting and are rapidly cleared. The half-life of SK and UK is approximately 15 minutes and is about 5 minutes for t-PA and reteplase. These medications are given intravenously or intraarterially and are excreted in the urine.[40,43]

For systemic therapy, these drugs are given via a peripheral vein (because it is compressible). For intraarterial use, they are administered via an angiographic catheter, inserted as close to the clot as possible. Urokinase is "laced" into the clot by pushing the angiogram catheter into the clot and infusing the drug as it is pulled back to the beginning of the clot.

Streptokinase and urokinase are given intraarterially for 12-16 hours but may be given longer. Streptokinase may be given for 24-72 hours and UK for up to 48 hours, depending upon the application. t-PA is given for shorter periods: 1 hour for cerebrovascular accidents,

BOX 8–6

Indications for Thrombolytic Agents[40-47]

Acute massive pulmonary embolism
Recent extensive deep venous thrombosis
Acute arterial graft occlusion
Central venous catheter occlusion
Superior vena cava syndrome
Acute arterial thrombosis and coronary artery occlusion following myocardial infarction
Identification of a cause of thrombosis so repair may be performed
To decrease the level of amputation if the clot cannot be removed completely
Prevention of arterial wall damage from thrombectomy
Acute arterial occlusion
Acute ischemic stroke

BOX 8–7

Contraindications to Thrombolytic Therapy

ABSOLUTE
Recent surgical procedures (less than 10 days)
Arteriogram
Lumbar puncture
Paracentesis
Renal or liver biopsy (less than 14 days)
Recent trauma (including cardiopulmonary resuscitation)
Pregnancy (including 10 days postpartum)
Visceral carcinoma
Ulcerative colitis
Severe hypertension (200 mm Hg systolic or 110 mm Hg diastolic)
Ulcerative wounds
Active tuberculosis
Defective hemostasis
Central nervous system surgery (2 months)
Gastrointestinal bleeding (6 months)
Allergic reaction

RELATIVE
Endocarditis
Atrial fibrillation (danger of bleeding into an unknown area of cerebral infarction)
Antibody formation—streptokinase only (such as after a recent streptococcal infection)

approximately 90 minutes in intracoronary applications, and 2 hours for pulmonary emboli.[40] The systemic loading dose for SK is 250,000 units/hour over 30 minutes followed by 100,000 units/hour. Intraarterial doses may be smaller, with a bolus of 20,000 units and a continuous infusion of 5000-10,000 units/hour. Intraarterial UK is administered with a dose of 250,000 units to lace the clot, 250,000 units over the next 2 hours, and then the dose adjusted to 10,000-60,000 units/hour until the clot is lysed. Some centers administer 100,000 units/hour after the initial dose.[39] Systemic UK (for pulmonary emboli) is started with a loading dose of 4400 units/kg for 10 minutes, followed by 4400 units/kg/hr for 12-24 hours.[39] The t-PA dose varies with use as does that of UK and may range from 80 mg in intracoronary use to 50 mg/hr in pulmonary emboli.

These drugs are administered at a fixed dose, unlike heparin and warfarin drugs. Heparin is given in conjunction with thrombolytic therapy. Thrombin times and/or fibrinogen levels may be ordered to be certain that the thrombolytic system has been activated. It is important to remember that no blood test is directly correlated to complications, and they may occur despite acceptable test results. The major complication of thrombolysis is bleeding. Febrile reactions to thrombolytic therapy may be due to contaminants with bacterial endotoxins or to the release of catabolic products of thrombolysis. Mild reactions to these drugs do not necessitate discontinuance of therapy. Alteplase has no antigenic properties because it occurs naturally in the body.

Nursing implications in thrombolytic therapy are very complex and are related to the stage of therapy—preinfusion, intrainfusion, and postinfusion. In the preinfusion state, the patient may be moved to a monitored area. Blood work should be performed to establish a baseline PTT, prothrombin time, hematocrit, white blood cell count, platelet count, thrombin time, and plasminogen level. These tests provide evidence of normal hemostasis and coagulation. If these results are abnormal for an unknown reason, the physician should be notified. If the bleeding time is greater than 15 minutes, therapy should not be instituted. Cross-matched blood should be available in case of bleeding. Aminocaproic acid (Amicar) and aprotinin (Trasylol) are antidotes for use if bleeding occurs. The thrombolytic solution must be administered via volumetric pump whose flow rate is not dependent on drop size.

In the pretherapy assessment of the patient, a good history is essential. Recent streptococcal infection may diminish the drug's effects. Use of antiplatelet drugs and oral or injectable anticoagulants should be recorded. Baseline pulses and/or pressures in each extremity must be obtained, using a Doppler transducer if necessary.

During infusion, vital signs are closely monitored in addition to extremity perfusion. Observation of the stool, urine, emesis, or dressings for bleeding is important. The nurse must be alert for hematoma formation, back pain, swelling, flank pain, and a falling hematocrit. If bleeding does occur, direct pressure is applied, infusion stopped, and the physician notified. Sandbags may be employed if necessary. Whole blood, fresh frozen plasma, or aminocaproic acid may be administered. Corticosteroids may be necessary for allergic reactions.

No intramuscular injections should be given within 24 hours of infusion, and no new medications initiated during therapy. No medications may be mixed with the thrombolytic drugs. Anticoagulants, antiplatelet agents, dextran, and phenylbutazone should be used with caution.

Invasive procedures may not be performed during therapy. If arterial blood gases are absolutely indicated, pressure must be applied to the site for 30 minutes and the site frequently observed for bleeding. A flow sheet of all doses and laboratory data should be kept. Thrombin times should be elevated 2-5 times, and the fibrinogen level should be approximately 100 mg/dl.

Post infusion, direct pressure by hand or sandbag should be applied to the infusion site. The patient should be on bed rest with the extremity immobile in straight alignment. Heparin is continued post infusion, and the usual precautions for heparin therapy apply.

Patient education regarding thrombolytic agents should include the purpose of therapy, possible side effects, and expected activity level both during and after therapy. Emotional support is essential. Patients are in a crisis situation and must be reassured that procedures are normal. It is important that the patient and the family be informed before the patient is transported to the radiology unit that if thrombolytic therapy is started, the patient will be transferred to intensive care or a monitored unit.

Pain is common in patients receiving thrombolytic therapy. Assessment of pain before initiation of therapy is essential, and the source must be determined. Accurate assessment can determine if distal embolization is the source of pain. Pulse rate and ankle-brachial index determination are standard measures of arterial flow; color, capillary return, and temperature may also be assessed. If pain becomes worse with reperfusion, analgesia should be given. Back pain from bed rest is common but must be differentiated from severe pain caused by retroperitoneal bleeding.

MISCELLANEOUS DRUGS

Dextran

Dextran is a polysaccharide first introduced as a plasma expander, for use when blood or blood products were not available. Its antithrombotic effect was a secondary finding and has been demonstrated in subsequent studies. This effect may be due to several factors: (1) increased blood volume, (2) decreased blood viscosity, (3) reduced platelet adhesiveness, (4) altered fibrin polymerization, and (5) interference with factor VIII antigen and the von Willebrand cofactor.[48]

One indication for dextran is prophylaxis against venous thrombosis. This is especially indicated in the patient at risk who, in addition, needs volume replacement. Controversy exists over its effectiveness.

Contraindications for dextran include known bleeding disorders, anuria, hypervolemic state, and drug-induced cardiac decompensation.[22] Care should be exercised in administering dextran to patients with cardiac or renal insufficiency or while heparin is administered. It is unknown whether the drug crosses the placental barrier, and therefore, dextran is not recommended in pregnancy.[22]

Dextran is given intravenously. Doses of dextran are begun with 10 mg/kg just prior to surgery and then increased to 500 ml/day for 2-3 days. It may be continued for up to 3 weeks with a dose of 500 ml every 2-3 days.

Dextran must be given slowly in patients with cardiac insufficiency. Central venous pressure must be monitored carefully. Oliguria or anuria should be reported to the physician. Complications of dextran include fluid overload, bleeding, decreased urine output, and anaphylactic reactions. Fluid overload and pulmonary edema can be avoided by limiting rate and volume in elderly patients or in patients with renal insufficiency. It is important to reassure the patient that urinary output problems are generally temporary. Anaphylaxis is a rare complication but occurs immediately after infusion. For this reason, the initial dose should not be given while the patient is under general anesthesia. Anaphylaxis is not related to a previous infusion history. Anaphylactoid reactions can be avoided with an intravenous injection of 20 ml of monovalent dextran.

Pentoxifylline

Pentoxifylline was introduced in the United States in the early 1980s. It is indicated for the treatment of intermittent claudication associated arterial occlusive disease. Pentoxifylline is structurally related to theophylline and caffeine. The drug's action may be related to inhibition of erythrocyte phosphodiesterase, resulting in improved erythrocyte flexibility, and a reduction in blood viscosity.[22,49] Pentoxifylline is contraindicated in patients with a history of intolerance to related drugs such as caffeine, theophylline, or theobromine. It should also be used with caution in the elderly, in patients at risk for bleeding, or in those having impaired renal or liver function.

Pentoxifylline is readily absorbed from the gastrointestinal tract. The drug is eliminated via complex metabolism and is eventually excreted in the urine. Medications and herbals that inhibit the metabolism of pentoxifylline should be avoided. Treatment may need to continue for up to 8 weeks of therapy in order to generate a therapeutic effect. Patients must be aware that results may not be noticeable for up to 2 months.

Dosage of the medication is 400 mg three times a day with meals. If stomach upset occurs, it may be reduced to twice a day. The caffeine-like side effects such as nausea, heartburn, dizziness, headache, and tremor are common. These are usually mild and improve after decreasing the dose.

The beneficial effects, if any, of pentoxifylline are unclear. A planned program of exercise alone may be more effective (see Chapter 10). This drug may be helpful to a few patients with impaired walking ability, but study results do not support the widespread use of this agent.[49,50]

Cilostazol

Cilostazol was introduced in the United States in 1999, approved for the treatment of claudication associated with arterial occlusive disease. Cilostazol has antithrombotic, antiplatelet, and vasodilator properties. It acts through inhibition of phosphodiesterase type III, inhibiting platelet aggregation, and promoting vasodilation.[21,49] The exact mechanism in peripheral arterial disease is unknown. Other phosphodiesterase type III inhibitors, such as milrinone, are associated with decreased survival in patients with heart failure. Because of this relationship, cilostazol is contraindicated (inadvisable) in patients with congestive heart failure of any severity. Cilostazol should also be avoided in women who are pregnant or breast-feeding. It should be used with caution in patients with cardiac disease, abnormal blood pressure, or those having impaired renal or liver function.

Cilostazol is administered orally and is best taken on an empty stomach. The drug is eliminated via complex and extensive metabolism and is eventually excreted in the urine. There are multiple medications and herbals that can inhibit the metabolism of cilostazol or interfere with coagulation, and they should be avoided. Consult with a pharmacist or Drug Information Center for an assessment of the risk of drug interactions.

Dosage of the medication is 100 mg twice a day. Lower doses may be necessary in patients taking interacting medications. Headache (34%), diarrhea, dizziness, and palpitations (all more than 10%) are common and troubling side effects.[21,49]

Beneficial effects of cilostazol include modest improvements in maximum walking distance and pain-free walking distance. Cilostazol also improved subjective assessments of quality of life as measured by questionnaire. Modest to moderate benefits can be expected in patients who are carefully screened for important contraindications and are monitored to avoid drug-drug and drug-diet interactions.

Ancrod

Ancrod is made of a purified portion of Malaysian pit viper venom. The introduction of the venom in the human body results in rapid defibrinogenizaion. Ancrod itself does not affect any other coagulation factors, but the defibrinogenation does. It produces anticoagulation, decreases blood viscosity, and enhances local clot thrombolysis. Ancrod has been used in Europe for years for prevention and treatment of various thrombotic disorders. In this application, ancrod is given intravenously in prescribed dosing. Plasma fibrinogen levels are monitored. It was recently tested for acute stroke and had a favorable risk-benefit ratio for these patients.[51] Future testing will determine its possible use in the United States. It is currently available in Canada.

SUMMARY

The nurse who is knowledgeable about the drugs most commonly used in vascular patients can enhance safety, monitor effects of medication, and educate the patient. The entire health care team must cooperate to recognize untreated and undertreated medical problems, to decrease medication complications, and to increase adherence to the prescribed routine.

REFERENCES

1. McLean J: Thromboplastic action of cephalin, *Am J Physiol* 41:250-257, 1916.
2. Murray D, Jacques L, Perrett T et al: Heparin and the thrombosis of veins following injury, *Surgery* 2:163-187, 1937.
3. Rosenfeld J, Estrada F, Orr R: Management of deep venous thrombosis in the pregnant female, *J Cardiovasc Surg* 31:678-682, 1990.
4. Fahey VA: Heparin-induced thrombocytopenia, *J Vasc Nurs* 13(4):112-116, 1995.
5. Matula P: Management of patients undergoing vascular surgery who are receiving epidural analgesia, *J Vasc Nurs* 11(4):104-107, 1993.
6. Nunnelee J: Low molecular weight heparin, *J Vasc Nurs* 15:94-96, 1997.
7. Falter H: Deep vein thrombosis in pregnancy and the puerperium: a comprehensive review, *J Vasc Nurs* 15(2):58-62, 1997.
8. Hirsh J, Warkentin TE, Shaughnessy SG et al: Heparin and low-molecular-weight heparin: mechanisms of action, pharmacokinetics, dosing, monitoring, efficacy, and safety, *Chest* 119(suppl 1):64s-94s, 2001.
9. Koopman M, Prandoni P, Piovella F et al: Treatment of venous thrombosis with intravenous unfractionated heparin administered in the hospital as compared with subcutaneous low molecular weight heparin administered at home, *N Engl J Med* 334:682-687, 1996.
10. Dolovich LR, Ginsberg JS, Douketis JD et al: A meta-analysis comparing low-molecular-weight heparins with unfractionated heparin in the treatment of venous thromboembolism: examining some unanswered questions regarding location of treatment, product type, and dosing frequency, *Arch Intern Med* 160(2):181-188, 2000.
11. Weitz JI: Low-molecular-weight heparin, *N Engl J Med* 337(10):688-698, 1997.
12. Hyers T, Agnelli G, Hull R et al: Antithrombotic therapy for venous thromboembolic disease, *Chest* 119(suppl):176s-193s, 2001.
13. The Columbus Investigators: Low molecular weight heparin in the treatment of patients with venous thromboembolism, *N Engl J Med* 337(10):657-662, 1997.

14. Harrington L, Hufnagel J: Heparin induced thrombocytopenia and thrombosis syndrome: a case study, *Heart Lung* 19:93-98, 1990.
15. AbuRahma A, Boland J, Witsberger T: Diagnostic and therapeutic strategies of white clot syndrome, *Am J Surg* 162:175-179, 1991.
16. Warkentin TE, Levine MN, Hirsch J et al: Heparin induced thrombocytopenia in patient treated with low molecular weight heparin or unfractionated heparin, *N Engl J Med* 332:1330-1335, 1995.
17. Aster R: Heparin induced thrombocytopenia and thrombosis, *N Engl J Med* 332:1374-1376, 1995.
18. Visentin G, Ford S, Scott J et al: Antibodies from patients with heparin induced thrombocytopenia/thrombosis are specific for platelet factor 4 complexed with heparin or bound to endothelial cells, *J Clin Invest* 93:81-88, 1994.
19. Wheeler H, Anderson F: Prophylaxis against venous thromboembolism in surgical patients, *Am J Surg* 161:507-511, 1991.
20. Hulin, M, Wakefield T, Andrews P et al: A novel protamine variant reversal of heparin anticoagulation in human blood in vitro, *J Vasc Surg* 26:1043-1048, 1997.
21. Clagett GP, Jackson MR: Antithrombotic therapy in peripheral arterial occlusive disease, *Chest* 119(1):283s-299s, 2001.
22. Hodgson B, Kizior R: *Saunders nursing drug handbook*, Philadelphia, 1998, WB Saunders, pp 1062-1064.
23. Hirsh J, Dalan J, Anderson DR et al: Oral anticoagulants, *Chest* 119(suppl):8s-21s, 2001.
24. Kurgan A, Nunnelee J: Upper extremity venous thrombosis, *J Vasc Nurs* 13(1):21-23, 1995.
25. Ansell J, Hirsh J, Dalen J et al: Managing oral anticoagulant therapy, *Chest* 119(Suppl 1):22s-38s, 2001.
26. Cole M, Mimifee P, Wolma F: Coumarin necrosis: a review of the literature, *Surgery* 103:271-277, 1988
27. Comp P, Elrod J, Karzenski S: Warfarin induced skin necrosis, *Semin Thromb Hemost* 16:293-298, 1990.
28. Kandrotas R, Detering J: Genital necrosis secondary to warfarin therapy, *Pharmacology* 3:351-354, 1998.
29. Leath M: Coumarin skin necrosis, *Tex Med* 79:62-64, 1983.
30. Heaton R, Wright L, Hargraves R et al: Coagulopathy and warfarin associated breast necrosis in a patient with a primary brain tumor, *Surg Neurol* 33:395-399, 1990.
31. Everett R, Jones F: Warfarin induced skin necrosis: a sign of malignancy, *Postgrad Med* 79:97-103, 1989.
32. Konrad P, Mellblom L, Berquist D et al: Coumarin associated skin necrosis, *Vasa* 17:208-215, 1988.
33. Conlan M, Bridges A, Williams E et al: Familial type II protein C deficiency associated with warfarin induced skin necrosis and bilateral adrenal hemorrhage, *Am J Hematol* 29:226-229, 1998.
34. Conn V, Taylor S, Kelley S: Medication regimen complexity and adherence among older adults, *Image J Nurs Sch* 23:231-235, 1991.
35. Fotis M, Patyk M, Fahey V: *Patient medication instructions—Warfarin*, Chicago, 1999, Northwestern Memorial Hospital.
36. Patronono C, Coller B, Dalen J et al: Platelet active drugs, *Chest* 119:39s-63s, 2001.
37. Diener HC, Cunha L, Forbes C: European Stroke Prevention Study. 2. Dipyridamole and acetylsalicylic acid in the secondary prevention of stroke, *J Neurol Sci* 143:1-13, 1996.
38. CAPRIE Steering Committee: A randomized, blinded trial of Clopidogrel versus Aspirin in Patients at Risk of Ischemic Events (CAPRIE), *Lancet* 348:1329-1339, 1996.
39. Apple S: New trends in thrombolytic therapy, *RN* 59(1):30-34, 1996.
40. Butler L, Fahey V: Acute arterial occlusion of the lower extremity, *J Vasc Nurs* 11(1):19-22, 1993.
41. Crouch M: Urokinase therapy in mesenteric venous thrombosis: a case study, *J Vasc Nurs* 11(4):99-103, 1993.
42. Ronayne R: Acute lower limb ischemia: a case study, *J Vasc Nurs* 10(3):14-19, 1992.
43. Anderson K: Thrombolytic therapy for treatment of acute peripheral arterial occlusion, *J Vasc Nurs* 10(3):20-24, 1992.
44. Gwynn M: TPA in acute stroke: risk or reprieve? *J Neurosci Nurs* 25(3):180-184, 1993.
45. Hacke E, Kaste M, Smith T et al: Intravenous thrombolytics with recombinant tissue plasminogen activator for acute hemispheric stroke, *JAMA* 224(13):1017-1019, 1995.
46. Kumpe D, Cohen M: Angioplasty/thrombolytic treatment of failing and failed hemodialysis sites: comparison with surgical treatment, *Prog Cardiovasc Dis* 34(4):263-278, 1992.
47. Weitz J, Byrne J, Clagett P et al: Diagnosis and treatment of chronic arterial insufficiency of the lower extremities: a critical review, *Circulation* 94(11):3026-3049, 1996.
48. Nehler MR, Taylor LM, Moneta GL et al: Natural history, nonoperative treatment and functional assessment in chronic lower extremity ischemia. In Moore WS, ed: *Vascular surgery: a comprehensive review*, Philadelphia, 1998, WB Saunders, pp 251-265.
49. Hiatt WR: Medical treatment of peripheral arterial disease and claudication, *N Engl J Med* 344(21): 1608-1621, 2001.

50. Williams LR, Ekers M, Collins PS et al: Vascular rehabilitation: benefits of a structured exercise risk factor modification program, *J Vasc Surg* 14:1636-1639, 1991.
51. Sherman D, Atkinson R, Chippendale T et al: Intravenous ancrod for treatment of acute ischemic stroke, The STAT study, a randomized controlled trial, *JAMA* 283(18):2395-2403, 2000.

9

Thrombotic Disorders in Vascular Patients

LISA BOGGIO □ DAVID GREEN

Blood is maintained in a fluid phase while it circulates through the vascular system. Upon injury to the blood vessel, a coagulum (blood clot) is formed to prevent exsanguination. This process is defined as hemostasis. Thrombosis refers to the abnormal formation of thrombi within the closed vasculature. Blood vessels, platelets, coagulation proteins, inhibitors of coagulation, and activators and inhibitors of fibrinolysis interact with each other in one of the most intricate and tightly controlled of biologic systems. The basic mechanism of hemostasis is divided into four phases:

Phase 1: Primary hemostasis involving the formation of a platelet thrombus that, within seconds, plugs the rent in the blood vessel wall
Phase 2: Activation of the coagulation cascade, leading to formation of fibrin that reinforces the platelet plug and creates the mature thrombus
Phase 3: The regulation of the extension of the thrombus by coagulation factor inhibitors and the fibrinolytic (blood clot dissolving) system
Phase 4: The remodeling and repair of the injury site after arrest of bleeding

The blood vasculature forms a circuit lined by a continuous layer of endothelial cells. Injury to endothelial cells exposes subendothelial supporting structures and adhesive proteins (collagen, von Willebrand factor, fibronectin, vitronectin), which provide binding sites for platelets. Platelets adhere to subendothelial proteins through specific receptors, become activated, and aggregate together to form a platelet plug.

Injury of the blood vessel endothelium and activation of platelets initiates the coagulation cascade that ultimately leads to the formation of fibrin, which constitutes a major portion of the mature clot. The coagulation system is composed of a series of serine proteinases and their cofactors, which react on the phospholipid surfaces of platelets and activated mononuclear and endothelial cells. The coagulation cascade is divided into an extrinsic pathway triggered by tissue factor–factor VII interaction and an intrinsic pathway initiated by surface contact factors. Recent evidence suggests that the extrinsic pathway is physiologically more relevant in the initial generation of fibrin.[1] Physiologic clotting is initiated when tissue factor, an intrinsic membrane protein, is expressed and exposed to circulating blood. The activated partial thromboplastin time (APTT) and prothrombin time (PT) substitute laboratory-prepared reagents for this critical step and, therefore, activate coagulation in a different fashion. Table 9-1 compares physiologic activation of coagulation, the APTT, and the PT.

Physiologic coagulation results in activation of factor VII and subsequently factor IX. However, the reagents used for the APTT mainly activate factor XII; factor VII is not involved. On the other hand, the reagent used for the PT activates factor VII so strongly that it is capable of directly activating factor X rather than factor IX; this results in the short clotting times typical of the PT test.

Coagulation processes are balanced by an elaborate system of naturally occurring inhibitors, including tissue factor pathway inhibitor, antithrombin (formerly called antithrombin III), protein C, and protein S that prevent excessive propagation of thrombus.

TABLE 9–1 The Physiologic Activation of Coagulation

Phase of Coagulation	Physiologic Clotting	Activated Partial Thromboplastin Time	Prothrombin Time
Initiation	Expose tissue factor (TF); TF/VIIa activates IX	Add a surface and lipid; activates XII	Add tissue factor (TF); TF/VIIa activates X
Propagation	IXa + VIIIa activate X	XII activates XI, IX; IXa + VIIIa activate X	Xa + V convert prothrombin to thrombin
	Xa + V convert prothrombin to thrombin	Xa + V convert prothrombin to thrombin	
Clot formation	Thrombin converts fibrinogen to fibrin	Thrombin converts fibrinogen to fibrin	Thrombin converts fibrinogen to fibrin

Deficiencies in these anticoagulants, or interference with their normal functioning, may increase the risk for the development of thrombosis. In this review, we will focus on hypercoagulability and thrombosis in vascular disease.

INHERITED THROMBOTIC DISORDERS

A number of genetic disorders predispose to thrombotic problems either in the newborn period or later on in life. Box 9-1 lists the most common of these disorders.

Antithrombin Deficiency

Antithrombin (AT) is a circulating anticoagulant that inhibits several coagulation proteases, including activated factors XI, X, IX, thrombin, and the tissue factor–factor VIIa complex. Its activity is greatly enhanced by the presence of heparin. Deficiency of AT is inherited in autosomal dominant fashion. Type I deficiency refers to a quantitative reduction in the level of AT. All clinically recognized patients are heterozygous for this disorder; homozygosity is probably lethal in utero. There have been more than 80 distinct mutations identified.[2] Type II deficiency describes qualitative abnormalities that reduce the functional activity of the molecule and can affect either the heparin-or thrombin-binding site.[3,4] It is estimated that the lifetime risk for the development of venous thromboembolism in an AT-deficient individual is about 50 percent.[5] Thrombotic episodes can occur spontaneously, but in 60 percent of patients they are associated with a predisposing risk factor such as surgery, trauma, pregnancy, or the use of oral contraceptives.[6] Patients with a known AT deficiency should undergo aggressive antithrombotic prophylaxis during high-risk situations; for example, in the immediate postoperative period. Treatment of an established thrombosis is accomplished with intravenous heparin or subcutaneous low-molecular-weight heparin followed by warfarin.

BOX 9–1

Inherited Disorders Predisposing to Thrombosis

Antithrombin (III) deficiency
Protein C deficiency
Protein S deficiency
Factor V Leiden
Prothrombin G20210A
Hyperhomocysteinemia

Occasionally, very high doses of heparin are required to achieve adequate anticoagulation.[7] In selected situations, commercially available AT concentrate can be infused to restore normal levels of this anticoagulant.[8]

Protein C Deficiency

Protein C is converted to its active form when thrombin is generated during clotting. The thrombin binds to an endothelial protein called thrombomodulin, and the thrombin-thrombomodulin complex activates protein C. Activated protein C cleaves activated clotting factors V and VIII; the reaction is greatly enhanced by a cofactor, free protein S. The synthesis of protein C and protein S requires vitamin K. Type I (quantitative) and type II (qualitative) deficiencies of protein C have been described. The gene for the protein is located on chromosome 2 and inherited in an autosomal dominant fashion. If mutant genes are inherited from both parents, the child is homozygous for this disorder and the levels of protein C are less than 1 percent of normal. Necrotizing skin and muscle lesions (purpura fulminans) appear shortly after birth, and the child will die unless protein C is provided. Patients who are heterozygous for protein C deficiency generally experience the first episode of thrombosis in early adulthood and are much more likely to have venous than arterial thrombosis. Approximately 70 percent of episodes of thrombosis develop spontaneously, and 30 percent are associated with known predisposing risk factors. Pregnant persons with proteins C and S deficiencies, AT deficiency, and factor V Leiden have an increased incidence of fetal loss.[9,10] Thromboses in patients with protein C deficiency are managed with heparin and warfarin, but the duration of warfarin therapy is unsettled; most clinicians would continue treatment for 6 to 12 months after a first episode of thrombosis and indefinitely in patients with recurrent thrombosis. Patients with protein C deficiency who have never had thrombotic events are not given anticoagulants as a routine but should receive antithrombotic prophylaxis when they undergo surgery or are exposed to other risk factors for thrombosis.

Protein C deficiency predisposes to an important complication called warfarin-induced skin necrosis. This syndrome may occur in patients with inherited deficiencies of proteins C or S, after large loading doses of warfarin, and in individuals with a nutritional deficiency of vitamin K. The latter have borderline-low protein C level and are susceptible to rapid reduction of protein C levels by warfarin. Because the half-life of protein C is shorter than that of several of the vitamin K–dependent procoagulants (factors II, IX, X), its levels fall more quickly than those of the other vitamin K–dependent procoagulants, creating an imbalance in favor of thrombosis during the first 24 hours of warfarin administration. This may cause skin and muscle necrosis, similar to that occurring in purpura fulminans. About 30 percent of patients with warfarin-induced skin necrosis have an underlying protein C deficiency.[11] Treatment of this complication includes prompt discontinuation of warfarin, intravenous heparin, and injection of vitamin K. In severe cases, infusion of plasma or protein C concentrate can rapidly restore levels of protein C.[12]

Protein S Deficiency

Protein S acts as a cofactor for protein C. The gene for this protein is found on chromosome 3. Its synthesis by the liver requires vitamin K and it circulates both free and bound to the C4b-binding protein. Since only the free form is active as the cofactor for protein C, disorders that increase the C4b-binding protein, such as infection and inflammation, decrease the amount of available free protein S and promote coagulation. The clinical manifestations and management of deficiency states are similar to those described for AT and protein C deficiencies. An association with thrombotic strokes has also been reported.[13]

Factor V Leiden Mutation

The factor V Leiden mutation is the most common of the inherited thrombophilias. It is caused by a single mutation in the factor V gene that results in substitution of arginine by glutamine at position 506 of the protein. This substitution renders factor V partially resistant to inactivation by activated protein C.[14,15] The prevalence of this trait is approximately

5-8 percent in persons of European extraction and is between 20 and 50 percent in various cohorts of patients with venous thrombosis. This is much more common than deficiencies of AT, protein C, and protein S, which combined are detected in only 5-10 percent of patients with thrombosis.

The risk of thrombosis for heterozygous carriers of factor V Leiden is estimated at 1.0 percent per year between the ages of 20 and 50, which is about 10 times higher than in the general population, but much lower than the thrombosis risk in persons with protein C, protein S, or antithrombin deficiency. The risk in women who are pregnant or on oral contraceptives is increased about 30-fold, although for women with factor V Leiden taking oral contraceptives the absolute additional number of persons affected is only 3 per 1000.[16] This is because the number of thrombotic events in such women is small compared to the number of oral contraceptive users. The odds ratio for thrombosis in individuals with mutations of both genes for factor V (homozygotes) is increased 30- to 140-fold.[17,18]

Patients with the factor V Leiden mutation have similar clinical manifestations as those with deficiencies of antithrombin, protein C, and protein S. While venous thrombosis is generally observed, there is an increased risk for stroke in the very young[19] and myocardial infarction in persons with additional risk factors such as cigarette smoking.[20]

Other defects in the factor V gene have been identified. Only factor V Cambridge, with a substitution of threonine for arginine at position 306, has been associated with increased risk of thrombosis.[21] Other mutations, such as the substitution of arginine by glycine in Hong Kong Chinese, are of uncertain significance.[22]

Acute thrombotic episodes are treated with heparin and warfarin. Studies[23] have shown about a twofold increased risk for recurrence of thrombosis if warfarin is discontinued within the first 6 months of thrombosis, but whether patients need to remain on treatment for longer than 6 months is unclear. Prophylaxis with adjusted doses of heparin or low-molecular-weight heparin is required at the time of increased risk for thrombosis such as during the perioperative period, while on prolonged bed rest, or pregnancy. Patients with recurrent or life-threatening thrombosis may need indefinite anticoagulant therapy.

Prothrombin G20210A Mutation

A mutation in the regulatory elements of the prothrombin gene leads to overproduction of this protein and an increase in the risk of venous thrombosis.[24] This mutation is a substitution of guanine for adenine at position 20210 in the prothrombin gene. It is observed in 18 percent of patients with a personal and family history of thrombosis. The thrombotic tendency is closely related to the level of plasma prothrombin; most affected patients have prothrombin concentrations in excess of 1.3 U/ml. The relative risk for thrombosis in persons with this mutation has been estimated at 2.8.[25] The prothrombin gene mutation is a risk factor for cerebral venous thrombosis particularly when oral contraceptives are used.[26,27]

Inherited Hyperhomocysteinemia

Homocysteine is an amino acid that is formed during the course of folate metabolism. It undergoes enzymatic conversion to methionine and cystathionine in a series of reactions requiring several enzymes as well as folic acid, vitamin B_{12}, and pyridoxine. In the rare disorder, homocystinuria, the activity of the enzyme cystathionine synthase is decreased, and high concentrations (>50 μmol/L) of homocysteine are present in blood and urine. Most commonly, a thermolabile form of the enzyme methylene-tetrahydrofolate reductase (MTHFR) is inherited, leading to mild hyperhomocysteinemia (10-20 μmol/L).[28] Defects in other enzymes such as cystathionine synthase and methionine synthase have also been reported.[29] More severe increases in homocysteine levels occur if there is concomitant deficiency of folic acid or B_{12}. On the other hand, dietary folate and B_{12} may decrease elevated homocysteine levels even in subjects homozygous for the MTHFR mutation. In fact, there is no statistically significant association between this mutation and venous or arterial thrombosis. What is important is the level of homocysteine itself. Elevated homocysteine concentrations injure the endothelium, decrease nitric oxide (NO) production and protein C activation, and enhance the binding of lipoprotein (a) to fibrin.[30,31] An analysis of 1041 elderly subjects in the Framingham Heart Study showed an increased risk of extracranial carotid artery stenosis when homocysteine levels were in the high normal range.[32] Hyperhomocysteinemia has been found in association with deep vein thrombosis and arterial occlusion, leading to stroke, myocardial infarction, and limb ischemia.[33-36] Patients with elevated levels of this amino acid, or those who have other risk factors for atherosclerosis and values in the high normal range, should receive a trial of treatment with folic acid with/without vitamins B_{12} and B_6.[37-39] This recommendation is supported by a recent study reporting that treatment with a combination of folic acid, B_{12}, and B_6 decreased homocysteine levels and reduced the rate of restenosis and the need for revascularization of the target lesion after coronary angioplasty.[40]

ACQUIRED THROMBOTIC DISORDERS

Acquired (noninherited) factors that predispose to thrombosis are age over 40, obesity, and cancer, as seen in Box 9-2. With regard to cancer, thrombosis occurs three to five times more frequently in cancer patients than in other patients undergoing surgery.[42] Multiple mechanisms are at play that predispose the cancer patient to thrombosis. Because of poor nutrition, the plasma concentrations of the anticoagulant proteins C and S are often decreased, but stress-related procoagulants such as fibrinogen and factor VIII are increased, thereby shifting the coagulation balance in favor of thrombosis. A potent inhibitor of fibrinolysis, plasminogen activator inhibitor-1, is another stress-related factor that is increased in cancer, enhancing clot formation over clot dissolution. Cancer cells may also activate clotting by exposing tissue factor and releasing specific cancer procoagulants. Lastly, tumor cells may injure endothelium and activate platelets and monocytes, encouraging thrombosis.

In patients with arterial thrombosis, the plasma lipid profile is usually examined; some fractions of low-density lipoproteins are particularly vasculopathic and promote thrombosis. In addition, lipoprotein (a) should be specifically measured. This lipid competes with plasminogen for binding sites on fibrin and is therefore thrombogenic.[43] Accelerated atherosclerosis in diabetes or renal failure may also predispose to arterial thrombosis.

Conditions associated with either venous or arterial thrombosis include the antiphospholipid antibody syndrome, hyperhomocysteinemia, myeloproliferative disorders, and heparin-induced thrombocytopenia with thrombosis (HITT) syndrome.

Antiphospholipid Antibody Syndrome

The antiphospholipid antibody syndrome is defined by two principal components: a positive laboratory test for an antiphospholipid antibody and certain characteristic clinical findings. These include venous and/or arterial thrombosis, neuropsychiatric disorders, valvular heart

BOX 9–2

Acquired Conditions Predisposing to Thrombosis[41]

Age over 40
Obesity
Surgery, trauma
Malignancy
Atherosclerosis (diabetes, hypertension, hyperlipidemia)
Antiphospholipid antibody syndrome
Hyperhomocysteinemia
Myeloproliferative disorders
Heparin-induced thrombocytopenia with thrombosis

lesions, thrombocytopenia, and recurrent fetal deaths due to placental infarcts. There are two forms of the syndrome: autoimmune and alloimmune.[44] The autoimmune form may be primary (idiopathic) or secondary to systemic lupus erythematosus or other connective tissue diseases, or associated with drugs such as chlorpromazine. The alloimmune form occurs after infections or in association with malignancies.

The antiphospholipid antibodies are thought to arise because of an event that exposes anionic (negatively charged) membrane phospholipids.[45] These phospholipids are normally located on the inside of cell membranes. When exposed to the flowing blood, they may initiate coagulation. To protect against thrombosis, circulating phospholipid-binding proteins such as ß$_2$-glycoprotein-1 form complexes with negatively charged phospholipids. In genetically susceptible persons, these complexes act as antigens and elicit the formation of antibodies. The antibodies cross-react with complexes of cardiolipin and ß2-glycoprotein-1 and are designated anticardiolipin antibodies (ACA). Antibodies may also develop to complexes of phospholipid and clotting factors (e.g., prothrombin), and these are called lupus anticoagulants (LA). Thus ACA and LA are distinct entities.

The mechanism of the thromboses in this syndrome is under intensive investigation. Most evidence favors the hypothesis that the antiphospholipid antibodies interfere with the protein C/protein S system. Protein C binds to the lipid bilayer of cell membranes and is activated by a complex of thrombin and membrane-bound thrombomodulin. With protein S as a cofactor, activated protein C inactivates factors Va and VIIIa. Resistance to activated protein C manifested by impaired inactivation of factor Va has been observed in patients with the lupus anticoagulant and one or more episodes of thrombosis.[46,47]

Other thrombogenic actions of antiphospholipid antibodies include the formation of immune complexes of antibody and phospholipid-binding protein. These may bind to and cross-link platelet Fc receptors, resulting in platelet activation. Activated platelets promote thrombosis and are consumed, resulting in thrombocytopenia. Another mechanism for thrombosis is based on the effects of the antiphospholipid antibodies on endothelial cells. The antibodies impair the release of prostacyclin, a potent endothelial cell inhibitor of platelet function.[48] Effects on antithrombin and fibrinolysis have also been described.[49]

A variety of clinical manifestations of the syndrome have been recorded. Most prominent among these is thrombosis, involving either arterial or venous vessels, or rarely, both. Men and women are affected equally, and often the thrombi appear before age 40. In patients with the lupus anticoagulant, the risk of thrombosis is increased 9.4-fold, whereas in patients with high titers of anticardiolipin antibody it is only increased 1.9-fold.[50] A typical patient will have recurrent strokes, peripheral arterial occlusion, and myocardial infarction. Others may present with repeated deep vein thromboses and pulmonary emboli. Livedo reticularis is a manifestation of thrombosis in superficial skin arterioles and has the appearance of tiny serpiginous lines in a map-like pattern. It may be seen on the back, arms, or legs and often occurs in association with stroke (Sneddon's syndrome). Other neurologic manifestations are episodes of transient blindness (amaurosis fugax), retinal artery occlusion, and psychoses.

The antiphospholipid antibody syndrome is often suspected in women who have recurrent miscarriages, usually in the second trimester. Examination of the placenta may disclose thrombosed vessels and placental infarcts. Other evidence of the syndrome in these women is thrombocytopenia. In patients with systemic lupus erythematosus, fibrin thrombi may be detected on heart valves using the technique of echocardiography. In a series of 35 patients, Asherson et al[51] detected venous thrombosis in 37 percent, arterial thrombosis in 29 percent, recurrent abortions in 17 percent, livedo reticularis in 37 percent, and valvular heart lesions in 65 percent.

The diagnosis of the antiphospholipid antibody syndrome depends on a characteristic clinical picture combined with a positive test for either the lupus anticoagulant or another antiphospholipid antibody such as anticardiolipin. Detection of the lupus anticoagulant relies on the prolongation of a phospholipid-dependent test of coagulation. Often, the patient will have a prolonged partial thromboplastin time that is not correctable with normal plasma, but shortened by the addition of platelets or phospholipids.[52] However, to detect this, it is necessary that fresh patient plasma be doubly centrifuged or filtered to remove residual platelets, since these may mask the effect of the lupus anticoagulant. Low-titer lupus anticoagulants may not prolong the partial thromboplastin time; it is often necessary to use a sensitive, phospholipid-dependent test such as the diluted Russell viper venom time to recognize them.[53] In patients who are being treated with heparin or warfarin, tests for lupus anticoagulants are altered; the laboratory must be informed of these treatments so that the testing can be modified.

Anticardiolipin antibodies are detected by enzyme-linked immunosorbent assays that are unaffected by patient treatment with anticoagulants. Antibodies of the IgG, IgA, and IgM class are detected and quantified using phospholipid (PL) units. Thus IgG antibodies would be recorded in GPL units and IgM antibodies in MPL units. Antibody titer is important, because low titers are found in 2 percent of blood donors and up to 12 percent of healthy elderly persons.[54] High titers predict the development of deep vein thrombosis,[55] with titers in excess of 30 GPL units associated with deep vein thrombosis.[56] Protein S concentrations decrease in patients with thrombosis and have been noted to vary inversely with the level of anticardiolipin antibody, with the lowest values in patients with the highest antibody titers.[57]

The treatment of patients with the antiphospholipid antibody syndrome is unsatisfactory. Despite the use of heparin and warfarin, patients often experience recurrent strokes and peripheral artery occlusion, resulting in progressive loss of function and disability. Repeated miscarriages despite intensive interventions are also common. Current therapeutic recommendations are mostly based on clinical experience rather than randomized, controlled trials.

Given these reservations, it has been suggested that acute thromboses be treated with heparin in full therapeutic doses, followed by warfarin to maintain the INR at 3-4[58] or warfarin plus aspirin at an INR of 2-3 (the latter is easier to manage and may have less risk of bleeding). While the risk of recurrence is high in patients with lupus anticoagulants, a significant difference was not observed after discontinuation of warfarin when those who were anticardiolipin positive were compared with those who were anticardiolipin negative.[50] While an early study suggested that steroids be used to prevent recurrent miscarriages,[59] only small numbers of patients were evaluated; more recent experience indicates that steroids may be associated with increased, rather than decreased, miscarriages.[60] Most authorities currently recommend the use of aspirin, 80 mg daily, combined with heparin or low-molecular-weight heparin given subcutaneously at therapeutic doses.[61,62]

Hyperhomocysteinemia

As described earlier, hyperhomocysteinemia is a risk factor for venous and arterial thrombotic disease, with odds ratios ranging from 2 to 13.[63] About 12 percent of the population have elevated levels of homocysteine, making this one of the more common risk factors. Patients having hyperhomocysteinemia as well as factor V Leiden, or other risk factors, are especially predisposed to thrombosis. Poor nutritional status associated with deficiencies of folic acid, pyridoxine (vitamin B_6), or vitamin B_{12} increases homocysteine levels. Some of the more important diseases associated with raised homocysteine levels are renal failure, hypothyroidism, pernicious anemia, and severe psoriasis. Supplementing the diet with folate, B_6, and B_{12} decreases homocysteine levels and may slow the progression of vascular disease, as suggested by the previously referenced study of coronary restenosis.[40]

Myeloproliferative Disorders

These conditions are defined by an increase in one or more of the blood elements: red cells (polycythemia), white cells (myeloid leukemia), or platelets (thrombocythemia). Thrombosis may be a presenting manifestation of these disorders, although in some patients bleeding is more prominent. Patients often have an enlarged spleen and almost always an abnormal blood count. Once the diagnosis is established, appropriate management is imperative, especially if an operative procedure is contemplated. For example, in patients with polycythemia, decreasing the hematocrit by phlebotomy may prevent intraoperative hemorrhage.

Perioperative thrombosis in persons with chronic myelogenous leukemia or essential thrombocythemia may be avoided by preoperative treatment with hydroxyurea, a drug that decreases leukocyte and platelet counts. Thus it is always important to review the preoperative blood count and, if abnormal, obtain hematology consultation prior to surgery.

Heparin-Induced Thrombocytopenia With Thrombosis Syndrome

The HITT syndrome occurs in about 1 percent of patients receiving heparin therapy.[64] In patients treated with heparin for longer than 5 days, or in patients re-exposed to heparin, antibodies may develop to a complex of heparin and platelet factor 4 clustered on the surface of the platelet. These complexes trigger the platelet to form microparticles, which promote platelet aggregation, thrombus formation, and thrombocytopenia.[65] Venous thrombosis is more common than arterial thrombosis, and thrombi may occur in the deep veins of the legs, in the pulmonary arteries, and in the axillary, internal jugular, and subclavian veins. Other manifestations are limb gangrene, anaphylactoid reactions, and skin necrosis at sites where heparin has been injected.

The HITT syndrome is significantly less frequent with low-molecular-weight-heparin than with unfractionated heparin, but once the syndrome develops, there is a high degree of cross-reactivity to low-molecular-weight heparins.[66,67] The diagnosis is suspected in patients receiving heparin who experience new thromboses during treatment or whose platelet counts acutely decline by 50 percent or more (Fig. 9-1) and is confirmed by performing tests to detect the presence of heparin-platelet antibodies. Suspicion of HITT should trigger an immediate discontinuation of heparin in all forms and by all routes, including heparin locked catheters and heparin flushes. Platelet transfusions worsen thrombosis and are contraindicated. Cessation of heparin alone may not be sufficient as these patients are at increased risk for thrombosis.[68] Patients with evidence of thrombosis should receive prompt treatment with

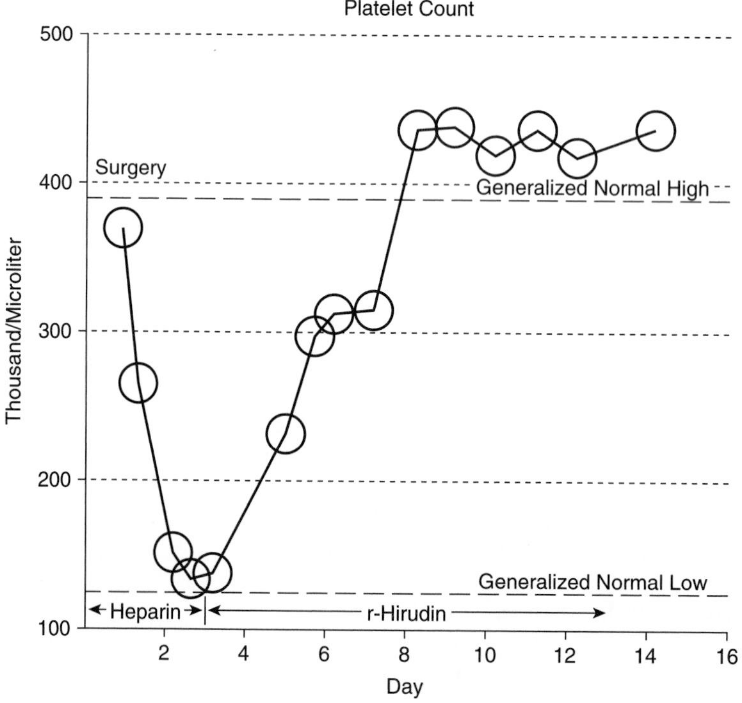

FIG. 9–1. Patient, with previous history of heparin exposure, received heparin for deep vein thrombosis prophylaxis after knee surgery. Postoperatively, he developed a deep vein thrombosis. Platelets were noted to have dropped by half of baseline (note that platelets did not drop below 100,000 per microliter). Heparin was stopped and r-Hirudin (lepirudin) begun with rapid increase in platelet count. Patient was discharged when therapeutic on warfarin.

a direct thrombin inhibitor such as lepirudin[69,70] or argatroban.[71] Therapeutic levels may be monitored by maintaining an APTT 1.5 times normal. Lepirudin is renally excreted, and argatroban is hepatically excreted; caution must be used when giving these agents in the setting of organ dysfunction. Warfarin therapy should be delayed until the patient is stable and the platelet count rises above 100,000 per microliter.[65,72]

PREOPERATIVE EVALUATION FOR HYPERCOAGULABILITY

Screening for hypercoagulability is indicated when there is strong clinical suspicion that a patient is at risk for thrombosis. Screening should not be performed indiscriminately, because the laboratory tests are expensive, test abnormalities require expertise in interpretation, and an abnormal result may stigmatize a patient, prejudicing future insurance coverage. However, persons with the risk factors shown in Box 9-3 should be further evaluated. Thrombosis in the young, especially when it is recurrent, demands explanation. Similarly, a patient with thrombosis of mesenteric, dural, or retinal veins needs evaluation. Many thrombotic disorders are inherited, and family studies are helpful in localizing the cause of the index patient's event. Recurrent fetal loss is often associated with the inherited thrombophilias as well as the antiphospholipid antibody syndrome.

Questions often arise about performing surgery in patients with a previous thrombotic event. Screening is probably not indicated if a thrombosis occurred in association with trauma or surgery and completely resolved with anticoagulant therapy. On the other hand, if the prior thrombosis was not associated with a precipitating event, screening is advisable.

In patients with a family history of venous thrombosis, molecular studies for factor V Leiden and prothrombin G20210A mutations should be requested; if not available, the activated protein C resistance test and prothrombin factor assay may be substituted.[74] In addition, laboratory tests of proteins C, S, and antithrombin should be obtained because deficiency of one of the naturally occurring anticoagulants may occur either in isolation or in combination with factor V Leiden. Homocysteine concentrations should also be measured. If all of the above are within normal limits, testing for abnormalities of fibrinogen, plasminogen, or deficiency of heparin cofactor II may be warranted.

When evaluating abnormal laboratory tests, it is important to consider the clinical setting. Thus, patients with underlying liver disease will have decreased levels of proteins C, S, and antithrombin, since these factors are synthesized by the liver. In persons with the nephrotic syndrome, protein C and antithrombin may be lost in the urine, and the plasma levels of these proteins are decreased. Patients who are pregnant or taking oral contraceptives usually have protein S levels below the normal range. Finally, intravascular clotting per se, manifested as pulmonary emboli, deep vein thrombosis, or disseminated intravascular coagulation (DIC), may be accompanied by a decrease in all of the anticoagulant proteins due to consumption of these factors. For example, a low value for protein S, recorded in a patient with a pulmonary embolus, should not be interpreted as evidence of inherited protein S deficiency. In most patients, repeating the test during convalescence will reveal normal values.

BOX 9–3

Characteristics of Hypercoagulable Patients: Indications for Further Investigation[73]

Venous thrombosis under age 45
Recurrent venous thrombosis
Thrombosis at unusual sites
Arterial thrombosis under age 30
Familial thrombosis
Unexpected neonatal thrombosis
Recurrent fetal loss

Other factors that may affect laboratory tests are the use of anticoagulants and the nutritional status of the patient. Heparin therapy alters most clotting tests, including antithrombin levels (usually slightly below the normal range), and assays for lupus anticoagulant. Warfarin decreases the levels of proteins C and S. The nutritional status of the patient is important because lack of vitamin K will not only prolong the prothrombin time, but also decrease proteins C and S. Low levels of vitamin K occur in patients who have poor food intake or vomiting or who are receiving antibiotics.

MANAGEMENT OF ANTICOAGULATION IN THE PERIOPERATIVE PERIOD

Patients with the above-described disorders may be on long-term anticoagulant therapy. Should operative procedures become necessary, the anticoagulant regimen must be modified. In patients receiving warfarin, an INR of 1.5 or less is considered safe for surgery.[75] Stopping the warfarin 4-5 days prior to operation will permit the INR to decline to this level. The warfarin may then be resumed the evening of operation, with the anticipation that the INR will be in the therapeutic range (2-3) in approximately 3 days. Therefore, for about 6 days (3 days before and 3 days after surgery) the INR will be less than optimal, but it will be below 1.5 for probably less than 2 days. Thus, the actual risk period for recurrence of thrombosis is brief, but the degree of risk depends on a variety of factors, including whether thrombi have been in the arteries or veins, how recently they have occurred, and whether atrial fibrillation or a mechanical heart valve is present. Kearon and Hirsh[75] recommend that patients with a history of recent venous thrombosis (within the previous 2-3 months) receive intravenous heparin postoperatively; for those with more distant thrombosis, the usual postoperative prophylaxis with subcutaneous heparin or low-molecular-weight heparin (LMWH) is advised. Postoperative subcutaneous LMWH is also given to patients with atrial fibrillation or mechanical heart valves. If at all possible, surgery should be avoided within the first month after an acute arterial or venous thrombosis. However, if an operation must be performed, intravenous heparin should be started when the warfarin is stopped, discontinued 6 hours preoperatively, and resumed 12 hours postoperatively as a continuous infusion without a bolus, providing there is no bleeding. LMWH may also be used; dalteparin has been shown to have undetectable anti–factor Xa levels 20 hours after dosing.[76] Therefore dalteparin may be given preoperatively and held on the day of the procedure (18-24 hours after the last dose) and resumed at half-dose 12 hours later with full-dose resumed the following day. When a patient requires emergency surgery within 2 weeks of having a thrombotic event, a vena cava filter is placed. In addition, intravenous heparin is given preoperatively and resumed 12 hours postoperatively unless the patient has an unusual bleeding risk.

REFERENCES

1. Saito H: Normal hemostatic mechanisms. In Ratnoff O, Forbes C, eds: *Disorders of hemostasis,* Philadelphia, 1996, WB Saunders, pp 23-52.
2. Lane D, Bayston T, Olds R et al: Antithrombin mutation databse: 2nd (1997) update—for the Plasma Coagulation Inhibitors Subcommittee of the Scientific and Standarization Committee of the International Society of Thrombosis and Haemostasis, *Thromb Haemost* 77:197-211, 1997.
3. Brunel F, Duchange N, Fischer A et al: Antithrombin III Alger: a new case of Arg 47—Cys mutation, *Am J Hematol* 25:223-224, 1987.
4. Ueyama H, Murakami T, Nishiguchi S et al: Antithrombin III Kumamoto: identification of a point mutation and genotype analysis of the family, *Thromb Haemost* 63:231-234, 1990.
5. Demers C, Ginsberg J, Hirsh J et al: Thrombosis in antithrombin III deficient persons: report of a large kindred and literature review, *Ann Intern Med* 116:754-761, 1992.
6. Thaler E, Lechner K: Antithrombin III deficiency and thromboembolism. In Prentice C, ed: *Clinics in hematology,* London, 1981, WB Saunders, pp 369-390.
7. Schulman S, Tengborn L: Treatment of venous thromboembolism in patients with congenital deficiency of antithrombin III, *Thromb Haemost* 68:634-636, 1992.

8. Bucur S, Levy J, Despotis G et al: Uses of antithrombin III concentrate in congenital and acquired deficiency states, *Transfusion* 38:481-498, 1998.
9. Brenner B, Blumenfeld Z: Thrombophilia and fetal loss, *Blood Rev* 11:72-79, 1997.
10. Preston F, Rosendall F, Walker I et al: Increased fetal loss in women with heritable thrombophilia, *Lancet* 348:913-916, 1996.
11. Teepe R, Broekmans A, Vermeer B et al: Recurrent coumarin-induced skin necrosis in a patient with an acquired functional protein C deficiency, *Arch Dermatol* 122:1408-1412, 1986.
12. Schramm W, Spannagl M, Bauer K et al: Treatment of coumarin-induced skin necrosis with a monoclonal antibody purified protein C concentrate, *Arch Dermatol* 129:753, 1993.
13. Green D, Otoya, J, Oriba H et al: Protein S deficiency in middle-aged women with stroke, *Neurology* 42:1029-1033, 1992.
14. Dahlback B, Carlsson M, Svensson P: Familial thrombophilia due to a previously unrecognized mechanism characterized by poor anticoagulant response to activated protein C: prediction of a cofactor to activated protein C, *Proc Natl Acad Sci USA* 90:1004-1008, 1993.
15. Zoller B, Dahlback B: Linkage between inherited resistance to activated protein C and factor V gene mutation in venous thrombosis, *Lancet* 343:1536-1538, 1994.
16. Vandenbroucke JP, Koster T, Briet E et al: Increased risk of venous thrombosis in oral-contraceptive users who are carriers of factor V Leiden mutation, *Lancet* 344:1453-1457, 1994.
17. Rosendaal F, Koster T, Vanderbroucke I et al: High risk of thrombosis in patients homozygous for factor V Leiden (activated protein C resistance), *Blood* 85:1504-1508, 1995.
18. Ridker P, Hennekens C, Lindpaintner K et al: Mutation in the gene coding for coagulation factor V and the risk of myocardial infarction, stroke and venous thrombosis in apparently healthy men, *N Engl J Med* 332:912-917, 1995.
19. Ganesan V, Kelsey H, Cookson J et al: Activated protein C resistance in childhood stroke, *Lancet* 347:260, 1996 (letter).
20. van der Born J, Bots M, Haverkate F et al: Reduced response to activated protein C is associated with increased risk for cerebrovascular disease, *Ann Intern Med* 125:265-269, 1996.
21. Williamson D, Brown K, Luddington R et al: Factor V Cambridge: a new mutation (Arg306 to Thr) associated with resistance to activated protein C, *Blood* 91:1140-1144, 1998.
22. Chan W, Lee C, Kwong Y et al: A novel mutation of Arg306 of factor V gene in Hong Kong Chinese, *Blood* 91:1135-1139, 1998.
23. Simoni P, Prandoni P, Lensing A et al: The risk of recurrent venous thromboembolism in patients with an Arg506 to Gln mutation in the gene for factor V (factor V Leiden), *N Engl J Med* 336:399-403, 1997.
24. Poort S, Rosendaal F, Reitsma P et al: A common genetic variation in the 3′-untranslated region of the prothrombin gene is associated with elevated plasma prothrombin levels and an increase in venous thrombosis, *Blood* 88:3698-3703, 1996.
25. van der Meer F, Koster T, Vandenbroucke J et al: The Leiden thrombophilia study, *Thromb Haemost* 78:631-635, 1997.
26. Martinelli I, Sacchi E, Landi G et al: High risk of cerebral vein thrombosis in carriers of a prothrombin gene mutation and in users of oral contraceptives, *New Engl J Med* 38:1793, 1998 (letter).
27. Reuner K, Ruf A, Grau A et al: Prothrombin gene G20210A transition is a risk factor for cerebral venous thrombosis, *Stroke* 29:1765-1769, 1998.
28. Rozen R: Genetic predisposition to hyperhomocysteinemia: deficiency of methylenetetrahydrofolate reductase, *Thromb Haemost* 78:523-526, 1997.
29. Gaustadnes M, Rudiger N, Rasmussen K et al: Intermediate and severe hyperhomocysteinemia with thrombosis: a study of genetic determinants, *Thromb Haemost* 83:554-558, 2000.
30. Rodgers G, Conn M: Homocysteine, an atherogenic stimulus, reduces protein C activation by arterial and venous endothelial cells, *Blood* 75:895-901, 1990.
31. Harpel P, Chang V, Borth W: Homocysteine and other sulfhydryl compounds enhance the binding of lipoprotein (a) to fibrin: a potential biochemical link between thrombosis, atherogenesis, and sulfhydryl compound metabolism, *Proc Natl Acad Sci USA* 89:10193-10197, 1992.
32. Selhub J, Jacques P, D'Agostino R et al: Association between plasma homocysteine concentrations and extracranial carotid-artery stenosis, *New Engl J Med* 332:286-291, 1995.
33. den Heijer M, Koster T, Blom H et al: Hyperhomocysteinemia as a risk factor for deep-vein thrombosis, *N Engl J Med* 334:759-762, 1996.
34. Perry I, Refsum H, Morris R et al: Prospective study of serum total homocysteine concentrations and risk of stroke in middle-aged British men, *Lancet* 346:1395-1398, 1995.
35. Clarke R, Daly L, Robinson K et al: Hyperhomocysteinemia: an independent risk factor for vascular disease, *New Engl J Med* 324:1149-1155, 1991.

36. Malinow M, Kang S, Taylor L et al: Prevalence of hyperhomocysteinemia in patients with peripheral arterial occlusive disease, *Circulation* 79:1180-1188, 1989.
37. Glueck C, Shaw P, Lang J et al: Evidence that homocysteine is an independent risk factor for atherosclerosis in hyperlipidemic patients, *Am J Cardiol* 75:132-136, 1995.
38. Franken D, Boers G, Blom H et al: Treatment of mild hyperhomocysteinemia in vascular disease patients, *Arterioscler Thromb* 14:465-470, 1994.
39. Brattstrom L, Israelson B, Bergqvist D et al: Impaired homocysteine metabolism in early onset cerebral and peripheral occlusive arterial disease: effects of pyridoxine and folic acid treatment, *Athersclerosis* 81:51-60, 1990.
40. Schnyder G, Roffi M, Pin R et al: Decreased rate of coronary restenosis after lowering of plasma homocysteine levels, *N Engl J Med* 345:1593-1600, 2001.
41. Carter C, Anderson F, Wheeler A: Epidemiology and pathophysiology of venous thromboembolism. In Hull R, Raskob G, Pineo G, eds: *Venous thromboembolism: an evidence-based atlas,* Armonk, NY, 1996, Futura, pp 8-12.
42. Donati M: Cancer and thrombosis: from phlegmasia alba dolens to transgenic mice, *Thromb Haemost* 74:278-281, 1995.
43. Scanu A, Lawn R, Berg K: Lipoprotein (a) and atherosclerosis, *Ann Intern Med* 115:209-218, 1991.
44. Triplett D: Antiphosopholipid antibody syndrome. In Seghatchian M, Samama M, Hecker S, eds: *Hypercoagulable states,* Boca Raton, Fla, 1996, CRC Press, pp 223-232.
45. Arnout J: The pathogenesis of the antiphospholipid syndrome: a hypothesis based on parallelisms with heparin-induced thrombocytopenia, *Thomb Haemost* 75:536-541, 1996.
46. Marciniak E, Romond E: Impaired catalytic function of activated protein C: a new in vitro manifestation of lupus coagulant, *Blood* 74:426-432, 1989.
47. Potzch B, Kawamura H, Preissner K et al: Acquired protein C dysfunction but not decreased activity of thrombomodulin is a possible marker of thrombophilia in patients with lupus anticoagulant, *J Lab Clin Med* 125:56-65, 1995.
48. Carreras L, Defreyn G, Machin S et al: Arterial thrombosis, intrauterine death, and "lupus" anticoagulant: detection of immunoglobulin interfering with prostacyclin formation, *Lancet* 1:244-246, 1981.
49. Chediak J: Lupus anticoagulants. In Green D, ed: *Anticoagulants: physiologic, pathologic, and pharmacologic,* Boca Raton, Fla, 1994, CRC Press, pp 143-156.
50. Ginsburg J, Wells P, Brill-Edwards P et al: Antiphospholipid antibodies and venous thromboembolism, *Blood* 86:3685-3691, 1995.
51. Asherson R, Khamashta M, Gill A et al: Cerebrovascular disease and antiphospholipid antibodies in systemic lupus erythematosus, lupus-like disease, and the primary antiphospholipid syndrome, *Am J Med* 86:391-412, 1989.
52. Triplett D, Brandt J, Kaczor D et al: Laboratory diagnosis of lupus inhibitors: a comparison of the tissue thromboplastin inhibition procedure with a new platelet neutralization procedure, *Am J Clin Pathol* 79:678-682, 1983.
53. Thiagarajan P, Pengo V, Shapiro S: The use of the dilute Russell viper venom time for the diagnosis of lupus anticoagulants, *Blood* 68:869-874,1986.
54. Love P, Santoro S: Antiphospholipid antibodies: anticardiolipin and lupus anticoagulant in systemic lupus erythematosus (SLE) and in non-SLE disorders, *Ann Intern Med* 112:682-698, 1990.
55. Ginsburg J, Liang M, Newcomer L et al: Anticardiolipin antibodies and the risk for ischemic stroke and venous thrombosis, *Ann Intern Med* 117:997-1002, 1992.
56. Ginsberg J, Wells P, Brill-Edwards P et al: Antiphospholipid antibodies I and venous thromboembolism, *Blood* 86:3685-3691, 1995.
57. Stahl C, Wideman C, Spira T et al: Protein S deficiency in men with long-term human immunodeficiency virus infection, *Blood* 81:1801-1807, 1993.
58. Khamashta M, Cuadrado M, Mujic F et al: The management of thrombosis in the antiphospholipid-antibody syndrome, *N Engl J Med* 332:993-997, 1995.
59. Lubbe W, Butler W, Palmer S et al: Fetal survival after prednisone suppression of maternal lupus-anticoagulant, *Lancet* I:361-363, 1983.
60. Boumpas D, Fessler B, Austin H et al: Systemic lupus erythematosus: emerging concepts, *Ann Intern Med* 123:42-53, 1995.
61. Danilenko-Dixon D, van Winter J, Homburger H: Clinical implications of antiphospholipid antibodies in obstetrics, *Mayo Clin Proc* 71:1118-1120, 1996.
62. Greaves M, Cohen H, MacHin S et al: Guidelines on the investigation and management of the antiphospholipid syndrome, *Br J Haematol* 109:704-715, 2000.

63. Selhub J, D'Angelo A: Hyperhomocysteinemia and thrombosis: acquired conditions, *Thromb Haemost* 78:527-531, 1997.
64. Warkentin T, Kelton J: A 14-year study of heparin-induced thrombocytopenia, *Am J Med* 101:502-507,1996.
65. Warkentin T, Hayward C, Boshkow L et al: Sera from patients with heparin-induced thrombocytopenia generate platelet-derived microparticles with procoagulant activity: an explanation for the thrombotic complications of heparin-induced thrombocytopenia, *Blood* 84:3691-3699, 1994.
66. Warkentin E, Levine M, Hirsh J et al: Heparin-induced thrombocytopenia in patients treated with low-molecular weight heparin or unfractionated heparin, *N Engl J Med* 332:1330-1335, 1995.
67. Greinacher A, Michels I, Mueller-Eckardt C: Heparin-associated thrombocytopenia: the antibody is not heparin specific, *Thromb Haemost* 67:545-549, 1992.
68. Warkentin T: Heparin-induced thrombocytopenia: yet another treatment paradox? *Thromb Haemost* 85:947-949, 2001.
69. Greinacher A, Volpel H, Janssens V et al: Recombinant hirudin (lepirudin) provides safe and effective anticoagulation in patients with heparin-induced thrombocytopenia: a prospective study, *Circulation* 99:73-80, 1999.
70. Greinacher A, Eichler P, Lubenow N et at: Heparin-induced thrombocytopenia with thromboembolic complications: meta-analysis of 2 prospective trials to assess the value of parenteral treatment with lepirudin and its therapeutic aPTT range, *Blood* 96:846-851,2000.
71. Lewis B, Wallis D, Berkowitz S et al: Argatroban anticoagulant therapy in patients with heparin-induced thrombocytopenia, *Circulation* 103:1838-1843, 2001.
72. Wallis D, Workman D, Steen L et al: Failure of early heparin cessation as treatment for heparin-induced thrombocytopenia, *Am J Med* 106:629-635, 1999.
73. Alving B: The hypercoagulable states, *Hosp Pract* 28:109-114, 119-121, 1993.
74. Lane D, Mannucci P, Bauer K et al: Inherited thrombophilia: part 2, *Thromb Haemost* 76:824-834, 1996.
75. Kearon C, Hirsh J: Management of anticoagulation before and after elective surgery, *N Engl J Med* 336:1506-1511, 1997.
76. Douketis J, Crowther M: Twice daily enoxaparin, but not once daily dalteparin, is associated with elevated anti-factor Xa heparin levels at the time of epidural catheter removal, *Blood* 98:707a, 2001 (abstract).

PART THREE

Arterial Diseases

10

Vascular Medicine and Peripheral Arterial Disease Rehabilitation

MITZI A. EKERS □ ALAN T. HIRSCH

Peripheral arterial disease (PAD) is a prevalent, chronic atherosclerotic disease that limits the functional capacity of affected individuals, adversely affects their quality of life, and is associated with a 3- to 10-fold increased risk of myocardial ischemic events or death.[1-4] Progression of PAD to its most severe stages, in which refractory claudication, ischemic rest pain, or nonhealing wound mandates surgical or percutaneous revascularization, is relatively rare, occurring in less than 5-8 percent of those with PAD.[5] When required, vascular surgical or percutaneous revascularization techniques can serve as effective interventions to alleviate disabling limb ischemic symptoms and may be essential to avoid the morbidity of amputation. However, the long-term benefits of successful limb revascularization may be limited if these interventions serve as the sole core of vascular care for this population. Limb revascularization does not modify the underlying atherosclerotic disease process, and long-term success of both endovascular and surgical revascularization is associated with optimal concomitant medical management. The successful long-term treatment of PAD requires the creation of a medical management program that may delay progression of disease, decrease cardiovascular ischemic events, and prolong life. The consistent, lifelong application of such medical therapeutic programs can be augmented by the development of a partnership between the patient, his or her family, and a devoted vascular health care team. A PAD rehabilitation program (PRP) can serve as an ideal environment for the creation of this partnership.

It is important for vascular clinicians to recognize the existence of potential barriers to the delivery of effective medical interventions for PAD. First, many primary care and vascular clinicians alike continue to believe that "conservative care" is an adequate care strategy for those who suffer from PAD. In the last decade, it has become clear that all individuals with PAD, whether symptomatic or asymptomatic, suffer high rates of stroke, myocardial infarction, and death. These outcomes can all be decreased by medical therapies but are too often left "unmanaged" by "conservative care." If global vascular health is our goal, then all vascular clinicians need to be familiar with the comprehensive lifestyle, exercise, and pharmacologic therapies that are proven to be effective in blunting rates of adverse ischemic events that frequently occur in PAD patients.

A second obstacle is the achievement of adequate patient compliance. The success of all medical therapies (e.g., smoking cessation and antiplatelet, lipid-lowering, antihypertensive, and diabetic therapies) requires a trusting, long-term therapeutic relationship. This relationship should encompass the physician, vascular nurse, rehabilitation staff, and other health care professionals. Long-term compliance with medical interventions often requires patients to initiate selected, but potentially major, behavioral and lifestyle modifications that may affect their vocation, relationships, and life goals. Patients with PAD are often among the most motivated to undertake such efforts, as long as they can rely on their vascular clinicians to provide guidance, the rationale for change, and specific tools for success. This chapter describes components of a comprehensive pharmacologic and behavioral approach to the treatment of PAD that can be utilized by all members of the vascular care team (Table 10-1).

TABLE 10–1 The Effects of Selected Medical Interventions on PAD Outcomes

Intervention	Improve Claudication Symptoms	Decrease CAD and Stroke Event Rates	Decrease Mortality
Tobacco cessation strategies	Minimal improvement	Yes	Yes
Antiplatelet therapies	Trend toward benefit (ticlopidine)	20-30%	Yes*
Lipid-lowering therapies	Unknown	Probable (as assessed in CAD cohorts)	Probable (as assessed in CAD cohorts)
Antihypertensive therapies	Unknown	20-35%	Yes

Modified from Hirsch AT, Treat-Jacobson D, Lando HA et al: The role of tobacco cessation, anti-platelet and lipid-lowering therapies in the treatment of peripheral arterial disease, *Vasc Med* 2:243-251, 1997.

*The effect of aspirin, ticlopidine, and clopidogrel on mortality has not yet been directly compared to placebo in a single clinical trial powered to detect such an effect. However, the data for each of these drugs on event-free survival strongly suggest that each agent is likely to be effective in achieving this critical endpoint.

PAD, Peripheral artery disease; *CAD,* coronary artery disease.

PAD is a chronic disease, and its long-term medical management has been reviewed elsewhere.[6,7] Therapeutic medical interventions and PAD rehabilitation can serve together as the fulcrum of vascular health for most individuals with PAD.

A COMPREHENSIVE VASCULAR MEDICINE APPROACH TO PERIPHERAL ARTERIAL DISEASE

Smoking

Tobacco use is the single most important cause of PAD. All forms of tobacco use are known to damage the vascular endothelium, promote intravascular coagulation, and accelerate progression of atherosclerosis. As delineated in Box 10-1, smoking is known to: (1) be the strongest risk factor for the development of de novo PAD, (2) foster progression of PAD from stable claudication to rest pain, (3) promote the failure of all surgical and percutaneous revascularization procedures, (4) increase rates of amputation, and (5) decrease profoundly patient survival.[8-11] The 5-year mortality rate for patients with claudication who continue to smoke is approximately 40-50 percent, predominantly due to myocardial infarction. The PAD patient must understand that continued tobacco use might shorten life so quickly that major life events will be missed (e.g., watching children grow, enjoying retirement, or maintaining

BOX 10–1

The Effects of Tobacco on PAD Disease Progression

- Progression from asymptomatic PAD to stable claudication
- Conversion of stable claudication to rest pain—such progression inevitably requires revascularization
- Increased failure rate of limb bypass grafts and limb angioplasty
- Increased amputation rate
- Accelerated rates of cardiovascular ischemic events—fatal and nonfatal MI, stroke
- Decreased survival

Modified from Hirsch AT, Treat-Jacobson D, Lando HA et al: The role of tobacco cessation, anti-platelet and lipid-lowering therapies in the treatment of peripheral arterial disease, *Vasc Med* 2:243-251, 1997.

PAD, Peripheral arterial disease; *MI,* myocardial infarction.

a meaningful, independent, ambulatory lifestyle). It is important to educate patients with PAD that successful abstinence from smoking is associated with markedly decreased rates of myocardial infarction and stroke, resulting in an impressive improvement in survival.[9,10] Therefore, therapeutic interventions must be invoked immediately because delay by the patient ("I'm not ready to quit this year") or the health care system ("We hope to offer a smoking cessation program next year") may permit death to supervene before the first effective attempt to quit is initiated.

Central to patients' long-term success in smoking cessation is their access to an understanding health care professional who can guide them through this difficult process. The members of the vascular team are ideally positioned to serve in this role. However, they must convey the right attitude in order to successfully facilitate smoking cessation efforts by their patients. There is a prevalent myth among some clinicians that individuals with PAD may be particularly reluctant to quit smoking, although there is no data to support this supposition. Furthermore, the presumption of failure begets continued failure. In contrast, current data confirm that a high percentage of PAD patients successfully quit smoking. For example, approximately only 20-40 percent of elderly individuals with stable claudication are current smokers, although most of this patient group had smoked previously.[11,12] In contrast, patients who present for surgical or percutaneous revascularization due to severe limb symptoms (e.g., severe claudication, ischemic rest pain, or gangrene) are characterized by a high (80-90 percent) rate of current smoking. This is not surprising inasmuch as continued tobacco use is known to accelerate the atherosclerotic and prothrombotic processes that convert stable PAD to limb-threatening ischemia. Health care providers can help those individuals with PAD quit smoking in order to blunt their disease progression to more serious disability or critical limb ischemia.[13,14] The principles and attitudes outlined in Box 10-2 are helpful in promoting successful smoking cessation.

An excellent resource for clinicians who are developing a smoking cessation program is the updated clinical practice guideline, *Treating Tobacco Use and Dependence*, available from the U.S. Department of Health and Human Services.[15] A key recommendation in this guideline is for practitioners to view tobacco use as a treatable chronic disease. From this perspective, it is then easier for clinicians to understand the nature of relapse into previous smoking behaviors and the need for continuing care. Relapse is seen as a recurrence of the disease rather than a failure on the part of the patient or practitioner. It also positions the role of pharmacologic therapy as standard of care so that patients more readily accept this approach instead of attempting to quit on their own.

This comprehensive guideline provides both behavioral and pharmacologic interventions. It includes the "Five As" strategies to help patients who are willing to quit (Table 10-2), effective

BOX 10–2

Attitudes to Consider When Facilitating Successful Smoking Cessation Interventions

- Do not blame the smoker. Recognize the patient as the victim of an addictive drug.
- Clarify the many specific links between the disease and smoking.
- Involve the whole family from grandparents through grandchildren.
- Set realistic expectations for the patient and yourself.
- Be a partner: Help create an individualized smoking cessation plan.
- Invoke action: The patient must set a quit date.
- Utilize both behavioral and pharmacologic adjunctive measures.
- Maintain a reassessment schedule, and utilize follow-up appointments.
- Approve and praise each passing success.
- Smoking cessation is a process and may require several attempts to achieve success.
- Patients with PAD can successfully quit smoking.

PAD, Peripheral arterial disease.

TABLE 10–2 Strategies for Smoking Cessation: The "Five As"

Action	Strategy for Implementation
ASK	Systematically identify all tobacco users at every visit.
ADVISE	Deliver a clear, strong, personalized message to every smoker to quit.
ASSESS	Determine patient's willingness to quit smoking.
ASSIST	Develop a quit plan with the patient using pharmacologic and behavioral techniques.
ARRANGE	Schedule frequent follow-up appointments either in person or by phone.

counseling and behavioral therapies, suggested pharmacotherapies, the "Five Rs" to help motivate patients to quit (Box 10-3), and strategies for relapse prevention. The guideline concludes that treatment for tobacco dependence is safe, clinically effective, and cost effective and as such should be a reimbursed treatment. Support from health plans and insurers will help ensure greater access to tobacco treatment programs.

Smokers who attempt to quit without medical intervention generally encounter a 7-10 percent 1-year success rate. Long-term success rates from behavioral treatment alone remain low. Only about 15-30 percent of smokers remain abstinent 1 year after treatment.[15-17]

BOX 10–3

The "Five Rs" for the Patient Unwilling to Quit at this Time

Smoking is a unique addiction and habit. Each patient has different reasons to smoke and different reasons and methods for quitting. As you try to motivate smokers to quit, help them identify their personal answers to the following:

RELEVANCE: WHY IS QUITTING SMOKING IMPORTANT FOR THIS PATIENT?

Relate smoking to the patient's current disease status and symptoms such as claudication or ulcerations and the impact of this on present lifestyle. Discuss the direct relationship of nicotine to pain from decreased oxygen in the blood, vasoconstriction, etc.

RISKS: WHAT ADDITIONAL HAZARDS FROM SMOKING MUST THIS PATIENT ACKNOWLEDGE?

Does the patient really believe there is substantial risk from smoking? Consider the following: failure of vascular surgery or angioplasty; greater tendency toward blood clotting; increased risk of heart attack, stroke, lung and other cancers; increased risk to spouse and others living in the same house.

REWARDS: WHAT BENEFITS FROM QUITTING SMOKING MEAN THE MOST TO THIS PATIENT?

Help the patient identify rewards that outweigh the risks. For example, better chance at controlling vascular diseases; setting a good example for children or grandchildren; food tastes better; less damage to blood vessels; save money; breath, home, car, clothes smell better; less guilt about exposing others to smoke.

ROADBLOCKS: WHAT IS KEEPING THIS PATIENT FROM QUITTING SMOKING?

Explore whatever barriers the patient identifies: fear of weight gain, belief that he or she cannot afford pharmacotherapy, real enjoyment of smoking, fear of failure, too much stress in his or her life, fear of losing friends.

REPETITION: IF AT FIRST YOU DON'T SUCCEED . . .

For clinicians: Each time you are with a patient who smokes, repeat your message regarding smoking cessation and offer continued assistance.

For patients: Those who have made previous unsuccessful attempts should be helped to learn from those experiences and to make a new plan. Remind them that most people make several attempts before they are successful.

Successful behavior change is a process. Smokers should be advised that it usually requires most people two or three attempts to successfully quit. Patients had to learn how to smoke and now must learn what to do instead of smoke. Smoking cessation is a major decision in their life, and like other major decisions, it should not be undertaken without a concrete plan and a support system to assist them with this process.

Essential components in most behavioral programs include assisting smokers with the following: (1) identification of reasons and benefits or incentives to quit smoking, (2) identification of events or situations that trigger the urge to smoke, (3) identification and practice of alternate coping skills, (4) discussion of the issue of relapse and development of a plan to deal with it ahead of time, and (5) development of a support system to help prepare for the quit date and for the months ahead. A behavior change of this magnitude usually requires frequent follow-up contact, especially soon after the quit date to congratulate success and offer continued encouragement.

Pharmacologic treatment of tobacco addiction includes nicotine replacement strategies and use of antidepressant therapy. Nicotine replacement therapy relieves or minimizes withdrawal symptoms by providing an alternative route to get the desired effects of nicotine while attenuating the reinforcing effects of continued nicotine self-administration.[18] There are four approved nicotine replacement therapies available: the transdermal patch, chewing gum, nasal spray, and inhalers. All of these methods report greater smoking cessation rates compared to placebo.[15] For example, use of the nicotine patch in the general population of smokers has elicited smoking cessation success rates of 23-27 percent at 6-12 months, which is superior to rates achieved with use of placebo.[15] There is also evidence that combining nicotine replacement methods, such as the patch and the gum, may increase long-term abstinence rates.[15] Nicotine patch therapy in patients with medical illnesses, such as smokers with cardiovascular disease, has been proven to be safe and does not increase angina, palpitations, or heart attacks.[19] Patients and families also need to be informed that nicotine replacement therapies do not accelerate any adverse limb events (e.g., worsened limb ischemia) in patients with PAD. This is not surprising because elevation in plasma nicotine levels that occur with nicotine replacement therapies are generally lower than those that occur with smoking. Thus nicotine replacement therapies are useful and safe.

Recent clinical trials have also demonstrated the efficacy of antidepressant therapies as an adjunct for smoking cessation. The use of these agents is based on the observation that nicotine may act as an antidepressant in some smokers.[20] Additionally, the development of a depressed affect or depression during smoking cessation may lead to a relapse.[21,22] In this context, Hurt et al have demonstrated that bupropion can promote a 44.2 percent tobacco abstinence rate at 7 weeks and a 23.1 percent abstinence rate at 1 year in smokers in a well-designed, placebo-controlled trial.[23] Bupropion (also available as Zyban) is safe, although it should not be used in patients with a history of seizures, who actively abuse alcohol, or in whom bupropion would be contraindicated due to the use of other psychotropic medications. Bupropion should be started at least 2 weeks prior to the "quit date" and can also be used as complementary therapy with nicotine replacement agents.

Vascular clinicians should inform their patients that tobacco is the single most important risk factor for PAD and may lead to worsened claudication, ischemic rest pain and ulceration, higher risk of amputation, as well as heart attack, stroke, or death. It is never too late to quit smoking. The entire family, including spouses and children, should be encouraged to participate in the smoking cessation intervention. Patients are not intrinsically self-destructive tobacco users; rather they are victims of a destructive, addictive drug (nicotine). Additional benefits of smoking cessation include decreased health care costs and improved patient survival.

Antiplatelet and Antithrombotic Strategies

PAD is but one overt manifestation of systemic atherosclerosis. Atherosclerosis is a disease that is characterized by disruption of the normal arterial architecture, by endothelial dysfunction, and by a propensity for plaque rupture and thrombosis. Platelet aggregation plays a central role in the progression of atherosclerosis as hemodynamically stable disease progresses to thrombotic occlusion. Such progression can be clinically recognized in patients with PAD in three clinical scenarios. Thrombosis in situ of a stenotic lower extremity artery may present as sudden worsening of previously stable claudication. Second, acute arterial occlusion may occur when thromboembolism suddenly obstructs a lower extremity artery. Third, the slow progression from severe claudication to critical limb ischemia (i.e., the development of rest pain or a nonhealing wound) can occur when thrombus obstructs the subdermal microcirculation. A worsened clinical outcome for patients with PAD can also be associated with the occurrence of thrombotic events in other circulations, as the patient with PAD suffers a coronary (myocardial infarction) or cerebrovascular ischemic (stroke) event. Thrombotic ischemic events in any arterial circulation portend a marked deterioration in the quality of life of the patient with PAD.

The natural history of PAD can be improved by antiplatelet therapies. The potential beneficial effects of aspirin and an aspirin/dipyridamole combination on femoral arterial atherosclerosis progression were reported by Hess et al in a small cohort of patients followed over 2 years.[24] Over this short period of observation, femoral atherosclerosis progression was diminished, with the greatest improvement in those patients who utilized dual antiplatelet therapy. The effects of long-term administration of aspirin on the natural history of atherosclerotic arterial disease have been reported from the Physicians Health Study.[25] This randomized, double-blinded, placebo-controlled trial evaluated the effects of low-dose aspirin (325 mg every other day) in 22,071 male physicians over an average of 60 months of treatment. Those individuals taking aspirin underwent only half as many surgical limb revascularization procedures as those taking a placebo. Aspirin use did not alter the incidence of claudication in the two treatment groups. These data suggest that aspirin decreased the frequency of those thrombotic events that convert stable claudication to critical limb ischemia. This is a remarkable result for a very inexpensive and safe pharmacologic intervention.

Although the benefits of aspirin use in the prevention of myocardial infarction and stroke are clearly defined (preventing as many as 20-30 percent of these ischemic events), many patients with atherosclerotic diseases still suffer recurrent events. There are individuals in whom aspirin use is not well tolerated, due to gastrointestinal bleeding or rarely allergy. This has provided an impetus to evaluate potentially more potent or safer antiplatelet therapies. Ticlopidine was evaluated in patients with PAD in the Swedish Ticlopidine Multicentre Study (STIMS) and smaller trials.[26-28] These studies demonstrated that this adenosine diphosphate (ADP)-receptor antagonist could decrease cardiovascular ischemic event rates, to perhaps improve claudication symptoms, and to improve patient survival. Picotamide, an investigational drug that is known to inhibit platelet thromboxane A_2 (TxA_2) synthase and to antagonize TxA_2 receptors, has also been shown to reduce cardiovascular ischemic events and to improve symptoms in patients with PAD.[29] A randomized, prospective clinical investigation of 2,304 patients treated with picotamide or placebo for 18 months demonstrated that event-free survival was improved in those individuals who were assigned to picotamide therapy. Preliminary evidence also suggested a beneficial effect of this antiplatelet drug on pain-free walking in patients with claudication, although this outcome has not been replicated.[30]

The relative benefits of aspirin and clopidogrel (a ticlopidine-like, ADP-receptor antagonist with potent antiplatelet properties) on rates of myocardial infarction, stroke, and death were reported from the Clopidogrel vs. Aspirin in Patients at Risk of Ischemic Events (CAPRIE) investigation.[31] CAPRIE recruited individuals with differing manifestations of systemic atherosclerosis by including patients who had suffered a recent myocardial infarction, ischemic stroke, or who suffered from established PAD. In CAPRIE, peripheral arterial disease was defined as either (1) self-reported claudication with an ankle-brachial index (ABI) less than 0.85 or (2) a history of prior lower extremity arterial revascularization procedures (either angioplasty or vascular surgery) or amputation. The hypothesis of CAPRIE was that individuals who present with stroke, myocardial infarction, or PAD all suffer comparably high rates of subsequent heart attack, stroke, and vascular death. The CAPRIE investigators recruited 19,185 patients from these three eligible cohorts. The inclusion of 6452 individuals with PAD in the CAPRIE study marks this investigation as one of the largest prospective trials ever performed to evaluate any medical therapy for peripheral arterial disease. Clopidogrel treatment was more effective than standard aspirin, achieving an overall relative risk reduction of 8.7 percent in preventing subsequent ischemic stroke, myocardial infarction, or vascular death in the total study population in this trial. Post hoc analysis demonstrated a more impressive risk reduction in those patients with peripheral arterial disease. Individuals with PAD enjoyed a 23.8 percent risk reduction for these morbid events with clopidogrel use as compared to aspirin treatment alone. The CAPRIE results suggest that PAD patients may be a population of individuals in which the atherosclerotic process can be effectively modulated by antiplatelet therapies.

Current clinical data therefore suggest that all patients with documented limb PAD should receive antiplatelet therapy unless otherwise contraindicated. These benefits of antiplatelet therapies for PAD have achieved broad acceptance by vascular clinicians. Nevertheless, as for many available and effective therapies, antiplatelet therapies remain in the "at risk" PAD population, as many PAD patients remain untreated. In the Minnesota Regional Peripheral Arterial Disease Screening Program, as many as 40 percent of patients with PAD were receiving no antiplatelet therapies.[12] These regional data were confirmed in the large national PAD Awareness Risk and Treatment: New Resources for Survival (PARTNERS) study of PAD standards of care. In PARTNERS, patients with PAD were consistently offered antiplatelet therapy at lower rates compared to individuals with other cardiovascular diseases. In particular, individuals with a new PAD diagnosis were no more likely to receive an antiplatelet medication than individuals with no atherosclerosis.[32] Thus, the potential benefits of antiplatelet therapies in preventing heart attack, stroke, and death in those with PAD will depend not only on the availability of these drugs at low cost, but on the commitment of both nurses and physicians to promote their long-term use in these patients.

Lipid-Lowering Strategies

Atherosclerosis is a complex, polygenic disorder that is modulated by serum lipids, in concert with a multitude of other factors that may damage the fragile endothelial lining of both large- and medium-sized arteries and arterioles. The penetration of lipoproteins across the endothelium permits the initial development of a fatty streak, especially at sites of altered shear stress, such as at arterial bifurcations. Oxidation of these lipoproteins within the arterial wall may serve as a central mechanism that promotes the subsequent release of chemoattractant proteins, causing monocytes to bind to the arterial wall, to undergo conversion to macrophages, and to continue the oxidation of low-density lipoproteins (LDL). The early atherosclerotic plaque continues to accumulate cholesterol, macrophages, and to initiate an inflammatory process that further promotes smooth muscle cell proliferation and inhibits endothelial healing of plaque ulcerations. Such complex atheromatous arterial lesions, regardless of the severity of the associated arterial stenosis, serve as the substrate upon which subsequent plaque fissuring can suddenly begin to attract platelets and initiate an aggressive thrombotic event.

Plasma lipids are transported in the blood attached to lipoproteins, which serve critical functions in modulating the efficient transfer of cholesterol and triglycerides from the gut, to the liver, and to peripheral tissues. Lipoproteins include easily measured components, such as LDL, high-density lipoproteins (HDL), and very low-density lipoproteins (VLDL), as well as a number of other intermediate particles. Elevated plasma levels of LDL and VLDL are associated with an increased risk of atheroma development and of ischemic events. In contrast, high HDL levels serve a protective role in transporting cholesterol from peripheral cells to the liver for processing and biliary excretion. Epidemiologic data confirm that elevations in LDL cholesterol are associated with an increased risk of cardiovascular disease, both in the general population as well as in individuals with PAD.[33] Patients with PAD may also demonstrate a pattern of lipid abnormalities that includes a low HDL–high triglyceride profile, which also confers cardiovascular risk.[34]

Effective lipid management should also be considered a mandatory component of the medical therapy of patients with PAD. This strategy has been sanctioned by the updated

National Cholesterol Education Program (NCEP) Adult Treatment Panel III (ATP III) guidelines that recommend that patients with objective evidence of atherosclerotic occlusive disease be treated by diet and pharmacologic therapy to achieve an LDL cholesterol less than 100 mg/dl.[35] For individuals with PAD, these guidelines apply whether the patient is symptomatic or asymptomatic. The implication is that any objective evidence of PAD (whether defined as a decreased ABI, by other noninvasive vascular laboratory or angiographic evidence of PAD, or by a prior limb arterial revascularization) defines a population at risk of cardiovascular ischemic events. This is logical inasmuch as some individuals with moderately severe PAD may not present with classic claudication symptoms. For example, some elderly individuals who at one time were limited by claudication may limit their activities of daily living to the point that claudication is no longer induced. Other individuals may have concomitant illnesses (e.g., degenerative joint disease, neuropathy) that also limit functional status, which may mask claudication. Finally, patients in whom limb revascularization strategies have been completely successful may have their claudication relieved, while remaining at risk of the coronary and cerebrovascular events that occur in patients with a systemic atherosclerotic disease.

Lipid-lowering strategies have been demonstrated to have beneficial, though small, effects on the progression of femoral atherosclerotic arterial disease. The Cholesterol Lowering Atherosclerosis Study (CLAS) of Blankenhorn et al assessed the rates of both coronary and femoral atherosclerosis disease progression in a cohort of 162 middle-aged, nonsmoking men in a double-blind, placebo-controlled study of dietary vs. aggressive lipid-lowering drug treatment.[36] Patients were treated either by combined dietary modification and colestipol and niacin therapy or by dietary management alone over a relatively brief 2-year study period. These data demonstrated that the rate of femoral arterial atherosclerosis progression, as assessed angiographically, was decreased and atherosclerosis regression was greater in those subjects who achieved optimal effective lipid lowering. These relatively short-term angiographic observations have been extended in the Program on the Surgical Control of the Hyperlipidemias (POSCH) study.[37] In these patients, lipid normalization was achieved by ileal bypass surgery in an era prior to the availability of statin medications. The observations of POSCH are unique due to the extended 10-year period of treatment and follow-up, which has yet to be replicated in any study of a pharmacologic intervention. As in the CLAS trial, the rate of femoral arterial atherosclerosis disease progression was diminished; more impressively, the rate of development of symptomatic claudication was also reduced by 27 percent. Finally, other data also suggest that the development of new claudication symptoms can be diminished by lipid normalization. In patients with coronary artery disease (CAD) who are treated aggressively to normalize LDL cholesterol, as was accomplished in the Scandinavian Simvastatin Survival Study (4S), the development of new symptomatic claudication was decreased.[38,39] There are as yet no published data to document any short-term beneficial effect of lipid lowering on claudication symptoms in patients with established PAD.

Data from coronary intervention trials has proven that survival is improved in high-risk patients with CAD in whom diet and/or drug intervention achieves an LDL cholesterol level of 100 mg/dl or lower (e.g., the Scandinavian Simvastatin Survival Study [4S], West of Scotland, PLAC I and II and CARE trials, and others).[38,40] Such lipid intervention trials have not yet been prospectively performed in any large cohort of individuals with PAD as the primary manifestation of atherosclerosis. The recently completed Heart Protection Study has provided the first prospective database to document that LDL lowering can markedly decrease cardiovascular event rates.[41] This landmark study of 20,536 individuals with prior myocardial infarction (MI), other manifestations of atherosclerosis (e.g., cerebrovascular disease or PAD), diabetes, or treated hypertension randomized patients to either simvastatin (40 mg), an antioxidant cocktail, or placebo. Use of the antioxidant vitamins did not alter any cardiovascular outcome. In contrast, use of simvastatin in the total study population was associated with a 25 percent risk reduction for all-cause stroke, 27 percent reduction in nonfatal myocardial infarction and coronary death, and 24 percent reduction in coronary and noncoronary revascularization procedures. This study included 2701 patients with PAD, who achieved a comparable risk reduction for each outcome as was observed in other risk cohorts in this trial. Thus, the evidence demonstrating the benefit of lipid normalization in general, and of LDL lowering in particular, is compelling.

Unfortunately, despite the potential benefit of lipid normalization (and perhaps because of the absence of many prospective trials in individuals with PAD), current data document that less than 8-15 percent of individuals with PAD in the United States in 1996 received lipid-lowering drug therapies.[12,32] This continued underrecognition by patients and clinicians of the ischemic risk of PAD and the associated undertreatment of hypercholesterolemia is a lost opportunity for cost-effective prevention.

Hypertension, Diabetes, and Estrogen Replacement Therapies

The progression of atherosclerosis is accelerated by the synergistic adverse effects of hypertension and diabetes. For women, epidemiologic data suggest that the clinical manifestations of atherosclerosis are delayed by approximately a decade, but accelerate in the postmenopausal state. Individuals with hypertension face approximately a twofold increased risk of developing claudication, and the risk of stroke, heart attack, and death from hypertension is magnified in individuals with PAD.[42] It is particularly important for all clinicians to be aware of the increased risk posed by isolated systolic hypertension, as well as diastolic hypertension. Treatment of elevated blood pressure, whether by lifestyle or pharmacologic means, should normalize both values in all hypertensive individuals.[43] Successful long-term treatment of high blood pressure should include a discussion with the patient of the specific goal blood pressure as well as an evaluation of the contribution of lifestyle factors (e.g., diet, weight, exercise, alcohol intake, stress) to high blood pressure and education regarding the use of both lifestyle and pharmacologic interventions. Most patients with PAD should achieve a blood pressure of less than 135/85 mm Hg, and a lower blood pressure is optimal in patients with hypertension and diabetes. While hypertension should be controlled in all patients, the choice of pharmacologic agents is generally not altered by the PAD diagnosis. In particular, beta-blocker medications (both selective and nonselective beta-antagonists) can be used without an adverse impact on claudication in patients with peripheral arterial disease.[44-46] There is increasing interest in the use of angiotensin-converting enzyme (ACE) inhibitors in patients at risk of cardiovascular ischemic events, as the blockade of angiotensin improves endothelial function and diminishes atherosclerotic events beyond that predicted by blood-pressure lowering. The Heart Outcomes Prevention Evaluation Study demonstrated that ACE inhibition in a high-risk population of 9297 patients reduced the primary endpoint of death from vascular causes, nonfatal myocardial infarction, or stroke.[47] This study included 4051 patients with PAD (44 percent of the study population), and event reduction by ramipril was comparable in patients with peripheral arterial disease as in the other populations at risk. Although successful treatment of hypertension is known to reduce the risks of ischemic coronary and cerebrovascular events, the effect of antihypertensive treatment on the symptomatic progression of PAD has not yet been evaluated.

Diabetes is associated with more premature, multisegmental, and rapid progression of PAD and involvement of more distal limb arterial sites. The neuropathy associated with diabetes increases the risk of development of foot ulcers and can either mask or mimic ischemic rest pain. The diagnostic sensitivity of the ankle-brachial index measurement can be decreased by medial arterial calcification, which may artifactually raise the ankle systolic blood pressure due to the noncompressibility of these arteries. Optimal achievement of tight glucose control in diabetics is associated with an improved natural history of microvascular disease (e.g., retinopathy and microalbuminuria). However, the effects of diabetic management on large vessel arterial occlusive disease in this population remain unclear in the absence of a controlled, prospective clinical trial. The Diabetes Control and Complications Trial evaluated 1441 patients with type 1 diabetes and compared the benefits of intensive and conventional insulin therapy. A trend toward a reduction of cardiovascular events ($p = 0.08$) was demonstrated in the intensive treatment cohort, but peripheral arterial disease endpoints were not changed.[48] The United Kingdom Prospective Diabetes Study evaluated 3867 patients with type 2 diabetes randomized to intensive drug treatment using sulfonylurea or insulin with dietary therapy.[49] A similar trend toward a reduction in myocardial infarction ($p = 0.05$) was observed in the intensive glycemic treatment group, but the rates of amputation due to peripheral arterial disease were not reduced in this study. In summary, optimal diabetic management in patients with either type 1 or type 2 diabetes has been proven to decrease cardiovascular ischemic events but has not yet been proven to decrease rates of amputation in patients with PAD.

Estrogen replacement therapy in postmenopausal women with overt atherosclerosis had long been assumed to offer a beneficial effect on cardiovascular ischemic event rates.[50,51] The Heart and Estrogen/Progestin Replacement Study evaluated the effects of estrogen therapy in 2763 postmenopausal women with coronary artery disease.[52] The administration of estrogen in this population did not alter the prospective incidence of aortic or carotid surgery, leg revascularization, or lower-extremity amputation. Postmenopausal use of estrogens may also decrease graft patency after femoropopliteal bypass surgery.[53] Although the decision to initiate estrogens must always include an individualized discussion of the relative benefits and risks, PAD alone in most women currently poses no major indication or contraindication to treatment. Postmenopausal women with PAD should be considered for estrogen replacement therapy by their primary care physician based on their global health care goals.

The Role of Pharmacologic Treatment of Claudication

Two medications are approved in the United States to relieve the symptom of intermittent claudication. These two drugs are pentoxifylline and cilostazol and are discussed in another chapter of this text (Chapter 8). Of these two, cilostazol has been shown to be the most effective in improving claudication symptoms. While pharmacotherapy is effective in offering symptom relief, supervised exercise has been proven to be more effective than either medication in patients who can comply with such an exercise program. While the potentially synergistic benefit of exercise and pharmacotherapy has not been objectively evaluated, it is common for patients to utilize both nonrevascularization options together. Once improvement is achieved after 3 months of dual treatment by exercise and medications, patients must be instructed to continue to exercise in order to maintain functional benefit. As well, patients who improve with pentoxifylline or cilostazol use alone may benefit from the improved atherosclerosis risk factor control that is often achieved in individuals who perform daily exercise. Exercise increases HDL cholesterol, lowers triglycerides, affords better control of glucose, blood pressure, and weight, and is an excellent aid in a smoking cessation program.

The Role of Exercise in Management of Peripheral Arterial Disease

Symptomatic individuals with PAD, whether presenting with claudication, rest pain, or ischemic ulceration, have usually restricted their activities of daily living prior to their seeking medical help. The discomfort of intermittent or persistent limb pain contributes to a profound deconditioning that can be detected even in community-based (nonreferred) individuals with PAD.[12] Reduced blood flow and lack of adequate oxygen to the legs may lead to a complex series of changes that affect muscle fibers. This results in a decrease in muscle strength, so patients with PAD experience a decline in walking ability, which perpetuates their disability[54] (Fig. 10-1). The postoperative bed rest required after successful surgical revascularization may also unavoidably induce iatrogenic deconditioning. Independent ambulation and freedom of mobility are the major end-organ functions of the lower extremities. This decreased mobility in patients with PAD represents a measurable factor that diminishes the quality of life of those with this disease.[55-58] Therefore, subjective, patient-derived indices of improved ambulation, whether assessed by treadmill distances or questionnaire (vs. angiographic patency rates), serve as the optimal patient-focused treatment goal for individuals with claudication. In this light, exercise training and rehabilitation can serve as vitally important treatment modalities, and as a mainstay of treatment, for patients with claudication.

The efficacy of claudication exercise training was established more than 30 years ago and has been reconfirmed by numerous investigations over the past decade.[54,59-65] Essentially all

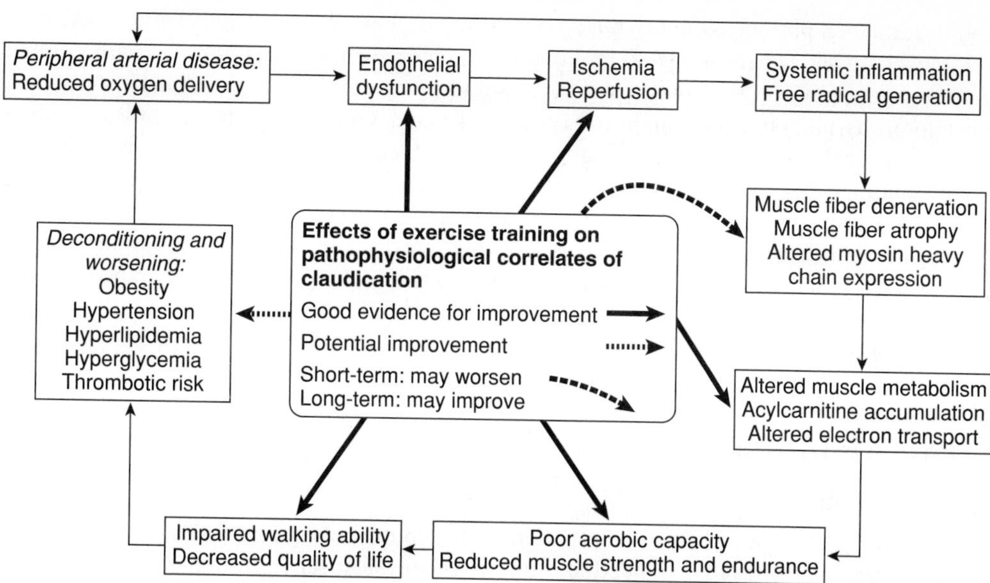

FIG. 10–1. The cycle of disability associated with peripheral arterial disease and claudication, and the potential role of exercise training to improve systemic and limb pathophysiology, functional capacity, and quality of life. The *boxes along the top and right side* of the figure represent potential pathophysiologic cellular and end-organ mechanisms that underlie the disability of peripheral arterial disease and claudication. The *boxes along the bottom and left side* represent the adverse consequences of peripheral arterial disease on patient functional capacity, symptoms, quality of life, and atherosclerosis risk factors. The *solid arrows* outline pathophysiologic mechanisms and patient outcomes for which there is good evidence for improvement with exercise training. The *short dashed arrow* represents the potential for improvement with exercise training that has yet to be studied prospectively in patients with claudication. The *curved dashed arrow* indicates that exercise training may potentially worsen these selected end-organ mechanisms in the short term. However, these potential deleterious short-term responses may be attenuated during the long-term adaptation to exercise training. (From Stewart KJ, Hiatt WR, Regensteiner JG et al: Exercise training for claudication, *N Engl J Med* 347(24): 1941-1951, 2002.)

studies of the efficacy of exercise training have demonstrated an improvement in both the pain-free walking time (the intermittent claudication distance, or ICD) and the maximal walking time (the absolute claudication distance, or ACD). Using a constant-load treadmill protocol, these investigations have demonstrated improvements that range from 50 percent to 300 percent. Similarly, exercise training may elicit improvements in maximal walking distance of 25 percent to 200 percent. The compliant patient in a supervised therapeutic program can expect to double the ICD and ACD. Although many clinicians continue to speculate that exercise training might improve performance in patients with claudication by augmentation of collateral blood flow, current data do not support this hypothesis. Alternative explanations remain plausible, such as exercise-induced decreases in blood viscosity, patients' learning to modify their walking techniques to involve more biomechanically efficient (and perhaps less ischemic) muscles, and increased ischemic pain tolerance.[54,66] It has been speculated that abnormal skeletal muscle oxidative metabolism, with accumulation of acylcarnitines, denervation of muscle bundles (as documented by both electrophysiologic and histopathologic studies), and/or a selective loss of type II myofibers in ischemic limbs could also underlie the disability of claudication and the mechanism of exercise-associated improvement.[67,68] However, while the contribution of any (or of all) of these mechanisms in response to exercise training remains uncertain, clinical data unambiguously support the conclusion that impressive improvements in pain-free and maximal walking distance can be consistently gained for patients in such programs.

Many clinicians and patients may derive a sense of wonder that such functional improvements can be obtained from supervised exercise programs in the absence of a readily explicable and documented physiologic mechanism. Nevertheless, there are many effective medical interventions that yield beneficial results and that have achieved "market acceptance" with minimal question (e.g., physical therapy for low back and knee injuries in lieu of surgical approaches). Therefore, vascular clinicians might reserve greater wonder, perhaps, that the clinical database supporting a role for exercise rehabilitation has not yet led to the widespread promulgation of the technique. Dissemination of effective medical interventions has historically first required widespread education of clinicians, who can then create such programs, as well as acceptance of the intervention by health care payers. Integrated medical approaches to common vascular diseases always seek to utilize the most effective and the most cost-effective therapeutic interventions that can safely improve patient-focused outcomes. Rehabilitation techniques can serve this role for individuals with PAD.

PAD REHABILITATION

Goals and Objectives

The ultimate goal of a PRP is to help patients gain control over their disease so that debilitating consequences may be avoided and improved physical function may be restored. This secondary prevention program uses a biopsychosocial approach to provide the crucial link between palliative and "curative" interventions to achieve this goal.

Improving functional capacity and controlling the progression of atherosclerosis demand major changes in behavior and lifestyle that patients often find difficult to make on their own. The staff of a PRP can empower patients to make these changes by focusing on three objectives: (1) to provide a sound knowledge base of vascular disease and its treatment, (2) to help patients discover their personal motivation to take action, and (3) to partner with patients in developing a personalized action plan that will work for them. A center-based rehabilitation program offers the direct and frequent supervision by professionals coupled with the peer support of other participants that promotes better compliance and ultimately greater success.

A Peripheral Arterial Disease Rehabilitation Model

Modeled after cardiac rehabilitation, most PAD rehabilitation programs are offered in a formal rehabilitation center. Some programs are integrated into existing cardiac rehabilitation facilities, while others may be developed as freestanding vascular rehabilitation programs. Reimbursement constraints have discouraged the proliferation of PRPs. After more than a decade of lobbying, Current Procedural Terminology (CPT) code 93668 was approved in 2001 for structured PAD rehabilitation sessions[69] (Box 10-4). This code has not yet achieved universal reimbursement, and it is yet to be determined what payers will honor the code and how much reimbursement will be provided. Vascular clinicians should use this code to initiate a

BOX 10–4

Summary of CPT Code 93668 for Peripheral Arterial Disease Rehabilitation

- Series of sessions lasting 45-60 minutes per session.
- Involves use of either a motorized treadmill or track.
- Patients walk to achieve symptom-limited claudication.
- Each session supervised by a nurse or exercise physiologist.
- Adjust workload to patient's claudication threshold and other cardiovascular limitations.
- Development of angina symptoms, new arrhythmias, or patient's inability to progress may require further physician review. These physician services are reported separately under appropriate level evaluation/mangement (E/M) code.

BOX 10–5

The Vascular Rehabilitation Model

PHASE I
Inpatient education
Introduction to Phase II

PHASE II
Outpatient physical reconditioning
In-depth patient education
Home exercise program

PHASE III
Maintenance program (at home or at the center)
Minimal supervision

care dialogue with insurance companies and Medicare officials in each state and should link use of the code with provision of data on the positive outcomes of these programs.

PRPs typically consist of three phases of instruction (Box 10-5). Each phase is independent of the others and is designed to meet the needs of patients at different stages of their disease process. The new CPT code is designed only for interventions described here as Phase II.

Phase I

Patients hospitalized for a revascularization procedure may be particularly receptive to advice about PAD and how to avoid further invasive treatment. In Phase I of PAD rehabilitation, a member of the rehabilitation staff, a vascular nurse specialist, or the hospital staff nurses can initiate the educational process through one-on-one or group instruction. Because patients may be hospitalized for as little as 8 hours for some interventions, it is not a Phase I objective to teach patients everything they need to know about vascular disease but merely to increase their level of awareness of several key points.

First, patients need to understand the etiology of the disease that necessitated their revascularization. The disease process and the symptoms it causes, the risk factors, and the revascularization procedure performed to alleviate those symptoms are discussed.[70] To facilitate this part of the instruction, excellent patient education information is available from the Society for Vascular Nursing and the Vascular Disease Foundation.[71,72]

Second, patients need to become more acutely aware of their circulatory system. What improvements have they noticed since the procedure? Perhaps rest pain has been alleviated, or a walk down the entire length of the hallway no longer produces calf pain. When they get home, they need to constantly evaluate and document their improved walking ability. Any decrease in this level of functioning or a return of previous symptoms must be reported immediately. Instruction should be given on how to safely care for themselves at home during their recuperation. Precautions include careful inspection and meticulous care of feet and incisions.

Third, patients need to understand that the surgical or interventional procedure does not cure the arterial disease, as well the necessity of significant lifestyle changes to control the disease process and to enhance the long-term success of the revascularization. In many cases, patients know what they need to do but not how to do it. Providing just a few initial actions such as a simple walking regimen, some basic dietary instruction, and tips on smoking cessation reinforces the importance of starting immediately to make changes.

An active Phase I program provides an unprecedented opportunity for hospital staff nurses, vascular nurse specialists, and rehabilitation staff to collaborate in secondary prevention teaching. It is at this stage when patients can be moved beyond merely contemplating behavior change to the action stage of "choosing a healthier lifestyle."[73] It is also an excellent method of identifying and initiating further discussions with potential candidates for Phase II of the PRP. While doing so, the vascular team conveys an understanding of the difficulty in making lifestyle changes and informs patients that expert help is available through the Phase II component. Careful follow-up of these initial patient contacts will ensure timely referral into Phase II.

Phase II

Phase II of the PRP provides initial and ongoing assessments, regular physical reconditioning sessions, and in-depth education on an outpatient basis. The long-term success of this phase depends on integration of the classroom information and techniques into the patient's daily home routine. Frequent evaluation, continuous encouragement, and consistent reinforcement of information facilitate this process.

Candidates for Phase II are referred by a physician or nurse practitioner and have a diagnosis of PAD manifested by intermittent claudication. This diagnosis should be based on a history and physical assessment and an objective hemodynamic evaluation such as Doppler pressures with a calculated ABI.

ASSESSMENT. Hemodynamic tests document the presence and severity of the arterial disease but do not always correlate well with functional status or exercise capacity. Conversely, participation in a PRP may improve both functional status and exercise capacity without noticeable improvement in hemodynamic measurements. Therefore, patients must undergo a comprehensive assessment using appropriate tests and evaluation tools to determine their entry-level status. These baseline values will be used to determine the effectiveness of the PRP in achieving the desired outcomes. Areas to be assessed include the following:

- Evaluation of coronary disease
- Clinical evaluation of exercise capacity
- Evaluation of daily functional status
- Impact on quality of life
- Presence and severity of atherosclerotic risk factors

Coronary Disease. Because PAD is a marker for coronary artery and other cardiovascular diseases, prospective Phase II patients should usually complete a monitored graded exercise test. This test is necessary to determine the clinical significance of any cardiac disease, to evaluate the relative risk of entering the program, and to assist in documenting the patient's exercise capacity. Information obtained is also used in calculating the individual exercise prescription.

It is beyond the scope of this chapter to discuss the various graded exercise testing protocols and clinical indications. The presence and severity of the patient's symptoms will determine the most appropriate protocol to use. For example, patients with asymptomatic PAD may be able to complete a treadmill evaluation using a standard Bruce protocol, but the patient with significant claudication will be severely limited, resulting in a submaximal test. In this case, a bicycle test or pharmacologic stress test might afford a more sensitive evaluation of cardiac status. Detection of significant myocardial ischemia may occasionally warrant further diagnostic evaluation and, perhaps, referral into a cardiac rehabilitation program.

Exercise Capacity. Historically, treadmill tests have been used to evaluate the severity of claudication and effectiveness of various interventions, such as exercise therapy, pharmacologic therapies, and revascularization procedures. Traditionally, a constant-load treadmill test was performed, using a fixed speed (1.5-2.0 mph) and an unchanging, predefined grade (0-12 percent). The objective assessment of functional capacity was defined by the time to the onset of claudication (the intermittent claudication distance, ICD) as well as the maximum or absolute claudication distance (or ACD). Several limitations to constant-load testing for PAD patients have been identified and the usefulness of the treadmill technique amplified by simple modifications.[74]

The objective functional assessment of patients with PAD may ideally be performed via application of treadmill protocols that can simultaneously assess both exercise capacity and cardiac status. Such simultaneous assessments often rely upon the use of graded treadmill protocols. There are two graded protocols in common use that offer practical alternatives to the traditional constant-load (fixed) protocol. For each protocol, the treadmill speed is held constant at 2.0 mph and patients are asked to walk at an initial 0 percent grade. The Hiatt protocol is characterized by sequential 3.5 percent increases in grade every 3 minutes, while the Gardner-Skinner protocol increases the grade by 2.0 percent every 2 minutes.[75,76] During these studies, patients are asked to indicate the location and time of onset of their claudication, and the maximum claudication distance is recorded. Any concomitant coronary ischemic symptoms are also recorded, and in many centers, simultaneous 12-lead cardiac monitoring may be performed in recognition of the coronary ischemic burden of the PAD population. These graded protocols have been validated in the PAD population, and initial data suggest that they demonstrate improved reproducibility as well as an ability to accommodate the patients of widely varied PAD functional limitations. A review of the sensitivity and specificity of fixed and graded treadmill protocols as an objective index of claudication treatment effectiveness has been reviewed elsewhere.[74] Results of objective exercise tests should be considered for inclusion as both baseline and outcome measures for patients enrolled in a Phase II PAD rehabilitation program. In addition to providing the rehabilitation program with objective efficacy data, such testing may provide patients with an index of their current functional status and make it easier to set specific therapeutic goals to be reached by the completion of the PRP. Inasmuch as successful vascular rehabilitation can provoke major improvements in exercise capacity, graded stress testing performed with cardiac monitoring can verify the safety of the exercise intervention when inducible coronary ischemia is not observed. In our experience, unmasking of major coronary ischemic symptoms or ST depression is rare. This added measure of safety can provide both the patient and the rehabilitation therapist alike a "green light" for a vigorous exercise program. Confidence in such a program by patient and therapist may well increase the likelihood of long-term success.

Functional Status. The treadmill provides information about claudication distance in a "clinical" setting but does not determine the impact of claudication on the patient's ability to perform daily activities. Improved physical function is one of the goals of a PRP; therefore, baseline functional status must be documented and used as the standard against which the patient's improvement will be measured. Use of appropriate questionnaires, such as the Walking Impairment Questionnaire and the Peripheral Arterial Disease Physical Activity Recall questionnaire, provide documentation of functional status before and after participation in the PRP.[74,77]

Quality of Life. Determining the impact of disease on quality of life may provide some of the most useful information from the entire assessment process. Resumption of those important activities that patients cannot enjoy due to limiting claudication becomes their motivation to make lifestyle changes and to comply with the exercise program. At present there is no quality of life questionnaire specific to PAD. However, the Medical Outcomes Study (MOS SF-36) is one questionnaire that has been used to evaluate the impact of disease on general health perceptions and of mental health, social function, and vitality domains.[78,79] Regardless of which questionnaire is used, it is recommended that such a subjective quality of life instrument be administered before starting Phase II and repeated at the completion of the program.

Atherosclerosis Risk Factors. During the assessment interview, the PRP should document the presence of all atherosclerosis risk factors (as outlined at the beginning of this chapter) and any risk factor treatments currently being provided and determine if risk factor goals have been achieved. From these data, the PRP and referring physician can develop a more aggressive risk factor intervention that can be implemented during the rehabilitation program. Too often cardiac and vascular rehabilitation programs focus solely on the exercise component of the program, with minimal attention to modification of risk factors. Physical reconditioning is only one intervention in the treatment regimen. Each contact with patients during the rehabilitation program must be fully utilized to reinforce teaching and monitor compliance with all aspects of treatment.

Once these physical parameters have been assessed, the assessment interview should focus on determining the patient's goals and expectations of the program. Patients benefit from a clear understanding of what the program does and does not offer. Some common misconceptions may include a presumption that participation in the program will ensure that surgery can be avoided, that the disease or symptoms will not worsen, or that a 12- or 24-week program of exercise is all that is necessary to "cure" the problem.

Goals must be realistic, safe, practical, and mutually acceptable to the patient and rehabilitation staff. Long-term goals (3-6 months) are important, but realistic short-term goals (1-3 weeks) appear more achievable, encourage patients to start immediately, and serve as early determinants of progress. Early goal attainment is also its own reward, providing the positive motivation patients need to continue with the program.

Allocating sufficient time (perhaps up to 2 hours) for this initial assessment interview cannot be overemphasized. Davis encourages us to convey a "healing attitude" for patients and refers to this interaction as the "helping interview."[80] She cautions practitioners that first impressions do count and that obtaining the patient's trust as early as possible is crucial to the rehabilitation process. She says that this initial interview " . . . is the cornerstone for the structure of care we give. Patients come to us worried and often in pain. They feel vulnerable and in need of our help and understanding. . . . As health professionals, the burden is on us to recognize that the patient feels at a distinct disadvantage and to reassure and support . . . At this initial meeting, interest, genuineness, acceptance and positive regard are critical to establishing a healing relationship."

By the end of the assessment, the interviewer should have some insight into the patient's level of commitment to the program. This should be discussed candidly. At this time, patients may be unsure of the depth of their commitment, but a willingness to try is essential. Without it, a successful rehabilitation course is dubious.

PHYSICAL RECONDITIONING

At the Rehabilitation Center. The cornerstone of Phase II of a PRP is the physical reconditioning instruction. The duration of the Phase II sessions varies from 12 to 24 weeks, although analysis of the literature shows optimal results achieved with a minimum of 24 weeks of therapy.[65] The results of the patient's graded exercise test and the guidelines established by the American College of Sports Medicine are used to calculate an individualized exercise prescription (Box 10-6).[81] The prescription includes the recommended time and intensity of exercise with a variety of equipment, as well as a target heart range to guide the patient's exercise. Proper use of the equipment as well as recording of the physical response to the exercise prescription is usually demonstrated before the first day of class, perhaps at the close of the initial assessment interview.

The actual format or degree of structure of the exercise sessions is not as important as making certain that the key elements of physical reconditioning—gradual warm-up, aerobic conditioning, and sufficient cooldown—are guided by safety and effectiveness. To reduce the

BOX 10–6

The Exercise Prescription

- Determined from the graded exercise test using the resting heart rate, maximum heart rate, and the maximum METs
- Calculations based on the American College of Sports Medicine Guidelines
- Entry training level set at 50 percent functional capacity
- Activity selected according to known energy expenditure at desired levels
- Subjective difficulty assessed with Borg's rate of perceived exertion

METs, metabolic equivalents.

risk of injury in this older group of patients, the importance of a gradual warm-up before more strenuous exercise cannot be overemphasized.[82,83] Patients may warm up by starting very slowly for 5 to 10 minutes. Another method that may also add interest and variety is to lead the entire group in a warm-up activity. This method makes it possible for proper techniques to be taught and observed and also provides a time of group interaction and support.

After sufficient warm-up, patients move to the various equipment stations. Walking provides the best exercise for improving claudication.[65] Patients with claudication should walk on the treadmill to the point of near-maximal pain (Fig. 10-2). Then, while claudication subsides, patients can continue exercising on other equipment that is less strenuous on the calf muscle, such as stationary bicycles, Airdyne bikes (Fig. 10-3), arm ergometers, stairs, (Fig. 10-4), and rowing machines. Use of a variety of equipment has the added advantage of improving total body fitness and preventing boredom. Patients should alternate back and forth from treadmill to other equipment so that several treadmill walks occur at each session.

The patient's tolerance of the prescribed exercise is recorded after each piece of equipment is used. This record includes the maximum heart rate achieved during exercise, the time to onset of claudication or other symptoms, the total exercise time on each piece of equipment, and at some centers, the patient's rate of perceived exertion according to the Borg scale.[81,84] Adjustments to the exercise prescription are made at appropriate intervals throughout the program until the patient reaches a minimum of 35-40 minutes of discontinuous aerobic exercise per session.

Improving exercise tolerance in patients who are experiencing pain is a constant challenge to the staff. Patients need to learn the specific parameters of their symptoms. With claudication, does their discomfort increase as they walk, forcing them to stop? Does it remain at a tolerable level or actually diminish, enabling them to walk through their pain[85,86]? Once patients understand that claudication does not injure their legs, they may be able to push themselves to walk longer. Then significant progress can be made.

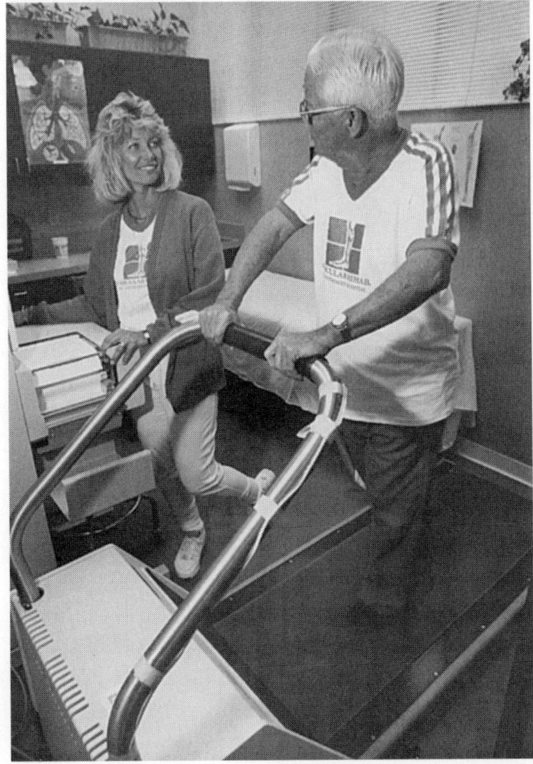

FIG. 10–2. Walking provides the best exercise for improving claudication.

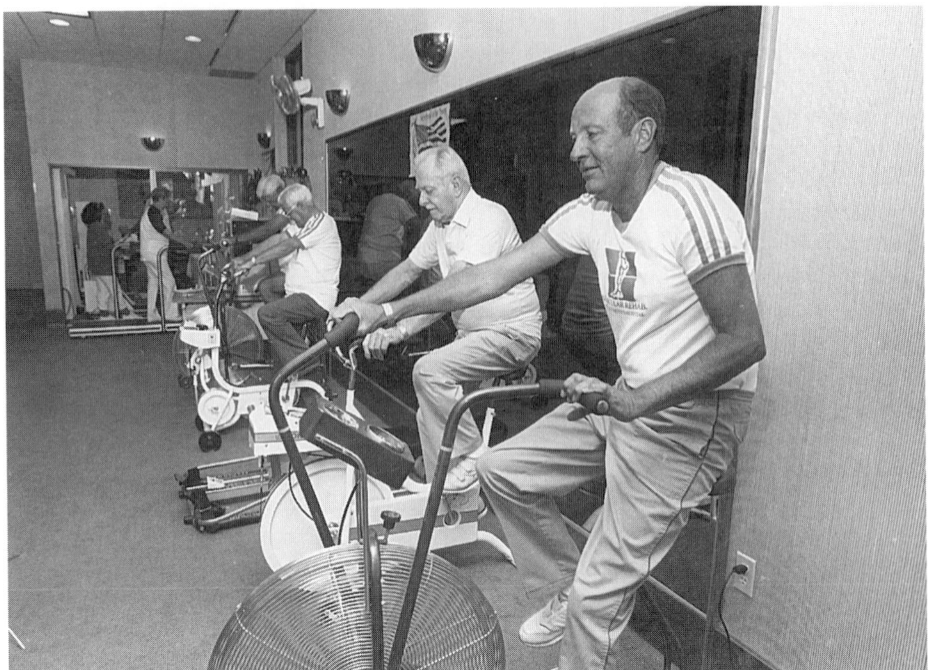

FIG. 10–3. Stationary bicycles are more sparing of the calf muscle and may allow patients to continue exercise while claudication subsides.

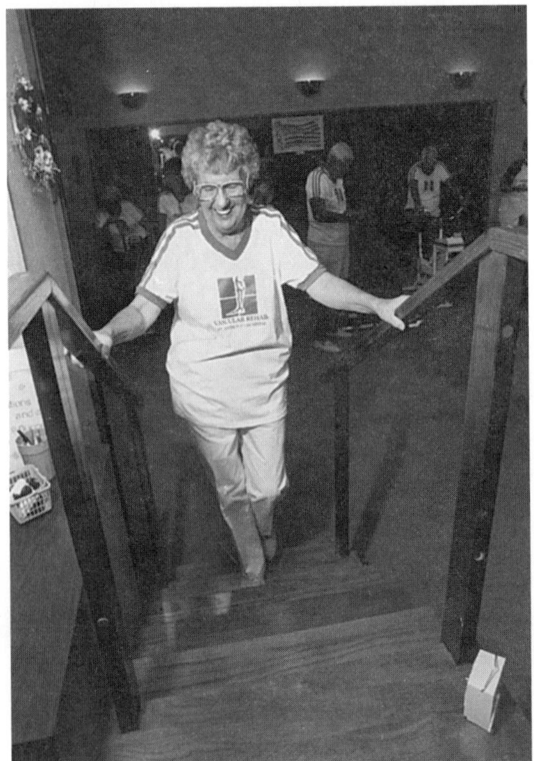

FIG. 10–4. Stair-climbing improves overall fitness and stamina.

Each exercise session should end with several minutes of activity that allows the body to cool down gradually.[82,83] This allows the heart rate and blood pressure to return to pre-exercise levels. Proper stretching at this time will improve flexibility and help prevent muscle soreness. As patients cool down and begin to relax, it may be helpful to incorporate stress-management techniques, such as guided imagery and total body relaxation.[87]

Even though a PRP can easily be incorporated into an existing cardiac program, utilizing common staff and equipment, it may be advisable for PAD patients to be treated in a distinct group, separate from others with coronary artery disease or heart failure, during the exercise sessions. Patients tend to identify and build supportive peer relationships more readily with others who have a similar diagnosis and symptoms. It is also easier for staff to manage a more homogeneous group. The exercise goals for PAD patients focus less on reaching target heart rates and more on walking beyond the initial onset of symptoms. This is not the goal with cardiac patients.

Supervised classes at a rehabilitation center are important in that they train patients in safe and effective guidelines for exercise to improve their stamina and fitness. These benefits continue only as long as the patient maintains a regular exercise program. To that end, patients are advised to begin a walking program at home on the days they are not at the center. This home walking regimen can then be the basis of their maintenance program once they have completed the program at the center. The development of such a program is essential to long-term success.

Exercise Training at Home. Whether patients with PAD are in supervised rehabilitation or not, each must understand the necessity of developing a pattern of daily exercise that can become an integral component of daily life. Many individuals with PAD may not be able or willing to participate in a structured center-based PRP. Various barriers to participation in a center-based program include the following:

- No center-based program may exist within the patient's health care system.
- There is a lack of reimbursement for a supervised program or other financial barriers to center-based participation.
- There may be no primary physician or vascular clinician to create a PAD rehabilitation referral.
- The PRP may be too far from the patient's home.
- Adequate (available and inexpensive) transportation to the center may not exist.
- Program times may conflict with their daily schedule.
- The patient may prefer exercising alone, instead of participating in group exercise.

In order for these patients to benefit from a secondary prevention program, and for graduates of a supervised program to continue a therapeutic exercise regimen, a home exercise program should be developed. Rehabilitation staff members assist patients in this endeavor during their Phase II program. They also can serve as an excellent resource to other vascular clinicians and primary care providers in the community as they work with their office patients in setting up similar programs.

Walking should be the major component of any exercise program to improve claudication, although alternative types of exercise can be added for variety and overall fitness. The clinician and patient must work together to plan the first stages of the home exercise plan, delineating specific steps for incorporating a regular exercise routine into the patient's day. Identify each patient's current level of exercise and activity in an effort to create a practical home program that is uniquely tailored to him or her. Many patients with PAD who are referred to a PAD rehabilitation program have never performed any regular, daily exercise and may doubt their ability to successfully initiate such a program at this stage of their lives. These patients may benefit from suggestions of various types of exercise, along with an exploration of different times and places in which such exercise might be most comfortable. Patients must develop their own practical regimen. Some patients find that exercising with a companion helps them follow their home program, whereas others prefer the introspection and relaxation that can be provided from such time alone. Patients should also be introduced to walking programs at local shopping malls and to various walking routes in their community, so as to

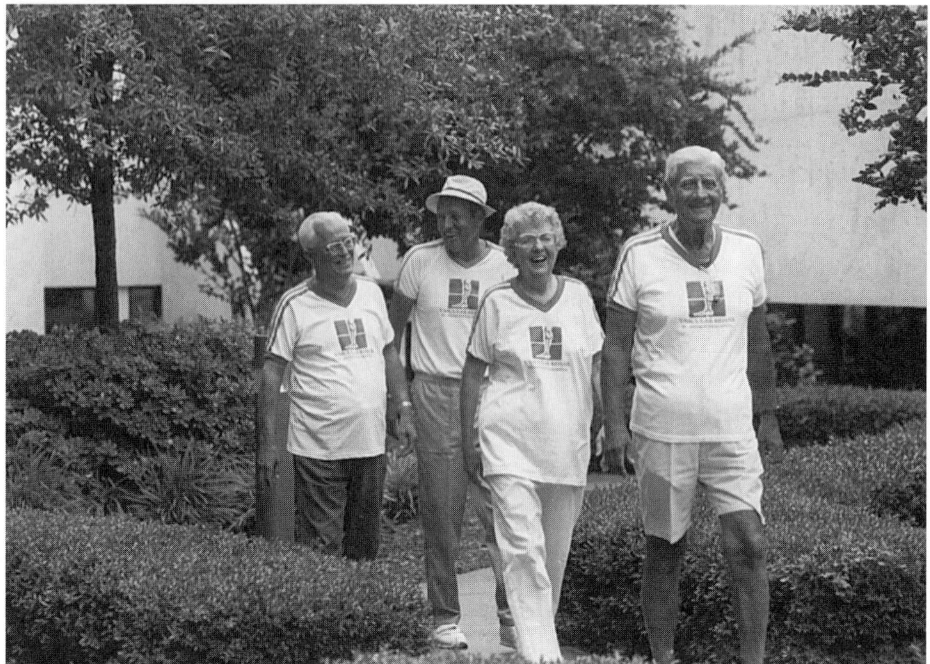

FIG. 10–5. Community walking clubs may improve compliance with a home exercise program.

lend variety and interest to the home program (Fig. 10-5). The home program should be considered a sign of a newly crafted independence, or as a "walk toward health."

Practitioners must plan home exercise individually. Prescribing too much could discourage the sedentary patient who has never exercised. Prescribing too little for a more active patient may cause him or her to lose interest. Regardless of the duration or intensity of exercise prescribed, the prescribed frequency should be the same for every patient, that is, to strive to exercise every day. If they follow this advice, patients can be sure of an adequate amount of exercise each week, even if they miss a day or two because of bad weather or unavoidable schedule conflicts. They also stand a better chance of developing a lifelong exercise habit.

A home exercise log is a useful tool for patients to record the home exercise experience. If they have to write it down, and know that it will be checked, they are more likely to exercise. Weekly review of this record by the staff allows appropriate changes in the program to be made and evaluated in a timely manner.[88] Those patients being followed in the office should be encouraged to bring the log to each office visit.

Home exercise programs assist patients in making exercise a part of their daily routine. However, the key to developing the exercise habit is helping patients identify their exercise motivation. Ekroth, Dahlof, Gundevall et al state that there are three types of exercise motives: body motives (look better, healthier body), psychologic motives (feel better, increased self-esteem), and social motives (exercise partners, social event). They believe that everyone has the motivation to exercise, although "it may be covered over by decades of suppression or accumulated fears about physical activity."[89] If vascular practitioners can encourage and assist patients in discovering exercise motives of all three types, there is a greater chance of long-term success.

PATIENT EDUCATION. Providing a sound knowledge base to patients means that clinicians must look for every opportunity to interact with patients, assess learning needs, and choose the best way to fill them. Increased understanding of the disease process and prognosis as well as the benefits of controlling risk factors may provide additional motivation for patients to modify behavior.

The rehabilitation program can offer a combination of formal and informal settings to enhance learning. A formal lecture series presented by the rehabilitation staff, vascular specialists, and allied health professionals is an excellent forum for delivering information on a selected topic to a large group of patients and their families. It also affords excellent visibility of the rehabilitation program and the hospital to the community if free lectures are offered and the public is invited to attend. The disadvantage of large-group instruction may be the varying levels of learning ability in the audience. Many people feel uncomfortable asking questions in front of a large group, so it may be difficult for the presenter to determine how well the information is understood. Follow-up time with each patient is needed to evaluate comprehension.

The physical reconditioning classes (usually a minimum of 24 sessions in a center-based program) provide ample follow-up time to reinforce classroom information. Informal discussions held with individual patients during these sessions enhance the patient-practitioner relationship and may serve two additional purposes. First, it is a good time to answer individual questions, personalizing and clarifying information. Second, it gives the patients something else to think about while exercising, keeping their eyes off the clock and perhaps allowing them to exercise longer.

Other informal teaching methods that reinforce classroom information include appropriate handouts, use of bulletin boards at the rehabilitation facility, DVD or video or audio tapes, a list of suggested reading material, Internet and community resources, and individual counseling sessions. Special presentations such as walking events, cooking classes, and restaurant expeditions provide practical "hands on" learning experiences where patients and families can put classroom information to use in real life.

Whether provided through formal classes at a rehabilitation center or one-on-one instruction in an office setting, educational content of PRPs should be similar. Patients need to hear basic information on the anatomy and physiology of the cardiovascular system, simple explanations of the pathophysiology of atherosclerosis and its associated symptoms, and the risk factors that contribute to the disease. Key points concerning each risk factor and how it contributes to the development of atherosclerosis, as discussed earlier in this chapter, should be incorporated into the patient education program. The importance of dietary changes, smoking cessation, and stress management can be introduced during the risk factor lectures; however, the actual techniques may be more effectively taught through separate, in-depth courses or individual counseling.

Although it is recommended that cardiac and PAD patients attend separate exercise sessions, it is entirely appropriate and perhaps even beneficial to include both groups of patients in the same education classes. They are facing the same disease with the same risk factors and need to understand the systemic nature of atherosclerosis. Cardiac patients need to know that they could experience leg symptoms, and PAD patients must realize that they may also have cardiac disease. Both groups need to know that they are at increased risk of having a stroke. Knowledge of these disease manifestations is essential for optimum management of this systemic disease.

Perhaps the one technique that has the greatest effect on behavior modification is that of role modeling. The more seasoned or "graduate" PAD rehabilitation patient serves as a role model for the novice, providing hope, empathy, and practical advice. Equally influential as role models are the members of the rehabilitation staff and the entire vascular team. They must be certain that the influence they exert on their patients is positive. Being a positive role model for health and fitness does not mean being "perfect." It does mean making a commitment to taking control and being responsible for one's own health. It also means being open, honest, and willing to share personal triumphs, defeats, strengths, and weaknesses.

PROGRESS EVALUATION. Progress is routinely discussed with patients during each exercise session, with more thorough evaluations scheduled halfway through the program. How much is accomplished in the final half of the program hinges heavily on this midpoint evaluation.

A graded treadmill walking test should be performed, following the same protocol that was used during the initial assessment. Doppler studies (e.g., the ABI) need not be repeated unless there has been deterioration in symptoms and/or walking ability. If lipid-lowering agents have recently been initiated, updated cholesterol profile data may be available from the physician and can be reviewed again with the patient. Particular attention is devoted to reviewing the home exercise records and planning the next stages of home exercise. Diet modifications are reviewed, and dietary consultations are arranged as needed. Progress with smoking cessation may be the most important aspect to evaluate, providing encouragement and adjusting interventions to help ensure success.

The staff member conducting this evaluation should candidly discuss the patient's performance in terms of attendance, commitment, attitude, physical improvement, and knowledge attained. This is the time to acknowledge every measure of improvement or success, no matter how small, and to be generous with praise where deserved. If the patient has not shown improvement, staff and patient should try to determine why. Has the patient been making a serious effort? If so, he or she may need to be reminded that improvement takes time. If the patient's attendance has been erratic, and no attempt has been made to exercise at home or to modify risk behaviors, this is the time for a frank discussion. There may be something in particular about the program that is upsetting and keeping the patient from participating. If no specific cause can be identified and the patient sincerely wants to continue, new goals and clear expectations should be identified for the remaining weeks of the program. Remember, lifestyle change is a process and patients progress and adapt at different rates.

Phase III

On completion of the Phase II program, patients usually are afforded two options regarding a maintenance program: continue with a home exercise program or continue in the third phase of PAD rehabilitation at the center. Ideally, most patients are well into their home exercise programs and are motivated enough to carry on without coming to the center for weekly supervised sessions. After these patients have been on their own for about 3 months, they should return for a repeat evaluation. At that time, if they continue to show satisfactory improvement and adherence to their home routine, evaluations can be scheduled at 6-month intervals.

Occasionally, there are patients who know they are not sufficiently disciplined to continue on a program by themselves. These patients are likely candidates for a Phase III maintenance program offered at the rehabilitation center. These sessions provide minimal supervision and are either offered on a set schedule, such as three times a week, or an open schedule allowing patients to attend anytime and as often as they like. Their evaluations are typically scheduled every 3 months. To participate in this phase of the program, patients must be able to function fairly independently on the equipment, continue to show improvement, and maintain regular attendance.

Results

The benefits of a structured PRP are significant for the vascular patient. A meta-analysis by Gardner and Poehlman of 21 programs confirmed that supervised PAD exercise training can be expected to offer an increase in pain-free walking distance and an increased maximal walking distance of 120-180 percent after exercise training.[65] This analysis also determined that the components most likely responsible for the improvement were using intermittent walking as the preferred exercise (in contrast to strength training or bicycle training), exercising to the point of near-maximal pain, and continuing the program for at least 6 months. Another study by Carter et al also demonstrated that improved treadmill walking distances might translate to even greater improvement during daily routine activities at home.[90] Overall, supervised PAD rehabilitation programs have been determined to be safe, beneficial, and cost effective.

CONCLUSION

The ideal management of patients with PAD encompasses the skills of a multidisciplinary team of vascular nurses, vascular internists, vascular surgeons, interventional radiologists, vascular technologists, dietitians, and rehabilitation professionals. During the past decade, new data have demonstrated that patients with PAD benefit from preventive, palliative, and therapeutic medical interventions that can improve the natural history of PAD (limb arterial disease progression and rates of myocardial infarction, stroke, and death), as well as functional outcomes (improved pain-free walking). Pharmacologic PAD interventions can now promote successful smoking cessation, normalize serum lipid levels, blunt the adverse effects of hypertension and diabetes, prevent thrombotic events, and improve symptoms of claudication. Exercise training can markedly improve pain-free and total walking distances. However, the promise of these approaches, which are integral to both vascular medicine and PAD rehabilitation, must now become part of the care for all patients with PAD (Fig. 10-6). The proposed integration of vascular medicine and rehabilitation can benefit all patients with PAD, inclusive of individuals with claudication and severe limb ischemic symptoms, both prior to and after effective revascularization procedures. All members of the health care team should view each clinical encounter with individuals with PAD as an opportunity to provide integrated vascular care. This opportunity is more than just a challenge; it defines our global responsibility as vascular clinicians for the long-term health of our patients.

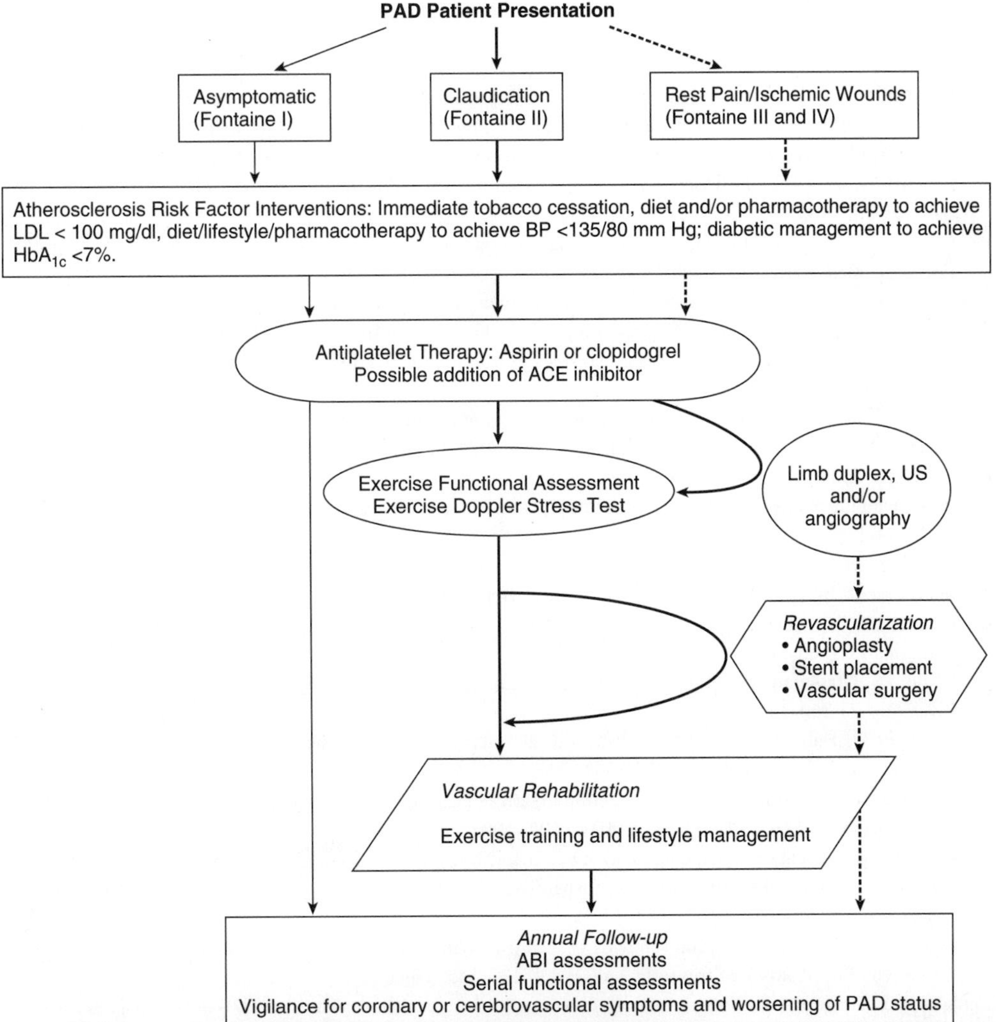

FIG. 10–6. An integrated vascular medical/rehabilitation approach for community-based peripheral arterial disease (PAD) care. *LDL*, low-density lipoproteins; *BP*, blood pressure; HbA_{1c}, glycosylated hemoglobin; *ACE*, angiotensin-converting enzyme; *US*, ultrasonography; *ABI*, ankle-brachial index.

REFERENCES

1. Criqui MH, Langer RD, Fronek A et al: Mortality over a period of 10 years in patients with peripheral arterial disease, *N Engl J Med* 326(6):381-386, 1992.
2. McKenna M, Wolfson S, Kuller L: The ratio of ankle and arm blood pressure as an independent risk factor of mortality, *Atherosclerosis* 87:119, 1991.
3. Newman AB, Siscovick DS, Manolio TA et al: Ankle-arm index as a marker of atherosclerosis in the Cardiovascular Health Study, Cardiovascular Health Study (CHS) Collaborative Research Group, *Circulation* 88(3):837-845, 1993.
4. Treat-Jacobson DT, Halverson SL, Ratchford A et al: A patient-derived perspective of health-related quality-of-life in peripheral arterial disease, *J Nurs Scholarsh* 34(1):55-60, 2002.
5. Weitz JI, Byrne J, Clagett P et al: Diagnosis and treatment of chronic arterial insufficiency of the lower extremities: a critical review, *Circulation* 94:3026-3049, 1996.
6. Hirsch AT, Reich L: Intermittent claudication, *Curr Treat Options Cardiovasc Med* 3:67-180, 2001.
7. Hiatt WR: Medical treatment of peripheral arterial disease and claudication, *N Engl J Med* 344(21):1608-1621, 2001.
8. Jonason T, Bergstrom R: Cessation of smoking in patients with intermittent claudication: effects on the risk of peripheral vascular complications, myocardial infarction and mortality, *Acta Med Scand* 221:253-260, 1987.
9. Faulkner KW, House AK, Castleden WM: The effect of cessation of smoking on the accumulative survival rates of patients with symptomatic peripheral vascular disease, *Med J Aust* 1:217-219, 1983.
10. Lassila R, Lepantalo M: Cigarette smoking and the outcome after lower limb arterial surgery, *Acta Chir Scand* 154:635-640, 1988.
11. Hirsch AT, Treat-Jacobson D, Lando HA et al: The role of tobacco cessation, anti-platelet and lipid-lowering therapies in the treatment of peripheral arterial disease, *Vasc Med* 2:243-251, 1997.
12. Hirsch AT, Halverson S, Treat-Jacobson D et al. The Minnesota Regional Peripheral Arterial Disease Screening Program: toward a definition of community standards of care, *Vasc Med* 6(2):87-96, 2001.
13. Quick C, Cotton L: The measured effect of stopping smoking on intermittent claudication, *Br J Surg* 695:S24-26, 1982.
14. Gardner AW: The effect of cigarette smoking on exercise capacity in patients with intermittent claudication, *Vasc Med* 1:181-186, 1996.
15. Fiore MC, Bailey WC, Cohen SJ et al: *Treating tobacco use and dependence, A clinical practice guideline,* AHRQ Publication No 00-0032, Rockville, Md, 2000, US Dept of Health and Human Services.
16. Lando HA: Toward a comprehensive strategy for reducing the health burden of tobacco, *Br J Addict* 86:649-652, 1991.
17. Power L, Brown NS, Makin GS: Unsuccessful outpatient counseling to help patients with peripheral vascular disease to stop smoking, *Ann R Coll Surg Engl* 74:31-34, 1992.
18. Jasinski DR, Henningfield JE: Conceptual basis of replacement therapies for chemical dependence. In Pomerleau OF, Pomerleau CS, eds: *Nicotine replacement: a critical evaluation*, New York, 1988, Alan R Liss, pp 13-34.
19. Working Group for the Study of Transdermal Nicotine in Patients With Coronary Artery Disease: Nicotine replacement therapy for patients with coronary artery disease, *Arch Intern Med* 154(9):989-995, 1994.
20. Hughes JR: Dependence potential and abuse liability of nicotine replacement therapies. In Pomerleau OF, Pomerleau CS, eds: *Progress in clinical evaluation*, New York, 1988, Alan R Liss, pp 261-277.
21. Covey LS, Glassman AH, Stetner F: Depression and depressive symptoms in smoking cessation, *Compr Psychiatry* 31:350-354, 1990.
22. Ginsberg D, Hall SM, Reus VI et al: Mood and depression diagnosis in smoking cessation, *Exp Clin Psychopharmacol* 3(4):389-395, 1995.
23. Hurt RD, Sachs DP, Glover ED et al: A comparison of sustained-release bupropion and placebo for smoking cessation, *N Engl J Med* 337(17):1195-1202, 1997.
24. Hess H, Miewtaschik A, Deischel G: Drug-induced inhibition of platelet function delays progression of peripheral occlusive arterial disease: a prospective, double-blind arteriographically controlled trial, *Lancet* 1(8426):415-419, 1985.
25. Goldhaber SZ, Manson JE, Stampfer MJ et al: Low-dose aspirin and subsequent peripheral arterial surgery in the Physicians Health Study, *Lancet* 340:143-145, 1992.
26. Janzon L, Bergquist D, Boberg J et al: Prevention of myocardial infarction and stroke in patients with intermittent claudication: effects of ticlopidine—results from STIMS, the Swedish Ticlopidine Multicentre Study, *J Int Med* 27:301-308, 1991.
27. Arcan JC, Blanchard J, Boissel J et al: Multicenter double-blind study of ticlopidine in the treatment of intermittent claudication and the prevention of its complications, *Angiology* 39:802-811, 1988.

28. Balsano F, Cocherri S, Libretti A et al: Ticlopidine in the treatment of intermittent claudication: a 21-month double-blind trial, *J Lab Clin Med* 114:84-91, 1989.
29. Balsano F, Violi F: Effect of picotamide on the clinical progression of peripheral vascular disease: a double-blind placebo-controlled study, The ADEP Group, *Circulation* 87(5):1563-1569, 1993.
30. Coto V, Cocozza M, Oliviero U et al: Clinical efficacy of picotamide in long-term treatment of intermittent claudication, *Angiology* 40(10):880-885, 1989.
31. CAPRIE Steering Committee: A randomized, blinded, trial of clopidogrel vs aspirin in patients at risk of ischaemic events (CAPRIE), *Lancet* 348(9038):1329-1339, 1996.
32. Hirsch AT, Criqui MH, Treat-Jacobson D et al: Peripheral arterial disease detection, awareness, and treatment in primary care, *JAMA* 286:1317-1324, 2001.
33. Stamler J, Wentworth D, Neatone JD: Is relationship between serum cholesterol and risk of premature death from coronary heart disease continuous and graded? Findings in 356,222 primary screenees of the Multiple Risk Factor Intervention Trial (MRFIT), *JAMA* 256(20):2823-2828, 1986.
34. Criqui MH, Wallace RB, Heiss G et al: Cigarette smoking and plasma high density lipoprotein cholesterol, The Lipid Research Clinics Program Prevalence Study, *Circulation* 62 (suppl IV):70-76, 1980.
35. Executive Summary of the Third Report of the National Cholesterol Education Program (NCEP) Expert Panel on Detection, Evaluation, and Treatment of High Blood Cholesterol in Adults (Adult Treatment Panel III), *JAMA* 285:2486-2497, 2001.
36. Blankenhorn DH, Azen SP, Crawford DW et al: Effects of colestipol-niacin therapy on human femoral atherosclerosis, *Circulation* 83:438-447, 1991.
37. Buchwald H, Varco RL, Matts JP et al: Effect of partial ileal bypass surgery on mortality and morbidity from coronary heart disease in patients with hypercholesterolemia: report of the Program on the Surgical Control of the Hyperlipidemias (POSCH), *N Engl J Med* 323:946-955, 1990.
38. Scandinavian Simvastatin Survival Study Group: Randomized trial of cholesterol lowering in 444 patients with coronary heart disease: the Scandinavian Simvastatin Survival Study (4S), *Lancet* 344:383-913, 1994.
39. Pedersen TR, Kjekshus J, Pyorala K et al: Effect of simvastatin on ischemic signs and symptoms in the Scandinavian Simvastatin Survival Study (4S), *Am J Cardiol* 81:333-335, 1998.
40. Sacks FM, Pfeffer MA, Moye LA et al: The effect of pravastatin on coronary events after myocardial infarction in patients with average cholesterol levels, The Cholesterol and Recurrent Events Trial Investigators, *New Engl J Med* 335:1001-1019, 1996.
41. MRC/BHF Heart Protection Study of cholesterol lowering with simvastatin in 20,536 high risk individuals: a randomized placebo-controlled trial, *Lancet* 360:7-22, 2002.
42. Kannel WB, McGee DL: Update on some epidemiologic features of intermittent claudication, *Lancet* 2:1093, 1996.
43. The Sixth Report of the Joint National Committee on Prevention, Detection, Evaluation and Treatment of High Blood Pressure, *Arch Intern Med* 137:2413-2446, 1997.
44. Hiatt WR, Stoll S, Nies AS: Effect of a-adrenergic blockers on the peripheral circulation in patients with peripheral vascular disease, *Circulation* 72:1226-1231, 1985.
45. Radack K, Deck C: Beta-adrenergic blocker therapy does not worsen intermittent claudication in subjects with peripheral arterial disease: a meta-analysis of randomized controlled trials, *Arch Intern Med* 151:1769-1776, 1991.
46. Heintzen MP, Strauer BE: Peripheral vascular effects of beta-blockers, *Eur Heart J* 15(suppl C):2-7, 1994.
47. The Heart Outcomes Prevention Evaluation Study Investigators: Effects of an angiotensin-converting-enzyme inhibitor, ramipril, on cardiovascular events in high-risk patients, *N Engl J Med* 342:145-153, 2000 (Errata, *N Engl J Med* 342:748, 1376, 2000).
48. Effect of intensive diabetes management on macrovascular events and risk factors in the Diabetes Control and Complications Trial, *Am J Cardiol* 75:894-903, 1995.
49. UK Prospective Diabetes Study (UKPDS) Group: Intensive blood-glucose control with sulphonylureas or insulin compared with conventional treatment and risk of complications in patients with type 2 diabetes, UKPDS 33, *Lancet* 352:837-853, 1998 (Erratum, *Lancet* 354:602, 1999).
50. Grodstein F, Stampfer MJ, Colditz GA et al: Postmenopausal hormone therapy and mortality, *N Engl J Med* 336(25):1769-1775, 1997.
51. Stampfer MJ, Colditz GA, Willett WC et al: Postmenopausal estrogen therapy and cardiovascular disease: ten year follow-up from the nurses' health study, *N Engl J Med* 325(11):756-762, 1991.
52. Hsia J, Simon JA, Lin F et al: Peripheral arterial disease in randomized trial of estrogen with progestin in women with coronary heart disease: the Heart and Estrogen/Progestin Replacement Study, *Circulation* 102:2228-2232, 2000.
53. Timaran CH, Stevens SL, Grandas OH et al: Influence of hormone replacement therapy on graft patency after femoropopliteal bypass grafting, *J Vasc Surg* 32:506-518, 2000.

54. Stewart KJ, Hiatt WR, Regensteiner JG et al: Exercise training for claudication, *N Engl J Med*, 347(24): 1941-1951, 2002.
55. Patterson RB, Pinto B, Marcus B et al: Value of a supervised exercise program for the therapy of arterial claudication, *J Vasc Surg* 25:312-319, 1997.
56. Ponte E, Cattinelli S: Quality of life in a group of patients with intermittent claudication, *Angiology* 47:247-251, 1996.
57. Regensteiner JG, Steiner JF, Hiatt WR: Exercise training improves functional status in patients with peripheral arterial disease, *J Vasc Surg* 23:104-115, 1996.
58. Khaira HS, Hanger R, Shearman CP: Quality of life in patients with intermittent claudication, *Eur J Vasc Endovasc Surg* 11:65-69, 1996.
59. Larsen O, Lassen N: Effect of daily muscular exercise in patients with intermittent claudication, *Lancet* 2:1093, 1966.
60. Dahloff A, Bjorntorp P, Holm J et al: Metabolic activity of skeletal muscle in patients with peripheral arterial insufficiency: effect of physical training, *Eur J Clin Invest* 4:9, 1974.
61. Dahloff A, Holm J, Schersten T et al: Peripheral arterial insufficiency: effect of physical training on walking tolerance, calf blood flow and blood flow resistance, *Scand J Rehabil Med* 8:18, 1976.
62. Hiatt WR et al: The valuation of exercise performance in patients with peripheral arterial disease, *J Cardiopulm Rehabil* 12:525, 1988.
63. Hiatt WR: Benefit of exercise conditioning for patients with peripheral arterial disease, *Circulation* 81:602, 1990.
64. Hiatt WR, Regensteiner JG: Exercise rehabilitation in the treatment of patients with peripheral arterial disease, *J Vasc Med Biol* 2:163, 1990.
65. Gardner AW, Poehlman ET: Exercise rehabilitation programs for the treatment of claudication pain: a meta-analysis, *JAMA* 274(12):975-980, 1995.
66. McDermott MM: Specific exercise training program for intermittent claudication. In Pearce WH, Yao JST, eds: *Advances in vascular surgery*, Chicago, 2002, Precept Press.
67. England JD, Regensteiner JG, Ringel SP et al: Muscle denervation in peripheral arterial disease, *Neurology* 42:994, 1992.
68. Regensteiner JG, Wolfel EE, Brass EP et al: Chronic changes in skeletal muscle histology and function in peripheral arterial disease, *Circulation* 87:413, 1993.
69. American Medical Association: *Current Procedural Terminology (CPT)*, Chicago, 2001, The Association.
70. Barnes M: Vascular rehabilitation update: components of a phase I program, *J Vasc Nurs* 10(4):31, 1992.
71. Society for Vascular Nursing, 7794 Grow Dr, Pensacola, FL 32514; website: www.svnnet.org.
72. The Vascular Disease Foundation, 3333 S Wadsworth Blvd #B104-37, Lakewood, CO 80227; website: www.vdf.org.
73. Landis BJ, Brykczynski KA: Employing prevention in practice, *Am J Nurs* 97(8):40-46, 1997.
74. Hiatt WR, Hirsch AT, Regensteiner JG et al: Clinical trials for claudication: assessment of exercise performance, functional status, and clinical end points, *Circulation* 92:614-621, 1995.
75. Hiatt WR, Nawaz D, Regensteiner JG et al: The evaluation of exercise performance in patients with peripheral vascular disease, *J Cardiopulm Rehabil* 12:525-532, 1998.
76. Gardner AW, Skinner JS, Cantwell BW et al: Progressive vs single-stage treadmill tests for evaluation of claudication, *Med Sci Sports Exerc* 23:402-408, 1991.
77. Regensteiner JG, Steiner JF, Panzer RJ et al: Evaluation of walking impairment by questionnaire in patients with peripheral arterial disease, *J Vasc Med Biol* 2:142-152, 1990.
78. Ware JE, Sherbourne CD: The MOS 36-item short-form health survey (SF-36). I. Conceptual framework and item selection, *Med Care* 30:473-483, 1992.
79. McHorney CA, Ware JE, Raczek AE: The MOS 36-item short-form health survey (SF-36). II. Psychometric and clinical tests of validity in measuring physical and mental health constructs, *Med Care* 31:247-263, 1993.
80. Davis CM: *Patient practitioner interaction: an experiential manual for developing the art of health care*, Thorofare, NJ, 1989, Slack.
81. American College of Sports Medicine: *Guidelines for graded exercise testing and exercise prescription*, ed 5, Philadelphia, 1995, Williams & Wilkins.
82. Pollock ML, Wilmore JH: *Exercise in health and disease: evaluation and prescription for prevention and rehabilitation*, ed 2, Philadelphia, 1990, WB Saunders.
83. Cooper KH: *The aerobics program for total well-being*, New York, 1982, Bantam Books.
84. Williams LR, Ekers, MA, Collins PS et al: Vascular rehabilitation: benefits of a structured exercise/risk factor modification program, *J Vasc Surg* 12:1636-1639, 1991.

85. Hubner C: Exercise therapy and smoking cessation for intermittent claudication, *J Cardiovasc Nurs* 1:50-58, 1987.
86. Taylor LM, Moneta GL, Porter JM: Natural history and nonoperative treatment of chronic lower extremity ischemia. In Rutherford R, ed: *Vascular surgery*, ed 5, Philadelphia, 2000, WB Saunders, pp 928-943.
87. Squires R, Gau GT, Miller TF et al: Cardiovascular rehabilitation: status 1990, *Mayo Clin Proc* 65:731-755, 1990.
88. Ekers MA: Vascular rehabilitation update, *J Vasc Nurs* 10(2):34, 1992.
89. Ekroth R, Dahlof AG, Gundevall B et al: Physical training of patients with intermittent claudication: indications, methods, and results, *Surgery* 84:640-643, 1978.
90. Carter SA, Hamel ER, Paterson JM et al: Walking ability and ankle systolic pressures, *J Vasc Surg* 10: 642-649, 1989.

11

Surgery of the Aorta

MARK K. ESKANDARI □ JON S. MATSUMURA □ LOUISE ANDERSON

Reconstructive surgery of the aorta has become a relatively safe and effective treatment of aortic aneurysms, aortoiliac occlusive disease, and aortic dissection. Previously, these diseases were incurable and often led to serious morbidity and the patient's rapid demise. Currently, approximately 60,000 patients per year in the United States benefit from procedures that have developed from experimental surgery into routine operations carried out in community hospitals. Perioperative mortality has fallen to single-digit levels in elective cases, and late complications are uncommon.[1-6] The great strides in the care of these patients have been possible because of advances in surgical and anesthetic techniques, graft materials, and perioperative care.

Nursing management of patients undergoing aortic surgery encompasses a wide breadth, ranging from preoperative teaching, intraoperative and intensive care, and postoperative support to recognition of complications. Knowledge of anatomy is key to understanding the manifestations of aortic diseases and the complications of aortic procedures. This chapter will first review aortic anatomy, then will discuss the three major diseases affecting the aorta with detailed discussion of presentation, diagnosis, and therapeutic options, and will finish with a description of short- and long-term complications.

ANATOMY AND FUNCTION

The aorta begins at the aortic valve, ascends in the anterior mediastinum, arches posteriorly, descends in the posterior mediastinum, and traverses the retroperitoneum to end at the bifurcation into the common iliac arteries (Fig. 11-1). The first branches are the left and right coronary arteries, which feed the myocardium. The arch vessels include the innominate artery, which branches into the right subclavian and right common carotid arteries, the left common carotid artery, and the left subclavian artery. The descending aorta gives off intercostal branches, some of which (usually in the T9 to L1 region) anastomose with the critical artery of Adamkiewicz, which feeds the spinal cord. Abdominal branches include the celiac artery, superior mesenteric artery, renal arteries, and inferior mesenteric artery.

Aortic diseases or surgical complications that impair the flow of blood to these branches affect the diverse functions of the corresponding organs. For instance, arch vessel embolism may manifest as transient ischemic attacks or hand ischemia, intercostal branch occlusion may precipitate paraplegia, and renal artery thrombosis may lead to hypertension or renal failure. Onset of clinical symptoms usually correlates with the pace of blood flow reduction. For example, in the Leriche syndrome, caused by aortoiliac occlusive disease, there is gradual onset of decreased femoral pulses, buttock claudication, and erectile dysfunction as a result of gradual distal aorta and common iliac artery occlusion. In contrast, with acute thrombosis of the infrarenal aorta or saddle embolization of the aortic bifurcation, aortic occlusion occurs without sufficient time for collateral development, and, hence, there is acute bilateral leg ischemia with myonecrosis and symptoms of pelvic arterial insufficiency such as rectal ischemia.

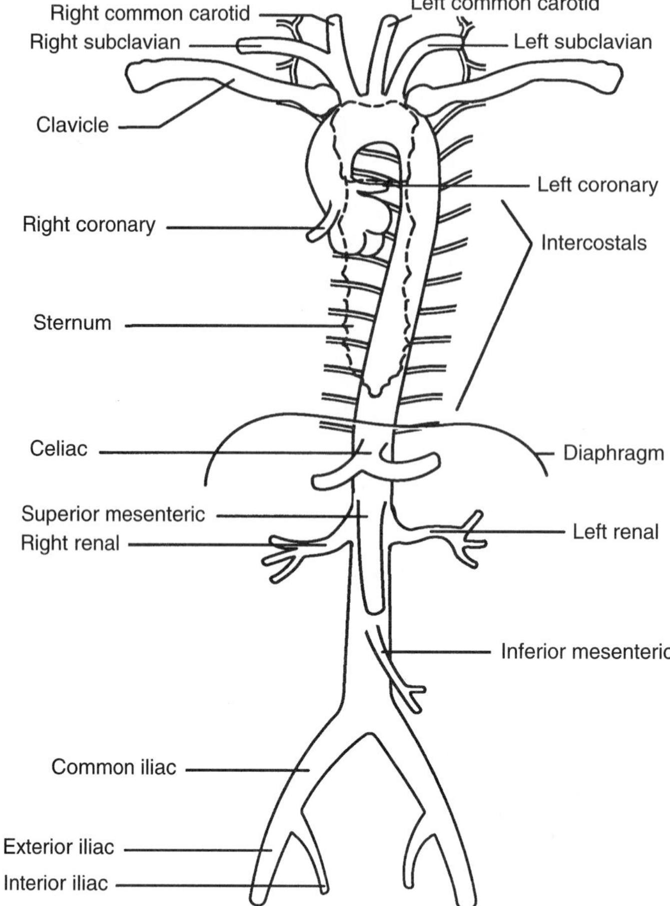

FIG. 11–1. Anatomy of the aorta and its major branches.

AORTIC ANEURYSM

Aneurysms are diseased areas of arteries that become dilated and thin walled. Mature elastin and collagen located in the layers of the aorta are the major structural proteins responsible for the integrity of the aortic wall. Elastin provides elasticity to the vessel, allowing its diameter to increase with changes in pressure and to recoil to its original diameter when pressure decreases. In contrast, collagen is responsible for mechanical strength and limits the amount of vessel distention and prevents rupture.[7] Both elastin and collagen have been shown to be present in decreased quantities in aneurysms.[8] Most of the research on aortic aneurysm formation has focused on structural changes that occur in the media. The specific mechanisms in the development of aneurysm formation are still poorly understood. However, current theory holds that two distinct pathophysiologic changes occur in their evolution. These are (1) elastin fragmentation, required for aneurysm formation, and (2) collagen deposition and degradation, responsible for aneurysm enlargement and rupture.[8] Recently, the role of the adventitia in aneurysm formation is being investigated.[9] A variety of theories related to aneurysm development have been proposed and are reviewed in Table 11-1.

Screening of unselected adults and men with peripheral vascular disease reveals a prevalence of 3.2-9.6 percent,[10] and about 15,000 Americans die from aortic aneurysms annually. They are more common in men than women with the onset at approximately age 50 for men and 60 for women. The incidence steadily increases with age and develops more frequently in smokers and people with coronary artery disease, hypertension, hyperlipidemia, and chronic obstructive pulmonary disease. Familial clustering of aortic aneurysms has been

TABLE 11–1 Theories of Aneurysm Pathogenesis

Etiology	Clinical Evidence	Theory
Genetic	Genetically linked enzyme deficiencies are associated with aneurysms Familial clustering is observed Male siblings have up to 25% lifetime risk of aneurysm	X chromosome linked and autosomal dominant inheritance pattern Specific defects in collagen
Atherosclerotic	Risk factors are similar to occlusive disease, including smoking, hypertension, and aging Aneurysm wall contains calcium and atherosclerotic lesions	Compensatory dilation of the artery becomes uncontrolled
Immunologic	A variant called *inflammatory aneurysm* is characterized by gross inflammation and microscopic leukocyte infiltrates	Antigen, possibly through molecular mimicry, precipitates autoimmune response
Degenerative	Disruption of normal aortic wall architecture Decreased amounts of elastin and collagen are found in aneurysms Hernias are common in patients with aneurysms	Elastin and collagen are aberrantly formed or digested
Hemodynamic	Aneurysms typically occur proximal to bifurcations or distal to stenoses	Wall tension, turbulence, vibration, and shear stress are increased dynamically in these areas
Iatrogenic	Occur at graft anastomosis, after endarterectomy, angioplasty, or fullthickness traumatic disruption	Structural injury, end-to-side anastomosis
Infectious	*Salmonella, Chlamydia pneumoniae, Streptococcus* species, *Staphylococcus* species, *Treponema pallidum* are associated with aneurysms	Microorganisms by direct extension, emboli, or infection from unknown primary site may stimulate inflammation or degradation

observed with an estimated 15-20 percent incidence occurring in first-degree relatives of the individual with the aneurysm.[11]

Potential consequences of aneurysms include (1) rupture, causing pain and internal hemorrhage; (2) thrombosis, leading to acute ischemia of all downstream branches; and (3) embolization, causing selective branch vessel symptoms. Most commonly, aortic aneurysms affect the infrarenal aorta and, if untreated, present with spontaneous rupture. Fortunately, many aneurysms are detected when they are asymptomatic, either on physical examination or by serendipitous findings on radiographic studies. An aortic aneurysm should be suspected when a peripheral aneurysm is present since at least one third of patients with a femoral or popliteal aneurysm will have an abdominal aortic aneurysm.[11]

Spontaneous rupture of an aortic aneurysm can be quite dramatic. Classically, patients complain of sudden onset of abdominal and lower back pain with associated physical findings consisting of shock and abdominal tenderness. Most patients do not survive the rupture long enough to get to a hospital. Survival is favored when a small leak is contained from either tamponade from adjacent structures or clot at the site of the leak. The majority of these patients present with transient hypotension, which progresses to shock over several hours. Because of the high mortality associated with aneurysm rupture, it should always be considered as a possible diagnosis in any elderly patient complaining of abdominal, back, or flank pain.[11] Hypovolemic shock and a pulsatile abdominal mass are diagnostic and mandate emergent surgical treatment without any additional radiologic studies. In cases of a contained rupture or rapidly enlarging aneurysm, symptoms may be rather vague and include scrotal pain referred from retroperitoneal irritation.

Fever and uremia may be indicative of an inflammatory aneurysm, which can cause hydronephrosis via the associated retroperitoneal inflammation that occurs near the ureters.

The classically described blue toe syndrome presents in patients with palpable pedal pulses and multiple ischemic toes, which are due to microembolization from a more proximally located aneurysm (Fig. 11-2, *A*). In rare cases, disseminated intravascular coagulation can occur among patients with exceedingly large aneurysms (Fig. 11-3). Computed tomography (CT) scans and abdominal ultrasound may be helpful in less obvious cases of acute symptoms and in chronic cases for planning treatment by assessing precise aneurysm size, location relative to branches, and ruling out multiple aneurysms.[12]

Risk of rupture is related primarily to the size of the aneurysm; hence, observation is recommended for most small (<4 cm) and asymptomatic aortic aneurysms. Although aneurysms expand at an average rate of 10 percent per year, many will remain stable for years. Despite the available data on aneurysm growth patterns, the rate of growth for an individual is unpredictable. Other risk factors identified with rupture are an abnormally elevated diastolic blood pressure and chronic obstructive pulmonary disease.[13]

Treatment is generally recommended for symptomatic aneurysms, rapidly enlarging aneurysms, and infrarenal aneurysms over 5 cm because the risk of rupture becomes excessive, although individual risk assessment is practiced.[14] The conventional operation is aneurysmorrhaphy (aneurysmal repair) and may be performed safely through a midline or transverse anterior approach or a retroperitoneal approach.[15] In the standard operation, the aorta is exposed and clamped above and below the aneurysm, and a graft is sutured inside of the aneurysm sac to restore continuity (Fig. 11-4). Mortality in large series at experienced centers is less than 4 percent and is 1.4 percent in the 25-year series by Crawford.[2,10] Some centers perform this operation through small (10-cm length) transperitoneal incisions and report a more rapid postoperative recovery time.[16]

Alternative strategies for repair of aortic aneurysms include retroperitoneal ligation of the aneurysm and bypass to restore distal perfusion,[17] laparoscopic ligation and axillobifemoral bypass,[18] and endovascular grafting. Endovascular treatment has received the greatest attention with multiple clinical trials in progress worldwide. Preliminary results suggest that mortality and hospital stay may be reduced, although complete evaluation will require long-term follow-up.[19-21] This topic is further discussed in Chapter 12.

Aneurysms that extend above the renal arteries and into the thoracic aorta are more difficult to repair (Fig. 11-5). Their presentation is less distinct because high back pain and chest pain may be mistaken for angina and pulmonary diseases. These patients require more extensive incisions into the chest cavity and have greater blood loss and coagulopathy, and their reconstruction must include additional attention to the important branches to the kidneys, bowel, and spinal cord. Because of the increased morbidity and mortality associated with these aneurysms, often a larger cutoff of 6-cm size is utilized as an indication for repair of thoracic and thoracoabdominal aneurysms. Specialized intraoperative techniques to prevent complications include cold renal artery perfusion, atrial-to-femoral cardiopulmonary bypass, spinal fluid drainage, and regional epidural hypothermia. Spinal fluid drainage is one modality used to reduce the incidence of spinal cord ischemia. It entails the placement of a small catheter within the spinal canal to allow for the free drainage of cerebrospinal fluid (CSF) at a predetermined pressure. Reduction in spinal cord pressure is most critical at times of systemic hypotension when spinal cord perfusion may be compromised; therefore, spinal drainage is typically most useful intraoperatively and during the first 3-4 days postoperatively. These techniques minimize organ metabolism and maximize collateral perfusion during the ischemic interval of aortic repair. Thoracoabdominal aneurysms are often treated in tertiary care institutions because of the higher rates of paraplegia, renal failure, and death.

AORTIC OCCLUSIVE DISEASE

Occlusive disease of the aorta is predominantly caused by atherosclerosis, with rare cases due to congenital coarctation, radiation injury, giant cell arteritis, Takayasu's disease, or "small aortic syndrome." Most symptomatic disease involves the infrarenal aorta and iliac arteries,

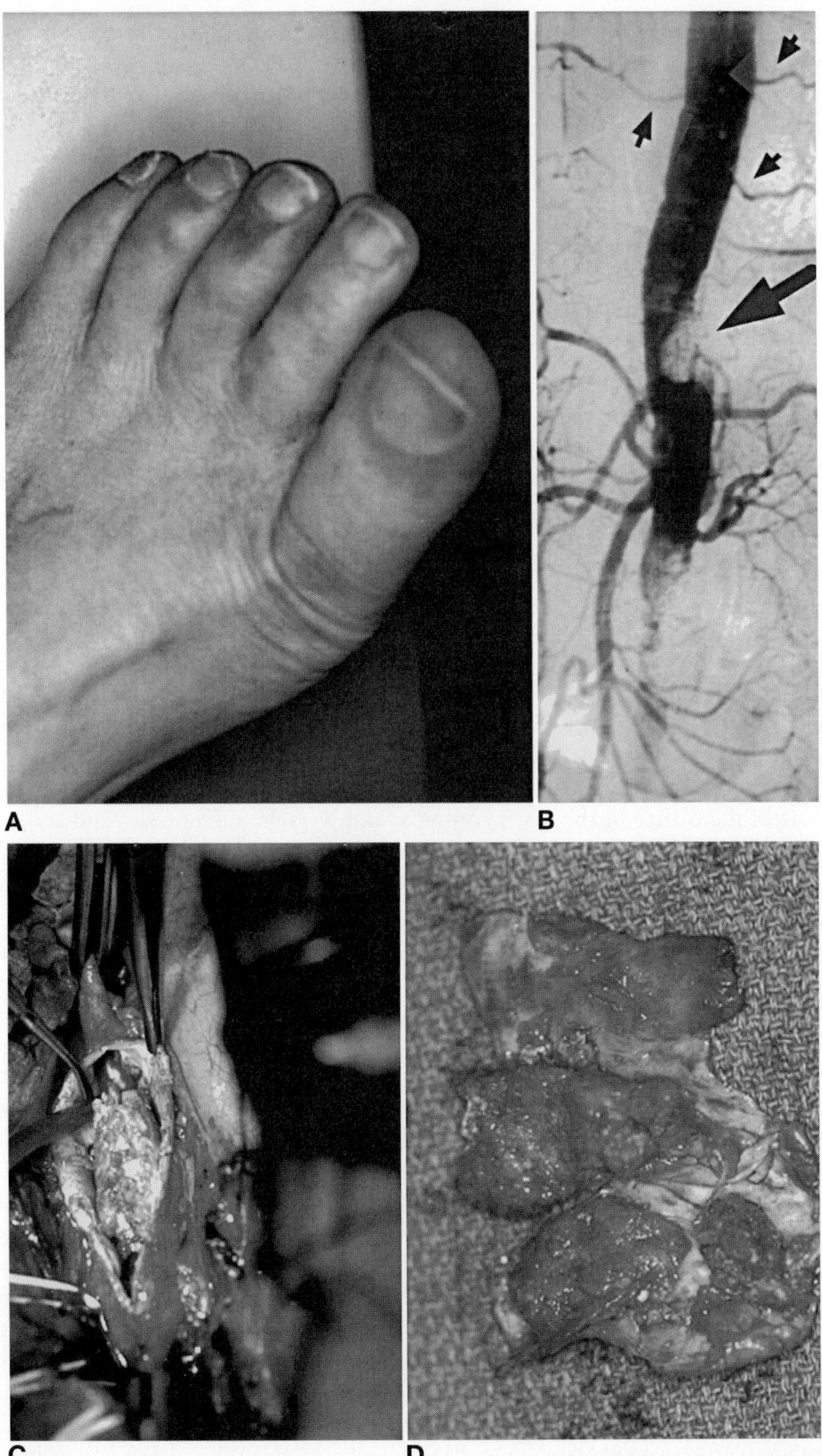

FIG. 11–2. Patient with blue toe syndrome. **A,** Mottling of distal aspects of toes. **B,** Digital subtraction angiogram of descending thoracic and abdominal aorta demonstrating plaque *(solid arrow)* with intercostal branches *(arrowheads)*. **C,** Aorta opened before endarterectomy. **D,** Close-up view of the specimen of "coral reef"–like plaque, which is the source of the distal emboli.

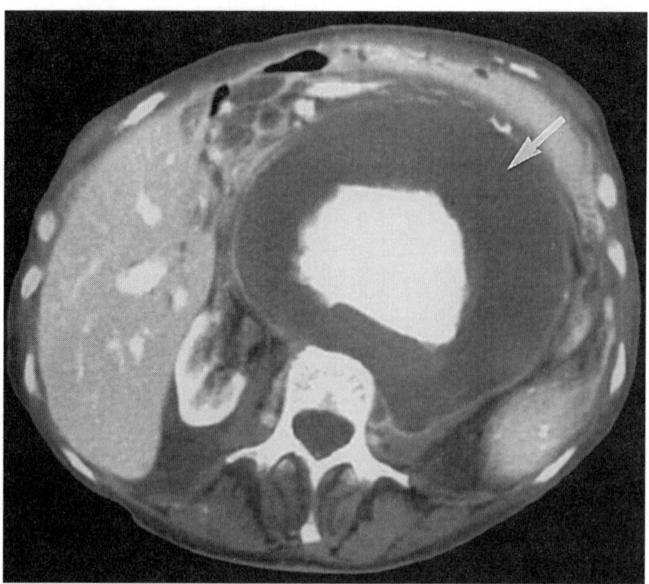

FIG. 11–3. Computed tomography (CT) scan of an enormous aortic aneurysm with lumen enhanced by white-appearing contrast and surrounded by thick intraluminal thrombus *(arrow)*.

and it is estimated that 1.8 percent, 3.7 percent, and 5.2 percent of adults less than 60 years old, 60 to 70 years old, and greater than 70 years old, respectively, experience claudication or intermittent leg pain with exercise.[22] Many of these patients' claudication symptoms are caused by aortoiliac disease. Aortic atherosclerosis can "spill over" into branch lesions, causing stenosis of the orifice of the main coronary, arch vessels, mesenteric, and renal arteries. These latter lesions and their treatment are covered in other chapters, although they are often treated with operations of the aorta that have similar complications.

Diagnosis of aortoiliac occlusive disease is by history and physical examination. Patients complain of lower-extremity muscle fatigue or cramping that occurs with a reproducible walking distance and is relieved by standing. This contrasts with similar pain of neurospinal etiology, which occurs at variable exercise levels, requires positional change for relief, and has an electrical or shooting quality. In men, erectile dysfunction may occur due to arterial insufficiency to the pelvis through the internal iliac arteries. With advanced occlusive disease, often at multiple levels, critical ischemia develops with rest pain or gangrene. Physical findings include abdominal bruits and diminished or absent femoral pulses. Occasionally, normal pulses are present at rest but "disappear" when the patient walks and vasodilates the distal vascular bed.

Initial treatment of patients with symptomatic aortoiliac disease begins with risk factor management. This includes counseling on the chronicity of the disease, smoking cessation, and an exercise program. Management of the patient's hypertension, diabetes, and hyperlipidemia should be optimized. In addition, patients must be instructed in the importance and the principles of meticulous foot care. Patients with persistent lifestyle-disabling symptoms and those with critical ischemia should be considered for revascularization. Aortobifemoral bypass is the gold standard and is performed through a combination of abdominal and femoral incisions (Fig. 11-6). Aortobifemoral bypass has a mortality of less than 3 percent and a remarkable 68 percent patency at 20 years according to the classic study by Szilagyi, which has been confirmed in over 20 other series.[23,24]

Many alternative procedures exist, each with purported specific benefits, including endarterectomy (see Fig. 11-2), which precludes the need for a prosthetic graft; axillobifemoral bypass, which avoids aortic cross-clamping and major cavity invasion (Fig. 11-7), and thoracofemoral bypass, with possible improved long-term patency[25] (Fig. 11-8). In the patient illustrated in Fig. 11-2, coral reef–appearing plaque not only impeded blood flow, but the irregular, ulcerated surfaces shed atheromatous debris, leading to the blue toe syndrome. Lately, laparoscopic aortobifemoral bypass has been explored and offers reduced recovery

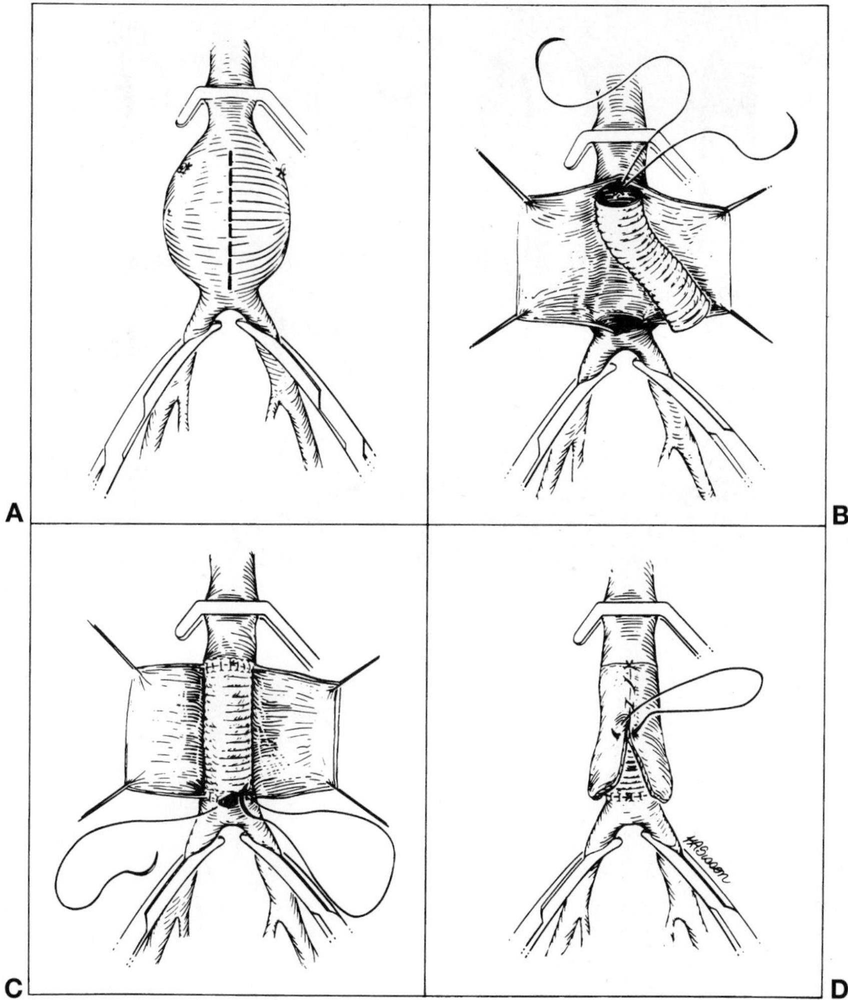

FIG. 11–4. Classic endoaneurysmal repair of an abdominal aortic aneurysm. **A,** Aorta is controlled with vascular clamps and opened. The prosthetic graft is sutured from within the aneurysm, attaching to the proximal **(B)** and distal **(C)** aorta. **D,** The aneurysm wall is closed over the graft to assist in hemostasis and prevent contact with the overlying bowel. (From Yao JST, Flinn WR, Bergan JJ: Technique for repairing infrarenal abdominal aortic aneurysm. In Nyhus LM, Baker RJ, eds: *Mastery of surgery*, Boston, 1984, Little, Brown & Co, pp 1361-1365.)

time while maintaining an anatomic revascularization.[26-28] The optimal choice of treatment should be based on balance between the durability of the procedure and its risks, considering each case individually.

Endovascular approaches have revolutionized the treatment of aortoiliac occlusive disease and are covered in detail in Chapter 6. Minimally invasive aortoiliac angioplasty has displaced bypass and endarterectomy as the primary procedure because of low complication rates and greatly reduced hospital stay and patient discomfort. Longer follow-up of randomized trials comparing angioplasty to conservative treatment has demonstrated improved arterial patency but equivalent patient satisfaction at 2 years.[29] Recent introduction of endovascular stenting and perhaps stent-grafting may provide improved long-term patency while maintaining the benefits of minimally invasive procedures.[30]

AORTIC DISSECTION

Dissection of the aorta is a condition in which the layers of the aortic wall have separated with a tear or opening into the lumen. Blood flows between the layers of the wall, “dissects”

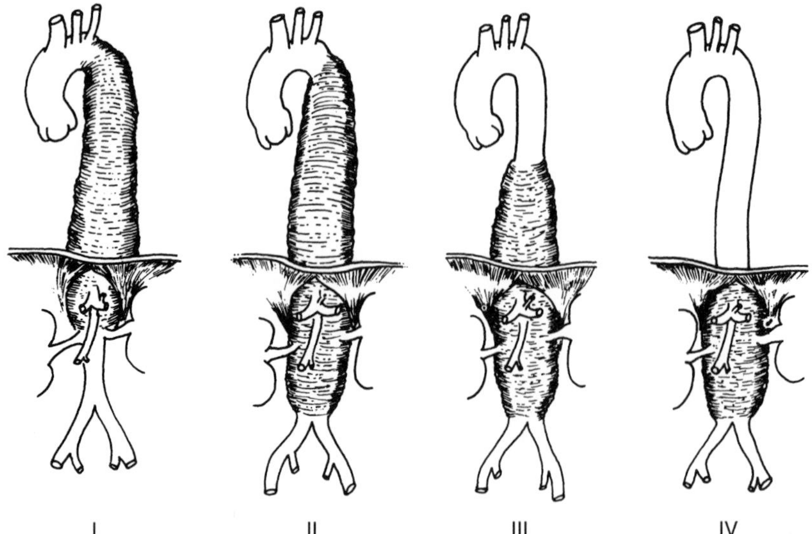

FIG. 11–5. Crawford classification of extent of thoracoabdominal aneurysms. Extent I and extent II aneurysms are associated with higher risks for paraplegia. (From Hamilton IN, Hollier LH: Thoracoabdominal aortic aneurysms. In Moore W, ed: *Vascular surgery: a comprehensive review*, ed 5, Philadelphia, 1998, WB Saunders, pp 417-434.)

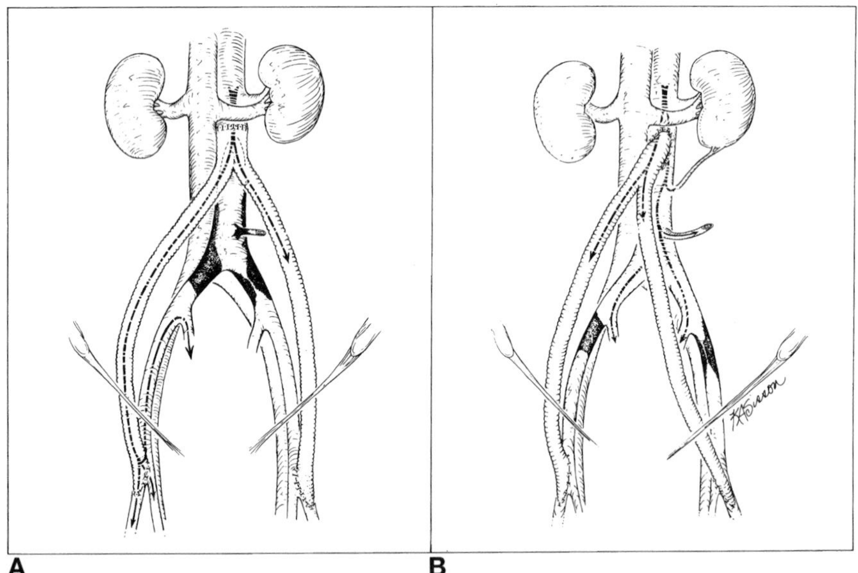

FIG. 11–6. Aortobifemoral bypass. **A,** End-to-end configuration for the aortic anastomosis. **B,** End-to-side configuration, which preserves native flow to the pelvis, inferior mesenteric artery, and inferior pole renal artery. (From Schuler JJ, Flanigan DP: Aortobifemoral artery bypass. In Nyhus LM, Baker RJ, eds: *Mastery of surgery*, Boston, 1984, Little, Brown & Co, pp 1419-1427.)

this space farther along the vessel, and creates a second blood-filled tube or "false lumen." In a dynamic process, differential blood flow and pressure occurs in the true and false lumen, resulting in sudden impaired perfusion to any of the aortic branches. In some hospitals, aortic dissection is a much more common emergency than ruptured aneurysm. Risk factors for dissection include hypertension, male gender, trauma (particularly deceleration injuries), cystic medial necrosis (Marfan's syndrome), and iatrogenic injury from catheter interventions and aortic clamping.

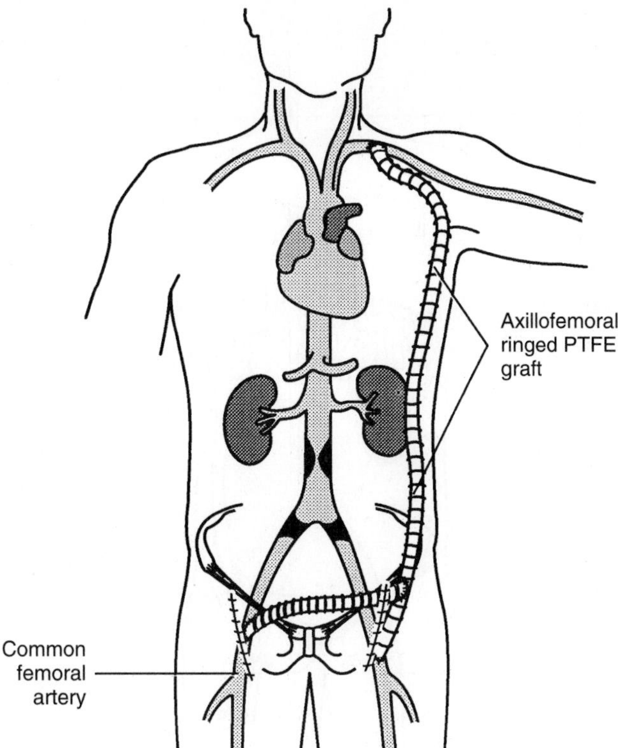

FIG. 11–7. Axillobifemoral bypass connects the axillary artery just beyond the clavicle to the femoral arteries along the side of the torso, avoiding invasion of major body cavities. This bypass can be performed under local and regional anesthesia. The externally supported grafts are usually palpable in the subcutaneous tunnels. *PTFE,* Polytetrafluoroethylene.

Aortic dissection typically presents with acute onset of "tearing" chest or back pain and can easily be mistaken for heart attack. Occasionally, patients will be pain free and present only with symptoms of branch artery occlusion, mimicking arterial embolism. Rupture of a dissection can cause internal hemorrhage akin to ruptured aortic aneurysm (Fig. 11-9). Because of the variety of presenting symptoms (Table 11-2), aortic dissection may be considered a great masquerader and is often misdiagnosed on admission. Physical examination of carotid, brachial, and femoral pulses with measurement of limb pressures must be performed and documented carefully, and continued surveillance for symptoms or change in pulse examination is a critical component to the care of these patients. A new cardiac murmur may be the earliest sign of aortic valve involvement.

Classification of aortic dissection is critical to predicting outcome and prescribing therapy. Acute dissection involving the ascending aorta may cause sudden death at a rate of 1-2 percent per hour because of the proximity to the coronary arteries, aortic valve involvement, or pericardial tamponade. These dissections are classified as Stanford type A (involves ascending) and DeBakey type I (ascending and descending) or type II (ascending only) and require immediate surgical treatment. Dissections limited to the descending aorta are classified as Stanford type B or DeBakey type III and are often initially treated with medical therapy (Fig. 11-10).[31]

Several tests are available to confirm the diagnosis of aortic dissection and classify its location. Helical CT scanning is widely available and, with proper timing of the contrast bolus, is a useful noninvasive screening test (Fig. 11-11). Transesophageal echocardiography has become the preferred test because it allows continued intensive care surveillance, is exceedingly accurate, and can provide additional information on ventricular function, aortic valve competency, and left main coronary patency.[32] Magnetic resonance imaging can be similarly helpful in an appropriate hospital setting.[33] Chest radiograms and electrocardiograms are

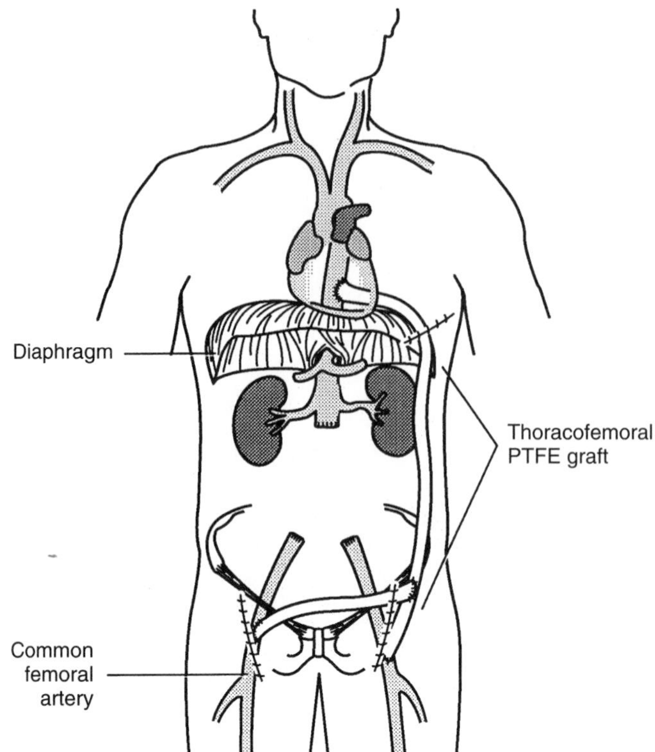

FIG. 11–8. Thoracofemoral bypass uses the descending thoracic aorta for inflow source. This bypass is also useful when there has been previous infection in the abdomen and the iliac arteries are ligated. *PTFE,* Polytetrafluoroethylene. (From McCarthy WJ, Rubin JR, Flinn WR et al: Descending thoracic aorto-to-femoral artery bypass, *Arch Surg* 121:681-688, 1986. Copyright 1986, American Medical Association.)

nonspecific and helpful mainly to exclude other diagnoses. Angiography, formerly the gold standard, is rarely performed because of the risk of worsening the dissection.

All patients with dissection require aggressive control of high blood pressure, usually in an intensive care unit with an arterial line. Beta-blockers have a theoretical advantage in reducing dp/dt (change in pressure over change in time) and wall stress, but several intravenous agents are available. As mentioned previously, constant surveillance for progression of dissection and branch vessel occlusion is necessary to detect peripheral ischemic complications rapidly. After the patient is pain free and clinically stable with blood pressure and pulse rate controlled to the desired parameters, the intravenous medications are gradually withdrawn and the patient is converted to oral antihypertensive agents and negative inotropic medications. Prior to discharge, it is imperative that patients understand their medication regimen and learn how to monitor their blood pressure and heart rate. After discharge, continued surveillance is required to ensure adequate blood pressure control, to monitor aortic size, and to detect progression of the dissection to an aneurysmal dilatation of the false lumen.

Surgical treatment is indicated in several circumstances: (1) location of dissection in ascending aorta, (2) development of ischemic complication, (3) poor response to medical management with continued pain, (4) aneurysmal degeneration, and (5) in selected Stanford type B patients dictated by local medical center experience.[34,35] Operations may include complete aortic replacement, fenestration of the intimal flap, interposition grafting, aortic valve resuspension, or extra-anatomic bypass. Fenestration involves making holes in the intimal flap to allow for communication of blood between the true and false lumens of a dissection plane. The procedure can be performed percutaneously or through an open operation.These patients have very high complication and death rates and are often referred to centers specializing in complex aortic operations. Endovascular interventions have also made a debut in

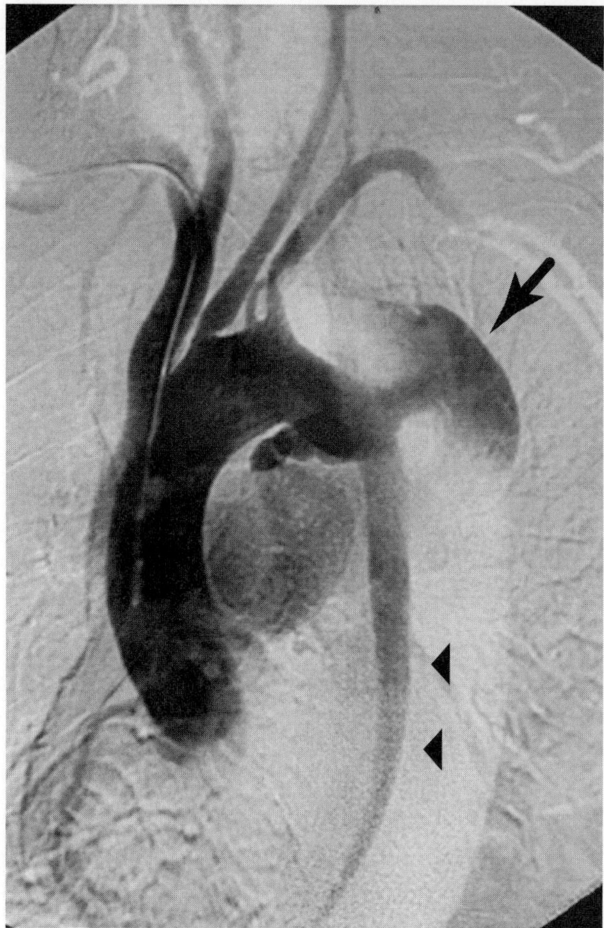

FIG. 11–9. Arteriogram demonstrating dissection flap *(arrowheads)* and impending rupture of false lumen *(solid arrow)*.

this disease process, with balloon fenestration and endovascular stenting, and offer hope of reduced morbidity and mortality in combination with standard surgical techniques.[36]

PERIOPERATIVE CARE

The preoperative evaluation of patients undergoing aortic operations includes a complete history and physical examination with attention to optimizing organ function in preparation for a major physiologic stress. Cardiac risk stratification is essential, as cardiac complications are the most frequent cause of early and late death, and aortic procedures are considered "high-risk" according to the American Heart Association guidelines.[2,37,38] There are varying opinions on the best way to evaluate cardiac risk preoperatively. However, there is agreement that using cardiac symptom severity in combination with a cardiac stress test provides adequate information to determine the patient's level of risk and the need for coronary angiography. The administration of beta-blockers, which decrease left ventricular workload, is a recommended procedure to use during the perioperative period to reduce the risk of myocardial ischemia in patients with cardiac risk.[11]

Equally important is preparing the patient mentally for the operation. This includes a thorough discussion of the indications and conduct of the operation, alternative treatments, discussion of risks of the operation and alternatives, setting reasonable expectations of recovery, providing preoperative teaching, and initiating discharge planning (Box 11-1).

TABLE 11–2 Symptoms and Pathogenesis of Aortic Dissection

Condition/Symptom	Frequency	Location/ Artery	Mechanism
Congestive heart failure	13-30%	Aortic valve	Ascending aortic tear results in deformation of aortic valve with acute valvular insufficiency and left heart failure
Hypotension	8-17%	Pericardium	False lumen ruptures through adventitia into pericardial space, causing pericardial tamponade; also may rupture into pleura or mediastinum with internal hemorrhage and shock
Myocardial ischemia	2%	Coronary	Dissection extends to coronary ostia, causing poor coronary perfusion and heart attack
Neurologic deficit	2-6%	Arch vessels Intercostal	Impaired perfusion to arch vessels causes stroke or to intercostal vessels causes paraplegia
Visceral ischemia	5%	Mesenteric	Branch occlusion causes ischemic liver and bowel
Hypertension, renal failure	5-10%	Renal	Decreased renal artery perfusion results in renin overproduction and renovascular hypertension; complete occlusion results in tubular necrosis and renal failure
Cold limb, pulse deficit	17%	Iliac Subclavian	Dissection continues down entire length of aorta into iliac vessels, and the cold foot is the most common peripheral ischemic complication
Aneurysm	20-50%	Aorta	Thinned aortic wall dilates, resulting in aneurysmal area; persistent patent tear and large initial diameter predict enlargement
Interscapular or substernal chest pain	90%	Aorta	Related to wall separation and often correlates to location and progression of dissection

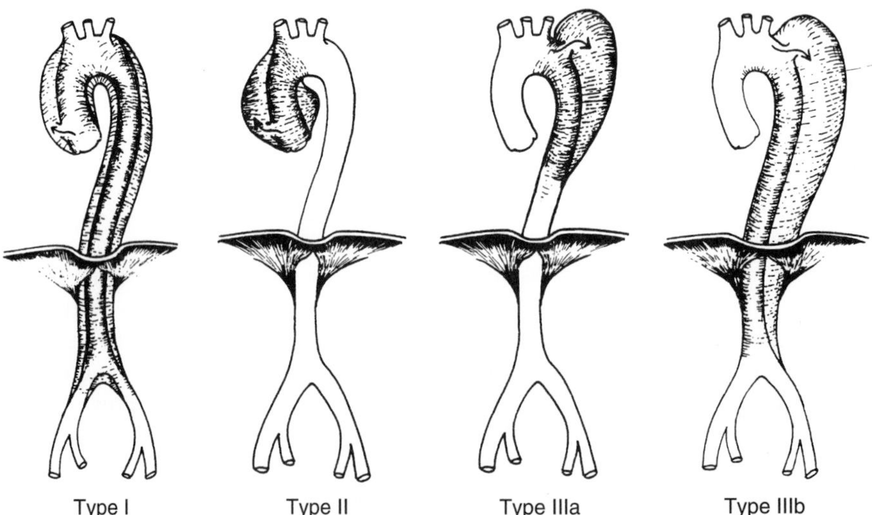

FIG. 11–10. Two popular classification schemes for aortic dissections. Diagnosis of involvement of ascending aorta has important prognostic and therapeutic implications. DeBakey types I and II are called type A in the Stanford classifications; DeBakey type III are equal to Stanford type B. (From Hamilton JN, Hollier LH: Thoracoabdominal aortic aneurysms. In Moore W, ed: *Vascular surgery: a comprehensive review*, ed 5, Philadelphia, 1998, WB Saunders, p 419.)

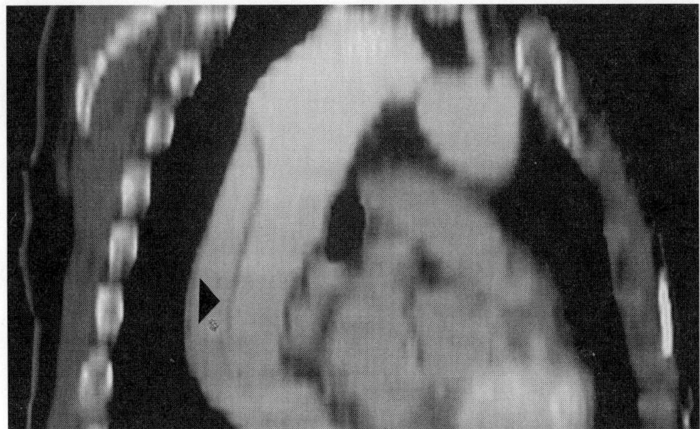

FIG. 11–11. Helical CT scan in sagittal plane demonstrating a Stanford type B dissection flap *(arrowhead)* limited to the descending thoracic aorta.

BOX 11–1

Teaching Plan (may vary from institution to institution)

PREOPERATIVE

Knowledge Deficit About Disease Process and Treatment

- Develop trusting relationship.
- Explain disease process and surgical procedure, using diagrams and written instructions when available.
- Teach and discuss with patient preop and postop routines; assess level of understanding and reinforce teaching.

POSTOPERATIVE

Activity

- Ambulate as tolerated, and increase activity gradually.
- Climbing stairs is acceptable in moderation.
- Going outdoors is acceptable.
- Regular exercise is important.
- No heavy lifting (more than 10 pounds) for 1 month after surgery.
- Sexual activity may be resumed in 3 to 4 weeks after discharge; discuss with physician if concerned.
- If leg swelling occurs, wear a 4-inch elastic bandage or elastic stockings when out of bed and elevate legs when sitting.

Bathing

- Bathing or showering is acceptable on the fifth day postop. Clean the incision with mild soap and water, and dry it well.

Driving

- Driving is usually permissible after the first check-up with the doctor and you can move legs normally. Do not drive if using narcotics or sleeping pills.

Wound Care

- No special care of wound is required unless otherwise indicated.

Avoiding Injury/Foot Care

- Inspect body daily, and be aware of how incisions, feet, and legs look and feel postop. This can help in recognition of early evidence of significant change.
- Wash feet regularly, and dry well; have a podiatrist care for corns, calluses, or ingrown toenails. Protect from excessive heat or cold by avoiding heating pads, heat lamps, and hot water bottles to feet and legs.
- Avoid cream hair removers or any chemicals on legs. Use lanolin creams to prevent skin cracking.

Continued

BOX 11–1

Teaching Plan (may vary from institution to institution)—cont'd

POSTOPERATIVE—cont'd

Avoiding Injury/Foot Care—cont'd

- Avoid clothes such as tight socks, garters, or panty hose that are constructing to the legs or feet.
- Wear shoes that fit well to avoid skin breakdown at pressure points. Wear socks or stockings with shoes at all times to prevent blistering, avoid walking barefoot, and inform physician if skin breakdown does occur.

Medications

- Explain medication, purpose of medication, dosage, and side effects.

Diet

- Inform patient that loss of appetite and changes in bowel habits may occur after surgery. One's appetite will slowly return to normal.
- Maintain a diet that prevents extra pounds. If patient requires special diet, obtain a dietitian consult.

Risk Factor Modification

- To control progression of atherosclerosis, it is important to make the following lifestyle changes:
  Control hypertension and diabetes.
  Stop smoking.
  Eat a low-fat, low-cholesterol diet.
  Reduce stress in your life.
  Exercise regularly.

Abdominal Aortic Aneurysms

- There is evidence that the risk of abdominal aortic aneurysm (AAA) is greater in first-degree relatives of patients with AAA. Both siblings and children may be at increased risk of developing aneurysms of the abdominal aorta. Please inform them so they can discuss this with their doctor.

Medical Regimen/Indications for Physician Notification

- Emphasize the importance of follow-up visits with physician.
- Notify the doctor of any changes in incision, new or unusual drainage, change in color or amount of drainage, increase in temperature, swelling at the incision site, inflammation or tenderness around incision, any unusual or severe increase in pain in back or legs, sudden weight gain or swelling of feet or legs, loss of sensation or movement, unusual tingling, coldness, or discoloration of the legs, or any skin breakdown on the foot. Inform patients to notify their physicians and/or dentists if they are undergoing any invasive procedure. Prophylactic antibiotics may be recommended during the first 6 months to 1 year after graft placement.

This counseling needs to be performed in an informative but also reassuring manner that integrates patients actively into their care.

Patients having elective surgery without the need for preoperative hospitalization are routinely admitted on the morning of the operation without apparent increased morbidity. Most patients receive general anesthesia for aortic procedures. Supplemental continuous epidural anesthesia is frequently used for its benefits of allowing a lighter level of general anesthesia as well as providing a delivery system for postoperative pain control.[11] Reduction in intensive care use can be implemented by establishing a designated vascular unit with concentration of nursing skills.[39,40] However, in most hospitals, patients undergoing aortic surgery are admitted to the intensive care unit after operation for invasive monitoring. This includes arterial pressure measurement, arterial blood gas analysis, electrocardiography, bladder catheterization, pulse oximetry, and physical examination including monitoring of neurologic status, central organ and limb perfusion and function, and ankle-brachial indices. Most patients require oxygen therapy and active topical warming. Postoperative cardiac enzymes and serial electrocardiograms are obtained based on signs or symptoms indicating myocardial ischemia.

The necessity and benefits of routine pulmonary artery catheters is being questioned; often only a central line is maintained for dependable intravenous access and infusion of vasoactive drugs.

Clinical pathways have become standard fare in medical centers. Clinical pathways with standardized order sheets may reduce unnecessary testing and, with intermittent data analysis, may identify areas of further quality improvement.[41] Shifting care to the ambulatory setting during the preoperative and postoperative stages reduces hospital charges but has an unknown effect on total costs.[39] A clinical pathway for open surgical repair of an abdominal aortic aneurysm is included in Table 11-3.

EARLY COMPLICATIONS AND NURSING INTERVENTIONS

Early complications and nursing interventions after aortic surgery are summarized in Table 11-4. The risk of myocardial stress is reduced by optimizing cardiac function during the perioperative period. This is accomplished by reducing cardiac afterload and maintaining adequate oxygenation, blood pressure control, volume balance, and a hematocrit of 28 percent.[11] Many complications such as embolization occur intraoperatively. Patient morbidity can be minimized with good postoperative support. Some problems such as intraabdominal bleeding and graft occlusion mandate immediate recognition and treatment to avoid a fatality. The hemodynamic changes and volume requirements that occur during aortic cross-clamping and declamping require delicate management of fluid and electrolyte balance, as many of the patients have compromised cardiac, pulmonary, and renal function that limits their reserve. Therefore, changes in cardiac function, acidosis, urine output, blood and fluid requirements, and limb perfusion are useful early markers of potential problems. Foremost in the care of these patients is a familiarity with the normal postoperative track so that departure from this course is quickly sensed and rectified. Extensive team experience is an important component of the postoperative care of patients after aortic operations.

LATE OUTCOME

Segmental aortic graft replacement does not influence the natural history of either more proximal aortic or distal iliac arterial disease. Typical, yet uncommon, late complications include development of secondary aneurysms, limb occlusion, graft infection, and pseudoaneurysms.[2,42-47] These complications often require reoperative aortic surgery several years after the first operation for correction of the presenting problem.

Subsequent Aneurysm

Rupture of a second aneurysm is a leading cause of death after abdominal aortic aneurysm repair.[2] In a recent survey of 10 years of reoperative aortic surgery at Northwestern, 67 secondary aneurysms were identified in 50 patients (Fig. 11-12). Presenting symptoms include rupture, limb ischemia, abdominal pain or mass, and hydronephrosis. One third of subsequent aneurysms are not palpable and are asymptomatic. Reoperations occur an average of 9 years after the first operation, and elective repair is safer compared to emergency operation. Similarly, of 26 patients presenting to the Mayo Clinic with rupture of a recurrent aneurysm, only 1 survived (4 percent).[48] This striking mortality after rupture requires that any patient fit to undergo an operation should have a secondary aneurysm repaired. Finally, routine radiographic imaging, usually a CT scan, is advisable at least every 5 years after aortic operations because these second aneurysms are often silent.[37,49]

Subsequent Occlusion

Graft occlusion presents as recurrent claudication or limb ischemia, usually in patients who had occlusive disease as the indication for their primary surgery. Progression of disease

TABLE 11–3 Clinical Pathway of Patient Undergoing Repair of Abdominal Aortic Aneurysm (Open)

	OR Day Date	ICU POD #1 Date	Floor POD #1 Date	POD #2 Date	POD #3 Date	POD #4 Date	POD #5 Date	POD #6 Date
Vital Signs/ Parameters	VS q 1 hour I/O q 1 hour	VS q 1 hour I/O q 1 hour Weight	VS q 4 hours I/O q 4 hours Weight	VS q 4 hours I/O q 4 hours Weight	VS q 4 hours I/O q 4 hours Weight	VS q 8 hours I/O q 8 hours Weight	VS q 8 hours I/O q 8 hours Weight	VS q 8 hours I/O q 8 hours Weight
Pulse/Doppler Assessment	Doppler tones/ ABI q 4 hours	Doppler tones/ ABI q 4 hours	Pulse/Doppler tones q 4 hours	Pulse/Doppler tones q 8 hours	Pulse/Doppler tones q 8 hours	Pulse/Doppler tones q 8 hours	Pulse/Doppler tones q 8 hours	Pulse/Doppler tones q 8 hours
Tests	SMA-8, CBC, PT/PTT Chest x-ray ECG ABG prn Isoenzymes prn	SMA-8, CBC, PT/PTT ECG ABG prn Isoenzymes prn			CBC, SMA-8	Arterial blood flow study (selectively)		
Consult/ Discharge Planning	PCA prn	PCA prn Transfer to floor	Physical therapy prn	Discharge planner/ social work prn Physical therapy prn	Discharge planner/ social work prn	Discharge planner/ social work prn May be discharged	Rx discharge instruction sheet completed May be discharged	Discharge skilled nursing unit prn
IV and PO Drugs	IV and A-line Antibiotic Pain medication prn Vasopressors prn	D/C A-line prn Pain medication prn Vasopressors prn	IV Pain medication prn	IV Pain medication prn	IV Pain medication prn	IV Pain medication prn	IV: D/C prn Pain medication prn	IV: D/C prn Pain medication prn
Activity	Bed rest	OOB × 1	OOB × 1 with assistance	Ambulate BID with assistance	Ambulate TID	Ambulate TID	Ambulate TID May shower	Ambulate TID May shower

Diet	NPO	NPO prn	NPO prn	NPO prn	Clear liquid diet after NG tube discontinued	Advance diet as tolerated	Low fat, low cholesterol	Low fat, low cholesterol
Treatment	NG tube prn Incentive spirometer TCDB q 2 hours O_2 prn Mouth care Incisional care Foley care	NG tube prn MD changes first dressing in AM Incentive spirometer TCDB q 2 hours Mouth care D/C Foley prn	NG tube prn Incentive spirometer TCDB q 2 hours Incisional care qd	NG tube prn Incentive spirometer TCDB q 2 hours Mouth care	Assess NG tube status Incisional care qd Mouth care	Assess NG tube status Incisional care qd Mouth care	Incisional care qd	Incisional care qd
Psychosocial	Provide support	Assess patient needs	Intervene with patient/family Psychosocial needs prn	Intervene with patient/family Psychosocial needs prn	Intervene with patient/family Psychosocial needs prn	Intervene with patient/family Psychosocial needs prn	Intervene with patient/family Psychosocial needs prn	Intervene with patient/family Psychosocial needs prn
Patient Education	Assess patient/family's level of under-standing Discuss post course with family	Assess patient/family's level of under-standing Discuss post course with family			Review patient education material including risk reduc-tion material	Discharge teaching	Discharge teaching	Discharge teaching

OR, Operating room; *ICU,* intensive care unit; *POD,* postoperative day; *VS,* vital signs; *q,* every; *I/O,* intake and output; *ABI,* ankle-brachial inex; *SMA,* Sequential Multiple Analysis; *CBC,* complete blood count; *PT/PTT,* prothrombin time/partial thromboplastin time; *ECG,* electrocardiogram; *ABG,* arterial blood gas; *prn,* as needed; *PCA,* patient-controlled analgesia; *Rx,* prescription (drugs and other medicaments); *DC,* discharge; *IV,* intravenous; *PO,* oral; *A-line,* arterial line; *D/C,* discontinue; *OOB,* out of bed; *BID,* twice a day; *TID,* three times a day; *NPO,* nothing by mouth; *NG,* nasogastric; *TCDB,* turn, cough, deep breathe; *MD,* physician; *qd,* every day.

TABLE 11-4 Potential Postoperative Complications, Causes, and Nursing Interventions

Complication	Pathogenesis	Nursing Interventions
Myocardial ischemia or infarction	Cardiac stress due to hemodynamic changes with aortic cross-clamping and declamping Pre-existing cardiac disease Supply: coronary thrombosis, hypoperfusion, anemia, hypoxemia; Demand: hypertension, tachycardia, hypothermia	Monitor vital signs; implement adequate analgesic regimen; monitor electrocardiogram; restart appropriate cardiac medications; active rewarming
Congestive heart failure	Fluid overload, myocardial ischemia Pre-existing cardiac disease	Monitor fluid balance; anticipate "mobilization" of third space fluids; initiate appropriate diuretic prescription
Dysrhythmia	Hypoxemia, myocardial ischemia, electrolyte imbalance, pulmonary artery catheter	Monitor oximetry, vital signs, and electrocardiogram; review chest radiogram and laboratory values
Atelectasis	Decreased lung function, incisional pain History of smoking and COPD	Implement analgesic regimen; encourage incentive spirometry/deep breathing; assist early mobilization
Renal failure	Embolization, renal artery damage, renal vein ligation, ureteral injury, dehydration, prolonged suprarenal clamp time, or rhabdomyolysis	Monitor blood pressure, urine output, creatinine, urine myoglobin, serum CPK, and fluid balance; check for hematuria
Ischemic colitis	Inferior mesenteric and hypogastric artery ligation, embolization, hypoperfusion	Maintain adequate hydration; monitor vital signs; monitor for abdominal distension, pain, or excessive third spacing, elevated white blood count, persistent tachycardia, worsening acidosis, bloody diarrhea
Prolonged ileus	Extensive operation, other postoperative complications	Maintain nasogastric drainage; monitor for abdominal tenderness; institute necessary nutritional support
Aortoenteric fistula	Erosion of graft into small bowel, most often involves the duodenum	Assess for signs of gastrointestinal hemorrhage
Leg ischemia	Embolization, graft occlusion, hypoperfusion	Monitor limb pulses, color, temperature, motor and sensory functions, and Doppler pressures; with axillo-to-femoral and femoral-femoral grafts, monitor donor limb pulses also
Graft occlusion	Technical error, hypotension, coagulopathy	Monitor limb perfusion and ankle pressures
Compartment syndrome	Prolonged ischemia from acute occlusion or clamp time	Assess for calf swelling and tenderness, tea-colored urine due to myoglobinuria

distal to the aortobifemoral bypass is the most common cause of late graft occlusion. Several options, including observation, extra-anatomic bypass, and thrombectomy with outflow revision are available as alternatives to reoperative aortic surgery for graft occlusion.[50] Whether widespread use of angioplasty and primary stenting for occlusive disease will reduce the need for reoperative aortic surgery or increase the use of aortic surgery for management of failure

TABLE 11-4 Potential Postoperative Complications, Causes, and Nursing Interventions—cont'd

Complication	Pathogenesis	Nursing Interventions
Hemorrhage	Technical error, coagulopathy, hypothermia, hypertension, thrombocytopenia, hypocalcemia	Monitor vital signs, complaints of abdominal or back pain, increase in abdominal girth; check laboratory values and notify physician if abnormal; check dressings and incisions for hematoma and bleeding; provide active rewarming and maintenance of euthermia, transfusion as necessary
Nosocomial infection	Invasive monitoring/tubes, aseptic technique break	Check dressings and observe quality of drainage; observe strict aseptic techniques; monitor for fever
Paraplegia	Spinal cord ischemia, hypotension, cord swelling	Monitor neurologic function; maintain spinal drainage as indicated
Erectile dysfunction	Disruption of periaortic sympathetic plexus	Document baseline status; provide preoperative patient counseling; make referral to urologist if necessary

COPD, Chronic obstructive pulmonary disease; *CPK,* creatinine phosphokinase.

of endovascular treatment is unknown. Nevertheless, mortality is 5 percent in elective reoperation, similar to primary surgery.[51]

Subsequent Infection

Fortunately, graft infections occur in less than 1 percent of patients after aortic operation. Antibiotic prophylaxis is recommended for dental procedures, gastrointestinal endoscopic

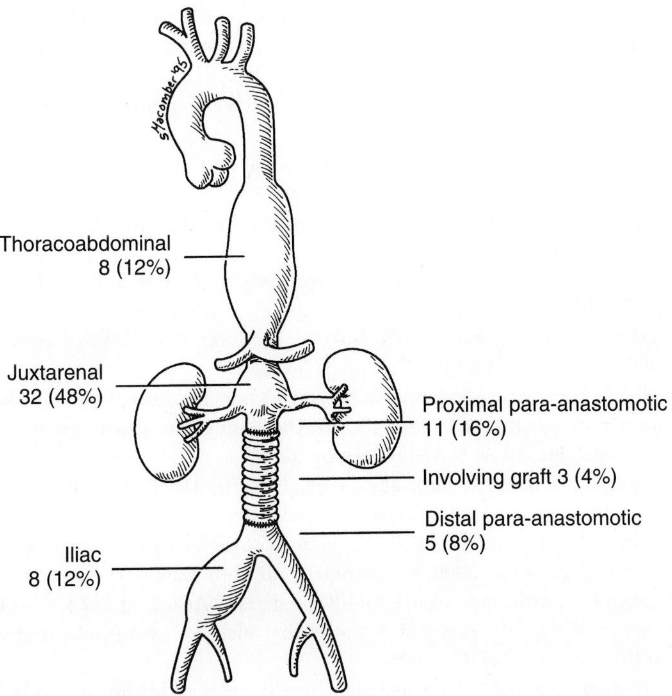

FIG. 11–12. Locations of 67 subsequent aneurysms.

procedures, and other interventions likely to result in bacteremia for the first year after prosthetic aortic graft placement. The interval between primary procedure and subsequent infection is shorter compared to other late complications after aortic operation. Presenting symptoms include fever, abdominal or groin mass, groin wound infection, and the dramatic aortoenteric fistula. The latter problem may manifest as exsanguinating gastrointestinal hemorrhage that requires emergent operation in an unstable patient. Graft infections often require total graft removal with extra-anatomic bypass and remain a challenging problem with high morbidity and mortality.[52] Other approaches in selected patients are in situ replacement with antibiotic-impregnated prosthetic grafts, cadaveric allografts, or autogenous femoral vein reconstructions, and improved results have been described with these techniques.[53-55]

Long-Term Mortality

Patient longevity after aortic surgery is reduced in some studies, primarily due to increased heart-related mortality,[56] although in others it was found to be comparable to age-matched controls.[57,58] These differences may be dependent on different utilization of coronary revascularization.[59] Overall survival is about 90 percent at 1 year and 65 percent at 5 years. Intensive study in this area is needed to evaluate whether strategies of coronary artery bypass grafting at the time of presentation with aortic disease will have significant benefits in long-term patient survival.

SUMMARY

Significant improvements over the past 50 years have resulted in the development of safe surgical procedures for aortic disease.[60] Early and late complications are well defined. Endovascular and other minimally invasive therapies are being developed, tested, and refined. Perioperative nursing care based on an understanding of the anatomic importance of the aorta remains an important component of quality patient care.

REFERENCES

1. Brewster DC, Darling RC: Optimal methods of aortoiliac reconstruction, *Surgery* 84:739-748, 1978.
2. Crawford ES, Saleh SA, Babb JW et al: Infrarenal abdominal aortic aneurysm: factors influencing survival after operation performed over a 25-year period, *Ann Surg* 193:699-709, 1981.
3. Kazmers A, Perkins AJ, Jacobs LA: Outcomes after abdominal aortic aneurysm repair in those ≥80 years of age: recent veterans affairs experience, *Ann Vasc Surg* 12:106-112, 1998.
4. Batt M, Staccini P, Pittaluga P et al: Late survival after abdominal aortic aneurysm repair, *Eur J Vasc Endovasc Surg* 17:338-342, 1999.
5. Williamson WK, Nicoloff AD, Taylor LM Jr et al: Functional outcome after open repair of abdominal aortic aneurysm, *J Vasc Surg* 33:913-920, 2001.
6. Huber TS, Wang JG, Derrow AE et al: Experience in the United States with intact abdominal aortic aneurysm repair, *J Vasc Surg* 33:304-311, 2001.
7. Zarins CK, Glagov S: Artery wall pathology in atherosclerosis. In Rutherford RB, ed: *Vascular surgery*, Philadelphia, 1989, WB Saunders, pp 178-193.
8. Goldstone J: Aneurysms of the aorta and iliac arteries. In Moore WS, ed: *Vascular surgery: a comprehensive review*, Philadelphia, 2002, WB Saunders, pp 457-480.
9. White JV, Scovell SD: Etiology of abdominal aortic aneurysms: the structural basis for aneurysm formation. In Calligaro KD, Dougherty MJ, Hollier LH, eds: *Diagnosis and treatment of aortic and peripheral arterial aneurysms*, Philadelphia, 1999, WB Saunders, pp 3-12.
10. Taylor LM Jr, Porter JM: Abdominal aortic aneurysms. In Porter JM, Taylor LM Jr, eds: *Basic data underlying clinical decision making in vascular surgery*, St Louis, 1994, Quality Medical Publishing, pp 98-100.
11. Cronenwett JL, Krupski WC, Rutherford RB: Abdominal aortic and iliac aneurysms. In Rutherford RB, ed: *Vascular surgery*, Philadelphia, 2000, WB Saunders, pp 1246-1280.
12. Crawford ES, Cohen ES: Aortic aneurysm: a multifocal disease, *Arch Surg* 117:1393-1400, 1982.
13. Cronenwett JL, Sargent SWK, Wall MH et al: Variables that affect the expansion rate and outcome of small aortic aneurysm, *J Vasc Surg* 11:260-268, 1990.
14. Cronenwett JL: Abdominal aortic aneurysms: predicting the natural history. In Yao JST, Pearce WH, eds: *Progress in vascular surgery*, Stamford, Conn, 1997, Appleton & Lange, pp 127-138.

15. Sicard GA, Reilly JM, Rubin BG et al: Transabdominal versus retroperitoneal incision for abdominal aortic surgery: report of a prospective randomized trial, *J Vasc Surg* 21:174-183, 1995.
16. Turnipseed WD, Carr SC, Tefera G et al: Minimal incision aortic surgery, *J Vasc Surg* 34:47-53, 2001.
17. Paty PSK, Darling RC III, Chang BB et al: A prospective randomized study comparing exclusion technique and endoaneurysmorrhaphy for treatment of infrarenal aortic aneurysm, *J Vasc Surg* 25:442-445, 1997.
18. Murayama KM, Grune MT, Baxter BT: Minimally invasive approaches to aneurysmal and occlusive disease of the aorta. In Yao JST, Pearce WH, eds: *Techniques in vascular and endovascular surgery*, Stamford, Conn, 1998, Appleton & Lange, pp 109-119.
19. Moore WS, Rutherford RB, for the EVT investigators: Transfemoral endovascular repair of abdominal aortic aneurysm: results of the North American EVT phase I trial, *J Vasc Surg* 23:543-553, 1996.
20. Matsumura JS, Pearce WH, McCarthy WJ III et al: Reduction in aortic aneurysm size: early results after endovascular graft placement, *J Vasc Surg* 25:113-123, 1997.
21. Ivancev K, Malina M, Lindblad B et al: Abdominal aortic aneurysms: experience with the Ivancev-Malmo endovascular system for aortomonoiliac stent-grafts, *J Endovasc Surg* 4:242-251, 1997.
22. McDaniel MD, Cronenwett JL: Basic data related to the natural history of intermittent claudication, *Ann Vasc Surg* 3:273-277, 1989.
23. Szilagyi DE, Elliott JP Jr, Smith RF et al: A thirty-year survey of the reconstructive surgical treatment of aortoiliac occlusive disease, *J Vasc Surg* 3:421-436, 1986.
24. de Vries SO, Hunink MGM: Results of aortic bifurcation grafts for aortoiliac occlusive disease: a meta-analysis, *J Vasc Surg* 26:558-569, 1997.
25. McCarthy WJ, Mesh CL, McMillan WD et al: Descending thoracic aorta-to-femoral artery bypass: ten years' experience with a durable procedure, *J Vasc Surg* 17:336-348, 1993.
26. Ahn SS, Clem MF, Braithwaite BD et al: Laparoscopic aortofemoral bypass, *Ann Surg* 222:677-683, 1995.
27. Dion YM, Katkhouda N, Rouleau C et al: Laparoscopy-assisted aortobifemoral bypass, *Surg Laparosc Endosc* 3:425-429, 1993.
28. Fabiani J-N, Mercier F, Carpentier A et al: Video-assisted aortofemoral bypass: results in seven cases, *Ann Vasc Surg* 11:273-277, 1997.
29. Whyman MR, Fowkes FGR, Kerracher EMG et al: Is intermittent claudication improved by percutaneous transluminal angioplasty? A randomized controlled trial, *J Vasc Surg* 26:551-557, 1997.
30. Marin ML, Veith FJ, Sanchez LA et al: Endovascular aortoiliac grafts in combination with standard infrainguinal arterial bypasses in the management of limb-threatening ischemia: preliminary report, *J Vasc Surg* 22:316-325, 1995.
31. Glower DD, Wolfe WG: Management of dissecting aortic aneurysms. In Yao JST, Pearce WH, eds: *Aneurysms: new findings and treatments*, East Norwalk, Conn, 1994, Appleton & Lange, pp 147-160.
32. Blanchard DG, Kimura BJ, Dittrich HC et al: Transesophageal echocardiography of the aorta, *JAMA* 272:546-551, 1994.
33. Nienaber CA, von Kodolitsch Y, Nicolas V et al: The diagnosis of thoracic aortic dissection by noninvasive imaging procedures, *N Engl J Med* 328:1-8, 1993.
34. Glower DD, Speier RH, White WD et al: Management and long-term outcome of aortic dissection, *Ann Surg* 214:31-41, 1991.
35. Fann JI, Smith JA, Miller DC et al: Surgical management of aortic dissection during a 30-year period, *Circulation* 92(suppl II):II113-121, 1995.
36. Slonim SM, Nyman U, Semba CP et al: Aortic dissection: percutaneous management of ischemic complications with endovascular stents and balloon fenestration, *J Vasc Surg* 23:241-253, 1996.
37. Edwards JM, Teefey SA, Zierler RE, et al: Intraabdominal paraanastomotic aneurysms after aortic bypass grafting, *J Vasc Surg* 15:344-353, 1992.
38. Eagle KA, Brundage BH, Chaitman BR et al: Guidelines for perioperative cardiovascular evaluation for noncardiac surgery: report of the American College of Cardiology/American Heart Association Task Force on Practice Guidelines (Committee on Perioperative Cardiovascular Evaluation for Noncardiac Surgery), *Circulation* 93:1278-1317, 1996.
39. Calligaro KD, Dandura R, Dougherty MJ et al: Same-day admissions and other cost-saving strategies for elective aortoiliac surgery, *J Vasc Surg* 25:141-144, 1997.
40. Bertges DJ, Rhee RY, Muluk SC et al: Is routine use of the intensive care unit after elective infrarenal abdominal aortic aneurysm repair necessary? *J Vasc Surg* 32:634-642, 2000.
41. Muluk SC, Painter L, Sile S et al: Utility of clinical pathway and prospective case management to achieve cost and hospital stay reduction for aortic aneurysm surgery at a tertiary care hospital, *J Vasc Surg* 25:84-93, 1997.
42. Stoney RJ, Albo RJ, Wylie EJ: False aneurysms occurring after arterial grafting operations, *Am J Surg* 110:153-161, 1965.

43. Mikati A, Marache P, Watel A et al: End-to-side aortoprosthetic anastomoses: long-term computed tomography assessment, *Ann Vasc Surg* 4:584-591, 1990.
44. den Hoed PT, Veen HF: The late complications of aorto-ilio-femoral dacron prostheses: dilatation and anastomotic aneurysm formation, *Eur J Vasc Surg* 6:282-287, 1992.
45. Szilagyi DE, Smith RF, Elliott JP et al: Anastomotic aneurysms after vascular reconstruction: problems of incidence, etiology, and treatment, *Surgery* 78:800-816, 1975.
46. Crawford ES, Manning LG, Kelly TF: "Redo" surgery after operations for aneurysm and occlusion of the abdominal aorta, *Surgery* 81:41-52, 1977.
47. Coselli JS, LeMaire SA, Büket S et al: Subsequent proximal aortic operations in 123 patients with previous infrarenal abdominal aortic aneurysm surgery, *J Vasc Surg* 22:59-67, 1995.
48. Plate G, Hollier LA, O'Brien P et al: Recurrent aneurysms and late vascular complications following repair of abdominal aortic aneurysms, *Arch Surg* 120:590-594, 1985.
49. Berman SS, Hunter GC, Smyth SH et al: Application of computed tomography for surveillance of aortic grafts, *Surgery* 118:8-15, 1995.
50. Brewster DC, Meier GH, Darling RC et al: Reoperation for aortofemoral graft limb occlusion: optimal method and long-term results, *J Vasc Surg* 5:363-374, 1987.
51. Erdoes LS, Bernhard VM, Berman SS: Aortofemoral graft occlusion: strategy and timing of reoperation, *Cardiovasc Surg* 3:277-283, 1995.
52. McCarthy WJ, McGee GS, Lin WW et al: Axillary-popliteal artery bypass provides successful limb salvage after removal of infected aortofemoral grafts, *Arch Surg* 127:974-978, 1992.
53. Bandyk DF, Bergamini TM, Kinney EV et al: In situ replacement of vascular prostheses infected by bacterial biofilms, *J Vasc Surg* 13:575-583, 1991.
54. Kieffer E, Bahnini A, Koskas F et al: In situ allograft replacement of infected infrarenal aortic prosthetic grafts: results in forty-three patients, *J Vasc Surg* 17:349-356, 1993.
55. Clagett GP, Valentine RJ, Hagino RT: Autogenous aortoiliac/femoral reconstruction from superficial femoral-popliteal veins: feasibility and durability, *J Vasc Surg* 25:255-270, 1997.
56. Johnston KW and the Canadian Society for Vascular Surgery Aneurysm Study Group: Nonruptured abdominal aortic aneurysm: six-year follow-up results from the Multicenter Prospective Canadian Aneurysm Study, *J Vasc Surg* 20:163-170, 1994.
57. Feinglass J, Cowper D, Dunlop D et al: Late survival risk factors for abdominal aortic aneurysm repair: experience from fourteen Department of Veterans Affairs hospitals, *Surgery* 118:16-24, 1995.
58. Stonebridge PA, Cullam MJ, Bradbury AW et al: Comparison of long term survival after successful repair of ruptured and nonruptured abdominal aortic aneurysms, *Br J Surg* 80:585-586, 1993.
59. O'Hara PJ, Hertzer NH, Krajewski LP et al: Ten year experience with abdominal aortic aneurysm repair in octogenarians: early results and late complications, *J Vasc Surg* 21:830-838, 1995.
60. Friedman SG: The 50th anniversary of abdominal aortic reconstruction, *J Vasc Surg* 33:895-898, 2001.

12

Endovascular Repair of Aortic Aneurysms

DIANA EASTRIDGE □ HERON RODRIGUEZ □ JON S. MATSUMURA

The treatment of abdominal aortic aneurysms (AAAs) has evolved through the years. In 1818, Sir Astley Cooper ligated the abdominal aorta to treat an iliac aneurysm. By the end of the nineteenth century, AAAs were treated by packing wire inside the aneurysm, in an effort to create thrombosis of the aneurysm. Rudolph Matas performed the first successful aortic ligation in 1923. In 1951, Charles Dubost accomplished a milestone in surgery by replacing the aneurysmal aorta with a cadaveric homograft.[1] The technique of aneurysm repair involving an open surgical method was refined, and by the end of the twentieth century, successful treatment of AAA was achieved with preoperative mortality rates under 2 percent and a high level of long-term efficacy.

During the last decade, the field of surgery experienced a revolution towards minimally invasive techniques. Aortic surgery was not the exception, and, in 1991, Parodi, Palmaz, and Barone[2] reported the treatment of an AAA with a novel technique: excluding the aneurysm from the circulation by inserting a covered stent through the femoral arteries.[2] In less than 10 years, the technique spread across the world.

This chapter will describe devices, techniques, complications, and nursing management associated with the emerging endovascular options in the treatment of AAA. It is important to note that the use of stent grafts for repair is a new technology and has not been explored in large, controlled clinical trials.

Case Report I

An 89-year-old man with back pain presented to an outside hospital with a ruptured infrarenal aneurysm. Computed tomography (CT) imaging showed a large retroperitoneal hematoma and extravasation of blood from his infrarenal aneurysm sac, which measured 8.0 cm in diameter. An endovascular repair was performed using a modular device. The patient survived, and subsequent CT scans showed no evidence of endoleak, gradual resolution of the retroperitoneal hematoma, and shrinkage of the aneurysm sac to 5.5 cm at 12 months (Fig.12-1).

Case Report II

A 35-year-old male with normal erectile function was treated with an endovascular stent graft for repair of a right common iliac artery aneurysm, associated with a focal dissection. The patient's case was remarkable for the fact that his twin brother had almost died from the rupture of a right iliac artery aneurysm. The patient had undergone preoperative coiling of his right hypogastric artery. CT imaging 1 month after surgery showed an excluded aneurysm without evidence of an endoleak (Fig. 12-2). He had no erectile or ejaculatory dysfunction and returned to work in 2 weeks.

Case Report III

Repeat endovascular procedures may need to be completed to achieve a satisfactory result after endovascular repair. A 74-year-old patient had a 6.2-cm aneurysm repaired 2½ years ago. During the intervening time from the initial repair, the aneurysm grew to 7.2 cm and the CT scan demonstrated a persistent endoleak (Fig. 12-3). The patient underwent three additional procedures,

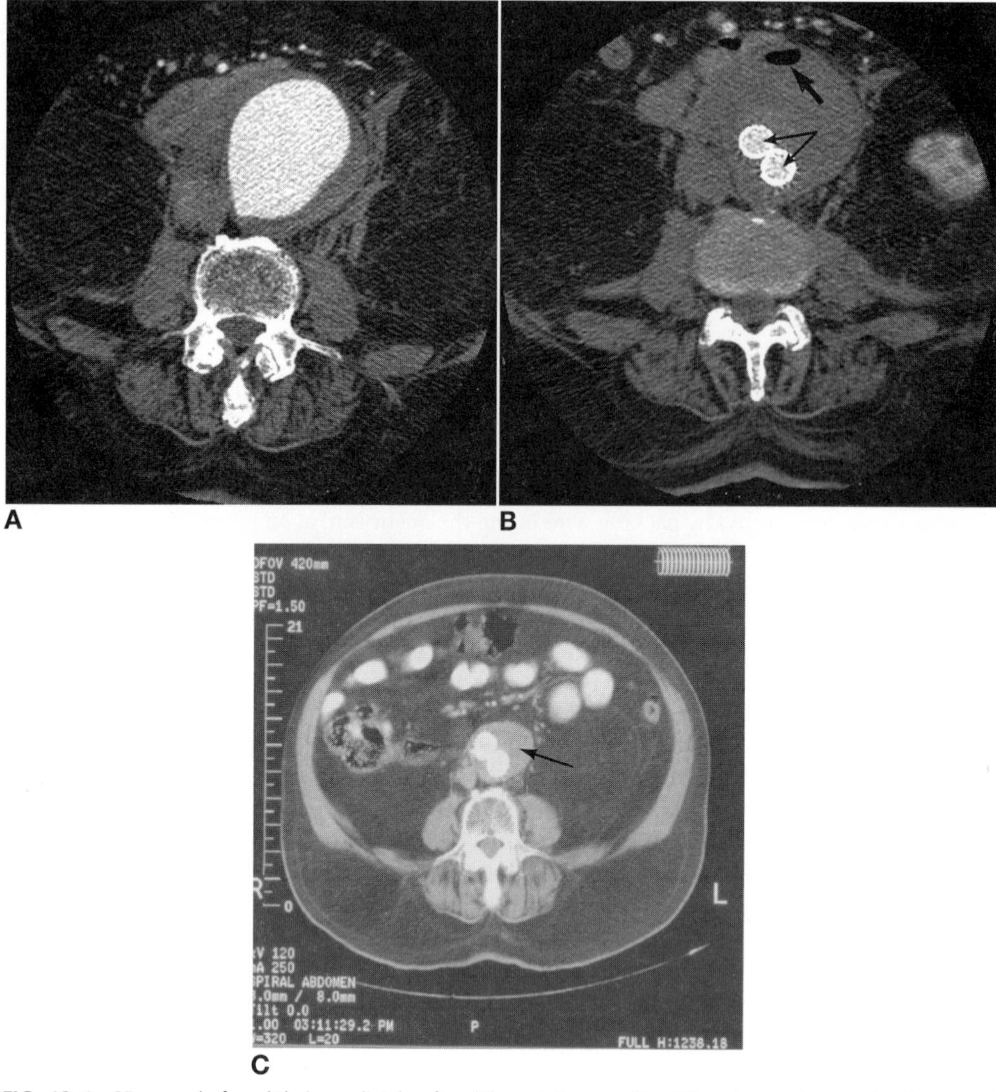

FIG. 12–1. CT scans before (**A**), immediately after (**B**), and 1 year after (**C**) endovascular repair of ruptured abdominal aortic aneurysm (AAA). **B,** Scan shows the limbs of the bifurcated endograft *(small arrowheads)*. Note the perigraft air shown within the aneurysm sac *(large arrowhead)*. These air bubbles are often seen in the sac after an endograft repair but disappear by approximately 2 weeks after repair. **C,** Scan shows the decrease in size in the aneurysm *(small arrowhead)*.

which included placement of supplementary modular device pieces and two coiling procedures. Three months after the third reintervention, the endoleak was still visualized, but at a reduced level and the aneurysm had decreased in size from the measurement on the previous CT scan.

These three cases illustrate the main benefits and problems with endovascular repair. This option allows safer treatment of patients with severe comorbidities and offers less invasive and less disabling treatment of highly functional patients. However, it does require chronic surveillance and relatively frequent reintervention after initial treatment.

PATIENT SELECTION

Diagnosis and Preoperative Imaging

Not all patients with abdominal aortic aneurysms can be treated with endovascular techniques. Suitability for an endograft repair depends on several factors, the most important of

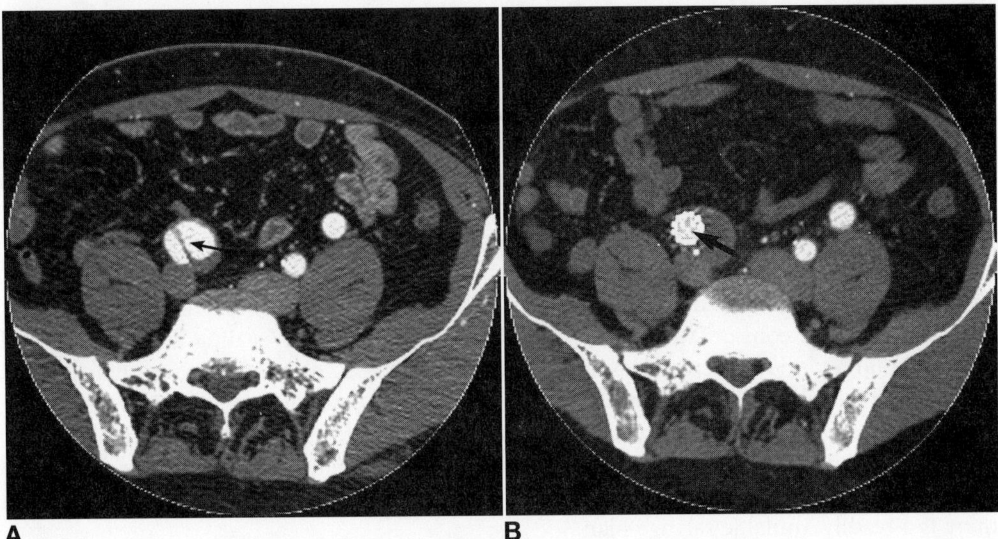

FIG. 12–2. CT scan before (**A**) and 1 month after (**B**) repair of right iliac artery aneurysm. **A,** Scan shows focal dissection *(arrowhead)*. **B,** Scan shows the flow of blood through the endovascular graft *(arrowhead)*, and the dissection is no longer seen.

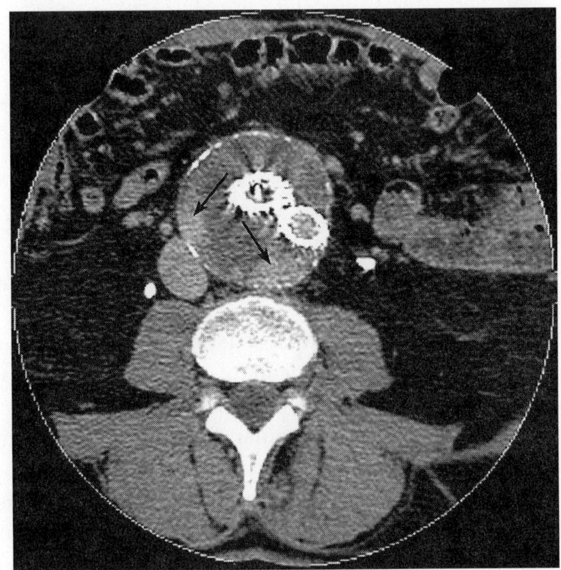

FIG. 12–3. Persistent endoleak *(arrowheads)* following endovascular repair of abdominal aortic aneurysm (AAA) and repeat interventions.

these being the anatomy of the aorta and iliac arteries. High-resolution CT scans, with 3-mm or thinner cuts, are used to obtain measurements of several anatomic structures. In the elective situation, a helical CT scan with dynamic radiocontrast infusion usually provides the required information on anatomic candidacy for endovascular repair. Length and diameter measurements are taken at various locations in the aorta to determine the sizing of the endograft and to select the appropriate endovascular device. Rarely, concern for the stenoses of internal iliac, mesenteric, or renal artery branches will prompt preoperative arteriography. In the emergent situation of a ruptured aneurysm or aortoenteric fistula, standard CT scans can provide enough information to undertake an endovascular repair as long as an adequate inventory of endografts is available.

The neck of the aneurysm (segment of the aorta between the lowest renal artery and the aneurysm) must be at least 15 mm in length and no more than 26 mm in diameter. Small, calcified, or tortuous iliac arteries are also relative contraindications for endovascular repair. Depending on the particular institution, 30-80 percent of patients may be candidates for endovascular repair. Other important factors influencing the decision to repair an aneurysm with endovascular grafts are the availability of a specific device and the local expertise and judgment of the vascular team.

Anatomic Assessment

Anatomic planning for endovascular repair of infrarenal aneurysms involves two main components. The first consideration is the identification of adequate sealing zones above and below the target lesion to ensure exclusion of the aneurysm. As stated earlier, there should be at least 15 mm of cylindrical neck, free of significant angulation, plaque, and thrombus, and a diameter such that 10-20 percent oversizing of the graft can be achieved. Endovascular exclusion without a type I endoleak is possible with neck anatomy less suitable than these ideal parameters but should be attempted only when the alternative options are poor or when there is a readily available salvage plan.

The second main consideration is a plan for endovascular access, and this requires a familiarity with various adjunctive procedures to overcome anatomic challenges. The combined assessment of iliac artery diameter, tortuosity, calcification, and stenoses is important for successful insertion and manipulation of large devices.

An individualized approach should be based on patient comorbidities, anatomic measurements, and the availability of open operative options. For example, an elderly patient with a 6.0-cm infrarenal aneurysm, a long, straight infrarenal neck, multiple previous retroperitoneal procedures, and a high cardiac risk would receive strong consideration for an endovascular repair.

DEVICES

Terminology

All endografts are made of three components: a fabric cover (the graft), a metallic frame incorporated to the graft (the stent), and a mechanism to attach the device to the aorta (the attachment system). Device designs vary on the characteristics of these three components. Some devices are unibody, and others are modular. Some devices are stented only at attachment sites, and others are fully supported.

A number of endograft configurations are available, and some comments specific to each type are warranted. The original Parodi aorto-aortic tube style endografts are not durable for primary treatment of infrarenal aortic aneurysms because of distal neck dilation but are often suitable for subsequent proximal aneurysms. Aorto-monoiliac devices (grafts with one iliac limb) offer versatility in the emergent situation when precise preoperative anatomic measurements are not possible. One-piece bifurcated endografts and modular-component endografts are the most popular choices. Modular systems often can overcome anatomic challenges of endovascular approaches because of the wide range of size combinations. Careful consideration of the sequence of placing modular grafts is important, in order to maximize sealing and fixation between components.

Food and Drug Administration–Approved Devices

At present, several different devices are being implanted in the United States. Three of these, the GORE EXCLUDER endoprosthesis (WL Gore, Fig. 12-4), the AneuRx (Medtronic, Fig. 12-5), and the Zenith (Coole), are approved by the Food and Drug Administration (FDA). There are other investigational devices, including the Talent (Medtronic) that are currently undergoing clinical trials and are not approved for use in the United States. Also, some insti-

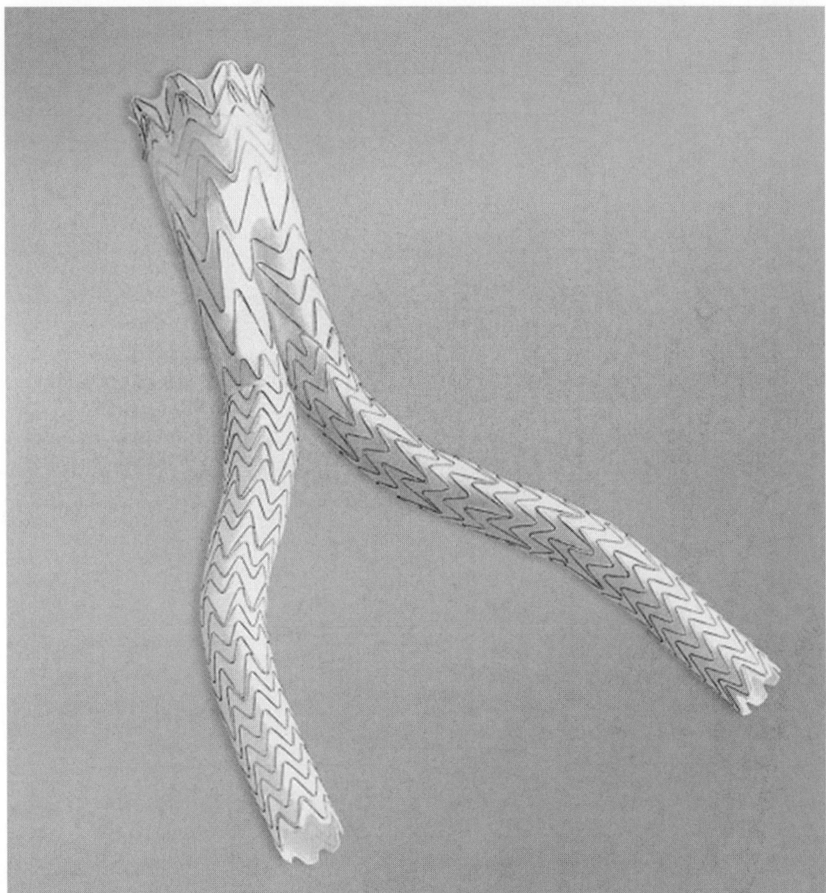

FIG. 12–4. GORE EXCLUDER endoprosthesis. (Reproduced with permission of WL Gore.)

tutions have designed their own endograft devices, which are currently being used to treat AAA.

ENDOGRAFT IMPLANTATION

Although each device is inserted with a particular technique, some steps are common to all endografts. The procedure can be done under general, regional, or local anesthesia. It can be performed with aseptic technique in a suite equipped with stationary fluoroscopic equipment, or it can also be done with a portable C-arm fluoroscope in an operating room. Some hospitals have constructed fully functional angiographic suite–operating room hybrids. The devices are inserted into the aorta through sheaths inserted in the femoral arteries, which may be exposed surgically (Fig. 12-6). Some devices can be placed by percutaneous technique. Using radiocontrast injection and digital subtraction angiography, the anatomy of the aorta is visualized and measured and the devices are deployed under fluoroscopic control. Fig. 12-7 is an illustration of the bifurcated GORE EXCLUDER endoprosthesis placed within the aorta.

COMPLICATIONS

Complications Related to Device Insertion

Some complications can occur during endograft deployment. Injury to the access arteries can occur while inserting or withdrawing the catheters and sheaths that contain the endograft. Calcification and tortuosity of these vessels increase the risk for rupture and dissection of

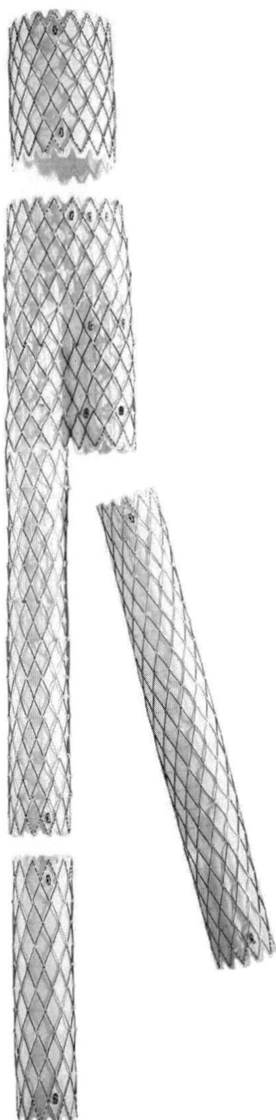

FIG. 12–5. Medtronic's AneuRx modular device. (Reproduced with permission of Medtronic AVE, Inc.)

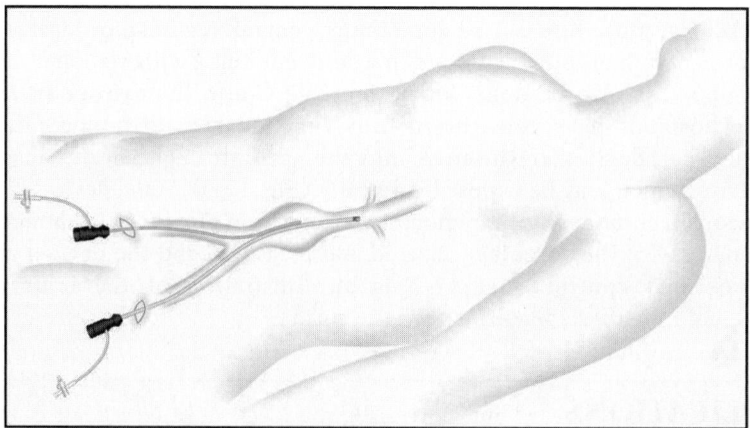

FIG. 12–6. Illustration showing bilateral groin incisions to expose femoral arteries and insertion of sheaths to deploy the endograft. (Reproduced with permission of Medtronic AVE, Inc.)

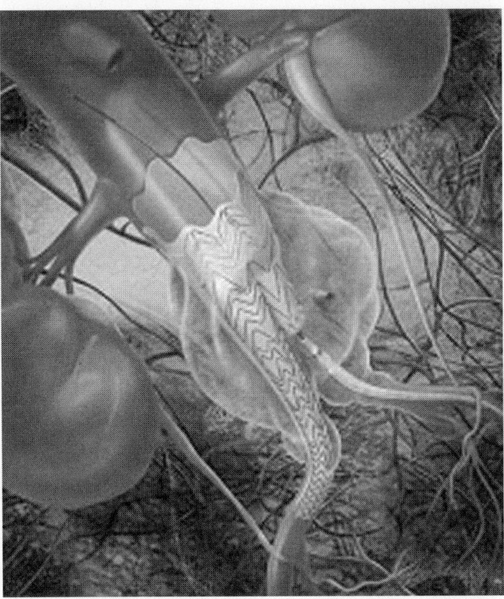

FIG. 12–7. Illustration of the GORE EXCLUDER endoprosthesis showing its placement within the aorta. (Reproduced with permission of WL Gore.)

the artery. Manipulation of the endovascular devices can produce embolization, causing lower extremity ischemia or renal failure. Common complications of endovascular repair are summarized in Table 12-1.

Endoleaks

Endoleaks are complications almost exclusively associated with the use of endografts. An endoleak occurs when there is failure to exclude the aneurysm from the circulation. In this situation, blood flows between the endograft and the aneurysm wall. Endoleaks are detected when contrast is observed outside the endograft. Meta-analysis of clinical studies has shown an average endoleak rate of 24 percent with a wide range of rates among the studies and the types of graft.[3]

Endoleaks are classified into four types. Type I endoleaks occur when there is an inadequate seal at the attachment sites. A type II endoleak occurs when a collateral vessel with retrograde flow remains patent and fills the aneurysm cavity. Type III endoleaks occur through the graft wall or union sites in the body of the graft, and type IV endoleaks are observed when blood diffuses through the porous fabric wall itself. A new term, *endotension*, has been coined and most commonly is used to refer to pressurization of an aneurysm sac without evidence of endoleak.[4]

Late Complications

Multiple studies have shown that the aneurysm size changes after endovascular graft placement.[5] In general, aneurysms without endoleak are associated with a reduction in the maximal transverse diameter. Those aneurysms with endoleak are associated with an increase in the maximal transverse diameter. Increase in diameter may vary with the type of endoleak.[6,7] One study has shown that new-onset endoleaks may lead to more rapid aneurysm growth than chronic endoleaks.[8] Shrinkage has also been noted in the length of the aneurysm post endograft repair,[9] and dilation of the distal neck of the aneurysm has been seen.[10] All of these changes could contribute to late complications, including migration of the graft, kinking of the graft, and rupture of the aneurysm.[11-14] In addition, thrombus formation has been noted inside of the endograft.[13,15] These late complications may lead to the need for

TABLE 12-1 Complications of Endovascular Repair

Complications	Manifestations	Prevention
EARLY COMPLICATIONS		
Bleeding	External bleeding, groin hematoma, back pain (retroperitoneal hematoma)	Meticulous technique during closure
Thrombosis	Decrease in ankle-brachial index (ABI), changes in neurovascular exam	Meticulous technique during closure
Infection	Skin erythema, fever, leukocytosis	Strict adherence to sterile techniques
Renal failure	Oliguria, elevated serum creatinine	Selection of patients with normal renal function; adequate perioperative hydration; limited use of contrast agents
ENDOLEAK		
Type I	Sac filling during completion arteriogram	Selection of patients with adequate anatomic characteristics; proper selection of graft size
Type II	Sac filling during completion arteriogram; aneurysm enlargement on follow-up CT scan	Embolization of large collateral branches
LATE COMPLICATIONS		
Graft migration	Sac filling, aneurysm enlargement on follow-up CT scan	Selection of patients with adequate anatomic characteristics; proper selection of graft size

secondary interventions, which would mean one or more additional surgical procedures for the patient.

PERIOPERATIVE NURSING CARE

This group of patients needs the same thorough preoperative evaluation as all patients who are undergoing open aortic surgery. Preoperative ankle-brachial indices (ABIs) are important in this group as a reference point for possible thromboembolic complications postoperatively. The teaching plan should address information about the disease process, treatment, and expectations concerning patients' expected recovery. The majority of the components presented in the teaching plan for aortic surgery patients apply to this group as well. Table 12-2 summarizes differences and similarities between endovascular and open repair.

Patients undergoing endovascular repair may suffer any of the postoperative complications that can occur after an open surgical repair of an AAA. However, special emphasis should be placed on the complications that are related to the endograft method of repair. Postoperative care involves patient assessment of complications related to thromboembolic and bleeding events due to the endovascular graft delivery. Extremity assessment must include a complete circulation assessment (pulses, ABIs, skin color, and skin temperature), movement, and sensation exam. A neurologic assessment should be done to rule out thromboembolic events such as a cerebrovascular accident or spinal cord ischemia. The abdomen is examined for signs of a retroperitoneal hematoma, and the groin wounds are examined for bleeding and signs of hematoma formation. Renal assessment should include comparison of postoperative blood urea nitrogen (BUN) and creatinine levels to the preoperative baseline levels. Nephrotoxicity may result from the large amount of angiographic contrast media that these patients receive during the procedure. Intake and output are measured to assure ade-

TABLE 12-2 Endovascular AAA Repair Compared to Open AAA Repair

	Endovascular Repair	Open Repair
Preop Evaluation	Imaging: fine-cut helical CT with IV contrast, possible angiogram Evaluate anatomy of aneurysm for suitability for endovascular repair, FDA-approved devices for infrarenal AAA only Stress need for frequent follow-up visits and long-term surveillance Consider strongly for candidates who are elderly, high cardiac risk, hx of COPD, hx of hostile abdomen	Imaging: CT with IV contrast; fine cuts, helical reconstruction, and angiogram usually not required Aneurysms that do not meet criteria for endovascular repair Consider strongly for candidates who are younger, low cardiac risk, fewer comorbidities, patients who are unable or unwilling to participate in long-term follow-up
Operative Venue	Surgical suite, set up for possible conversion to open repair Some institutions use special radiographic suites for repair	Surgical suite
Anesthesia	Most commonly general; regional anesthesia or local anesthesia with IV sedation possible	General
Incision	Two groin incisions, percutaneous access possible with some cases	Transperitoneal or retroperitoneal
ICU	Often no intensive care unit (ICU) stay needed	Standard of 1-day stay
Pain Control	IV pain medications immediately postop, frequently patient able to tolerate oral pain medications on day of OR	PCA or epidural infusion, advance to oral pain medications with return of bowel motility
Diet	Frequently able to tolerate a minimum of clear liquids on day of OR, advance diet prior to discharge	Usually NPO for 3-4 days, advance diet prior to discharge
Activity	Up with assist on OR day, ambulate on POD # 1	Bed rest on OR day, up with assist on POD # 1-2, PT evaluation often necessary
Length of Stay	Discharge on day 1 possible, average length of stay 2-3 days	Average length of stay: 6 days
Postop Recovery	Most patients have returned to prior level of activity within 1 month of operation	Most patient have returned to prior level of activity within 3-6 months of operation; stay at rehab facility or home PT possible
Patient Follow-up	Seen in the clinic 1 month postop; CT scan and/or abdominal duplex Repeat scans at 6 months and 1 year and then yearly if no imaging concerns Lifelong surveillance may be needed	Seen in the clinic 2 weeks after discharge Clinic visit at 1 year and yearly Repeat CT scan q 5 years or sooner if concerns

AAA, Abdominal aortic aneurysm; *CT,* computed tomography; *IV,* intravenous; *FDA,* Food and Drug Administration; *hx,* history; *COPD,* chronic obstructive pulmonary disease; *ICU,* intensive care unit; *OR,* operating room; *PCA,* patient-controlled analgesia; *NPO,* nothing by mouth; *POD,* postoperative day; *PT,* physical therapy; *q,* every.

quate renal function and hydration. Monitoring for symptoms of cardiac ischemia is essential given the high incidence of heart disease in this patient population.

Fever and leukocytosis are often seen in this group of patients after surgery and, in almost all cases, is not related to an infectious source.[16,17] It is postulated that this is an inflammatory response to the graft material and does not need to be treated with antibiotic agents.

Patients should be warned about the possibility of this occurrence and advised to report this to their surgeon to see if further evaluation of the fever is necessary.

In most cases, these patients are transferred to the regular surgical unit after their stay in the recovery room and do not require an intensive care unit (ICU) admission. The average length of stay varies from institution to institution but may be as short as 1 day postoperatively. With a shortened length of stay, it is necessary to recognize complications promptly and to provide extensive teaching prior to hospitalization.

PATIENT FOLLOW-UP

Endovascular repair of AAA is a new technology, and long-term durability of the grafts has not yet been established. Thus, the need for ongoing follow-up in this group of patients is imperative.

A protocol in which to follow these patients needs to be established in each institution. Fig. 12-8 is an example of a flow chart to aid in the decision process for patient reimaging and possible reintervention with angiography or additional endovascular procedures. Fine-cut contrast-enhanced CT scans (with precontrast, dynamic, and delayed images) allow for the measurement of the aneurysm sac and an evaluation for endoleak, seal zone (length of aorta covered by the graft before the aorta becomes aneurysmal), and graft migration. Four-view abdominal x-rays offer additional information about the stent structure and intercomponent migration. These x-rays allow visualization of the graft components and are used to check for breaks in the wire skeletons, the movement of graft pieces, and kinking of graft limbs.

Certain patients may not be able to undergo contrast-enhanced CT scans due to renal problems or severe contrast dye allergies. In these patients, noncontrast CT scans and four-view abdominal films provide a portion of the information for follow up. However, these modalities cannot check for endoleak. Color duplex ultrasound scan has been shown to be an acceptable alternative to evaluate for endoleak when it is performed by an experienced registered vascular technologist.[18,19] The results of these scans, however, may be influenced by the patient's body habitus, patient movement, and the presence of bowel gas.

In an optimal situation, the patient would return to the institution where the device was implanted for follow-up examinations. However, this is not always possible due to the age and comorbidities of the patient and the travel distance. Alternative strategies may have to be developed in order to provide follow-up imaging for some patients. The availability of good-quality CT scans is increasing, and it is helpful to establish contacts with other institutions where these scans can be performed. The films can then be sent to the original institution, where they can be reviewed by the surgeon and his or her staff.

It is imperative to stress the importance of follow-up and the necessary requirements prior to the implantation of the endovascular device. Establishing an early relationship with patients is beneficial when coordinating future care. This can be accomplished by preoperative teaching and listening to the concerns of both the patients and their families. Establishing an individual as a contact person for each patient ensures that his or her concerns are addressed and that patients are not lost to follow-up. Other useful strategies include keeping a database with the details of subsequent examinations and reimaging results along with a schedule for future follow-up examinations.

COST OF ENDOVASCULAR REPAIR

Developing new technology is expensive, and the need to continue to improve and refine this technology contributes to high costs. In the case of endovascular devices, the cost of the device itself contributes to a total hospitalization fee that has been shown to be considerably higher than the fee for a standard open repair.[20,21] The cost of diagnostic imaging is also

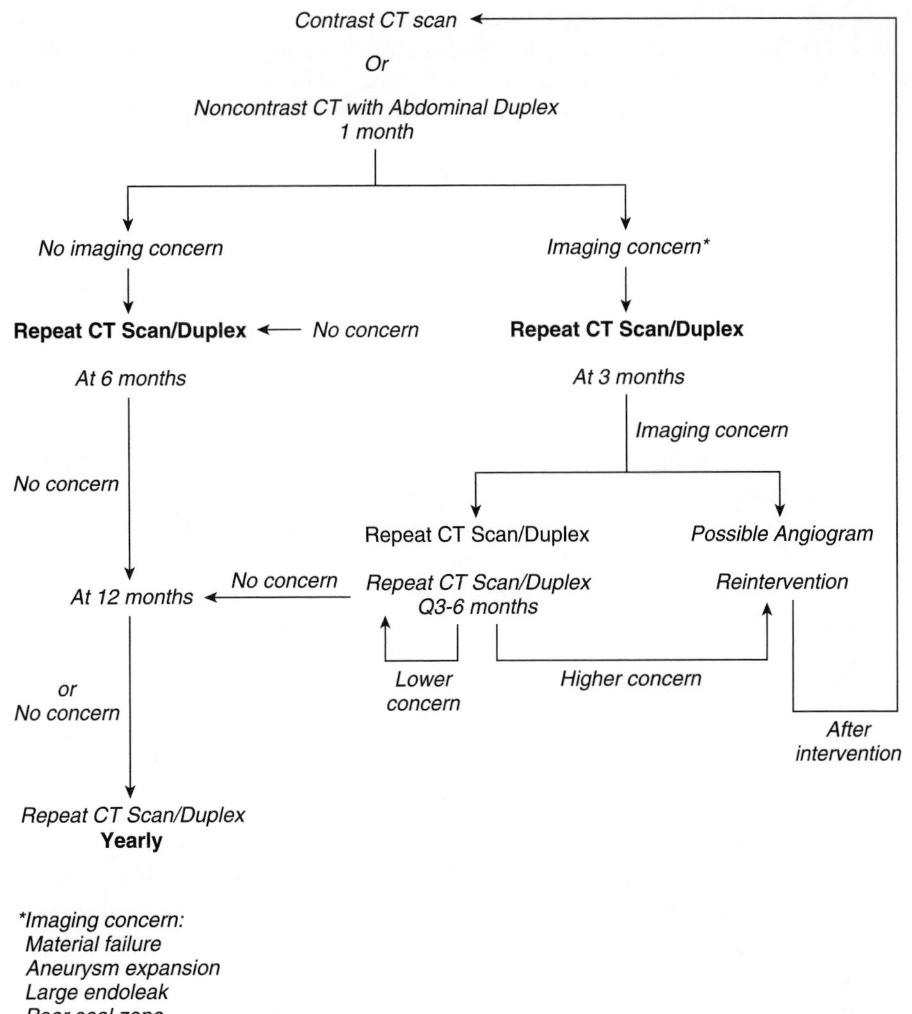

FIG. 12–8. Patient follow-up for endovascular repair.

higher in the endovascular patient, both preprocedure and postprocedure. Cost savings have been realized from decreased lengths of stay, decreased ICU stays, and decreased utilization of other hospital services.

In evaluating costs, the cost of aneurysm repair in high-risk patients must also be considered. Elective open repair in high-risk patients has been shown to be more expensive than in low-risk patients, and emergent open repairs contribute to large financial losses for hospitals.[22] In this group, endovascular repair may reduce both perioperative mortality and morbidity, as well as the need for an emergent repair at some later point.[23] Decision making for the use of this type of repair should take into consideration the long-term costs, quality of life, and outcomes for a given patient, in addition to the initial costs and outcomes.[24]

ADDITIONAL USES OF AORTIC ENDOVASCULAR REPAIR

Endovascular grafts have been used in the repair of ruptured abdominal aortic aneurysms.[25,26] This method for repairing ruptured AAAs should become more widespread as an increasing number of institutions have the capability to implant these devices. This type of repair may offer the best option for high-risk patients who are not likely to survive an open operation to repair the ruptured aneurysm. Investigation is also ongoing for the use of endovascular grafts for the repair of descending thoracic aortic aneurysms.[27-29] However, none of the devices for this type of repair has obtained FDA approval.

CONCLUSION

Endovascular repair of AAA remains an evolving technology with many unanswered questions and uncertain outcomes. Long-term follow-up is not available to assess how these patients will fare in a time frame of 10 years or greater. With the evolution of new endografts, the results from previous studies may not be completely valid due to the varying outcomes that have been recorded from device to device. In addition, many deployment systems and devices undergo refinement as often as every year. Outcomes may also be related to the experience of the surgeon, and authors with extensive endovascular experience have commented on a learning curve with improving outcomes related to higher level of experience.[23,30,31] Additionally, careful patient selection based on experience has an influence on outcomes.

Patients in today's health care environment are increasingly educated and seek out alternative treatments to traditional modalities. The demand for endovascular AAA repair will no doubt increase due to the shortened hospital stay and decreased period of recovery. With a large number of patients having an endovascular repair, the follow-up of these patients will become increasingly burdensome and the mechanism of surveillance must be addressed. At this point, there is no mandatory registry in place in the United States to monitor follow-up and outcomes.

Questions also remain concerning the correct venue for this procedure and which medical specialty should do the repair. Should it be done only in a surgical suite so that a conversion to an open repair is possible, or is an angiographic suite a reasonable alternative? Are infection rates different between the two settings? Should endovascular aneurysm repair be left to the province of the vascular surgeon, or are interventional radiologists and cardiologists qualified to perform this procedure unassisted? How will the training and continuing medical education of these medical professionals be conducted?

The future of endovascular repair should become clear over the next decade. The input of numerous groups will be necessary to help establish a consensus on where, when, and how these devices are best used. Management of these patients may best be handled by a team approach due to their complicated histories, the complex technical and imaging requirements of the procedure, and the need for long-term follow-up. As a part of this team, nursing must be involved to provide education and care to these patients and their families.

REFERENCES

1. Dubost C, Allary M, Oeconomos N: Reconstruction of an aneurysm of the abdominal aorta, *Arch Surg* 34:512, 1952.
2. Parodi JC, Palmaz JC, Barone HD: Transfemoral intraluminal graft implantation for abdominal aortic aneurysm, *Ann Vasc Surg* 5:491-499, 1991.
3. Schurink GW, Aarts NJ, van Bockel JH: Endoleak after stent-graft treatment of abdominal aortic aneurysms: a meta-analysis of clinical studies, *Br J Surg* 86:581-587, 1999.
4. White GH, May J, Petrasek P: Endotension: an explanation for continued AAA growth after successful endoluminal repair, *J Endovasc Surg* 6:308-315, 1999.
5. Matsumura JS, Chaikof EL: Anatomic changes after endovascular grafting for aneurysmal disease, *Semin Vasc Surg* 12:192-198, 1999.
6. Schunn CD, Krauss M, Heilberger P et al: Aortic aneurysm size and stent graft behavior after endovascular stent-grafting: clinical experiences and observations over 3 years, *J Endovasc Ther* 7:167-176, 2000.
7. Zarins KC, White RA, Hodgson KJ et al: Endoleaks as a predictor of outcomes after endovascular aneurysm repair, *J Vasc Surg* 32:90-107, 2000.

8. Wolf YG, Hill BB, Rubin GD et al: Rate of change in abdominal aortic aneurysm diameter after endovascular repair, *J Vasc Surg* 32:108-115, 2000.
9. Harris PL, Brennen J, Martin J et al: Longitudinal aneurysm shrinkage following endovascular aortic aneurysm repair: a source of immediate and late complications, *J Endovasc Surg* 6:11-16, 1999.
10. Matsumura JS, Chaikof EL for the EVT Investigators: Continued expansion of aortic necks after endovascular repair of abdominal aneurysms, *J Vasc Surg* 28:422-431, 1998.
11. Harris PL, Vallabhaneni SR, Desgranges P et al: Incidence and risk of late rupture, conversion, and death after endovascular repair of infrarenal aortic aneurysms: the EUROSTAR experience, *J Vasc Surg* 32:739-749, 2000.
12. Kramer SC, Seifarth H, Pamler R et al: Geometric changes in aortic endografts over a 2-year observation period, *J Endovasc Ther* 8:34-38, 2001.
13. Laheji RJ, Buth J, Harris PL et al: Need for secondary interventions after endovascular repair of abdominal aortic aneurysms: intermediate-term follow-up results of a European collaborative registry (EUROSTAR), *Br J Surg* 87:1666-1673, 2000.
14. Zarins CK, White RA, Fogerty TJ: Aneurysm rupture after endovascular repair using the AneuRx stent graft, *J Vasc Surg* 31:960-970, 2000.
15. Wegner M, Gorich J, Kramer S et al: Thrombus formation in aortic endografts, *J Endovasc Surg* 8:372-379, 2001.
16. Blum U, Voshage G, Lammer J et al: Endoluminal stent-grafts for infrarenal abdominal aortic aneurysms, *N Engl J Med* 336:13-22, 1997.
17. Velazquez OC, Carpenter JC, Baum RA et al: Perigraft air, fever, and leukocytosis after endovascular repair of abdominal aortic aneurysms, *Am J Surg* 178:185-189, 1999.
18. Sato DT, Goff CD, Gregory RT et al: Endoleak after aortic stent graft repair: diagnosis by color duplex ultrasound scan versus computed tomography scan, *J Vasc Surg* 28:657-663, 1998.
19. Wolf YG, Johnson BL, Hill BB et al: Duplex ultrasound scanning versus computed tomographic angiography for postoperative evaluation of endovascular abdominal aortic aneurysm repair, *J Vasc Surg* 32:1142-1148, 2000.
20. Clair DG, Gray BG, O'Hara PJ et al: An evaluation of the costs to health care institutions of endovascular aortic aneurysm repair, *J Vasc Surg* 32:148-152, 2000.
21. Sternbergh WC, Money SR: Hospital costs of endovascular versus open repair of abdominal aortic aneurysms: a multicenter study, *J Vasc Surg* 31:237-244, 2000.
22. Breckwoldt WL, Mackey WC, O'Donnell TF: The economic implications of high-risk abdominal aortic aneurysms, *J Vasc Surg* 13:798-804, 1991.
23. Chuter TAM, Reilly LM, Faruqi RM et al: Endovascular repair in high-risk patients, *J Vasc Surg*31: 122-133, 2000.
24. Patel ST, Haser, PB, Bush HL et al: The cost-effectiveness of endovascular repair versus open surgical repair of abdominal aortic aneurysms: a decisional analysis model, *J Vasc Surg* 29:958-972, 1999.
25. Ohki T, Veith FJ: Endovascular grafts and other image-guided catheter-based adjuncts to improve the treatment of ruptured aortoiliac aneurysms, *Ann Surg* 232:466-479, 2000.
26. Noel AA, Gloviczki P, Cherry KJ et al: Ruptured abdominal aortic aneurysms: the excessive mortality of conventional repair, *J Vasc Surg* 34:41-46, 2001.
27. Greenberg R, Resch T, Nyman U et al: Endovascular repair of descending aortic aneurysms: an early experience with intermediate-term follow-up, *J Vasc Surg* 31:147-156, 2000.
28. White RA, Donayre CE, Walot I et al: Edovascular repair of descending thoracic aortic aneurysms and chronic dissections: initial clinical results with the AneuRx device, *J Vasc Surg* 33:927-934, 2001.
29. Burks JA, Faries PL, Gravereaux EC et al: Endovascular repair of thoracic aortic aneurysms: stent-graft fixation across the aortic arch vessels, *Ann Vasc Surg* 16:24-28, 2002.
30. May J, White GH, Waugh R et al: Adverse events after endoluminal repair of abdominal aortic aneurysms: a comparison during two successive period of time, *J Vasc Surg* 29:32-39, 1999.
31. Zarins CK, White RA, Schwarten D et al: AneuRx stent graft versus open surgical repair of abdominal aortic aneurysms: multicenter prospective clinical trail, *J Vasc Surg* 29:292-308, 1999

13

Arterial Reconstruction of the Lower Extremity

VICTORA A. FAHEY □ NANCY SCHINDLER

The lower limbs are the most common site of involvement of peripheral artery occlusive disease.[1] More than 6 million Americans over age 50 have significant peripheral arterial disease (PAD), resulting in more than 400,000 hospitalizations per year.[2] The prevalence is five times greater in those over 70 years of age. It affects men and women equally.

Lower-extremity arterial occlusive disease is often a chronic process and when it becomes symptomatic, it can alter a person's lifestyle with reduced functional capacity and possible limb loss that limits one's ability to perform daily activities and decreases quality of life. As there is no cure for PAD, outcomes must be measured in terms of relief of symptoms, return of ambulatory function, and preservation of limb.[3] Acute arterial occlusion can be limb- as well as life-threatening.

Peripheral arterial disease is an important predictor of systemic atherosclerosis. There is a 3- to 10-fold increased risk of myocardial infarction, stroke, or death in patients with PAD.[4,5]

Recognition and understanding of PAD is important in providing optimal management. This chapter will discuss chronic and acute arterial disease of the lower extremity. Because patients with PAD are usually elderly and often have many complicated medical problems due to multisystem involvement of atherosclerosis, they are at high risk and present many challenging problems to nursing.

ANATOMY

The abdominal aorta bifurcates into the common iliac arteries, each of which divides into an internal iliac artery, to supply the pelvis, and an external iliac artery. Anatomically the aortic bifurcation is at the level of the umbilicus. The external iliac artery becomes the common femoral artery when it passes under the inguinal ligament into the upper leg. The common femoral artery gives rise to the superficial femoral artery and the profunda femoris artery, which supplies the muscles of the thigh.

The superficial femoral artery becomes the popliteal artery as it passes through the adductor hiatus in the distal thigh. The popliteal artery gives rise to the anterior tibial artery. Several centimeters below the origin of the anterior tibial artery are the origins of the posterior tibial and peroneal arteries. The posterior tibial artery continues down the medial aspect of the leg, passing behind the medial malleolus into the foot. The anterior tibial artery lies in the anterior compartment of the leg and continues onto the dorsum of the foot as the dorsalis pedis artery. The peroneal artery courses through the center of the leg and terminates in the distal leg, giving rise to two major branches capable of serving as collateral circulation to the pedal arch. Fig. 1-3 in Chapter 1 illustrates lower-extremity arterial anatomy.

DIAGNOSTIC EVALUATION

The history and physical examination of the patient with lower-extremity arterial disease are discussed in Chapter 4. In addition to eliciting a description of the patient's chief complaint, a complete evaluation includes assessment of risk factors for atherosclerosis, a history of arterial occlusion in other systems (e.g., cerebrovascular disease, cardiac disorders, renal failure), an occupational profile, and a medication history. The physical examination can often determine the proximal site of involvement by pulse deficits and the presence of bruits.

The noninvasive laboratory plays an important role in the evaluation of patients with lower-extremity arterial disease. Segmental arterial pressures and/or pulse volume recordings provide an objective assessment of lower-extremity circulation by localizing the occlusive lesion and determining the degree of ischemia. They also provide a baseline against which future changes can be measured. Noninvasive testing is also helpful in predicting the possibility of healing following a toe amputation or other surgical procedures involving the foot.[6]

The ankle-to-brachial index (ABI) can quantitatively stratify PAD severity in nearly all individuals. Yao, Hobbs, and Irvine[7] determined the ABI in normal individuals to be slightly greater than 1.0; in patients with intermittent claudication, the ABI averaged 0.6; and in patients with rest pain or gangrene, the ABI was less than 0.3.[7] It is important to obtain bilateral brachial pressures, because in order to determine the correct ratio, the ankle pressure must be divided by the highest brachial pressure. If a difference between the right and left arm pressures is greater than 20 mm Hg, a subclavian stenosis may be present. The ABI has limitations; in diabetics with calcified arteries and patients with prosthetic grafts, the readings may be falsely elevated.

The ABI is a predictor of mortality usually due to cardiovascular events. A person with a low ABI (<0.4) has a 5-year probability of survival of only 44 percent.[8-10]

Occasionally, the need arises to perform segmental arterial blood flow measurements after the patient has exercised. This is because patients with claudication may have ankle pressures near normal at rest but develop a significant blood pressure drop following exercise. This decrease occurs as the lower-extremity muscular demand for blood outstrips the ability of the proximal diseased arterial segment to supply it. Routine exercise arterial blood flow studies are conducted by measuring ankle pressures before and after a standard walk on a motorized treadmill.

Ultrasonic duplex scanning may be used in assessing arterial disease. However, the routine use of duplex ultrasound as the sole preoperative imaging study for planning lower-extremity bypass is debatable.[11] Duplex scanning is also used to assess the presence of an adequate saphenous or upper-extremity vein for bypass grafting. The course of the veins may be mapped on the skin to guide the surgeon in the operating room. The aforementioned tests are discussed in greater detail in Chapter 5.

Other diagnostic tests may be required for patients with pain in the lower extremities that does not appear to be due to arterial occlusive disease. For example, electromyography, measurements of nerve conduction velocity, and lumbar spine x-rays may be useful in patients with diabetic neuropathy or neurogenic claudication caused by spinal stenosis. Laboratory testing for coagulopathies should be analyzed in patients with atypical arterial thrombosis (see Chapter 9). In the case of acute arterial occlusion, echocardiography, transesophageal echocardiography, Holter monitoring, and computed tomography (CT) scanning may be performed to identify a proximal source of emboli.[12]

Once the diagnosis of arterial insufficiency has been demonstrated by noninvasive testing and therapeutic intervention is contemplated, angiography or magnetic resonance angiography (MRA) may be performed. Angiography, which demonstrates the location and extent of arterial disease, is the most precise diagnostic tool for the assessment of arterial anatomy in the lower extremity and is used to depict the aorta, iliac, femoral, popliteal, and tibial arterial segments.

Because the etiology, clinical manifestations, and treatment vary between chronic and acute arterial ischemia, further discussion will be divided into chronic and acute problems.

Chronic Arterial Ischemia Etiology

The multiple etiologies of PAD of the lower extremity are included in Box 13-1, atherosclerosis being the most common cause of PAD. The risk factors for atherosclerosis of the lower extremity are the same as for the other vascular beds: advanced age (over 40), male sex, diabetes mellitus (four times the risk), cigarette smoking, hypertension, hyperlipidemia, and hyperhomocysteinemia (see Chapter 1).[1,4,13,14]

The superficial femoral and proximal popliteal arteries are the most susceptible to atherosclerosis; however, the aortoiliac segment and the tibial and peroneal arteries are also commonly affected. The arterial stenosis or occlusion that occurs reduces the blood flow to the lower limb during exercise or at rest.

Clinical Manifestations and Natural History

Patients with chronic arterial occlusive disease most often complain of cramping pain in the muscles of the lower extremity during exercise that disappears after rest. This condition is known as intermittent claudication. The distance a patient can walk before the onset of pain is usually consistent for that patient. The occluded arterial segment is the one just proximal to the symptomatic muscle group; thus, superficial femoral artery occlusion causes calf pain, external iliac artery disease produces thigh pain, and aortic disease is heralded by cramping of the buttock muscles (see Fig. 4-5). Most patients with claudication will remain stable throughout their lifetime, with approximately 20 percent of patients deteriorating to the extent that incapacitating symptoms require surgical intervention.[15] Only 5-10 percent of claudicators will go on to amputation, most commonly those who smoke or have diabetes.[16]

When arterial occlusive disease progresses to involve multiple arterial segments, patients may complain of continuous pain even at rest. *Rest pain* is a specific term referring to discomfort in the forefoot, often across the metatarsal heads, that is aggravated by elevation and diminished by hanging the foot in a dependent position. It usually begins as an isolated nocturnal event reflecting a patient's decreased cardiac output while asleep and the effect of the relative elevation of the extremity in the supine position. It occurs when resting blood flow is insufficient to meet the maintenance metabolic requirements for nonexercising tissue.[17]

BOX 13–1

Etiology of Arterial Occlusive Disease of Lower Extremity*

ATHEROSCLEROSIS
Atherosclerotic arterial occlusive disease
Atheroembolism

THROMBOEMBOLISM
Cardiac disease
Aortic aneurysm/peripheral aneurysm

ANATOMIC OR DEVELOPMENTAL ANOMALIES
Popliteal entrapment syndrome
Adventitial cystic disease of popliteal artery
Fibromuscular dysplasia
Persistent sciatic artery

INFLAMMATORY CONDITIONS
Buerger's disease
Vasculitis (collagen vascular disease)
Repetitive trauma

VASOSPASTIC CONDITIONS
Raynaud's phenomenon
Ergotism
Illicit drug infusion

HYPERCOAGULABLE STATES
Anticoagulant deficiency
Procoagulant excess

*References 3, 14, 16, 64, 68, 87, 88.

Tissue necrosis and gangrene may also be present with severe disease. Areas of an ischemic foot subject to local pressure that may develop skin necrosis include the medial and lateral metatarsal heads and the tip of the heel. Skin ulcerations heal slowly, if at all, in the ischemic limb. Areas of tissue necrosis may degenerate to wet or dry gangrene. Dry gangrene is a mummification of tissue, which, if left untreated, may progress slowly to involve the entire foot or leg. Wet gangrene manifested by blebs, bullae, and violaceous discoloration implies significant underlying tissue infection and is often complicated by a rapid progression. Critical limb ischemia, as evidenced by rest pain or tissue necrosis, is associated with inevitable amputation for most patients unless surgical correction is undertaken.

One of the hallmarks of chronic arterial insufficiency is the dusky, purplish discoloration of the foot and leg when the foot is placed in a dependent position. This "dependent rubor" changes to a characteristic chalky white "pallor on elevation" of the extremity. Changes in the skin related to insufficient delivery of nutrients by the inadequate blood flow result in atrophy and dryness, with thin, shiny skin and diminished or absent hair growth. The toenails become brittle and opaque, and the affected extremity is often cooler to touch than the opposite foot (see Chapter 4).

Medical Treatment

The treatment of lower-extremity ischemia is based on the severity of the patient's symptoms and the overall medical condition of the individual. Full medical evaluation is necessary prior to arterial surgery. Some patients may require carotid endarterectomy or coronary artery bypass grafting before femoral reconstruction is undertaken. The majority of patients with claudication are managed conservatively with an exercise program and modification of associated risk factors, especially smoking cessation (see Chapter 10).

Exercise Therapy

Exercise therapy designed to increase exercise tolerance has been found to be the most consistently effective medical treatment for claudication.[4] Patients are advised to walk to the limit of their discomfort on a daily basis to develop collaterals in the affected leg. The precise mechanism accounting for the improvement in pain-free walking capacity remains unknown but probably involves adaptation of skeletal muscle to hypoxic conditions.[1]

Exercise therapy may also be used in conjunction with bypass surgery. Additive beneficial effects of bypass surgery and subsequent exercise training when compared with operation or exercise training alone have been reported. Exercise therapy may be part of a vascular rehabilitation program (see Chapter 10).

Risk Factor Modification *(see Chapter 10)*

Because of the systemic nature of atherosclerosis and the high risk of cardiovascular ischemic events in patients with PAD, aggressive risk factor modification should be attempted in all patients.[4,18] Hypertension, hypercholesterolemia, and diabetes should be aggressively treated. All patients should be strongly encouraged to stop smoking and be given needed support to do so.

Pharmacologic Therapy *(see Chapters 8 and 10)*

The role of pharmacologic therapy in the treatment of chronic lower-extremity arterial occlusive disease is yet to be defined. In the last few years, there has been increased development of some new potentially useful pharmacologic agents. These include antithrombotic agents (anticoagulants, antiplatelet agents, thrombolytic agents, and dextran), rheologic agents, prostaglandins, calcium channel blockers, lipid-lowering agents, and others.[7,10] In addition to enhancing lower-extremity graft patency, antiplatelet drugs are effective at reducing the risk of fatal and nonfatal ischemic events (myocardial infarction and stroke) in patients with PAD. Thus, aspirin or clopidogrel should be considered in all patients with PAD.[19,20] Cilostazol and pentoxifylline are the only two medications currently approved by the Food and Drug Administration (FDA) for the treatment of claudication and may result in improved walking distances in some patients with PAD.[21]

Thrombolytic therapy has been used selectively for the treatment of chronic lower-extremity arterial occlusion. The Surgery versus Thrombolysis for Ischemia of the Lower Extremity (STILE) trial was designed to investigate the results of traditional surgical revascularization compared with those of thrombolytic therapy. This trial concluded that surgical revascularization for lower-extremity native artery occlusion is more effective and durable than thrombolytic therapy. Thrombolysis used initially provides a reduction in the extent of the surgical procedure for a majority of patients; however, long-term outcome is inferior, particularly for patients who have a femoropopliteal occlusion, diabetes, or critical ischemia.[22]

Interventional Procedures (see *Chapter 6*)

Percutaneous transluminal angioplasty (PTA) and stenting have become an accepted therapy for certain iliac artery stenoses and are selectively used in more distal arteries.[23,24] Results of arterial dilation/stenting below the inguinal ligament are not as promising as those at the iliac level. The primary limitation of PTA and stenting remains restenosis.[16] A direct comparison of PTA and bypass surgery series is difficult because of the heterogenecity of the lesions treated. Angioplasty may be used in conjunction with surgery, such as with the stenting of a proximal iliac lesion prior to a femoral-to-popliteal artery bypass.[25] Lesions best suited to angioplasty and stenting are those that are proximal, short, focal, and stenotic rather than totally occluded. Longer, distal, or totally occluded arterial lesions respond less favorably to PTA and are usually better treated with bypass procedures.

The use of endovascular grafts for the treatment of PAD continues to evolve. They may be used in high-risk patients with medical comorbidities who are unfit for conventional open repair. Further refinement, increasing experience, and long-term follow-up with regard to durability and complications will establish the role of endovascular grafts in the treatment of arterial occlusive disease.[26]

Surgical Treatment

Patients with claudication may be candidates for bypass surgery if the disability severely limits their lifestyle or occupational activity or if continued disability exists despite appropriate medical management. In the presence of rest pain, a nonhealing ulceration, gangrene of the toes or foot, or embolization from a peripheral aneurysm, surgical revascularization is usually necessary to restore and/or maintain limb viability. After bypass surgery, rest pain is relieved, ulcerations heal with standard attention, and gangrenous tissue can usually be amputated with prompt healing. An arterial reconstruction may thus allow substitution of a minor toe or forefoot amputation for an inevitable below-the-knee or above-the-knee amputation. Patients with limb-threatening ischemia with no potential for rehabilitation or who are bedridden with limited life expectancy may be treated conservatively.

Because arterial disease is often present in several areas, it is essential to determine the arterial segment with the hemodynamically significant stenosis responsible for the patient's problems. For example, the stenosis may be at the aortoiliac level, affecting arterial inflow to the legs. It is a fundamental principle that the inflow should be corrected before the outflow to the foot is repaired. This prevents a newly placed bypass graft from thrombosing because of inadequate blood flow through the graft.

If the aortoiliac segment is diseased as well as the femoral/popliteal/tibial arteries, an aorto-femoral artery graft (see Fig. 11-6) or angioplasty may be necessary to improve inflow prior to femoral bypass surgery. Patients who cannot tolerate an abdominal operation may undergo an axillofemoral reconstruction (see Fig. 11-7). This operative procedure supplies the legs with blood flow using one of the axillary arteries as inflow through a graft tunneled in the subcutaneous tissue. If iliac blood flow to the noninvolved leg is adequate, a femoro-femoral bypass graft is sometimes used.

After it is ascertained that the inflow to the femoral system is adequate, femoral reconstruction can be undertaken. The two traditional approaches for revascularization of the lower extremity are (1) to position a bypass around the obstruction (most common procedure) and (2) to open the artery and remove the obstruction by performing an endarterectomy.

The choice of surgical procedure depends on the level of arterial disease. Selecting the proper bypass involves determining the best proximal site for inflow and the best distal site for outflow (Fig. 13-1). Generally, the proximal anastomosis is anastomosed to the common femoral artery. Under unusual circumstances, the graft may be attached to the limb of an aortobifemoral graft, the superficial femoral artery, the popliteal artery, or the deep femoral artery. The distal graft is anastomosed to the most cephalic portion of the leg that allows unobstructed blood flow to the foot.

Femoropopliteal Bypass

The most common point of arterial occlusion in the leg is at the lower portion of the superficial femoral artery as it passes through the medial adductor muscles just above the knee. Therefore, a femoral-to-above-knee popliteal graft is frequently performed. If the upper popliteal artery is diseased, the graft may be sewn to the below-knee popliteal artery. A popliteal aneurysm is ligated above and below the aneurysm with the bypass placed around the ligatures to eliminate it from the circulation (Fig. 13-2).

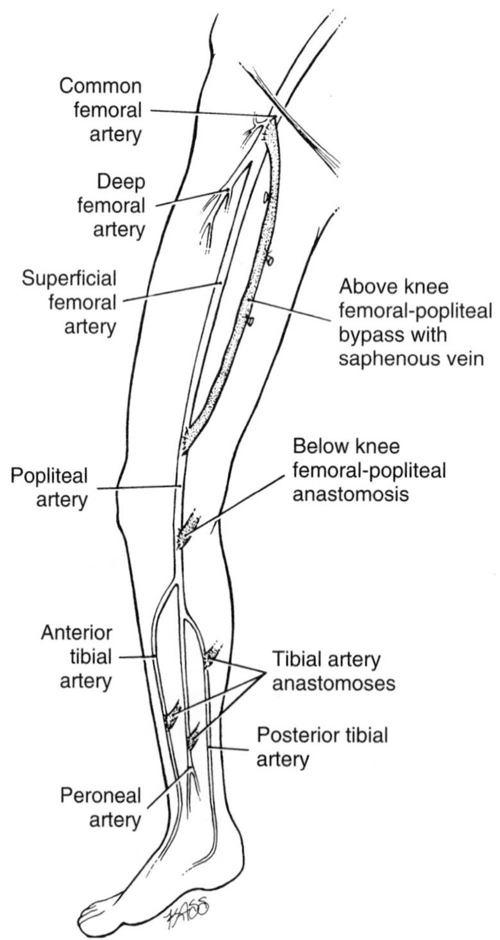

FIG. 13–1. Femoral artery bypass grafts may be anastomosed to the popliteal or any one of the three tibial arteries. (From McCarthy WJ, Williams LR: Femoral artery reconstruction, *Critical Care Quarterly* 8:43, 1985. Reprinted with permission of Aspen Publishers, Inc, © 1985.)

Infrapopliteal Bypass

In the event that there are no tibial branches remaining in continuity with the popliteal artery, the graft may be sewn directly to one of the three tibial/peroneal arteries. The tibial vessel of largest diameter with the least disease and the best outflow to the foot should be selected for the distal anastomosis.

If the tibial vessels are poorly visualized on the preoperative arteriogram, an arteriogram may be performed in the operating room at the time of surgery. After completion of the bypass, an arteriogram is usually performed in the operating room to identify technical problems or an arteriovenous fistula that may be present after an in situ bypass. A duplex scan may also be used in assessing the bypass at this time. If a technical flaw is discovered, it can be corrected while the bypass is still exposed.

Axillopopliteal Bypass

An axillopopliteal bypass (Fig. 13-3) is used when amputation is otherwise imminent and a more standard arterial reconstruction is not feasible because of groin infection, previous scarring, or very rarely because of extensive bilateral atherosclerosis of the femoral arteries, when the femoral vessels would not provide sufficient outflow to support a graft limb.[27] Polytetrafluoroethylene (PTFE) is usually used for these grafts, and there may be an advantage to using a ringed (externally supported) graft.

Obturator Foramen Bypass

The obdurator foramen bypass (Fig. 13-4) is used to revascularize an extremity in which the femoral area is infected or inappropriate for dissection because of previous surgery or previous irradiation. The graft originates in the retroperitoneum at a point proximal to the infection and is sewn to the iliac artery. It is then brought through the obturator foramen in a clean field and anastomosed to a distal uninvolved artery.[28]

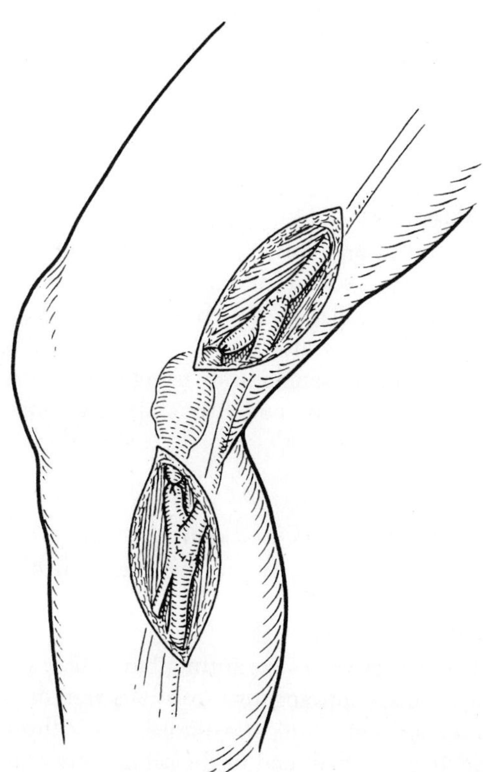

FIG. 13–2. Popliteal artery aneurysm repair. (From Clyne CA: Aneurysm of the popliteal artery. In Bell PR, Jamieson CW, Ruckley CV, eds: *Surgical management of vascular disease,* Philadelphia, 1992, WB Saunders, p 880.)

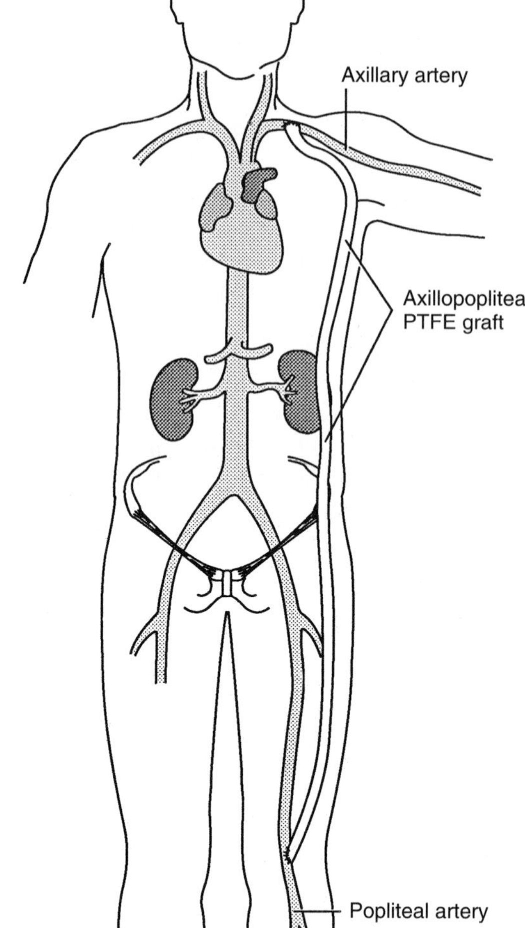

FIG. 13–3. Axillopopliteal bypass with polytetrafluoroethylene (PTFE).

Endarterectomy/Profundaplasty

Endarterectomy may be useful as an adjunct to bypass grafting or alone in the repair of a stenotic profunda femoris artery (the deep femoral artery). The profunda femoris artery is the main component of an important collateral system that provides arterial flow when there is occlusive disease of inflow arteries and also provides alternative flow to the foot in presence of superficial artery occlusion. A patch angioplasty using vein or prosthetic material may also be used to widen the lumen of the profunda after endarterectomy; this is called a profundaplasty.[29]

Graft Material

A variety of conduits are available for bypass grafting to the lower-extremity arteries. Two types of conduits are used: autogenous (vein) and synthetic (artificial) grafts.

Reversed Greater Saphenous Vein

The saphenous vein has a series of valves permitting blood flow only in the direction of the heart. The traditional way of using autologous saphenous vein tissue as an arterial bypass is to reverse the vein, which allows blood to flow unobstructed through the vein valves. This reversal necessitates attaching the small end of the saphenous vein to the common femoral artery at the proximal anastomoses and the large end of the saphenous vein to a smaller-diameter popliteal or tibial artery at the distal anastomosis.

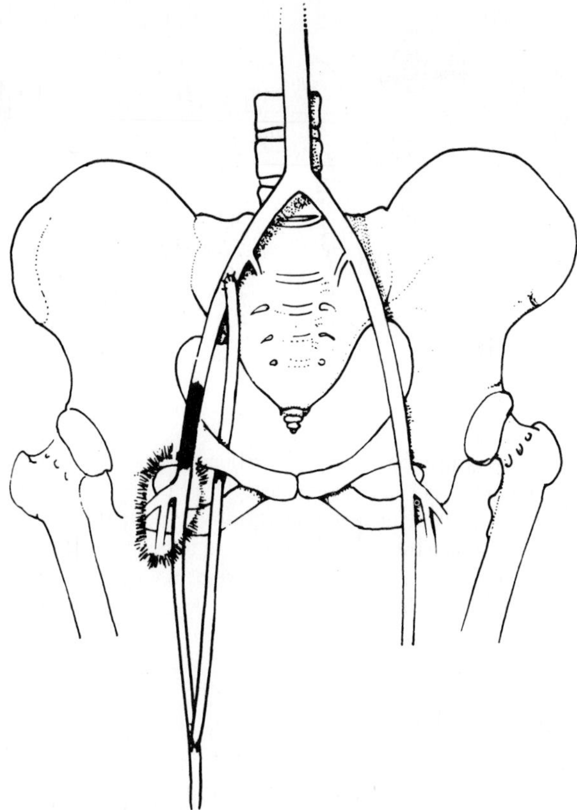

FIG. 13-4. Obturator foramen bypass. (From Brief DK, Brener BJ: Extraanatomic bypass. In Wilson SE, Veith FJ, Hobson RW II et al, eds: *Vascular surgery principles and practice,* New York, 1987, McGraw-Hill, p 422.)

In Situ Saphenous Vein

The inevitable size mismatch of the reversed vein graft prompted the development of a technique using the vein in its natural position without reversal; this is known as the in situ technique. Besides the obvious advantage of anastomotic size match, the in situ technique provides physiologic preservation of venous endothelium. This is because the long saphenous vein is not entirely removed from its bed in the subcutaneous position, and, therefore, it retains its adventitial blood supply. Deprivation of a vein's blood supply for longer than 30-40 minutes creates a flow surface that is conducive to thrombus deposition, particularly in low-flow states. In addition, this technique allows more frequent use of small veins and thus a higher vein utilization rate.[30] Limitations of the in situ technique include problems with rendering valves incompetent (retained valve cusps), the size and quality of the vein, the learning curve of the surgeon, and difficulty in locating and controlling arteriovenous (AV) fistulae.[31]

In situ surgery entails mobilization of the vein's ends for construction of the proximal and distal arterial anastomoses, removal of the valvular obstructions to arterial flow by rendering the valves incompetent, and interruption of the venous branches to prevent AV fistulae (Fig. 13-5).[32] The vein may be exposed through multiple interrupted (closed) or continuous (open) incisions (Fig. 13-6). Angioscopic guidance providing direct visualization for valve interruption and localization of AV fistulae has increased the use of the closed technique (see Chapter 7).[33] The use of such minimally invasive techniques has resulted in fewer wound complications, diminished pain, and possibly decreased length of hospital stay. However, the superiority of any one in situ technique over another has not yet been clarified.[34,35]

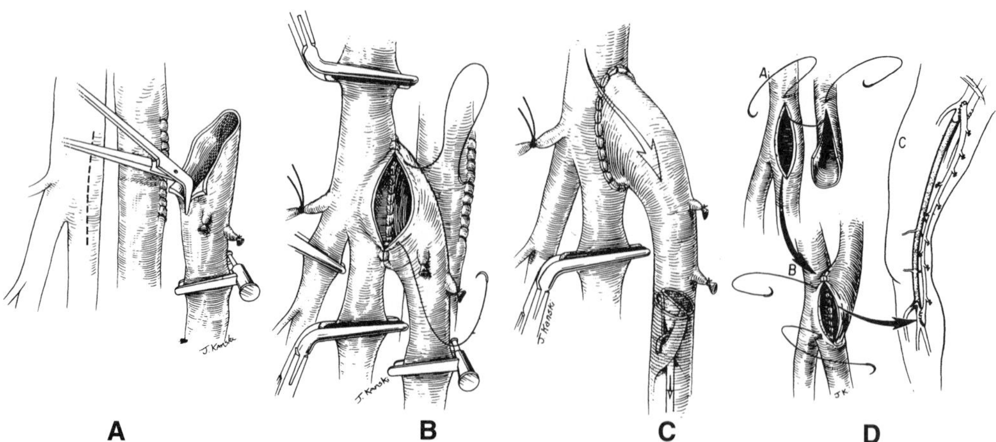

FIG. 13–5. A, In the in situ method, the saphenofemoral junction is transected in the groin, the venotomy in the femoral vein oversewn, and the proximal end of the saphenous vein prepared for anastomosis. **B,** After the first venous valve is excised under direct vision, the graft is anastomosed end to side to the femoral artery. **C,** Flow is then restored through the vein graft and the valvulotome inserted through side branches at appropriate intervals to lyse residual valve cusps. **D,** The distal anastomosis is completed, in this case at the level of the distal tibioperoneal trunk. (From Whittemore AD: Infrainguinal bypass. In Rutherford RB, ed: *Vascular surgery,* ed 5, Philadelphia, 2000, WB Saunders, pp 998-1018.)

Nonreversed Greater Saphenous Vein

The use of a nonreversed greater saphenous vein graft provides optimal size match between the artery and vein at each anastomosis. The most common indication for use of this graft is when a contralateral greater saphenous vein is required for a long bypass graft. One study produced results equivalent to those achieved in a series of in situ bypass procedures.[36]

Lesser Saphenous Vein

Although the lesser saphenous vein may be used, it has limitations because it extends only from the ankle to the knee.

Arm Vein

Cephalic and basilic veins (Fig. 13-7) from the upper extremity constitute viable alternatives for use as infrapopliteal bypass grafts when other sources of autogenous vein are unavailable (utilized for coronary artery or peripheral bypass surgery, a vein stripping, or the vein is inadequate, e.g., with phlebitis, variations in venous anatomy, chronic venous insufficiency, or a small saphenous vein). The preferred arm vein for grafting is the forearm cephalic vein. When a single arm vein is not long enough to span blocked segments, two or three veins can be

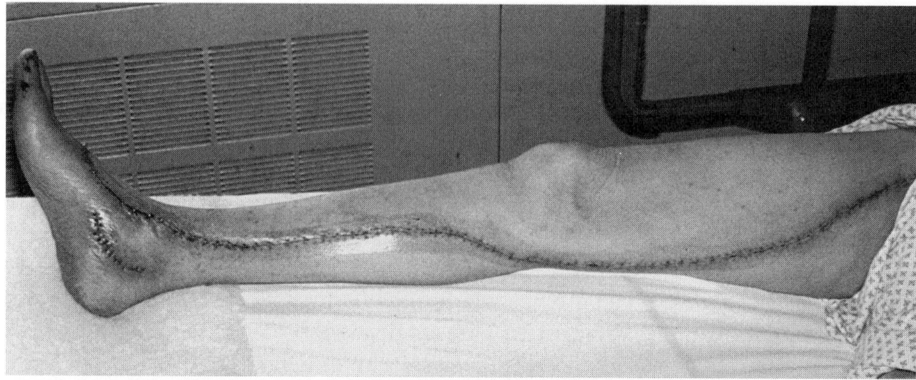

FIG. 13–6. Incision of in situ bypass along the entire leg to expose and ligate arteriovenous (AV) fistulae.

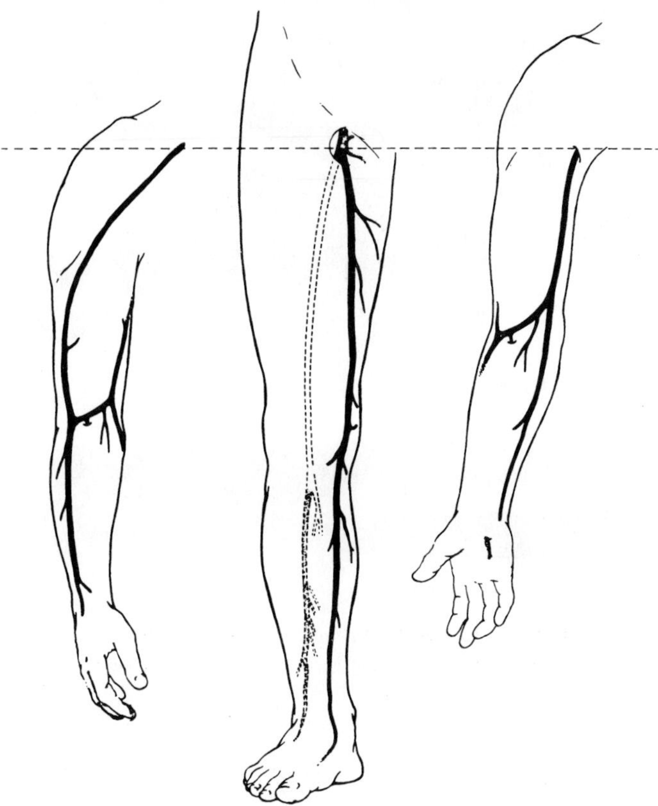

FIG. 13–7. Relative lengths of the cephalic and basilic veins as potential bypass grafts in the lower extremity. (From Andros G, Harris RW, Dulawa LB et al: The use of arm veins as lower extremity arterial conduits. In Kempczinski RF, ed: *The ischemic leg,* Chicago, Year Book Medical Publishers, 1985, p 427.)

spliced to create a composite arm vein graft. Disadvantages of arm veins are that they tend to be thin walled, thus requiring careful dissection and increased time to harvest the vein; their use is associated with an increased incidence of aneurysmal change; the vein diameter is small; multiple segments may be necessary to provide adequate length; and they are prone to intimal fibrosis.[6, 37]

There are several recommendations for the successful use of arm veins as conduits. These include protocols to preserve arm veins, the education of patients and health care professionals, and the training of surgical nurses related to the maneuvers for arm vein implantation. Use of physician orders, periodic in-service training programs, signage in patient rooms, and protection of the patient's arm with gauze can be helpful. The protection of arm veins from venipuncture or intravenous therapy is essential to prevent phlebitis.

Synthetic Prosthetic

The conduit of choice in the absence of adequate vein is made of expanded PTFE.[38] Dacron may also be used. Prosthetic grafts can also be used for extended conduits such as axillary-to-femoral (see Fig. 11-7) or axillary-to-popliteal artery bypasses (see Fig. 13-3). Potential advantages of a prosthetic bypass are decreased dissection in an ischemic limb and decreased time of operation.

Because results achieved with distal PTFE grafts have proved to be less than optimal, several modifications of the standard approach have been attempted. A collar of vein may be interposed between the distal arteriotomy and the distal PTFE graft (Miller cuff) (Fig. 13-8, *A*) or a vein patch across the distal anastomosis (Taylor patch) may be used (Fig. 13-8, *B*). Also, an AV fistula may be used at the distal anastomosis. These techniques hopefully augment flow through the prosthetic graft and enhance graft patency.[6,39,40,41]

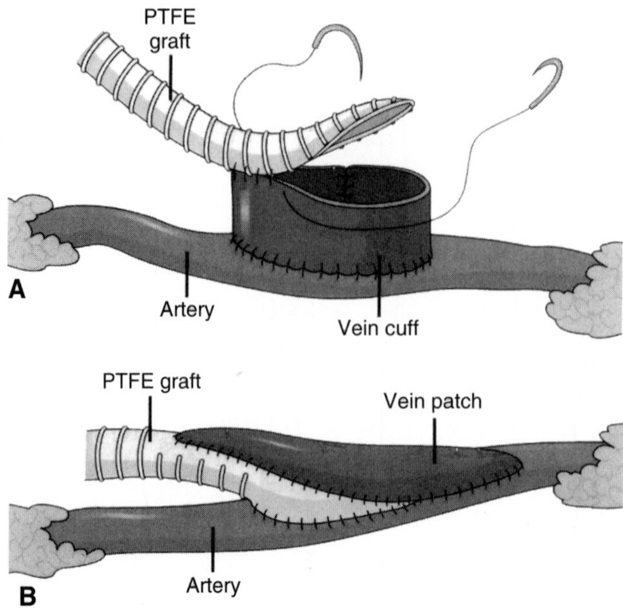

FIG. 13–8. A, Miller vein cuff technique for creating an autogenous vein cuff at distal anastomosis of PTFE bypass. **B,** Taylor vein patch technique for widening a distal PTFE graft anastomosis to an artery. (From Donaldson MC, Whittemore AD: Lower limb arterial occlusive disease. In Corson JD, Williamson R, eds: *Surgery,* London, 2001, Mosby, p 4-11.8. Reprinted with permission.)

Human Umbilical Vein

Grafts constructed from human umbilical cord vein may be used for arterial bypass surgery. Umbilical veins are treated with glutaraldehyde, which acts as a tanning agent, increasing strength and also preventing antigenic recognition and rejection by the graft recipient. They are wrapped with a polyester mesh to help prevent aneurysm formation. Although the patency rate compares to that of PTFE grafts, there remains a high incidence of aneurysmal degeneration with these grafts.[42] Also, the time required for operative preparation is lengthy.

Cryopreserved Vein Graft

Cryopreserved vein (CPV) from cadaveric harvest may be an alternative conduit for limb salvage when no autogenous tissue is available, such as in the presence of infection. It is very expensive, and in addition to low patency, it has incidence of aneurysm formation.[43,44]

Composite Sequential Bypass Graft

When adequate vein is unavailable for a bypass graft, a composite sequential bypass graft made up of autogenous vein and prosthetic material may be used. A prosthetic graft, usually PTFE, is used from the femoral to the popliteal level, and a vein graft is then placed directly onto the PTFE material and brought down through an anatomic tunnel to the selected site for tibial outflow (Fig. 13-9).[45]

Results

Technical advances in the last decade have contributed to improved success with several studies documenting the ability of surgical revascularization to provide durable salvage of ischemic limbs. The long-term patency and success of these grafts are influenced by a variety of factors, including the indications for surgery, the bypass conduit, the anatomic and hemodynamic characteristics of the inflow artery, the site of the distal anastomosis and associated outflow, distal arterial anatomy, diabetes, smoking, the use of anticoagulation, primary or secondary procedure, the progression of atherosclerosis, and the development of fibromuscular

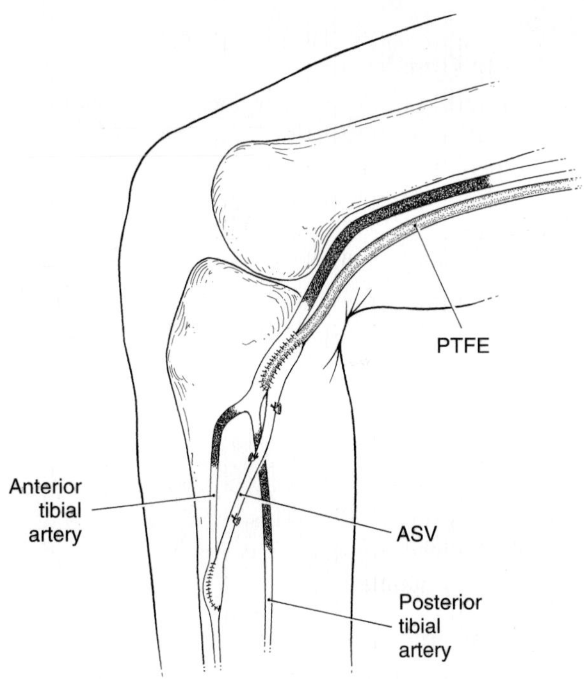

FIG. 13–9. Composite-sequential bypass graft. *PTFE,* Polytetrafluoroethylene; *ASV,* autogenous saphenous vein. (From McCarthy WJ, Pearce WH, Flinn WR et al: Long-term evaluation of composite sequential bypass for limb threatening ischemia, *J Vasc Surg* 15[5]:765, 1992.)

hyperplasia. Unless patients have been stratified for these factors, it is difficult to draw meaningful conclusions from the results of numerous studies of lower-extremity bypass surgery.[1]

Despite the multitude of studies, one conclusion is clear. Intact greater saphenous vein is the conduit of choice for most infrainguinal bypasses.[1] The superior patency of vein grafts over PTFE prosthetic conduit was well documented by a multicenter randomized trial. At 5 years, the primary patency rate for all autogenous vein grafts to the popliteal artery was 68 percent compared to 47 percent for PTFE.[46] When placed in the femoral to above-knee popliteal position, no statistically significant difference was observed; however, in grafts to the infrapopliteal artery, the 5-year patency rate for vein was 49 percent compared to 12 percent patency rate for PTFE.[46-48] The use of an all-autogenous graft appears to provide the best long-term patency and limb salvage in below-knee grafts.[37]

Results of a multicenter randomized prospective trial demonstrated there was no statistically significant difference in observed primary or secondary patency rates between PTFE and Dacron grafts used in the above-knee position.[49]

The question of which vein graft is the best conduit remains an unanswered question requiring further study.[6] With autogenous conduit, the vein type, size, and quality are important determinants for long-term patency. In several studies, long-term outcome of femoropopliteal bypass was satisfactory using both in situ and reversed vein grafts.[50,51] The results achieved with alternate autogenous vein grafts (arm veins, lesser saphenous veins) are generally inferior to those achieved with intact ipsilateral greater saphenous vein. One study demonstrated that the patency results of the alternate vein bypass graft to infrapopliteal arteries are superior to those achieved with prosthetic grafting.[52] However, the results of alternate autogenous vein bypass are not clearly superior to those achieved with prosthetic grafting, especially in view of recently reported improved results of prosthetic grafting using modified anastomotic techniques and long-term anticoagulation with warfarin.

Composite sequential bypass grafts have better patency than an all-prosthetic bypass to the tibial level.[45] Benefits are compounded if the venous graft crosses the knee joint.

Additional Procedures

Bypass and Free Tissue Transfer

Patients may present with such extensive tissue loss that primary wound healing is not expected even after successful arterial reconstruction. This situation, seen frequently in diabetic patients with severe peripheral neuropathy, occurs most often on the weight-bearing plantar surface of the foot. The performance of distal arterial reconstruction and microvascular tissue transfer provides an opportunity for limb salvage in these patients, who would normally be candidates for amputation. Advantages to free tissue transfer include (1) adequate debridement of infected tissue is possible, (2) adequate bulk is restored to weight-bearing surface, (3) local infection is better controlled, and (4) neovascularization from the free flap may improve local tissue perfusion. Close collaboration between the plastic and vascular surgeons is necessary.[53,54]

Amputation

In certain cases, extensive gangrene with major foot destruction, infection, or osteomyelitis is best handled by a primary leg amputation. This approach also is used if no distal arteries remain for a bypass. All effort is made to preserve as much of the extremity as possible so that the potential for rehabilitation is optimal.

Adjunctive Medical Management

The variable patency of all lower-extremity arterial bypasses, regardless of the type of conduit, suggests the need for adjunctive postoperative antithrombotic therapy. A number of agents are used, including aspirin, dipyridamole, dextran, low-dose heparin, intravenous heparin, low-molecular-weight heparin (Lovenox), and warfarin.[20] There is no consensus as to the optimal form of pharmacotherapy that should be used to prevent graft failure.[55]

Antiplatelet drugs are believed to inhibit platelet aggregation, preventing their deposition on the surface of thrombogenic grafts, and may help prevent perianastomotic fibrous hyperplasia. Aspirin, 325 mg/day, may be useful in patients undergoing vein and prosthetic lower-extremity grafts.

Warfarin has been used in patients undergoing infrainguinal bypass surgery in an attempt to decrease the incidence of graft failure. It may be recommended for patients undergoing prosthetic bypasses, long bypasses to small arteries, composite bypass grafts, redo of a failed bypass graft, and after a compromised operation, i.e., with poor distal runoff or a very small diameter vein graft.[20,56] It may also have a role in patients with hypercoagulable states. The effectiveness of warfarin varies among studies, and its exact role remains unanswered.[57] Warfarin may be used in conjunction with a platelet inhibitor in patients at highest risk who have undergone complex revascularizations to preserve graft patency.[58] Hemorrhagic complications remain, and risk needs to be addressed.

In the Dutch study, oral anticoagulants were significantly more effective in prevention of vein graft occlusion, whereas aspirin prevented more nonvenous graft occlusion.[59] This is not universally accepted; thus, there is an important need for additional clinical trials evaluating warfarin and aspirin in the treatment of these patients.

The principal difference between thrombotic occlusion of vein and prosthetic bypass grafts has to do with surface thrombogenicity. Because vein grafts are lined with endothelium, they are inherently less thrombogenic than prosthetic grafts. Vein grafts may lose variable amounts of their endothelial lining during harvesting and implantation, which may contribute to early occlusion. This suggests the rationale for early antithrombotic therapy that could be discontinued after healing at anastomotic sites and repavement of graft with endothelium. Prosthetic grafts, however, remain highly thrombogenic.[20]

When perioperative anticoagulation is recommended, low-molecular-weight heparin (LMWH) provides a safe and effective alternative to intravenous heparin for infrageniculate PTFE bypass graft procedures. LMWH may reduce the number of postoperative hospital days and coagulation studies by allowing discharge before therapeutic anticoagulation with warfarin.[60] LMWH should be avoided or used with extreme care in patients with renal insufficiency.

Dextran 40 may also be beneficial in preventing postoperative thrombosis following lower-extremity bypass. It should not be used routinely because of its side effects and cost and should be reserved for complex cases.[20]

Refer to Chapter 8 for additional information.

ACUTE ARTERIAL ISCHEMIA

Acute arterial occlusion (AAO) of the lower extremity refers to the sudden interruption of arterial blood supply. Regardless of etiology, AAO differs from chronic occlusion in that good collateral circulation is lacking. With chronic occlusion, symptoms develop slowly because as the artery narrows, collateral vessels develop around the blockage. With abrupt occlusion, critical ischemia of the extremity results within hours. AAO represents a vascular emergency that may result in loss of both limb and life.

Etiology

Embolism, thrombosis, and trauma are the primary causes of acute arterial occlusion in the lower extremity. Venous outflow obstruction, including phlegmasia cerulea dolens and compartment syndrome, and low-flow states may also result in acute occlusion (Box 13-2).

Embolism

Emboli are fragments of thrombus, atheromatous debris, tumor, or other material that have migrated from another source. Causes of embolism are included in Box 13-2. Many patients with embolization of cardiac origin are in atrial fibrillation or recently converted from fibrillation to a sinus rhythm (Fig. 13-10). Mitral stenosis produces a high left atrial pressure, and stasis predisposes the affected person to thrombus formation. Following myocardial infarction, thrombotic debris forms on the surface of the injured endocardium. Thrombus may embolize from the sewing rings of a prosthetic valve or from deposits on the valve leaflets. With appropriate anticoagulation and the introduction of tissue valves, there has been a reduced incidence of embolization from these sources.[61]

Noncardiac (artery to artery) emboli originate from proximal aortic plaque, such as an ulcerated aortic atheroma or thrombotic debris from an aneurysm (see Fig. 13-10).[62] Paradoxical emboli, in which venous thrombus embolizes into the arterial circulation, can occur in the presence of an intracardiac right-to-left shunt such as a patent foramen ovale. The source of embolism remains unknown in a small percentage of acute ischemia cases.

Most emboli lodge where the vessel suddenly tapers or branches and consequently are located most often in the lower extremities (Fig. 13-11). An embolus that lodges at the bifurcation of the aorta is known as a saddle embolus.

Thrombosis

Acute arterial thrombosis may be the result of local arterial factors and/or a consequence of systemic conditions such as alterations in plasma coagulation (see Box 13-2). High-grade stenosis of an artery alone is not necessarily an indicator of adverse outcomes; it is the occlusive thrombus that causes acute events. Thrombus formation occurs when plaques fissure, crack, and rupture and do not stabilize. More than half of acute ischemic events occur in vessels with mild to moderate stenosis. Stabilized plaque may lead to stenosis resulting in claudication, but not necessarily to acute events.[63-66]

Popliteal aneurysms, which account for 70 percent of all peripheral aneurysms, contain intraluminal clot and may thrombose or embolize to the tibial circulation.[67] Patients with a popliteal aneurysm have a significant chance of having a popliteal aneurysm in the contralateral leg.[68]

Trauma

Trauma resulting in arterial injury may be responsible for acute arterial occlusion. Fractures of the femur and tibial plateau, posterior dislocations (knee), and crushing and penetrating

BOX 13–2

Etiology of Acute Arterial Ischemia[12,61-68,70]

EMBOLIC
- Heart
  - Atherosclerotic heart disease
    - Coronary heart disease
    - Acute myocardial infarction
    - Dysrhythmia
  - Valvular heart disease
    - Rheumatic
    - Degenerative
    - Congenital
    - Bacterial
    - Prosthetic
- Artery-to-artery
  - Aneurysm
  - Atherosclerotic plaque
  - Paradoxical embolus
- Idiopathic

THROMBOSIS
- Arterial factors
  - Atherosclerosis
  - Aneurysm of popliteal artery
  - Arterial dissection
  - Arterial graft occlusion
  - Arterial entrapment
- Systemic factors
  - Hypercoagulable states (inherited and acquired) (see Boxes 9-2 and 9-3)
  - Antithrombin III, protein C, or protein S deficiency, hyperhomocysteinemia
  - Heparin-induced thrombocytopenia with thrombosis (HITT)
  - Polycythemia vera
  - Collagen vascular disease
- Vascular grafts
  - Progression of disease
  - Intimal hyperplasia
  - Mechanical failure

TRAUMATIC
- Penetrating trauma
  - Direct vessel injury
  - Indirect injury
  - Missile emboli
  - Proximity
- Blunt trauma
  - Fracture of femur and tibial plateau/posterior knee dislocation
    - Intimal flap
    - Spasm
  - Iatrogenic
    - Intimal flap
    - Dissection
    - Presence of medical device
    - Space-occupying thrombosis
  - Clot propagation
- External compression
- Drug abuse
  - Intraarterial administration leading to mycotic aneurysm
  - Drug toxicity
  - Contaminant
  - Microembolization

OUTFLOW VENOUS OCCLUSION
- Compartment syndrome
- Phlegmasia cerulea dolens

LOW-FLOW STATES (DECREASED CARDIAC OUTPUT)
- Cardiogenic shock
- Hypovolemic shock
- Myocardial infarction
- Congestive heart failure
- Sepsis
- Vasopressors

injuries are all common problems that can lead to arterial occlusion from direct transection or secondary to intimal disruption with subsequent thrombosis of the artery (Fig. 13-12).[64] Although laceration and transection of the artery are most frequent, mural contusion and isolated intimal injury of an intact artery also are encountered, sometimes leading to a delayed arterial occlusion.

With increased use of percutaneous catheters for diagnostic and therapeutic procedures, iatrogenic trauma from arterial catheterization has become a more frequent source of acute arterial occlusion.[61] Large catheters, extended catheterization, and underlying arterial disease are just a few of the contributing factors. Clinical manifestations may appear during a procedure while indwelling arterial catheters are in place or after the catheter has been removed.

Outflow Venous Occlusion

Venous outflow may be impeded by compartment syndrome or phlegmasia cerulea dolens. Compartment syndrome, a condition that exists when a rise in intracompartmental pressure

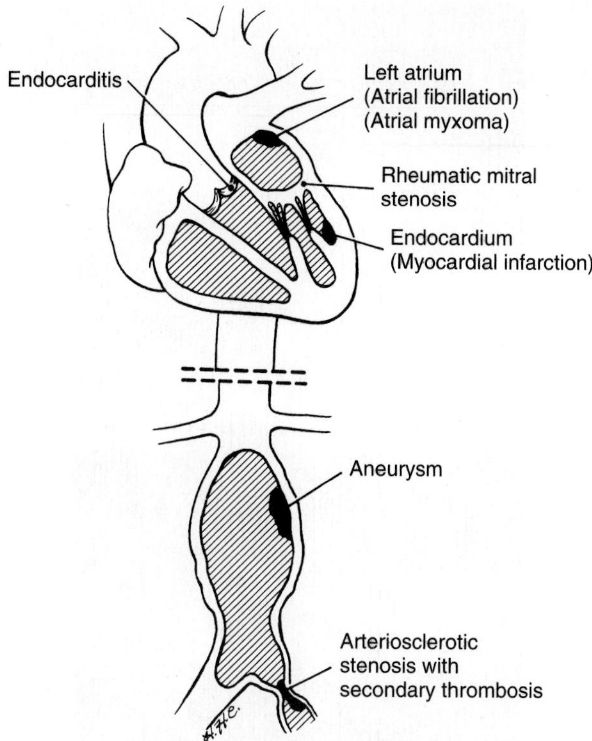

FIG. 13–10. Sources of emboli. Most emboli originate in the diseased heart, but they may also represent debris from an aneurysm or atherosclerotic arteries. (From Zimmerman JJ, Fogarty TJ: Acute arterial occlusion. In Moore WS, ed: *Vascular surgery: a comprehensive review,* New York, 1983, Grune & Stratton, p 694.)

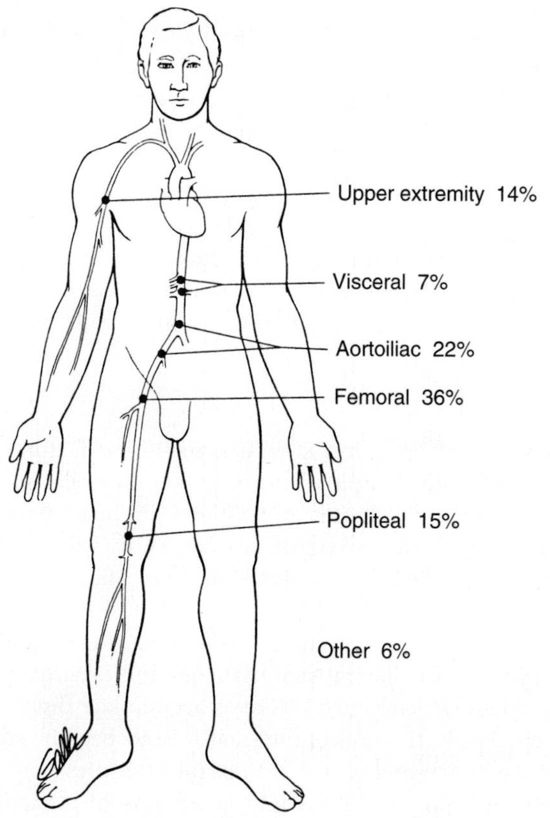

FIG. 13–11. Incidence of embolic occlusion at different sites. (From Greenburg RK, Ouriel K: Arterial thromboembolism. In Rutherford RB: *Vascular surgery,* ed 5, Philadelphia, 2000, WB Saunders, pp 822-835.)

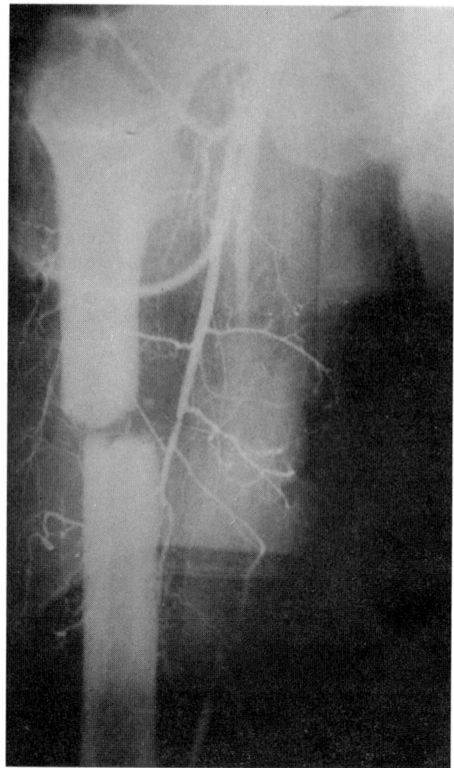

FIG. 13–12. Fracture of femur resulting in acute arterial occlusion of the superficial femoral artery.

exceeds capillary filling pressure, may compromise the neurovascular structures (artery, vein and nerves) within that space. If this process goes unchecked, arterial inflow may eventually be restricted, leading to permanent nerve injury and muscle ischemia. Phlegmasia cerulea dolens, the most severe form of iliofemoral venous thrombosis, can also lead to acute arterial occlusion and limb ischemia.[64]

Low-Flow States

Low-flow states (i.e., low cardiac output) can potentiate ischemia, especially when superimposed on pre-existing atherosclerotic disease. This occurs because of peripheral vasoconstriction with resultant decrease in blood flow through collateral circulation (see Box 13-2).[12,64]

Pathophysiology

The impact of sudden arterial occlusion is related to several factors, including the site of obstruction, extent of thrombus propagation, adequacy of collateral circulation, and the hemodynamic state of the patient. Because of differences in tissue tolerance to ischemia, severe and sometimes irreversible anoxic injury occurs in skeletal muscle or peripheral nerves about 4-6 hours after the onset of ischemia; skin and subcutaneous tissue remain viable for longer.[12,64]

Three events occur during acute arterial occlusion. First, the arterial thrombus may propagate, occluding the orifices of collateral side branches and eventually the collateral vessels themselves. Then, ischemic skeletal muscle tissues accumulate fluid and swell, resulting in compartment syndrome. Lastly, the cells of the small vessels become edematous, causing significant narrowing of the lumen and obstruction of the arterioles, capillaries, and venules or a bypass graft and nerve injury.[12,64] Signs and symptoms of compartment syndrome are included in Box 13-3.

BOX 13–3

Signs and Symptoms of Compartment Syndrome

- Decreased sensation or anesthesia of nerves in the compartment
- Pain out of proportion to injury
- Tenseness and fullness of compartment
- Pain on passive muscle stretching
- Decreased muscle strength within the compartment
- Decreased simple touch perception
- Pulses: normal or diminished or absent in late stage

Systemic metabolic consequences of ischemic myopathy can occur during the acute phase of occlusion or after revascularization of skeletal muscle.[12] These include metabolic acidosis, hyperkalemia, elevated muscle enzymes, and myoglobinuria. The venous effluent from the revascularized limb may contain high concentrations of lactic acid, potassium, creatine phosphokinase (CPK), and lactate dehydrogenase (LDH). Severe hyperkalemia and acidosis are most dangerous because they can result in cardiac depression and dysrhythmia. Myoglobin and metabolic products released from ischemic muscle may have nephrotoxic effects (renal failure) when myoglobin is deposited in the renal tubules, also known as myoglobinuria.[69]

Clinical Manifestations

Clinical manifestations of AAO, which occur distal to the site of arterial occlusion, will vary depending on the level and severity of obstruction and the adequacy of collateral circulation.[12] The patient may exhibit signs of pain, pallor, pulselessness, and poikilothermy (coolness) in the affected extremity. The extent of paresthesia and paralysis is a good index of the degree of ischemic injury to nerves and muscle and correlates well with the ultimate prognosis. Preservation of sensitivity to light touch is often the best guide to viability. Its absence and paralysis are grave signs with potential irreversibility.[61]

Irreversible nerve damage manifested as a foot drop may also occur.[12] An ischemic blue toe, known as blue toe syndrome, may result from distal embolization from a proximal source such as an aneurysm, heart, or any proximal atherosclerotic lesion.[70]

Diagnosis

An accurate diagnosis of an arterial occlusion as embolic or thrombotic in origin is necessary in order to initiate appropriate treatment (Box 13-4). When arterial thrombosis occurs in a nonatherosclerotic artery, signs and symptoms are similar to those of embolism. When there is no question that embolism is the cause of acute ischemia and the patient is suspected to have normal baseline arterial flow, an arteriogram may not be needed before surgery. If the diagnosis is unclear, then an arteriogram is usually performed immediately.

BOX 13–4

Acute Arterial Occusion (AAO): Embolism vs. Thrombosis

EMBOLISM

Sudden onset of pain in an extremity without prior symptoms of arterial insufficiency
Loss of pulses in one leg with normal pulses in contralateral extremity
Presence of likely source of emboli, (e.g., atrial fibrillation, valvular heart disease, recent myocardial infarction, ventricular aneurysm)

THROMBOSIS

Gradual to acute onset of symptoms in affected extremity
Symptoms of arterial insufficiency, (e.g., claudication, rest pain)
Contralateral disease
No proximal source of emboli

It is important to determine the severity of ischemia so that an appropriate plan for treatment can be made. Evaluation of the consistency of skeletal muscle is an important part of the physical exam to determine the severity of ischemia. With increased ischemia, cellular swelling occurs and the muscle no longer feels soft but becomes thick, inelastic, and necrotic. As this worsens, the extremity becomes stiff and firm. This rigidity, which may occur many hours before clinical and laboratory abnormalities become apparent, is an ominous sign.[64,69]

Treatment

Initial Treatment

The approach to acute leg ischemia varies significantly from treatment used in the chronic situation, because immediate intervention is usually required. Because a delay in or inadequate treatment may result in limb loss, damage to vital organs, or death, prompt treatment of the patient is crucial to successful management. The cause and severity of ischemia and the underlying cardiopulmonary status of the patient play a significant role in the choice of treatment and the patient's outcome.[71]

After the diagnosis of acute leg ischemia has been confirmed, if there are no immediate life-threatening contraindications, systemic anticoagulation with heparin is initiated with a 10,000-unit bolus followed by a continuous drip of 1000 units each hour. This helps to prevent thrombus propagation, which can impair collateral circulation and thrombosis of arteries distal to the occlusion as well as prevent proliferation of new emboli.[20,61,64]

Thrombolytic Therapy

Thrombolytic therapy may be used to treat recently formed arterial and bypass graft occlusions. Thrombolysis can help dissolve platelet fibrin aggregates in the microcirculation and thrombi in collateral vessels and expose underlying disease that may be treated with less extensive interventions. Research is ongoing to define the exact role of thrombolytic therapy in the treatment of acute arterial occlusion.[72] Recent data suggest that bypass graft occlusions may be associated with a better thrombolytic response than native arterial occlusions. Only in rare cases of embolic events or prosthetic graft occlusion will thrombolysis be sufficient as the sole intervention.[73]

A multicenter trial of thrombolysis or peripheral arterial surgery (TOPAS) was organized to compare the use of recombinant urokinase (rUK) with surgery for the initial treatment of acute lower-extremity ischemia.[74] The preliminary results suggested that an initial rUK dose of 4000 IU/min is safe and efficacious in the treatment of acute limb-threatening ischemia in native arterial or bypass graft. Therapy with rUK is associated with limb salvage and patient survival rates similar to those achieved with surgery, concurrent with a reduced requirement for complex surgery after thrombolytic intervention.[74,75] For patients without diabetes who have older vein grafts, thrombolysis may provide significant improvement in patency rates. However, in diabetics, thrombolytic therapy is unlikely to result in durable patency or limb salvage even if newly discovered disease is corrected.[74,76]

Thrombolytic therapy may be used alone or in conjunction with surgical intervention (see Chapter 6). Selective intraarterial delivery of a thrombolytic agent has been used with the advantage of local thrombolysis and minimizes risk of systemic effects.[61] Thrombolytic therapy may require 8-72 hours to be successful and can be used only in patients who do not require immediate restoration of blood flow. For patients with severe ischemia, surgical exploration may afford a more expeditious restoration of blood flow. Thrombolytic therapy is associated with a higher frequency of hemorrhagic complications and is contraindicated in patients with other risk factors for bleeding, including recent surgery or stroke and severe uncontrolled hypertension.

Surgical Intervention

Embolism

Arterial embolism can often be corrected by an embolectomy, the extraction of the embolus using a Fogarty embolectomy catheter with a small balloon at one end (Fig. 13-13).[12]

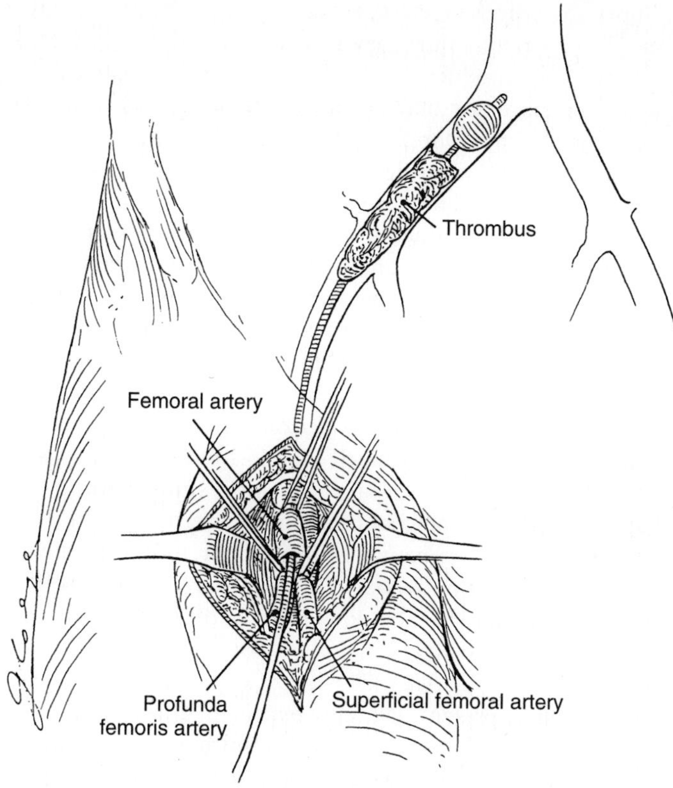

FIG. 13–13. Operative technique for femoral embolectomy. (From Quinones-Baldrich WJM: Acute arterial and graft occlusion. In Moore W, ed: *Vascular surgery: a comprehensive review,* ed 5, Philadelphia, 1998, WB Saunders, p 679.)

Through an opening in the artery, the catheter is passed down the affected arterial segment with the balloon deflated. When the tip is beyond the obstruction, the balloon is inflated and the catheter and embolus are withdrawn. This procedure can often be performed using local anesthesia. If an embolus is present in a badly diseased artery, an embolectomy may fail and a bypass graft may be required. Most patients are maintained on heparin and warfarin postoperatively.

Thrombosis

Arterial thrombosis is treated in much the same way as is chronic ischemia, with a bypass procedure to the appropriate nonoccluded arterial segment. Depending on the location of thrombosis, aortofemoral, femoro-femoral, or femoral-to-popliteal or distal artery bypass may be performed. Ligation of a popliteal aneurysm may also be necessary. With an arterial graft thrombosis, thrombectomy of the graft may be adequate or a new bypass graft may be necessary. However, the surgical management of a failed graft depends on the cause of the failure.

Trauma (*see Chapter 22*)

After the evaluation of an injured patient, if there is any suggestion of arterial injury, a careful pulse exam and an ABI must be obtained in the affected leg. In blunt trauma, following crush injury, fracture, or major dislocation, an arteriogram should be obtained when the Doppler examination suggests a blood pressure drop in the affected extremity, even if the palpated pulses are normal. Certain types of blunt trauma are so likely to produce arterial injury that an arteriogram is recommended even without any Doppler evidence of arterial injury. These injuries include dislocation of the knee, which causes popliteal artery injury in about one third of all cases. Patients with an associated fracture and arterial obstruction may need external fracture stabilization or reduction at the time of arterial repair.[64]

Blunt arterial injury sometimes precipitates leg ischemia chronologically remote from the initial accident. An arterial stretch injury may produce intimal tearing that slowly progresses and occludes the vessel. This produces severe leg pain hours or even days after the initial injury, at a time when the extremity may be surrounded by a well-fitted plaster cast. These painful complaints demand rapid Doppler assessment of ankle pressure and must not be attributed to inadequate analgesia or benign swelling beneath the plaster. Delays under these circumstances often result in leg amputation.

Penetrating leg wounds may produce severe leg ischemia similar to that seen in blunt trauma from arterial contusion, or the patient may present with massive external bleeding from the wound. Injured patients should always be examined with a stethoscope to detect an arteriovenous fistula between the injured artery and adjacent vein.

Leg injuries caused by bullet wounds or stabbing require liberal evaluation with arteriography if occult vascular injuries are to be avoided. Arterial injuries of the thigh and leg require an attempt at direct vascular reconstruction because arterial ligation frequently leads to amputation. Information from World War II, before arterial repair was commonly used, reminds us that leg amputation is necessary following simple ligation in 81 percent of common femoral arteries and in 55 percent of popliteal arteries.[77]

Arterial reconstruction in blunt or penetrating arterial trauma is usually undertaken using a saphenous vein graft from the uninjured leg. Experience has shown that if the adjacent vein is also injured, it should be repaired at the time of initial reconstruction.

Compartment Syndrome

If a compartment syndrome is present or highly expected, a fasciotomy may be performed, which allows expansion of the edematous muscle, resulting in decompression of the compartment and relief of pressure. Incisions are made over the leg compartments, and the underlying fascia is opened from the knee to the ankle (Fig. 13-14). Immediate identification of compartment syndrome and prompt fasciotomy can reduce the sequelae of muscle necrosis, nerve damage, and possible limb amputation.

Muscle debridement may be necessary until healthy granulation tissue is present. A fasciotomy wound can either be closed once swelling resolves or may be covered with a skin graft.[61] Complications after fasciotomy result from infection, bleeding from anticoagulation, or peroneal nerve injury. Vigorous physical therapy and a splint to prevent foot drop may be necessary.[78]

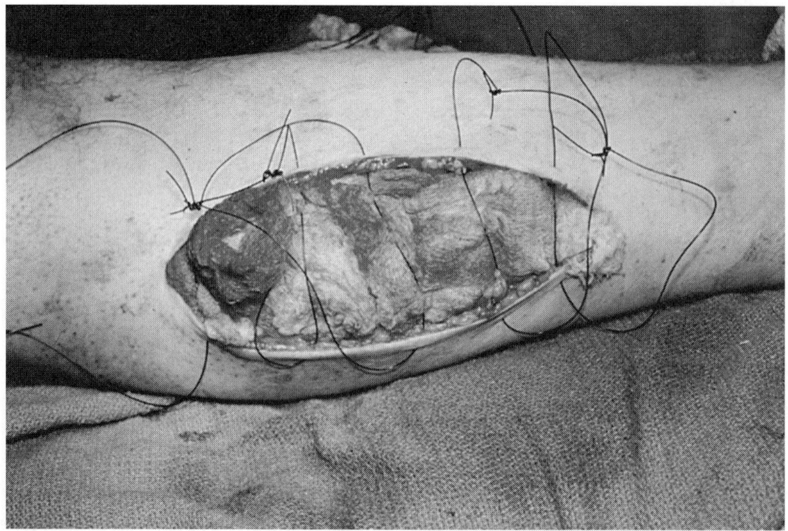

FIG. 13–14. Fasciotomy performed for compartment syndrome.

Amputation

Amputation may be an acceptable alternative under certain circumstances. Attempted revascularization can be inappropriate and potentially dangerous due to metabolic complications. Primary amputation may be urgent if advanced tissue ischemia has led to systemic toxicity or the leg is irreversibly anesthetic or paralytic.

Treatment of Metabolic Complications

As discussed previously, serious systemic complications including acidosis, hyperkalemia, and renal failure can occur. Treatment is directed at maintaining normal physiologic functions and ameliorating systemic effects caused by metabolic derangements. Dysrhythmias need to be corrected. Aggressive fluid resuscitation and careful attention to cardiac and renal function is needed. Metabolic acidosis should be anticipated and can be treated with sodium bicarbonate during the early stages of reperfusion. Leakage of potassium during cell death leads to hyperkalemia. Administration of glucose and insulin drives potassium into the cells, thus controlling hyperkalemia. Oral or rectal administration of exchange resins or even hemodialysis may be necessary. This may be aggravated by acute renal failure secondary to myoglobin precipitation in the collecting tubules. Maintaining a high urine output with alkaline urine is the best way to prevent myoglobinuria and potential renal failure. The systemic administration of mannitol to promote osmotic diuresis and bicarbonate to maintain alkaline urine may also be used.[12]

Treatment of Underlying Conditions

In addition to restoring blood supply to an extremity, underlying medical conditions leading to emboli or thrombosis also require treatment. If the patient is at risk for further embolization from a proximal source, the source must be treated. Warfarin may be prescribed in the case of atrial fibrillation or arrhythmias, and cardiac surgery may be indicated to replace diseased valves. An abdominal aortic aneurysm or popliteal aneurysm should be repaired if it is the cause of embolism. If heparin-induced thrombocytopenia occurs, heparin must be stopped promptly.

Because renal or mesenteric infarction can also occur, the patient should be monitored for abdominal, flank, or back pain, hematuria, gut emptying, and an elevated white blood count. These may be indicative of acute renal or visceral ischemia.

POTENTIAL COMPLICATIONS AND NURSING MANAGEMENT

Nursing management of complications and additional nursing care of patients with chronic and lower-extremity arterial ischemia are included in Box 13-5.

Cardiac

Patients with lower-extremity ischemia have significantly higher mortality because atherosclerotic disease is multifocal, in most instances including the coronary or cerebral vessels. The clinically silent or apparently stable coronary disease is unmasked by the stress of surgery. Myocardial ischemia in this patient population occurs more often postoperatively than during surgery.

Graft Stenosis and Thrombosis

Failure of a graft will result in an acutely ischemic limb or a return to its preoperative status. The causes of graft thrombosis are multifactorial (Box 13-6). Early recognition and aggressive treatment of failed bypass grafts may result in successful restoration of graft patency in most patients. The appropriate treatment of graft failure depends on several variables, including the timing of the occlusion, the cause of occlusion, type of graft material, limb viability, the patient's ability to tolerate reoperation, continued validity of original indications for operation or new indication, the condition of the proximal and distal arteries, and likelihood of success of reoperation.

BOX 13–5

Nursing Management

LOWER-EXTREMITY ISCHEMIA

- Check pedal pulses and ankle-brachial indices (ABIs) every hour for 24 hours, then every shift or as ordered. Report decrease in ABI greater than .15.
- Monitor pain status of leg.
- Check sensory and motor function and color of extremities.
- Monitor for heparin-induced thrombocytopenia with thrombosis syndrome (HITT): Drop in platelet count less than 100,000/mm^3, systemic thrombosis (myocardial infarction, stroke, deep vein thrombosis), increased requirements for heparin.

SYSTEMIC THROMBOSIS

- Monitor for mesenteric ischemia (abdominal pain, elevated white count, or gut emptying [vomiting or diarrhea]) and renal ischemia (flank or back pain, decreased urine output, elevated creatinine).
- Monitor for myocardial infarction and transient ischemic attack (TIA) and stroke.

HEMATOMA AND/OR HEMORRHAGE

- Observe for signs of shock, including increase in pulse, decrease in blood pressure, anxiety, restlessness, pallor, cyanosis, thirst, oliguria, clammy skin, venous collapse, and level of consciousness.
- Check incision for the presence of a hematoma and excessive drainage, and for a tense calf or thigh; a pulsatile mass at the incision site may be indicative of a false aneurysm.
- Assess pulmonary artery pressures and/or cardiac output when parameters are available.
- Check daily weights; monitor intake and output closely.
- Check lab values, e.g., hematocrit, hemoglobin, and notify physician if abnormal.

COMPARTMENT SYNDROME

- Assess extremity for motor and sensory function, the presence of foot drop, and for pain out of proportion to the situation.
- Assess extremity for hematoma, severe swelling and/or a tense calf, and consistency of muscle (doughy gastrocnemius muscle indicative of compartment syndrome). Severe swelling may impede blood flow through the graft.
- Use sterile technique for dressing changes of fasciotomy.
- Monitor fasciotomy site for infection.
- The extremity with a compartment syndrome should be positioned at a level no higher than the heart.

RENAL FAILURE/MYOGLOBINURIA

- Monitor urine output and creatinine level.
- Maintain urine output at 100 ml/hr.
- Monitor for myoglobinuria indicated by a change in color (reddish brown) and presence of red blood cells in urine.

METABOLIC COMPLICATIONS

- Monitor for hyperkalemia and acidosis secondary to increased concentrations of potassium and lactic acid.
- Monitor creatine phosphokinase (CPK) level.
- Monitor arterial blood gas (ABG).
- Monitor for arrhythmias.

WOUND INFECTION/WOUND CARE

- Observe for fever, cellulitis, increase in white blood count, or drainage from wound.
- Remove initial dressing postoperative day 1. If wound is sealed and dry, no further dressing is needed. If drainage is present, paint incision with betadine (or equivalent) one to two times daily. Apply dry gauze over the incision. Change dressing as often as necessary.
- Use aseptic technique during dressing changes.

Continued

BOX 13–5

Nursing Management—cont'd

EDEMA
- Elevate the extremity.
- Provide appropriate elastic support when indicated.
- Restrict ambulation.
- Treat cardiac failure when indicated.
- Use diuretic therapy when needed.

PREVENTION OF TISSUE DAMAGE
- Avoid tape on the skin below the knee to prevent skin damage.
- Separate toes that press on each other with dry gauze (see Fig. 13-15) or lambswool.
- Use sheepskin to reduce friction under the heels as the patient moves in bed.
- Elevate the heels off the bed.
- Remove pressure on the toes from bed linen.
- If a bed cradle is used, position it properly.
- Provide good skin care.

IMPAIRED PHYSICAL MOBILITY
- Assess for the presence of neurologic deficits or foot drop.
- Assess causative factors for immobility, the patient's range of motion, and ability to ambulate.
- Encourage progressive ambulation and range of motion while in bed.
- Request physical therapy consult when appropriate.
- Encourage independence in activities of daily living.

PAIN
- Assess patient's level of pain, type, duration, and location.
- Avoid elevation of limb.
- Provide comfort measures and means of distraction.
- Medicate with prescribed analgesics as needed (prn).
- Evaluate effectiveness of pain medication after each administration.

DISTURBANCE IN SELF-CONCEPT/CHANGE IN BODY IMAGE
- Establish a trusting relationship with patient.
- Encourage patient to verbalize feelings.
- Promote social interaction.
- Make appropriate referrals if indicated.

If graft failure is secondary to a problem with anticoagulation, graft thrombectomy or thrombolytic therapy may be adequate to restore blood flow. Neointimal hyperplasia usually requires a new bypass or revision of the distal anastomosis with a patch angioplasty. Progression of distal disease may require a completely new or an extended graft with a new distal anastomotic site.

Following femoral artery bypass, the dorsalis pedis and posterior tibial artery pulses should be assessed frequently to assess graft patency. However, the ABI provides the best means for monitoring the patency of femoral artery bypasses. These pressures vary postoperatively depending on the type of graft, the location of the distal anastomosis, and the degree of arterial disease beyond the bypass graft. In cases of severely calcified distal arteries, the ankle vessels may be noncompressible and thus the ABI may be falsely elevated.

Patients with normal arteries distal to the bypass, or with bypasses extending to near the ankle, should have ABIs of approximately 1.0. Arterial occlusive disease distal to the bypass will not permit an elevation in ankle-level blood pressure to a systemic level. A reduction in the ABI of greater than 0.15 may be indicative of a graft occlusion and warrants prompt physician notification. Ankle pressure measurements are not recommended when a bypass to the dorsalis pedis or posterior tibial artery has been performed.

BOX 13–6

Causes of Graft Failure

IMMEDIATE TO EARLY (WITHIN 30 DAYS OF SURGERY)

Technical defects
- Anastomosis
- Sewing vein shut with suture
- Intimal flap
- Retained valve cusp
- Compression/twisting of graft

Hypercoagulability/clotting disorder
- Inadequate anticoagulation
- Hypercoagulable state
  - Decreased antithrombin III
  - Heparin-induced thrombocytopenia

Decreased cardiac output (i.e., hypotension/ myocardial infarction)
Poor runoff (outflow)
Poor patient selection
Unexplained

INTERMEDIATE (30 DAYS TO 2 YEARS)

Graft stenosis
Myointimal hyperplasia
Embolization
Inadequate/failure of anticoagulation
Unexplained

LATE (GREATER THAN 2 YEARS)

Progression of disease (inflow/outflow)
Thrombosis of proximal reconstruction
Embolization from proximal source
False aneurysm
Inadequate/failure of anticoagulation
Graft infection
Valvular fibrosis

Although discomfort is expected after a femoral artery bypass, this must be differentiated from the extreme pain of lower-extremity ischemia or compartment compression. Severe pain in the foot across the metatarsal heads may be the first sign of graft occlusion. Sudden motor weakness or limb anesthesia may also reflect graft occlusion.

Sustained graft patency is enhanced with graft surveillance and intervention before graft thrombosis occurs.[49,79,80] Duplex scan surveillance is usually recommended 3-6 months after surgery, and yearly thereafter, depending upon whether it is a vein or prosthetic graft. Any significant change in pressure, or new symptoms, warrants further evaluation.

Hematoma/Hemorrhage

Any bleeding from the wounds following surgery is cause for concern. Suture line disruption, pseudoaneurysm formation, or failed ligature must be corrected in the operating room promptly. A tense hematoma can present as a compartment syndrome and compromise arterial blood flow and nerve function. Hematomas related to femoral grafts should be evacuated in the operating room to prevent skin damage and graft infection.

Renal Failure

A complication of compartment syndrome is the release of myoglobin by the damaged muscle cells. Patients with preoperative muscle paralysis or rigor should have urine checked for the presence of myoglobin. If myoglobinuria is anticipated, alkalinization of the urine with sodium bicarbonate, as well as osmotic diuresis using mannitol, is employed.[69]

Edema

Leg edema following femoral revascularization is common. The exact etiology is not clear but is believed to be a result of interstitial fluid accumulation, dissection around perivascular lymphatics, lymphatic obstruction, and a loss of subcutaneous venous channels. Edema can inhibit wound healing, and a mild diuretic may sometimes be necessary. An elastic bandage applied below the knee when the patient is out of bed can help to control edema; however, elastic bandages may not be recommended if an in situ vein bypass has been performed because of the graft's location (Fig. 13-15). Patients should understand that edema usually resolves within the first 8-12 postoperative weeks but can last many months after surgery.

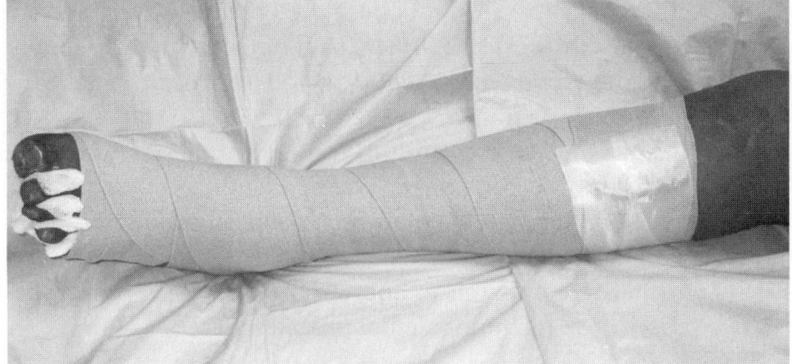

FIG. 13–15. Elastic bandage wrapped from toe to below the knee with dry gauze placed between the toes.

If swelling continues, the patient may be fitted for an elastic stocking. Leg elevation is also beneficial to control the edema. In addition, any cardiac failure needs to be treated.

Wound Complications

Wound infection usually is related to persistent hematoma, lymphocele, or superficial necrosis. Wounds that develop evidence of infection should be cultured and appropriate antibiotics ordered. Close observation and local wound care are needed. Local incision and drainage of wound with debridement may be necessary. Minor amputation wounds may not be completely healed at the time of discharge but should be clean and granulating well. Wound dehiscence or exposure of the graft necessitates immediate readmission of the patient to the hospital. Wound complications will develop in 10-40 percent of patients with infrainguinal bypass.[81]

Lymphatic Complications

Vascular surgical wounds, especially in the groin, may develop lymphatic collections between the arterial dissection and the skin. Lymphoceles (injury to lymphatic pathway) often appear between the fifth and seventh postoperative days with the discharge of clear, pale yellow fluid. The lymphatic fistula usually heals after treatment with bed rest, antibiotics, and dressing changes. If it persists, direct operative exploration with lymphatic suture and the use of a suction drain may be necessary. Prosthetic graft infection can result secondary to a prolonged lymph leak. In rare cases, a lymphocele may develop after the patient is home when the wound is well healed.

A perigraft seroma may be seen along the length of a subcutaneous synthetic graft; this usually is benign and resolves over time. Owing to increased risk of infection, these collections of fluid usually should not be aspirated. The late appearance of a fluid collection may also indicate graft infection.

Graft Infection

Graft infection is one of the most serious complications of bypass surgery and threatens both limb and life. Causes of graft infection include contamination of the graft during insertion, penetrating injury from an angiography catheter, or blood-borne inoculation. Treatment of these infections has evolved in recent years, reflecting improvements in antibiotics, wound care, and more liberal use of local or distal free flap transfer.[82]

It is no longer standard practice to remove all infected prosthetic grafts. Graft preservation may be indicated for patients with a patent vein or prosthetic graft, no evidence of systemic sepsis, and no graft hemorrhage. Wound debridement, wet to dry dressings, intravenous antibiotics, and a myocutaneous tissue flap as soon as possible may be sufficient. Muscle flaps are helpful in reducing the incidence of complications. Placing a healthy muscle over infected wounds may not only prevent graft desiccation and rupture, but may promote healing of the wound, promote earlier discharge, and decrease the need for debridement. Graft preservation eliminates the need for a major operation with associated risks and results in almost universal limb salvage as long as the graft is patent.[82,83]

Broad-spectrum antibiotic coverage should be started preoperatively and continued for at least the first postoperative day. Postoperatively, patients are carefully monitored for low-grade fever, an elevated white blood count, septic emboli, or hemorrhage, which are all suggestive of infection.

Poorly nourished patients appear to be most prone to wound disruption, graft infection, and possible graft thrombosis.[84] These patients may be identified preoperatively by their low serum albumin levels. Dietary supplementation by enteral or parenteral routes is beneficial in patients with delayed wound healing. Because of the severe consequences of graft infection, patients with prosthetic grafts require appropriate antibiotic prophylaxis during any subsequent invasive procedures, including dental procedures.

Nerve Injury

Following bypass grafting, a saphenous neuropathy may occur. The patient may complain of pain along the medial aspect in the lower part of the thigh and medial aspect of the leg. The severity of the pain varies from patient to patient.[85] This pain is related to an operative injury to the nerve or may result from nerve entrapment in the scar tissue in the lower thigh. It may appear as a mild transient discomfort or may assume a burning character or more rarely may be persistent and disabling. Most injuries resolve within 3-6 months.[16]

Pharmacologic Management

Depending on the type of anticoagulation therapy used postoperatively, patients may require frequent monitoring of their partial thromboplastin time/prothrombin time (PTT/PT) or international normalized ratio (INR). With heparin therapy, the platelet count should be checked before any heparin is administered and every day starting on day 5 to monitor for heparin-induced thrombocytopenia. A drop in platelet count to less than $100,000/mm^3$ can be indicative of this problem. Observe patients for skin breakdown or necrosis, called Coumadin necrosis, which can result from warfarin therapy. Patients who are anticoagulated should be assessed for signs of bleeding, including local as well as systemic problems, including mental status changes. Patients receiving thrombolytic therapy must have fibrinogen levels and coagulation parameters monitored regularly (see Chapter 8).

Foot Care

Because of the importance of skin integrity in vascular patients, particularly those with diabetes, it is imperative to establish a detailed plan for foot maintenance. The patient must be educated about specific maintenance steps and their significance, so that foot problems can be avoided. Foot care, footwear, and steps to avoiding injury are included in Box 13-7. Diabetics have peripheral sensory neuropathy and retinopathy, which limits their ability to detect lesions early. Foot care must include preventative measures to avoid pressure sores in patients who may have compromised sensation or mentation. It is important to remember that the contralateral limb is also at risk because it will usually have compromised sensation and blood flow.

The nurse should inform the patient of the hazard of cutting skin during nail care and should assess the patient's visual acuity to perform this task. A tiny break in the skin can allow a host of organisms to penetrate it. With impaired arterial flow, the potential for infection is high and the results can be limb threatening.

Psychosocial Needs

Delivery of comprehensive care to a person with vascular disease is based on an understanding of disease pathophysiology, associated risk factors, and an awareness of the patient's response to the disease. Vascular patients and their families vary greatly in their responses to the diagnosis and chronicity of arterial insufficiency. Although some patients may express a positive outlook, others express anger, anxiety, depression, guilt, uncertainty, or helplessness. Psychosocial variables can affect the patient's ability to adapt to altered function and

BOX 13–7

Postoperative/Discharge Teaching Plan (May Vary From Hospital to Hospital)

GRAFT PATENCY

- Review disease process and surgical procedure with patient and family. Use diagram and written information when available.
- Teach the patient/family how to palpate pulses in the foot.
- Teach the patient signs and symptoms of graft failure that need to be reported to the physician.

ACTIVITY

- Regular exercise is important, and climbing stairs, going out of doors, and bending knee are acceptable. There is no danger of disrupting an anastomosis by normal convalescent activity.
- Avoid heavy lifting.
- Sexual activity may be resumed in 2 weeks; discuss with physician if concerned.

BATHING

- Bathing or showering is acceptable on the fifth day after surgery or on an individual basis if there are open wounds or skin lesions.
- Clean incision gently with mild soap and water; dry it well.

PRESENCE OF PROSTHETIC GRAFT

- Inform patient if a prosthetic graft is used; patient should notify other physicians and dentist if undergoing any invasive test or procedure or extensive dental work.
- Inform patient that prosthetic graft is not rejectable.

WOUND CARE

- Instruct patient that no special care of wound is required unless otherwise indicated. If oozing from the incision is present, the area should be covered with dry gauze. If sutures are subcuticular, the patient should be informed that sutures do not require removal.
- Avoid tape on the skin below the knee. Use gauze such as Kling or Kerlix, and tape the gauze. Physicians' opinions on dressing material for open wounds or ulcers vary widely. Saline, Betadine ointment, Silvadene, Garamycin ointment, Neosporin, Polysporin, hydrogels, enzymatic products, and Betadine solution are some of the choices. The first six keep the wound moist while exerting a bacteriostatic action on the wound. Betadine solution has a drying effect unless kept constantly wet as a wet dressing. It exerts a debriding effect each time the gauze is changed.
- Instruct patient about importance of eating nutritiously to assist with proper wound healing.

FOOT CARE

- Inspect body on a daily basis for cuts, blisters, ingrown toenails, between toes and be aware of how incisions, feet, and legs look and feel after surgery. This can help in the recognition of early evidence of significant change. Use a mirror if necessary. If poor vision, have someone else check.
- Wash feet and clean between toes daily, and dry well. Mild soap and warm water should be used. Check the water temperature with the hand or a thermometer each time the feet are bathed. A warm, moist washcloth will remove dry, scaly skin.
- Apply a lubricating, lanolin-based cream to the feet, except between the toes and near open ulcers. Apply especially over the heels. The lubricant should be used sparingly and rubbed into the skin. Avoid perfumed preparations.
- If the feet perspire excessively, a hypoallergenic, nonmedicated talcum powder should be lightly dusted on the feet twice a day. Avoid powder in the presence of cracked skin or ulcerations.
- Nail care should be performed under good lighting while the nails are softened from the bath. If nail care cannot be performed then, soak the feet for 5-10 minutes before to soften the nails. Do not trim nails if they are hypertrophic, badly ingrown, infected, or painful. Toenails are to be cut straight across. The corners are filed slightly to rid the edges of sharp points, but they should not be cut back. See a podiatrist for assistance, especially with corns, calluses, or ingrown toenails. Make sure the podiatrist is aware of the vascular status of the patient.

Continued

BOX 13–7

Postoperative/Discharge Teaching Plan (May Vary From Hospital to Hospital)—cont'd

- Corns and calluses should not be trimmed or cut. A pumice-impregnated soap bar used regularly on the heels and the bony prominences during bathing can help impede callus formation.
- Dry gauze, cotton, or lambswool may be placed between the toes to prevent pressure (see Fig. 13-15). The bony prominences of each toe put pressure on the adjoining toe, which can result in a pressure ulcer. Change the padding daily or when it becomes wet.
- Report skin breakdown to the physician.

FOOTWEAR/AVOIDING INJURY

- Wear properly fitting shoes to avoid skin breakdown at pressure points. It is best to buy shoes midday to take into account some edema that may develop.
- Shoes should be soft, flexible leather. Manmade materials such as patent leather and plastic should be avoided because they prevent evaporation and may contribute to fungal infections. Since athletic shoes have become more popular, more styles with proper support are available. Avoid sandals.
- Break new shoes in gradually.
- Wear socks or stockings with shoes at all times to prevent blistering.
- Socks should be clean, preferably cotton or wool, nonmended, and without seams, to prevent skin breakdown.
- Stockings should not be held up with garters or by twisting at the knee. Men's socks should not constrict the ankle or the leg below the knee.
- Inspect shoes for foreign objects, holes, or nail points in the soles. Decreased sensory perception in the diabetic foot makes it possible for patients to be unaware of sharp objects, stones, or other debris for extended periods of time. Any potential area of damage should be eliminated because pressure may result in skin breakdown with subsequent infection and potential limb loss.[64]
- Avoid clothes such as tight socks, garters, or panty hose that constrict the legs or feet.
- Wear protective shoes or slippers when out of bed. Avoid walking barefoot. Simple debris or splinters on the floor or in the carpet can go unnoticed in a foot that lacks sensory perception or be noticed only after the injury is inflicted.
- Protect feet/legs from excessive heat or cold by avoiding heating pads/cold packs, heat lamps, or hot water bottles, and cream hair removers, adhesive corn pads, or any harsh chemicals.
- Use sheepskin and foot cradle when needed.

ELASTIC SUPPORT

- Inform patient that leg swelling is normal after surgery. Because of decreased postoperative activity and immobilization during the surgical procedure, fluid accumulates in lower leg.
- If ordered, instruct patient how to wrap 4-inch elastic bandage snugly from the toe to just below the knee (see Fig. 13-15), to apply bandage before ambulation, to remove at night, to wear bandage for 2 weeks or until swelling disappears. Elastic bandages can be washed with mild soap and water and can be reused. They can be purchased at most drug stores. Elastic bandages are usually not recommended with in situ bypass grafts.

MEDICATIONS

- Instruct patient regarding medications with which he or she will be discharged, their purposes, dosages, and side effects. Document teaching (see Chapter 8).

DRIVING

- Driving may be possible after returning to first office visit or when patient has returned to baseline in terms of mobility.

BOX 13–7

Postoperative/Discharge Teaching Plan (May Vary From Hospital to Hospital)—cont'd

RISK FACTOR MODIFICATION (SEE CHAPTER 10)

MEDICAL FOLLOW-UP/INDICATIONS FOR PHYSICIAN NOTIFICATION

- Instruct patient regarding importance of follow-up visits with physician and arterial blood flow studies on regular basis.
- Inform patient to notify physicion of any changes in incision, new or unusual drainage, change in color or amount of drainage, increase in temperature, swelling or pulsatile mass at the incision site, inflammation or tenderness around incision, any unusual or severe increase in pain in leg especially when it is severe enough to prevent sleep, sudden weight gain or swelling of feet or legs, fever, loss of sensation or movement of legs, unusual tingling, coldness, or discoloration of the feet or legs, and any skin breakdown on the foot.

comply with the prescribed medical regimen. Nursing interventions can be enhanced by an understanding of how the disease affects feelings, coping capabilities, self-esteem, and psychosocial resources of the person, all of which are reflected in general well-being.

Traditionally, the outcome of surgery has been based on patency and limb salvage rates. Quality of life (pain, sleep, physical mobility) analysis has become increasing important as an outcome measure in vascular surgery. Studies have shown that the treatment of PAD has resulted in an immediate and relatively lasting improvement in patients' quality of life.[86]

Patient Education

Nurses play a significant role in the care and education of the patient and the family. Every patient should be informed that PAD is a marker for heart disease and stroke and that risk modification is essential.

Box 13-7 outlines a postoperative/discharge teaching plan. A clinical pathway of the patient undergoing lower-extremity bypass surgery is outlined in Table 13-1.

TABLE 13–1 Clinical Pathway of Patient Undergoing Lower-Extremity Bypass Surgery (May Vary From Institution to Institution)

	OR DAY: Postop Date	POD #1Date	POD #2 Date	POD #3-5 Date
Vital Signs/ Parameters	VS q 2 hr I/O 2 hr	VS q 4 hr I/O q 8 hr	VS q 4 hr I/O q 8 hr	VS q 4 hr I/O q 8 hr
Pulse/Doppler Assessment	Pulse/Doppler tones q 1-2 hr ABI q 4 hr	Pulse/Doppler tones q 4 hr ABI q AM	Pulse/Doppler tones q 4 hr ABI q AM	Pulse/Doppler tones q 8 hr ABI q AM
Activity	Bed rest	Ambulate with assistance 1-2x	Ambulate 2-3x	Ambulate 3x May shower POD 5
Medication	IV; A-line prn	IV Antibiotic prn	IV: D/C prn Antibiotic prn	
	ASA or anticoagulation	ASA or anticoagulation Monitor for HIT	ASA or anticoagulation Monitor for HIT	ASA or anticoagulation Monitor for HIT
	Pain meds prn	Pain meds prn	Pain meds prn	Pain meds prn

Continued

TABLE 13–1 Clinical Pathway of Patient Undergoing Lower-Extremity Bypass Surgery (May Vary From Institution to Institution)—Cont'd

	OR DAY: Postop Date	POD #1 Date	POD #2 Date	POD #3-5 Date
Tests	Chemistry panel prn, CBC, PTT/PT Platelet count if on heparin ECG prn	Chemistry panel prn, CBC, PTT/PT/INR Platelet count if on heparin	PTT/PT/INR Platelet count if on heparin	PTT/PT/INR Platelet count if on heparin
Consult/ DC Planning		DC planner/SW prn Physical therapy	DC planner/SW Physical therapy	DC planner/SW Physical therapy May be discharged to home/rehab or skilled unit
Diet	NPO	Low fat, low cholesterol	Low fat, low cholesterol	Low fat, low cholesterol
Treatment	Observe for bleeding, hematoma q 2 hr TCDB q 2 hr	Wound/incisional care: Observe for bleeding, hematoma q 4 hr/4-inch bandages below knee (not in situ grafts) rewrap q 8 hr	Incisional care qd Elastic bandages rewrap q 8 hr	Incisional care qd Elastic bandages rewrap q 8 hr
Psychosocial needs	Provide support	Assess pt/family needs	Intervene with pt/family psychosocial needs prn	Intervene with pt/family psychosocial needs prn
Patient Education	Assess family's level of understanding Discuss postop course with family	Assess pt/family's level of understanding Discuss postop course with pt /family	Discuss pt progress with pt and family Begin DC teaching, anticoagulation therapy teaching prn	DC teaching including risk reduction, elastic bandage application, anticoagulation therapy prn

OR, Operating room; *POD,* postoperative day; *VS,* vital signs; *q,* every; *I/O,* intake and output; *ABI,* ankle-brachial index; *BID,* twice a day; *TID,* three times a day; *IV,* intravenous; *A-line,* arterial line; *prn,* as needed; *ASA,* acetylsalicylic acid (aspirin); *HIT,* heparin-induced thrombocytopenia; *D/C,* discontinue; *CBC,* complete blood count; *PTT/PT,* partial thromboplastin time/prothrombin time; *ECG,* electrocardiogram; *DC,* discharge; *SW,* social worker; *NPO,* nothing by mouth; *TCDB,* turn, cough, deep breathe; *qd,* every day; *pt,* patient.

SUMMARY

Nurses play a significant role in the care of patients with lower-extremity arterial disease. High-quality patient care includes the early identification of potential problems and appropriate nursing action as well as provision for patient education. Nurses must also take an active role in educating patients about risk factor modification.

REFERENCES

1. Weitz JI, Byrne J, Clagett P et al: Diagnosis and treatment of chronic arterial insufficiency of the lower extremities: a critical review, *Circulation* 94(11):3026-3049, 1996.
2. American Heart Association: *2001 Heart and stroke: statistical update,* Dallas, 2001, The Association.
3. Donaldson MC, Whittemore AD: Lower limb arterial occlusive disease. In Corson JD, Williamson E, eds: *Surgery,* London, 2001, Mosby, Section 4, pp 11.1-11.11.
4. Hiatt WR: Drug therapy: medical treatment of peripheral arterial disease and claudication, *N Engl J Med* 334:1608-1621, 2001.
5. Criqui MH, Langer RD, Fronek A et al: Mortality over a period of 10 years in patients with peripheral arterial disease, *N Engl J Med* 326:381-386, 1992.
6. Sanchez LA, Veith FJ: Femoral-popliteal-tibial occlusive disease. In Moore WS, ed: *Vascular surgery: a comprehensive review,* ed 5, Philadelphia, 1998, WB Saunders, pp 497-520.
7. Yao JST, Hobbs JT, Irvine WT: Ankle systolic pressure measurements in arterial disease affecting the extremities, *Br J Surg* 56:677-683, 1969.
8. McKenna M, Wolfson S, Kuller L: The ratio of ankle and arm arterial pressure as an independent predictor of mortality, *Atherosclerosis* 87:119-128, 1991.
9. Dormandy JA, Heeck L, Vig S: The fate of patients with critical leg ischemia, *Semin Vasc Surg* 12:142-147, 1999.
10. Vogt MT, McKenna M, Anderson SJ et al: The relationship between ankle-arm index and mortality in older men and women, *J Am Geriatr Soc* 41:523-530, 1993.
11. Proia RR, Walsh DB, Nelson PR et al: Early results of infragenicular revascularization based solely on duplex arteriography, *J Vasc Surg* 33:1165-1170, 2001.
12. Quinones-Baldrich WJM: Acute arterial and graft occlusion. In Moore W, ed: *Vascular surgery: a comprehensive review,* ed 5, Philadelphia, 1998, WB Saunders, pp 667-689.
13. Dormandy JA, Rutherford RB: Management of peripheral arterial disease (PAD), TASC Working Group, TransAtlantic Inter-Society Concensus (TASC), *J Vasc Surg* 31(1 pt 2):S1-S296, 2000.
14. Graham IM, Daly LE, Refsum HM et al: Plasma homocysteine as a risk factor for vascular disease, The European Concerted Action Project, *JAMA* 277(22):1775-1781, 1997.
15. Whittemore AD, Belkin M: Infrainguinal bypass. In Rutherford RB, ed: *Vascular surgery*, ed 5, Philadelphia, 2000, WB Saunders, pp 998-1018.
16. Hallet JW, Brewster DC, Rasmussen TE: *Handbook of patient care in vascular diseases,* Philadelphia, 2001, Lippincott, Williams & Wilkins.
17. Taylor LM, Moneta GL, Porter JM: Natural history and nonoperative treatment of chronic lower extremity ischemia. In Rutherford RB, ed: *Vascular surgery*, ed 5, Philadelphia, 2000, WB Saunders, pp 928-943.
18. Rasmussen D, Barnason S, Smith J et al: Patient outcomes after peripheral revascularization surgery, *J Vasc Nurs* 14(4):108-114, 2001.
19. A randomized, blinded trial of clopidogrel versus aspirin in patients at risk of ischaemic events (CAPRIE), CAPRIE Steering Committee, *Lancet* 348(9038):1329-1339, 1996.
20. Jackson MR, Clagett GP: Antithrombotic therapy in peripheral arterial occlusive disease, *Chest* 119(suppl 1):283S-299S, 2001.
21. Dawson DL, Cutler BS, Meissner MH et al: Cilostazol has beneficial effects in treatment of intermittent claudication, *Circulation* 98:678-686, 1998.
22. Weaver FA, Comerota AJ, Youngblood M et al: Surgical revascularization versus thrombolysis for nonembolic lower extremity native artery occlusions: results of a prospective randomized trial, The STILE Investigators, Surgery versus Thrombolysis for Ischemia of the Lower Extremity, *J Vasc Surg* 24:513-523, 1996.
23. Dalsing MC, Harris VJ: Intravascular stents. In White RA, Fogarty TJ, eds: *Peripheral endovascular interventions,* St Louis, 1996, Mosby, pp 315-339.
24. Zarge JI, Duke DN, White JV: Balloon angioplasty. In White RA, Fogarty TJ, eds: *Peripheral endovascular interventions,* St Louis, 1996, Mosby, pp 258-275.
25. Brewster DC: Staged inflow angioplasty and femoral bypass. In Yao JST, Pearce WH, eds: *Techniques in vascular and endovascular surgery,* Stamford, Conn, 1998, Appleton & Lange, pp 361-366.
26. Ramaswami G, Marin ML: Stent grafts in occlusive arterial disease, *Surg Clin North Am* 79:597-609, 1999.
27. McCarthy WJ, McGee GS, Lin WW et al: Axillary popliteal artery bypass provides successful limb salvage after removal of infected aortofemoral grafts, *Arch Surg* 127:974-978, 1992.
28. Rutherford RB,: Extra-anatomic bypass. In Rutherford RB, ed: *Vascular surgery,* ed 5, Philadelphia, 2000, WB Saunders, pp 981-997.
29. Deaton DH, Quinones-Baldrich WJ: Infrainguinal revascularization to the popliteal and proximal tibial arteries. In Callow AD, Ernst CB, eds: *Vascular surgery: theory and practice,* Stamford, Conn, 1995, Appleton & Lange, pp 689-705.

30. Leather RP, Veith FJ: In situ vein bypass. In Haimovici H, Ascer E, Hollier LH et al, eds: *Vascular surgery,* ed 4, London, 1996, Blackwell Science, pp 632-641.
31. Rosenthal D: Endovascular in situ bypass. In Whittemore AD, Bandyk DF, Cronenwett JL, eds: *Advances in vascular surgery,* St Louis, 1999, Mosby, pp 137-146.
32. Towne JB: In situ saphenous vein grafting for lower extremity occlusive disease. In Ernst CB, Stanley JC, eds: *Current therapy in vascular surgery,* ed 4, St Louis, 2001, Mosby, pp 463-465.
33. Rosenthal D, Piano G, Martin JD et al: Angioscopic-assisted in situ vein graft. In Yao JST, Pearce WH, eds: *Techniques in vascular and endovascular surgery,* Stamford, Conn, 1998, Appleton & Lange, pp 259-264.
34. Iafrati MMD: Less invasive saphenous harvest, *Surg Clin North Am* 79:623-644, 1999.
35. Rosenthal D, Martin JD, Kirby LB et al: Minimally invasive in situ bypass, *Surg Clin North Am* 645-652, 1999.
36. Belkin M, Magruder DC, Whittemore AD: Nonreversed saphenous bypass graft for infrainguinal arterial reconstruction. In Yao JST, Pearce WH, eds: *Techniques in vascular and endovascular surgery,* Stamford, Conn, 1998, Appleton & Lange, pp 233-242.
37. Faires PL, LoGerfo FW, Arora S et al: A comparative study of alternative conduits for lower extremity revascularization: all-autogenous conduit versus prosthetic grafts, *J Vasc Surg* 32:1080-1090, 2000.
38. Suggs WD, Kashyap VS, Moore WS: Expanded polytetrafluoroethylene and Dacron grafts for atherosclerotic lower extremity occlusive disease. In Ernst CB, Stanley JC, eds: *Current therapy in vascular surgery*, ed 4, St Louis, 2001, Mosby, pp 471-473.
39. Neville RF, Tempesta NP, Sidway AN: Tibial bypass for limb salvage using polytetrafluoroethylene and a distal vein patch, *J Vasc Surg* 33:266-272, 2001.
40. Cronenwett JL: What's new in vascular surgery, *J Am Coll Surg* 192(2):255-275, 2001.
41. Parkinson K, Wijesinghe LD, Scott DJ: Polytetrafluoroethylene femorodistal grafts: can the use of a vein collar offer patients a reasonable chance of success? *J Vasc Nurs* 16:6-10, 1998.
42. Haddad F, Johnson W: Human umbilical vein grafts for atherosclerotic lower extremity occlusive disease. In Ernst CB, Stanley JC, eds: *Current therapy in vascular surgery,* St Louis, 2001, Mosby, pp 473-476.
43. Harris L, O'Brien-Irr M, Ricotta JJ: Long-term assessment of cryopreserved vein bypass grafting success, *J Vasc Surg* 33:528-532, 2001.
44. Buckley CJ, Abernathy S, Lee SD et al: Suggested treatment protocol for improving patency of femoral-infrapopliteal cryopreserved saphenous vein allografts, *J Vasc Surg* 32:731-738, 2000.
45. Sullivan MW, McCarthy WJ: Composite sequential bypass for lower extremity occlusive disease. In Ernst CB, Stanley JC, eds: *Current therapy in vascular surgery*, ed 4, St Louis, 2001, Mosby, pp 465-467.
46. Veith FJ, Gupta SK, Ascer E et al: Six-year prospective multicenter randomized comparison of autologous saphenous vein and expanded polytetrafluoroethylene grafts in infrainguinal arterial reconstructions, *J Vasc Surg* 3(1):104-114, 1986.
47. Veterans Administration Cooperative Study Group 141: Comparative evolution of the prosthetic, reversed, and in situ vein grafts in distal popliteal and tibial peroneal revascularization, *Arch Surg* 123:434-438, 1988.
48. Quinones-Baldrich WJ, Prego AA, Ucelay-Gomez R et al: Long-term results of infrainguinal revascularization with polytetrafluoroethylene: a ten year experience, *J Vasc Surg* 16:209-217, 1992.
49. Abbott WM, Green RM, Matsumoto T et al: Prosthetic above-knee femoropopliteal bypass grafting: results of a multicenter randomized prospective trial, *J Vasc Surg* 25:19-28, 1997.
50. Leather RP, Veith FJ: In situ vein bypass. In Haimovici H, ed: *Vascular surgery*, ed 4, London, 1996, Blackwell Science, pp 632-641.
51. Watelet J, Soury P, Menard J et al: Femoropopliteal bypass: in situ or reversed vein grafts? Ten-year results of a randomized prospective study, *Ann Vasc Surg* 11:510-519, 1997.
52. Calligaro KD, Syrek JR, Dougherty MJ et al: Use of arm and lesser saphenous vein compared with prosthetic grafts for infrapopliteal arterial bypass: are they worth the effort? *J Vasc Surg* 26:919-927, 1997.
53. McCarthy WJ, Matsumura JS, Fine N et al: Combined arterial reconstruction and free tissue transfer for limb salvage, *J Vasc Surg* 29:814-820, 1999.
54. Illif KA, Moran S, Serlette J et al. Combined free tissue transfer and infrainguinal bypass graft: an alternative to major amputation in selected patients, *J Vasc Surg* 33:17-23, 2001.
55. Sarac TP, Huber TS, Back MR et al: Warfarin improves the outcome of infrainguinal vein bypass grafting in high risk for failure, *J Vasc Surg* 28:446-457, 1998.
56. Liem TK, Silver D: Options for anticoagulation. In Whittemore AD, Bandyk DF, Cronenwett JL et al, eds: *Advances in vascular surgery*, St Louis, 1997, Mosby, pp 201-221.
57. Kretschner GJ, Holzenbein: The role of anticoagulation in infrainguinal bypass surgery. In Yao JST, Pearce WH, eds: *The ischemic extremity: advances in treatment,* Norwalk, Conn, 1995, Appleton & Lange, pp 447-454.
58. Halperin JL: *Antithrombotic therapy for peripheral arterial disease,* http://www.svmb.org/medpro/cme/p2/ptll_hal.pdf.

59. Efficacy of oral anticoagulants compared with aspirin after infrainguinal bypass surgery (The Dutch Bypass Oral Anticoagulants or Aspirin Study): a randomised trial, *Lancet* 355(9201):346-351, 2000.
60. McMillan WD, McCarthy WJ, Lin SJ et al: Perioperative low molecular weight heparin for infragenicu-late bypass, *J Vasc Surg* 25:796-802, 1997.
61. Greenberg RK, Ouriel K: Arterial thromboembolism. In Rutherford RB, ed: *Vascular surgery*, ed 5, Philadelphia, 2000, WB Saunders, pp 822-835.
62. Tunick PA, Perez JL, Kronzon I: Protruding atheromas in the thoracic aorta and systematic embolization, *Ann Intern Med* 115(6):423-427, 1991.
63. Deitcher SR, Carman TL, Sheikh MA et al: Hypercoagulable syndromes: evaluation and management strategies for acute limb ischemia, *Semin Vasc Surg* 14:74-85, 2001.
64. Ouriel K: Acute limb ischemia. In Rutherford RB, ed: *Vascular surgery*, ed 5, Philadelphia, 2000, WB Saunders, pp 813-821.
65. Killewich LA: Intrinsic and arterial thrombosis, *Vasc Surg* 34:193-199, 2000.
66. Earnshaw JJ: Demography and etiology of acute leg ischemia, *Semin Vasc Surg* 14:86-92, 2001.
67. DeWeese JA, Shortell C, Green R et al: Operative repair of popliteal aneurysms. In Yao JST, Pearce WH, eds: *Long term results in vascular surgery,* Norwalk, Conn., 1993, Appleton & Lange, pp 287-293.
68. Buth J: Lower extremity arterial aneurysms. In Corson, JD, Williamson E, eds: *Surgery,* London, 2001, Mosby, Section 4, pp 12.1-12.6.
69. Haimovici H: Metabolic complications of acute arterial occlusions and skeletal muscle ischemia: myonephropathic-metabolic syndrome. In Haimovici H, Ascer E, Hollier LH et al, eds: *Vascular surgery*, ed 4, London, 1996, Blackwell Science, pp 509-530.
70. Kaufman JL: Atheroembolism and microthromboembolic syndromes (blue toe syndrome and disseminated atheroembolism). In Rutherford RB, ed: *Vascular surgery* ed 5, Philadelphia, 2000, WB Saunders, pp 836-845.
71. Eslami MH, Ricotta JJ: Operation for acute peripheral arterial occlusion: is it still the gold standard? *Semin Vasc Surg* 14:93-99, 2001.
72. Korn P, Khilnana NM, Fellers JC et al: Thrombolysis for native arterial occlusions of the lower extremi-ties: clinical outcome and cost, *J Vasc Surg* 33:1148-1157, 2001.
73. Ouriel K: Current status of thrombolytic therapy in occlusion of native arteries and bypass grafts. In Yao JST, Pearce WH, eds: *Progress in vascular surgery,* Stamford, Conn, 1997, Appleton & Lange, pp 277-285.
74. Ouriel K, Veith FJ, Sasahara AA: Thrombolysis or peripheral arterial surgery: phase I results, TOPAS Investigators, *J Vasc Surg* 23(1):64-75, 1996.
75. Ouriel K, Veith FJ, Sasahara AA: A comparison of recombinant urokinase with vascular surgery as initial treatment for acute arterial occlusion of the legs, *N Engl J Med* 338:1105-1111, 1998.
76. Nackman GB, Walsh DB, Fillinger MF et al: Thrombolysis of occluded infrainguinal vein grafts: predic-tors of outcome, *J Vasc Surg* 25:1023-1032, 1997.
77. DeBakey ME, Simeone FA: Battle injuries of the arteries in World War II, *Ann Surg* 123:534-579, 1946.
78. Lyden SP, Shortell CK, Illig KA: Reperfusion and compartment syndromes: strategies for prevention and treatment, *Semin Vasc Surg* 4(2):107-113, 2001.
79. Gibson KD, Caps MT, Gillen D et al: Identification of factors predictive of lower extremity vein graft thrombosis, *J Vasc Surg* 33:24-31, 2001.
80. Visser K, Idu MM, Buth J et al: Duplex scan surveillance during the first year after infrainguinal autolo-gous vein bypass grafting surgery: costs and clinical outcomes compared with other surveillance pro-grams, *J Vasc Surg* 33:123-130, 2001.
81. Tukianinen E, Biancari F, Lepantalo M: Deep infection of infrapopliteal autogenous vein grafts: immedi-ate use of in leg salvage, *J Vasc Surg* 6:680-688, 1995.
82. Treiman GS, Copland S, Yellin AE et al: Wound infections involving infrainguinal autogenous vein grafts: a current evaluation of factors determining successful graft preservation, *J Vasc Surg* 33:948-954, 2001.
83. Calligaro KD, Veith FJ, Schwartz ML et al: Management of infected lower extremity autologous vein grafts by selective graft preservation, *Am J Surg* 164:291-298, 1992.
84. Casey J, Flinn WR, Yao JST et al: Correlations of immune and nutritional status with wound complica-tions in patients undergoing vascular operations, *Surgery* 93:822-827, 1983.
85. Veith FJ, Haimovici H: Femoropopliteal arteriosclerotic occlusive disease. In Haimovici H, ed: *Vascular surgery*, ed 4, London, 1996, Blackwell Science, pp 605-631.
86. Klevsgard R, Risberg BO, Thomsen MB et al: A 1-year follow-up quality of life study after hemodynamically successful or unsuccessful surgical revascularization of lower limb ischemia, *J Vasc Surg* 33:114-122, 2001.
87. Fowl RJ, Kempczinski RF: Popliteal artery entrapment. In Rutherford RB, ed: *Vascular surgery,* ed 5, Philadelphia, 2000, WB Saunders, pp 1087-1093.
88. Vevien LJ, Bergan JJ: Adventitial cystic disease of the popliteal artery. In Rutherford RB, ed: *Vascular sur-gery,* ed 5, Philadelphia, 2000, WB Saunders, pp 1079-1087.

14

Extracranial Cerebrovascular Disease

MARK D. MORASCH □ WILLIAM H. PEARCE

Stroke is the leading cause of disability in the United States and the third leading cause of death, behind heart disease and cancer. It is estimated that each year 500,000 Americans will suffer a stroke. The mortality rate following a stroke ranges from 26 to 52 percent. According to the most recent American Heart Association statistics, it is estimated that stroke accounts for half of all hospital admissions for acute neurologic disease. In addition, 28 percent of annual stroke victims are under the age of 65.[1] Although stroke may be caused by a variety of diseases, atherosclerosis is the most common contributing factor. The focus of this chapter will be the anatomy, pathophysiology, diagnosis, treatment, and nursing management of patients with extracranial cerebrovascular disease.

ANATOMY OF THE EXTRACRANIAL VASCULAR SYSTEM

Blood is supplied to the brain through paired carotid and vertebral arteries. These arteries are present in nearly constant configuration across the population. The unique anatomy and collateral blood supply to the brain is such that loss of a single or several vessels is tolerated. However, stroke is unavoidable with embolization.

The supra-aortic vessels usually arise as three separate trunks from the aortic arch within the superior mediastinum. Anatomic variations are seen in about 15 percent of patients. The right common carotid artery takes its origin from the innominate artery (brachiocephalic trunk), which is the first major branch of the aortic arch. The left common carotid artery originates directly from the arch. The left subclavian is the third trunk vessel. The conventional definition of the supra-aortic trunk (SAT) vessels includes the innominate artery, the subclavian arteries up to the origins of the vertebral arteries, and the common carotid arteries up to their bifurcations. In general and in nondiseased states, the blood supply to the anterior two thirds of the brain is provided by the carotid circulation while the posterior third is supplied by the vertebral arteries (Fig. 14-1).

At the angle of the jaw and the superior border of the thyroid cartilage, the common carotid artery bifurcates into the internal and external carotid arteries. The external carotid artery lies anterior to the internal carotid artery (ICA) and branches immediately to supply the face and soft tissues of the head and neck. The first section of the internal carotid artery is dilated and is known as the carotid bulb or sinus. This region is heavily innervated and bears both baroreceptors for sensing and controlling blood pressure and chemoreceptors that detect CO_2 levels in the blood. The ophthalmic artery is the first branch of the internal carotid artery, and atheroemboli to this branch can result in amaurosis fugax (transient monocular blindness). The internal carotid arteries end at the base of the brain and give rise to the vessels of the circle of Willis.

The vertebral arteries supply the posterior third of the brain and originate from the posterior aspect of the subclavian arteries bilaterally to provide blood to the brain stem, cerebellum,

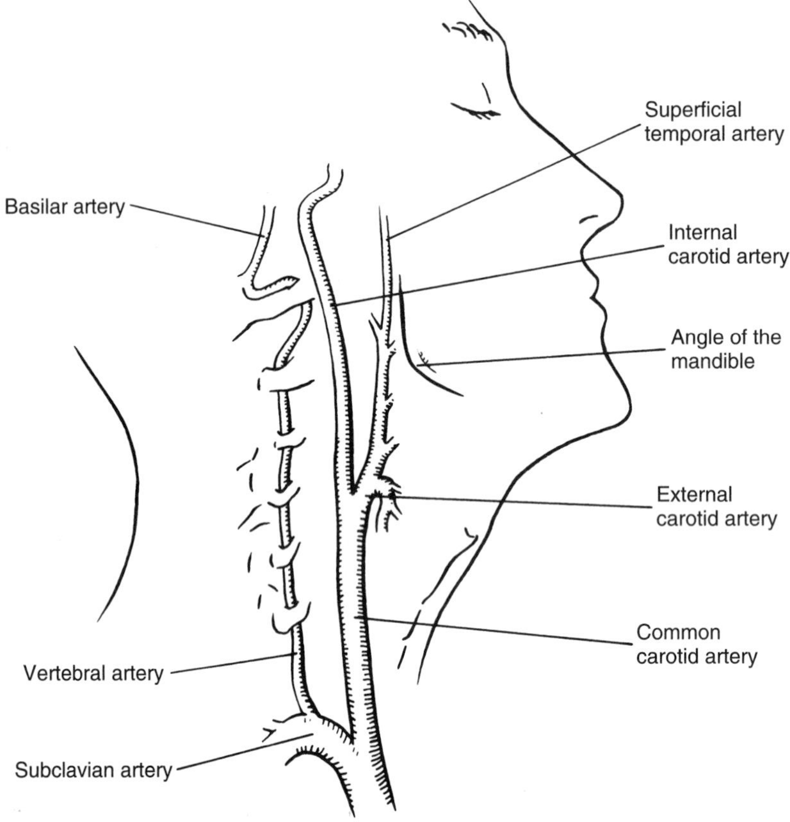

FIG. 14–1. Arterial anatomy of the neck. (Reprinted from *Critical Care Nursing Quarterly,* Vol 8, No 2, p 12, with permission of Aspen Publishers, Inc, © 1985.)

and occipital lobes. The vertebrals are surgically accessible for a short distance in the neck before entering the bony canal at the C6 vertebra and again at the base of the skull (C2). The vertebral arteries enter the skull and fuse in the midline to form the basilar artery. Before fusing, the vertebrals give off branches that supply the spinal cord (anterior spinal artery) and the cerebellum (posterior inferior cerebellar arteries). The basilar artery supplies branches to the remainder of the cerebellum, the brain stem, and the occipital lobes. This posterior circulation communicates with the carotid circulation via the posterior communicating arteries and through the circle of Willis.

The four extracranial vessels—two vertebral (via the basilar) and two carotid arteries—join at the base of the brain and form the anastomotic network known as the circle of Willis. The anterior, middle, and posterior cerebral arteries arise from this network (Fig. 14-2). The circle provides compensatory collateral flow anteriorly or posteriorly as necessary. There is also the potential for "crossover flow" from one hemisphere to the other through the anterior communicating arteries. Unfortunately, the circle of Willis may be incomplete, either congenitally or because of atherosclerotic occlusion, in as much as 50 percent of the population.[2]

PATHOPHYSIOLOGY OF THE EXTRACRANIAL VASCULAR SYSTEM

The most common cause of cerebrovascular disease in the United States is atherosclerosis, which accounts for 90 percent of all cases.[2,3] The causes of the remaining 10 percent of cases of extracranial cerebrovascular disease include fibromuscular dysplasia, radiation or Takayasu's arteritis, carotid dissection, and traumatic injury. In any case, symptoms occur whenever arterial flow to an area is insufficient to support neuronal function.[2]

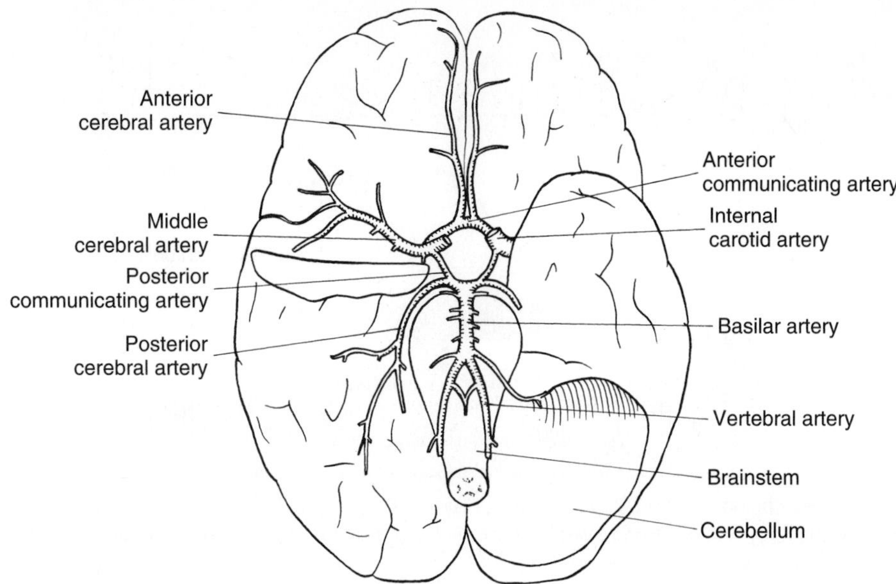

FIG. 14–2. Cerebral blood supply. (Reprinted from *Critical Care Nursing Quarterly,* Vol 8, No 2, p 13, with permission of Aspen Publishers, Inc, © 1985.)

Atherosclerosis

The pathologic characteristics of atherosclerosis are described in Chapter 1 of this text. As in other areas of the body, most extracranial lesions occur at branch points and areas in which the artery is either fixed by the surrounding structures or curved. In arteriographic studies of patients with cerebrovascular insufficiency, Hass et al[4] found that 75 percent of patients with symptoms had extracranial, surgically correctable lesions. Nearly 34 percent of all the extracranial lesions were at the common carotid bifurcation. Occlusive disease of the branches of the aortic arch is fairly common. The Joint Study of Arterial Occlusions reported that a third of patients undergoing arteriography have significant lesions involving one or more of the proximal vessels supplying blood to the head and arms.[1] Lesions of the vertebral arteries were most common at the origin and proximal one third of the arteries. The same study population demonstrated a 40 percent rate of intracranial lesions. These were most common at the carotid siphon, the basilar artery, and the terminal portion of the vertebral artery. This is significant because it can be difficult to determine whether symptoms are due to the intracranial or extracranial lesions when both are present.

The major mechanisms by which atherosclerosis causes ischemic symptoms are embolization and thrombosis.[5] Ulcerated lesions occur when the lining of the artery (endothelium and fibrous cap) ruptures, exposing cholesterol deposits, which may become emboli to the brain (Fig. 14-3). At Northwestern Memorial Hospital in Chicago, the carotid plaques from 44 patients undergoing carotid endarterectomy were studied. Plaque rupture occurred in 74 percent of symptomatic patients as compared with 32 percent of asymptomatic patients. With plaque rupture and high-grade stenosis with greater than 90 percent occlusion of the internal carotid artery, thrombosis may occur because of sluggish flow across the lesion (Fig. 14-4). In patients with an incomplete circle of Willis, thrombosis of a carotid artery will produce a significant stroke.

The most common disease affecting the SAT is atherosclerosis. Nonatherosclerotic diseases such as Takayasu's or radiation-induced arteritis, dissections, aneurysms, and congenital lesions account for less than 20 percent of the cases that require intervention. The most common disease affecting the vertebral artery is also atherosclerosis. Less common pathologic processes include trauma, fibromuscular dysplasia, Takayasu's disease, osteophyte compression, dissections, aneurysms, and other arteritides.

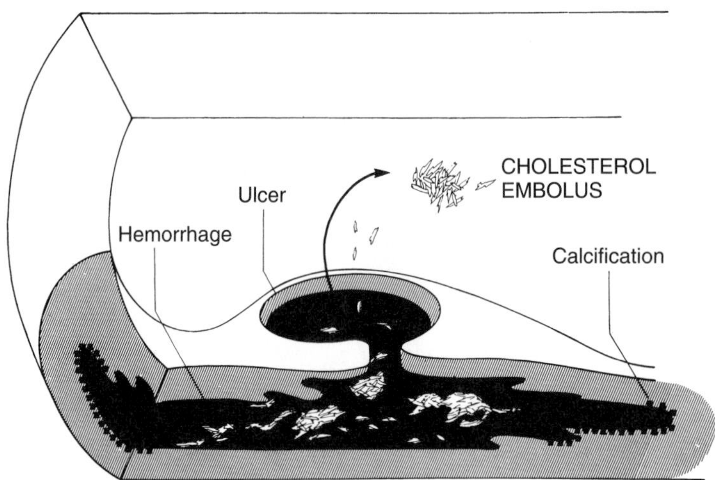

FIG. 14–3. Cholesterol embolization. (From Lugsby RJ, Farrell LD, Wylie EJ: The significance of intraplaque hemorrhage in the pathogenesis of carotid atherosclerosis. In Bergan JJ, Yao JST, eds: *Cerebrovascular insufficiency,* New York, 1983, Grune & Stratton, p 450.)

Fibromuscular Dysplasia

Fibromuscular dysplasia (FMD) occurs primarily in white females and involves larger arteries (renal, iliac, internal carotid arteries). The disease is usually bilateral and is characterized by fibromedial or intimal hyperplasia, which leads to focal stenosis and dilation of the artery. Of the extracranial vessels, the internal carotid artery is most often affected, although the vertebral arteries may demonstrate the disease as well.

Most patients have no symptoms; however, cerebral embolization may occur. Since fibromuscular dysplasia is well above the carotid bifurcation, arteriography is needed to make the diagnosis. In these cases, first-line therapy involves the use of antiplatelet agents. In general, percutaneous transluminal angioplasty (PTA) and stenting of the carotid artery or surgery is needed to correct the problem.[6] Anticoagulation is required for those few persons who continue to have ischemic symptoms.

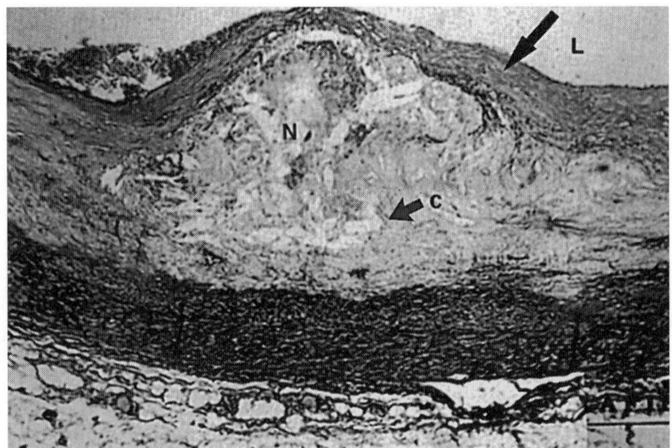

FIG. 14–4. Histologic section of diagram in Fig. 14-3. Mature atherosclerotic plaque with an intact fibrous cap (*arrow* near *L*) covering the necrotic core *(N)*. The shoulder of the fibrous cap contains many inflammatory cells and is thought to represent a weak point in the plaque. *L,* Lumen; *C,* cholesterol in plaque, which can become an embolus. (From Carr SC, Cheanvechai V, Virmani R et al: Histology and clinical significance of the carotid atherosclerotic plaque: implications for endovascular treatment, *J Endovasc Surg* 4:322, 1997.)

Cervical Irradiation

External beam radiation for head and neck malignancy can damage the entire vessel wall and may accelerate atherosclerosis. Endarterectomy in these vessels is possible, although the lesions are longer. Wound problems may occur as a result of prior scarring and fibrosis of neck tissue. An increased probability of postoperative airway compromise in this population has been reported.[7]

Carotid Artery Dissection

Blunt trauma, sudden extension of the neck, or even paroxysms of coughing or vomiting may cause intimal tearing with subsequent carotid artery or vertebral artery dissection. This entity is more common in persons under the age of 50 years, those with hypertension, and those with fibromuscular dysplasia.[8] Arteriographically, the result is a tapered stenosis in the shape of a bird's beak.

Most commonly, these patients present with ipsilateral headaches, ocular or cerebral ischemic events, and Horner's syndrome. Less frequent symptoms include a variety of cranial nerve disturbances such as slurred speech, facial nerve palsy, and dysphagia.[6] Commonly, the arterial dissection passes into the bony canal, making surgery impossible. Observation and anticoagulation constitute the treatment of choice. In the majority of the patients, the dissection will heal without consequence.[9]

Arteritis

Takayasu's arteritis is a vasculitis of the giant-cell type, often involving the aortic arch and its supra-aortic branches. Young women, especially those of Asian descent, are most commonly affected. Symptoms of carotid artery involvement can include transient ischemic attacks (TIAs), stroke, and cranial neuropathies. Corticosteroids are usually given for acute disease. Some patients with aggressive disease have been reported to benefit from the addition of the cytotoxic agent cyclophosphamide (Cytoxan).[10] However, there are no controlled studies to confirm this combined approach. For upper-extremity or cerebral ischemia that has not responded to medical therapy, arterial bypass may be required. Surgery is not usually performed during the active phase of the disease.

CLINICAL MANIFESTATIONS

The symptoms related to carotid artery disease may be divided into several broad categories. The first group is patients without symptoms. Atherosclerotic occlusion of the carotid artery may build up slowly without symptoms. The remaining three blood vessels increase blood flow to accommodate the decrease in blood flow in the diseased artery. When followed over long periods of time, patients with asymptomatic stenosis may develop symptoms (3-5 percent per year). The natural history of these lesions is often erratic, and a minor stenosis may rapidly progress to plaque hemorrhage and rupture.

However, the majority of patients present with symptoms, which can be divided into focal, global, and vertebrobasilar. Focal symptoms are any that produce discrete, unilateral findings. Embolic debris from the proximal carotid artery may lodge in the retinal artery, producing visual field deficits and visual loss. Ocular examination may detect a Hollenhorst plaque, which results from cholesterol emboli to the retinal vessels. Emboli to the retinal artery may also result in total occlusion, producing monocular blindness. If the embolic debris passes into the brain and lodges within one of the terminal branches of the middle cerebral artery, the patient may experience hemiparesis, hemiplegia, or aphasia.

If the neurologic deficit lasts less than 24 hours, it is termed a transient ischemic attack (TIA). If the event lasts greater then 24 hours, it is called a stroke. Clinical manifestations of stroke may resolve quickly or leave the patient with long-lasting residual neurologic deficits. Ischemic damage can be detected by magnetic resonance imaging (MRI) or by computed tomography (CT) in patients suffering a stroke. Patients with diffuse extracranial vascular disease may also present with focal symptoms when the responsible ("watershed") area of the brain becomes more ischemic than others. Watershed infarcts are usually in the terminal branches of the cortex and are best detected by MRI scans. Finally, there are a few patients who have multiple-vessel occlusions leading to ocular ischemia of the eye, producing the "red-eye syndrome." The red-eye syndrome is extremely rare but should not be missed because of the potential for eventual blindness.

Patients may also present with global symptoms reflecting decreased perfusion to all areas of the brain. These patients most often have multiple-vessel occlusions and present with dizziness, syncope, and occasional ocular manifestations. These patients may be difficult to separate from patients with vertebrobasilar ischemia (VBI). Patients with vertebrobasilar symptoms have decreased perfusion to the brain stem and as a result may complain of dizziness, syncope, ocular symptoms, and neurologic deficits of the arms and legs. The patients with global and vertebrobasilar symptoms are most difficult to separate from those with nonspecific neurologic diseases. Such patients often require neurologic evaluation in addition to assessment of the cerebral circulation.

The manifestations of vertebrobasilar ischemia are varied and vague, often making the diagnosis difficult. A number of medical conditions may mimic vertebrobasilar ischemia, thus confounding the selection of patients in need of posterior circulation treatment. These include inappropriate use of antihypertensive medications, cardiac arrhythmias, anemia, brain tumors, and benign vertiginous states. The classic symptoms of vertebrobasilar ischemia are dizziness, vertigo, diplopia, perioral numbness, alternating paresthesias, tinnitus, dysphasia, dysarthria, drop attacks, and ataxia. Ischemia affecting the temporo-occipital areas of the cerebral hemispheres and segments of the brain stem and cerebellum characteristically produce bilateral symptoms.

PATIENT EVALUATION

History

Evaluation of the patient with known or suspected extracranial cerebrovascular disease includes a thorough history and physical examination along with noninvasive vascular testing. For the patient with symptoms, the goals of history taking are to characterize the neurologic event and identify any coexisting medical problems. The ischemic event should be described in detail, including symptoms and findings noted by others at the time of the incident. Family members may provide details that the patient is unable to recall. The assessment should include questions about speech difficulties, visual disturbances, motor weakness or paralysis, vertigo, syncope, and confusion and memory loss. Timing of the incident would include time of day, activity the patient was involved in at the time, the duration of symptoms, and the frequency of episodes.

Because atherosclerosis accounts for the majority of ischemic episodes, the patient should be evaluated for risk factors that may be modified. Risk factors include tobacco use, hypertension, diabetes mellitus, hyperlipidemia, and family history of disease. Other evidence of the systemic nature of the disease includes intermittent claudication, angina, congestive heart failure, myocardial infarction, prior cardiac or vascular surgery, or known aneurysms.

Any indication of cardiac disease should be carefully evaluated. Hertzer et al[11] found that more than half of all persons with peripheral arterial disease had clinically suspected coronary artery disease. This included 57 percent of those evaluated for cerebrovascular disease. Severe coronary artery disease was demonstrated by angiography in 35 percent of the cerebrovascular patients. Detection is essential for proper management of the cardiac disease as well as for determining whether the patient may be a candidate for surgery. Some patients may require either staged or combined repair of both the coronary and extracranial cerebrovascular disease.

Physical Examination

Extracranial artery disease can be assessed through careful evaluation of the head and neck. Bilateral pulse examination should include the superficial temporal artery, which can be palpated just anterior to the ear. The carotid artery should be palpated low in the neck to avoid dislodging plaque from the bifurcation. Massage of the carotid sinus may also lead to bradycardia or asystole. The neck should be evaluated for the presence of bruits, which are best heard with the bell of the stethoscope. The location of the bruit should be described as being at the angle of the jaw, in the midportion of the neck, or low in the neck. Particular attention should be paid to carotid bruits heard in both systole and diastole, as they indicate severe stenosis. However, severe stenosis may not be associated with a bruit. Bruits heard in the supraclavicular fossa may indicate subclavian stenosis, which can affect vertebral perfusion, and vertebral artery bruits may be heard posterior to the sternocleidomastoid muscle.[12] A variety of clues to vascular disease may be found during the fundoscopic examination. Signs of hypertension, diabetic retinopathy, Hollenhorst plaque (atheromatous debris), and retinal ischemia can be seen on the funduscopic exam.

In addition to the vascular exam, a complete neurologic examination should be performed. This includes an evaluation of sensory and motor function, visual acuity, speech, memory, level of consciousness, and comprehension. In some cases, deficits may help to identify the areas of the brain affected and indicate the location of the diseased arterial segment. The initial neurologic examination will also serve as a baseline to detect postoperative complications.

The remainder of the evaluation should focus on the degree of arterial insufficiency in other areas of the body. Bilateral upper-extremity blood pressures are measured to detect hypertension and occlusion of either the innominate or subclavian arteries. Cardiac evaluation should include auscultation for rhythm, murmurs, and the presence of abnormal heart sounds. Peripheral edema, shortness of breath, and jugular vein distention may also point to cardiac dysfunction. Finally, the extremities should be observed for the presence of ulcers, ischemic skin changes, and peripheral pulses.

Noninvasive Testing

Further evaluation of the patient is based on the findings from the history and physical examination. The primary tool for the evaluation of the neck arteries is duplex ultrasonography. The duplex scan is accurate in quantifying carotid artery stenosis and is described in detail in Chapter 5. Duplex can also be used as a screening tool for supra-aortic trunk vertebral artery disease. Because of the high accuracy of the duplex scanning of the carotid bifurcation, many surgeons are performing surgery based solely upon the duplex scan itself in order to avoid the risks of contrast angiography. Noninvasive testing is used for routine follow-up of the patient to detect recurrent stenosis after carotid endarterectomy.

CT scanning may be performed to identify those patients whose symptoms are due to tumors, hemangiomas, intracranial vascular disease, or subdural hematomas. The scan is also used to detect stroke and is used postoperatively for any neurologic complication. Preoperative CT results rarely influence the operative decisions, however, and rarely do preoperative results correlate with postoperative neurologic events.

Recent developments in magnetic resonance angiography (MRA) show great promise for safe, noninvasive, detailed evaluation of both the extracranial and intracranial vasculature. Newer MRI techniques, some commercially available but many still under investigation, now make possible fast, accurate, and safe assessment of not only the carotid bifurcation but also the aortic arch and great vessels, the vertebrobasilar system, the intracranial vasculature including the branches of the circle of Willis, and brain parenchyma in both the anterior and posterior fossae, all without moving the patient from the scanner. Additional MRI protocols have been developed that can measure atherosclerotic plaque burden and quantify blood flow through the carotid artery. Functional magnetic resonance imaging now practically permits the assessment of local intracranial vasoreactivity and autoregulation, which can help identify the limits to cerebrovascular reserve in disease states. New imaging sequences have been designed that can delineate components within atherosclerotic plaque, putting the "Holy Grail" of plaque characterization within our reach. This research will help to refine the indications for medical and surgical intervention for stroke prevention and help to make these interventions safer (Fig. 14-5).

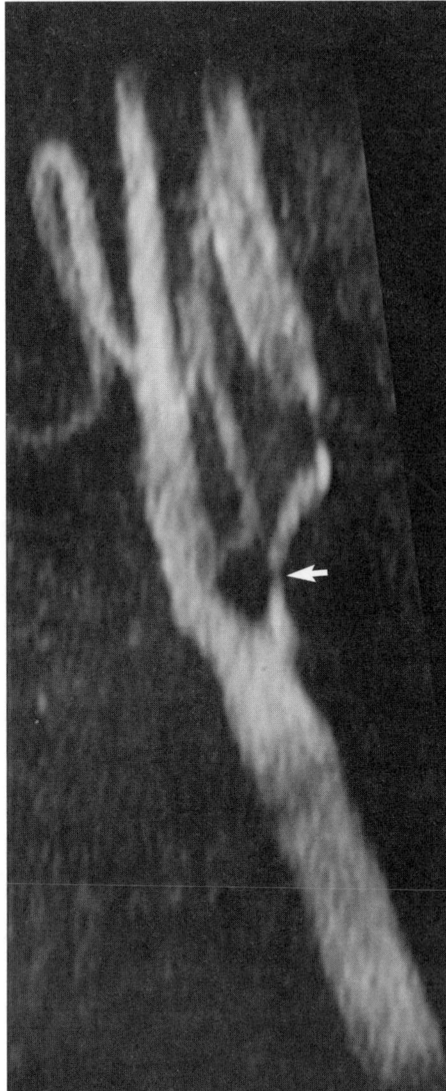

FIG. 14–5. Magnetic resonance angiography (MRA) demonstrating stenosis of the internal carotid artery (*arrow*) in the same patient as Fig. 14-6.

Invasive Diagnostic Studies

Invasive testing is usually reserved for patients in whom the cause of the neurologic event is questioned or when the results of duplex or MRA are inadequate or do not coincide, as clearly cerebral angiography is not a benign procedure, carrying up to a 1 percent risk of causing stroke.[2] Arteriography of the aortic arch, neck vessels, and cerebral circulation identifies the exact location and extent of disease (Fig. 14-6). Arteriography is particularly helpful in the identification of lesions in the vertebral circulation. Angiography is more fully described in Chapter 6.

Conventional arteriography has been enhanced by the addition of digital subtraction techniques. Digital subtraction angiography (DSA) is a computerized fluoroscopic method that subtracts the bone and soft-tissue structures from a stored summation of all of the contrast that has circulated in the arterial tree. The information is displayed on a screen and can be printed as other arteriograms are. Although DSA can be performed intravenously, the images are usually inferior to those obtained with an intraarterial injection. Also, the arterial route allows for the use of less contrast material.

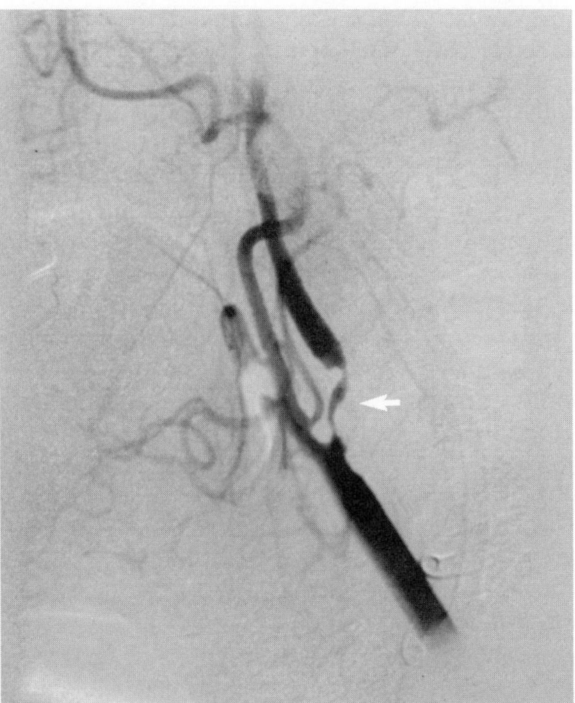

FIG. 14–6. Carotid angiogram demonstrating stenotic lesion of the internal carotid artery (*arrow*) in the same patient as Fig. 14-5.

MEDICAL AND SURGICAL MANAGEMENT

Carotid endarterectomy (CEA) is currently the most frequently performed noncardiac vascular surgical procedure in the United States.[13] The goal of this surgery is to prevent stroke. In the mid 1980s the efficacy of CEA in preventing stroke was questioned. As a result, a number of randomized prospective studies were performed comparing surgery with best medical management in both symptomatic and asymptomatic patients. The two most significant symptomatic trials are the North American Symptomatic Carotid Endarterectomy Trial (NASCET)[13] and the European Carotid Surgery Trial (ECST).[14] Both studies demonstrated a significant benefit of carotid endarterectomy for patients with symptoms in whom there was more than 70 percent stenosis of the internal carotid artery. Endarterectomy in patients with symptomatic moderate carotid stenosis of 50 to 69 percent also yielded moderate reduction in the risk of stroke.[15] For patients with less than 30 percent stenosis, however, surgery was not beneficial.

Asymptomatic carotid disease, as mentioned earlier, does not always remain asymptomatic. In a large Veterans Affairs Cooperative Study, carotid endarterectomy reduced the incidence of an ipsilateral neurologic event in men without symptoms and a greater than 50 percent stenosis. The incidence of ipsilateral neurologic event was 8 percent in the surgical group as compared with 20.6 percent in the medical group ($p < 0.001$).[16] In the Asymptomatic Carotid Atherosclerosis Study (ACAS), asymptomatic patients with a stenosis of 60 percent or greater had a reduced 5-year risk of ipsilateral stroke with carotid endarterectomy, provided they were good surgical candidates and aggressively managed modifiable risk factors.[17]

The natural history of disease must be weighed against the risks of mortality and morbidity associated with surgery. Carotid endarterectomy is now recommended for symptomatic patients with more than 50 percent stenosis if the operation can be done with little risk.[13,17-19] Also, asymptomatic patients with greater than 60 percent stenosis may benefit if the perioperative stroke risk can be kept very low (less than 2 percent).

Indications for revascularization of the supra-aortic trunk vessels are multiple. Symptomatic disease may manifest as ocular, hemispheric, or vertebrobasilar TIA or stroke as well as upper-extremity symptoms. More commonly, patients will present with a combination of both anterior and posterior circulation ischemic symptoms. Patients may also develop varying degrees of arm ischemia ranging from arm fatigue observed in patients with subclavian steal to limb-threatening ischemia secondary to extensive arterial occlusion or emboli. A third, less common problem is that of myocardial ischemia in patients who develop innominate or subclavian disease proximal to an internal mammary revascularization of the coronary arteries (coronary steal). Finally, asymptomatic severe (greater than 75 percent) lesions of the innominate or common carotid arteries should be repaired in patients who present a reasonable risk for the same reasons we repair asymptomatic severe carotid bifurcation stenoses. Asymptomatic lesions in the proximal subclavian artery should also be repaired in patients contemplating myocardial revascularization via an internal mammary artery. Repair should also be considered in patients with bilateral subclavian artery disease in order to permit blood pressure management. Lesions of the supra-aortic trunks can be repaired surgically through the sternum as an aortic-based bypass (Fig. 14-7), or isolated lesions can be reconstructed through an isolated cervical approach as a transposition (Fig. 14-8) or bypass.

Once the diagnosis of vertebrobasilar ischemia has been confirmed, vertebral artery reconstruction may be considered. The mere presence of vertebral artery stenosis in an asymptomatic patient is rarely an indication for surgery. Surgical reconstruction is based on the specific etiology. The indication for surgery in patients with hemodynamic symptoms depends on the ability to demonstrate insufficient blood flow to the basilar artery. In other words, a single normal caliber vertebral artery can supply sufficient blood flow into the basilar artery regardless of the status of the contralateral vessel. In this particular subset of patients, surgical intervention is indicated only in the presence of a severely stenotic (greater than 75 percent) vertebral artery and an equally diseased or occluded contralateral vessel. Surgical reconstruction is not indicated in an asymptomatic patient with the aforementioned

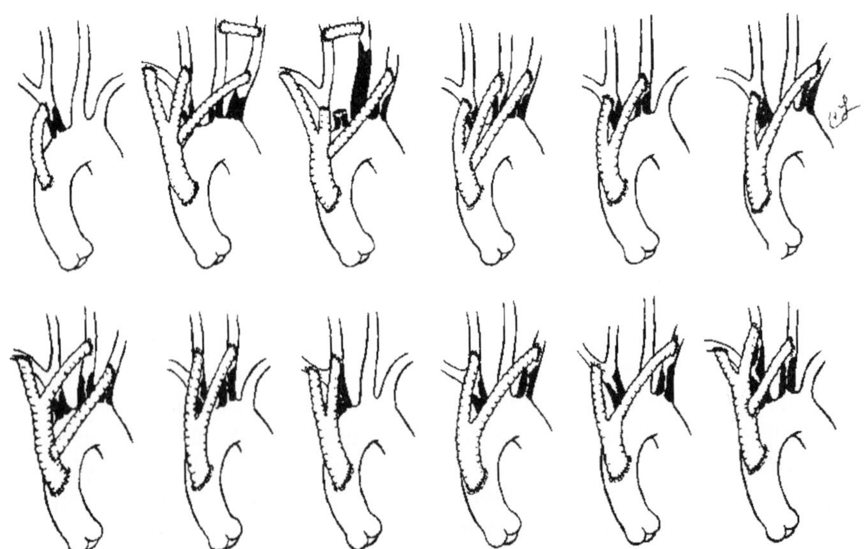

FIG. 14–7. Schematic drawings of the various types of vascular reconstruction used in 27 patients who underwent revascularization of the innominate artery and accompanying lesions by means of a transthoracic approach and bypass grafting at the Texas Heart Institute. In patients with innominate artery lesions alone, when the transthoracic bypass technique was used, a bypass was placed from the ascending aorta to the innominate, right carotid, or right subclavian artery depending on the degree of distal vessel involvement and exposure. (From Reul GJ, Jacobs MJ, Gregoric ID et al: Innominate artery occlusive disease: surgical approach and long-term results, *J Vasc Surg* 14:405, 1991. Reproduced with permission.)

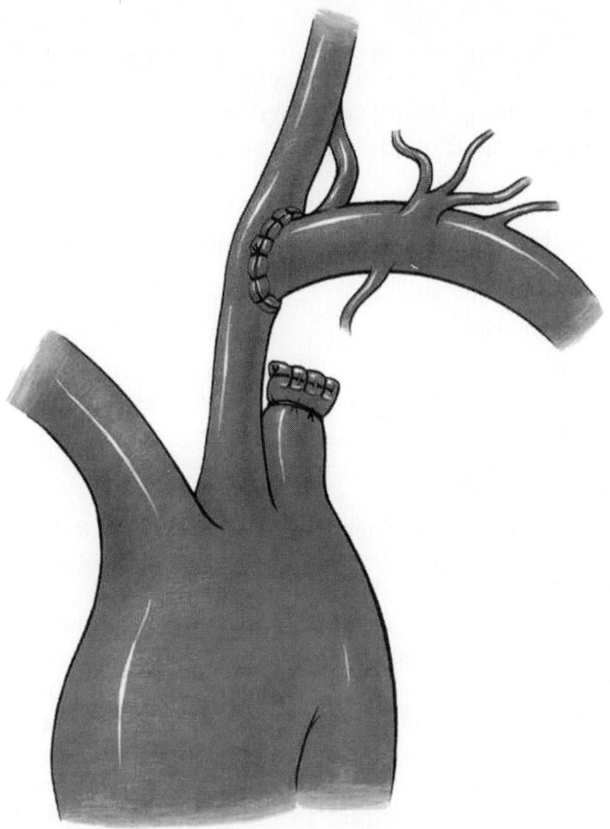

FIG. 14–8. Left subclavian-to-carotid transposition. (From Berguer R, Kieffer E: *Surgery of the arteries to the head,* New York, 1992, Springer-Verlag. Reproduced with permission.)

radiographic findings, as these patients are well compensated from the carotid circulation through the posterior communicating vessels.

In contrast, patients with symptomatic vertebrobasilar ischemia due to emboli are candidates for surgical correction of the offending lesion regardless of the condition of the contralateral vertebral artery. However, as in the hemodynamic group, surgical intervention is not indicated in asymptomatic patients with suspicious radiographic findings.

Previous experience has shown that, with appropriate diagnosis and surgical correction, complete resolution of hemodynamic and embolic symptoms can occur predictably. Vertebral artery reconstruction can be successfully performed with fewer ischemic complications than carotid artery surgery and with durable long-term results. The location of disease will dictate the type of surgical reconstruction that is required.

Medical Management

Aspirin, other antiplatelet agents, and anticoagulants have been studied for their effectiveness in preventing stroke in cases of carotid and vertebral atherosclerosis. Recent research indicates that daily doses of aspirin after TIA result in a 15-30 percent reduction in stroke rate.[17] Research doses have ranged from 40 to 1300 mg daily. Doses of 325 mg daily have been shown to be as effective as higher doses and to have fewer side effects.[18] The role of aspirin has yet to be clarified in the treatment of women, patients with ulcerative carotid artery lesions, and persons with asymptomatic disease.[17] It is important to remember that aspirin does not change the progression of the arterial plaque. Also, it is not likely to prevent thrombosis of highly stenotic lesions.[2]

Ticlopidine is another antiplatelet agent that has recently received attention. Patients who received ticlopidine after a stroke demonstrated a 30.2 percent lower risk of subsequent stroke, myocardial infarction, and vascular death than similar patients who received a placebo. This effect was the same for both men and women.[20] However, ticlopidine has significant side effects, including white blood cell abnormalities and thrombotic thrombocytopenic purpura (TTP). Other antiplatelet agents given with aspirin, such as sulfinpyrazone and dipyridamole, have shown little additional benefit over aspirin alone.[2, 18]

Anticoagulation with heparin or warfarin has been studied with varying results. Although some studies would advocate this treatment for certain patients, others indicate that anticoagulation may actually be harmful.

Surgical Management

Indications for CEA are given in Box 14-1. When surgery is being considered, the risk of stroke must be weighed against the risk of mortality and morbidity associated with the operation in the specific institution.

Perioperative Care

Each patient should have an intraarterial catheter to monitor blood pressure during extracranial cerebrovascular surgery so that cerebral perfusion can be maximized. Wide fluctuations in the patient's blood pressure are common, and excessive hypertension or hypotension may produce stroke. Carotid endarterectomy may be performed with local, regional, or general inhalation anesthesia. Trunk and vertebral reconstruction require a general anesthesia. The risk of stroke during surgery is related not to the type of anesthesia but rather to the surgeon's qualifications and experience. Because the benefit of surgery is based on a low perioperative stroke rate, the surgeon performing these procedures must be very experienced, with an operative stroke rate of less than 3 percent in asymptomatic patients and less than 6 percent in the symptomatic patient for all types of procedures.

A carotid endarterectomy incision is made either along the anterior border of the sternocleidomastoid muscle or transversely in a skin crease. All of the dissection is performed gently to avoid atheroembolization. Once the vessels are controlled, the patient is given heparin to prevent thrombosis. A longitudinal arteriotomy is performed. The plaque and arterial intima, along with portions of the media of the artery, are then removed. A patch of autogenous vein or prosthetic material may be used if primary closure of the carotid artery will cause narrowing of the artery or when the endarterectomy is being repeated

BOX 14–1

Indications for Carotid Endarterectomy (CEA)

SYMPTOMATIC

Proven

- Surgical morbidity and mortality <6%
- Transient ischemic attack (TIA) or mild stroke with ≥70% stenosis

Acceptable

- TIA or mild stroke with 50-69% stenosis
- Progressive stroke ≥70%
- CEA ipsilateral to TIA or stenosis ≥70% and associated coronary artery surgery

ASYMPTOMATIC

- Surgical morbidity and mortality <3%
- 60% or greater stenosis (primarily men)

Data from Moore WS, Barnett HJM, Beebe HG et al: Guidelines for carotid endarterectomy: a multidisciplinary consensus statement from the ad hoc committee, American Heart Association, *Circulation* 91:566-579, 1995.

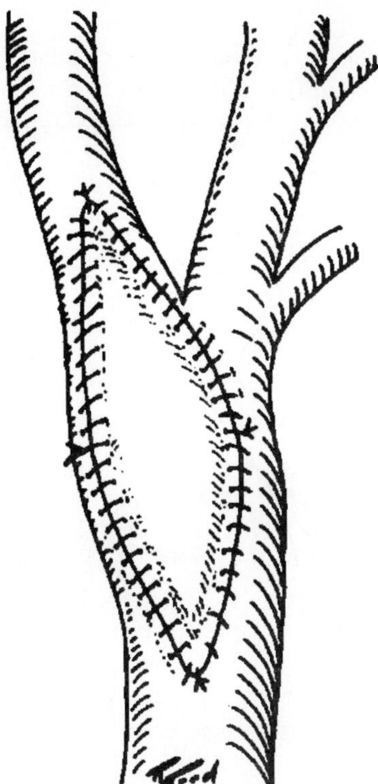

FIG. 14–9. Vein patch angioplasty. (From Painter TA, Hertzer NR, O'Hara PJ et al: Symptomatic internal carotid thrombosis after carotid endarterectomy, *J Vasc Surg* 5:445, 1987. Reproduced with permission.)

(Fig. 14-9). Alternatively, eversion endarterectomy can be performed by transecting the ICA from the bifurcation, removing the plaque, and reimplanting the vessel to shorten a redundant ICA. During CEA, cerebral perfusion is a primary concern. Theoretically, this should occur via collaterals and the circle of Willis. However, collateral flow is not always adequate and an intraluminal shunt is placed (Fig. 14-10). Some surgeons use shunting routinely, whereas others use it selectively, and some not at all. Methods of monitoring cerebral perfusion during clamping include transcranial Doppler, spectrophotometry, continuous electroencephalography (EEG) monitoring, and the use of the stump pressures (Fig. 14-11).

The choice of vertebral reconstruction is based upon the site of disease. The two main options for treating offending ostial vertebral lesions (V1 segment) are transposition of the proximal vertebral artery onto the common carotid artery or vertebral artery bypass, both of which are performed through an incision in the base of the neck above the clavicle (Fig. 14-12). The bypass can originate from either the common carotid artery or the adjacent subclavian artery. Choices of conduit include either saphenous vein grafts or prosthetic material (polytetrafluoroethylene [PTFE] or Dacron). Less commonly performed is a subclavian-vertebral artery endarterectomy.

The V2 segment, which ascends within the foramina of the cervical vertebrae, is the site of a wide variety of disorders. External compression is most likely to occur in this segment due to osteophytes, the edge of the transverse foramina, or the intervertebral joints. Positional changes, rotation or extension of the neck, usually trigger compression of the vertebral artery in this segment. The V2 segment is also the site of aneurysmal degeneration, fibromuscular diseases, and embolizing atherosclerotic plaques. Elective surgical reconstruction is very rarely undertaken within this segment; however, ligation (at the C1-C2 level) and bypass to the distal (V3 segment) vertebral artery may be indicated. Extrinsic lesions can be corrected to relieve kinking or compression of the artery. The most common indication for

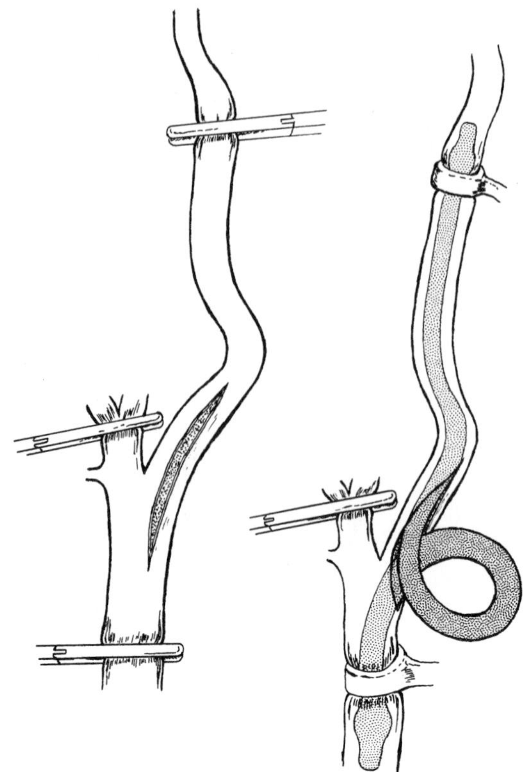

FIG. 14–10. Intraluminal shunt placement during carotid endarterectomy. (Reprinted from *Critical Care Nursing Quarterly,* Vol 8, No 2, p 18, with permission of Aspen Publishers, Inc, © 1985.)

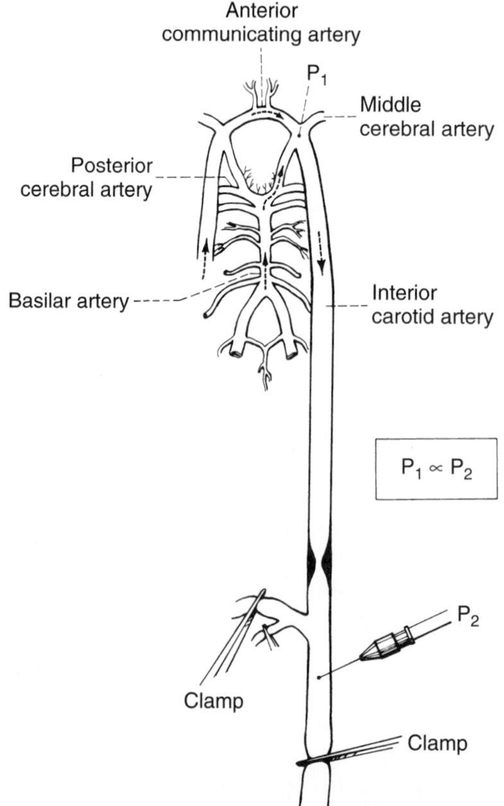

FIG. 14–11. Stump pressure measurement. (From Moore WS, Hall CD: Carotid artery back pressure, *Arch Surg* 99:705, 1969. © 1969, American Medical Association.)

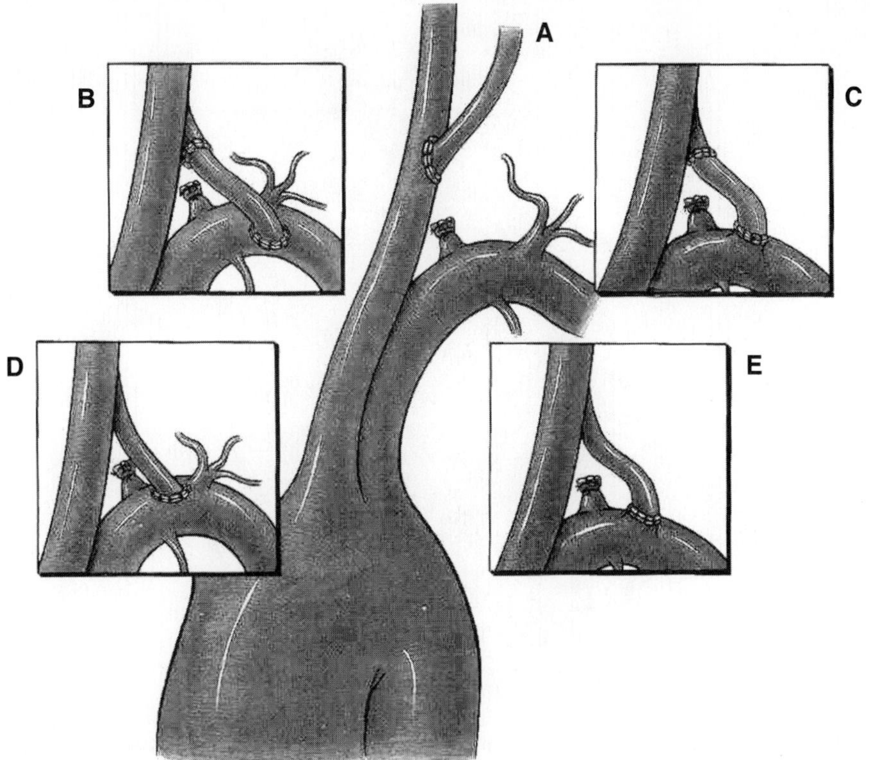

FIG. 14–12. Modalities for reconstructing the proximal vertebral artery. Transposition to the common carotid artery is the usual technique ***(A)***. A subclavian vertebral bypass may take origin in the subclavian artery ***(B)*** or in the divided thyrocervical trunk ***(C)***. A redundant vertebral artery may be transposed to a new subclavian site ***(D)*** or to the divided thyrocervical trunk ***(E)***. (From Berguer R, Kieffer E: *Surgery of the arteries to the head,* New York, 1992, Springer-Verlag. Reproduced with permission.)

exposure of this segment of the artery is for control of hemorrhage, which is best relieved with proximal and distal ligation of the artery. This has not been associated with worsening neurologic sequelae.

Reconstruction of the distal (V3 segment) vertebral artery is usually performed through an incision similar to that for CEA. The techniques most often used to reconstruct the distal vertebral artery at the C1-C2 level include (a) saphenous vein bypass from the common carotid, subclavian, or proximal vertebral artery (Fig. 14-13), (b) transposition of the external carotid or hypertrophied occipital artery to the distal vertebral artery, and (c) transposition of the distal vertebral artery to the side of the distal internal carotid artery. More distal pathology can be accessed surgically above the level of the transverse process of C1. At this level, the vertebral artery is vulnerable to direct trauma and stretch injuries that can lead to intimal damage, thrombosis, embolization, and dissection. This segment is also prone to arteriovenous fistula formation and aneurysmal degeneration. Surgical exposure at the suboccipital segment requires resection of the C1 transverse process and part of its posterior arch. Reconstruction at this level is limited to saphenous vein bypass from the distal internal carotid artery.

Results following both proximal and distal vertebral artery reconstructions are generally equal to or better than those reported for other forms of cerebrovascular revascularizations. In experienced hands, the combined stroke and death rates are 4 percent or less. Long-term patency of the reconstructions is excellent. Greater than 80 percent of patients will have relief of their symptoms following surgical reconstruction.[21] The perioperative complication rates differ for proximal and distal vertebral artery repairs. The technically easier proximal operations have been reported to have a combined morbidity/mortality rate

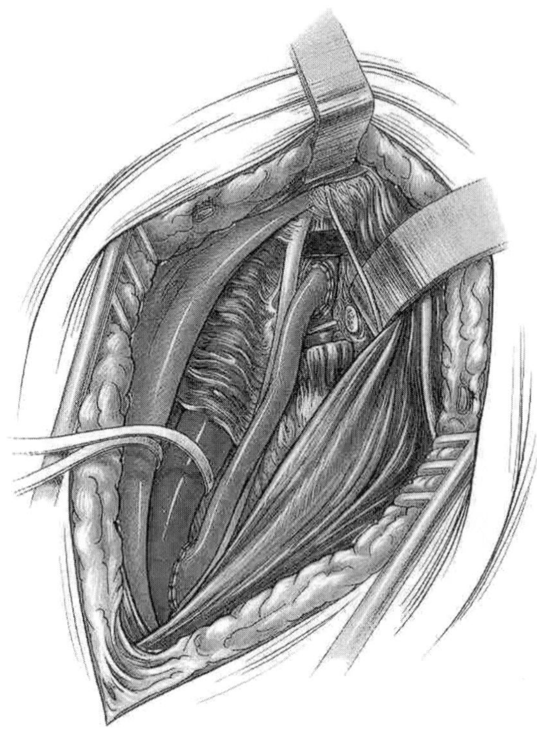

FIG. 14–13. Common carotid to distal vertebral artery vein bypass. (From Berguer R, Kieffer E: *Surgery of the arteries to the head,* New York, 1992, Springer-Verlag. Reproduced with permission.)

of 0.9 percent. Distal reconstructions have been met with a combined morbidity/mortality rate of 3-4 percent.[22]

POSTOPERATIVE NURSING CARE

Following carotid endarterectomy or vertebral reconstruction, the patient may recover on a surgical unit or may require an intensive care unit (ICU) bed. A patient requiring close monitoring can remain up to 4 hours in the recovery room and in an ICU for 8-24 hours. Frequent neurologic and hemodynamic assessments will be required in either setting. New neurologic deficits require prompt attention and sometimes reoperation. Thorough assessment and timely treatment can aid in preventing undesirable outcomes. Standard nursing care after CEA is described in Box 14-2.

Because of the shortened length of stay, nurses are required to provide comprehensive teaching in a shorter period of time. Discharge teaching is directed toward a return to normal activities and modification of risk factors for atherosclerosis. Control of risk factors and behavioral modification is critical for optimal long-term outcome.[23,24] Specific instructions regarding driving, bathing, and other activities may vary with physician preference. In general, there are very few limitations in the uncomplicated postoperative course. Box 14-3 provides further teaching information. A duplex scan may be recommended 6 months to a year after surgery to assess any restenosis of the carotid arteries. The scan may then be performed on an annual basis. For the unfortunate person who has sustained a perioperative stroke, more extensive planning and placement may be required.

In this time of increased health care costs, cost containment, and increased utilization of ICU beds, nurses are striving to find methods for efficient utilization of resources without compromising the quality of patient care. Clinical pathways are one tool utilized to streamline the patient's hospital course.[25] Table 14-1 presents a clinical pathway for care of a patient undergoing carotid endarterectomy. Two studies have demonstrated that the introduction of clinical pathways reduced cost without increasing risk in patients undergoing CEA.[26,27]

BOX 14–2

Potential Postoperative Complications and Nursing Management

BLOOD PRESSURE DEVIATION

- Monitor for hypotension and hypertension. Administer appropriate medication as ordered.

HYPERPERFUSION SYNDROME

- Monitor for severe headache postoperatively.

NEUROLOGIC PROBLEMS

- Monitor patient for increased blood pressure, decreased heart rate, and Cheyne-Stokes respiration (increased intracranial pressure secondary to hemorrhage); decreased blood pressure, increased heart rate and respirations (due to cerebral ischemia); symptomatic bradycardia (due to vagal nerve stimulation).
- Assess level of consciousness. Is patient oriented to time, date, place, and person? Does patient respond appropriately to command and/or pain? Check response to auditory and tactile stimuli.
- Assess pupils. Are they equal in size? Do they respond to light equally and briskly? Is the resting position of the eyes at midline?
- Assess motor function. Can patient move all extremities in response to command (flexion and extension)? Are hand grips equal in strength?

CRANIAL NERVE INJURY

See Table 14-2 for summary of nerve injuries and presenting symptoms.

HEMATOMA/RESPIRATORY DISTRESS

- Monitor for excessive bleeding, swelling at incisional site, or sudden increase in neck circumference. Observe for signs of respiratory distress, shortness of breath, changes in vital signs, anxiety, restlessness, pallor, cyanosis, or changes in level of consciousness.

Other studies have attempted to determine a predictable postoperative course in patients undergoing CEAs. In the past 5 years, dramatic strides have been made in both reducing ICU bed need and decreasing hospital stay after carotid endarterectomy. Hirko et al[28] reduced the ICU stay from 94.8 percent in 1990 to 12.5 percent in 1993. This study also revealed a significant decrease in length of stay. The total length of stay was reduced from an average of 6.18 days to 2.0 days. This study also confirmed that these changes have not adversely affected the safety of the operation.

POSTOPERATIVE COMPLICATIONS

Postoperative problems include perioperative stroke, cranial nerve injuries, and wound complications. Cardiac events are the major cause of the few deaths that occur following surgery.

Perioperative Stroke

Because of improvements in anesthesia, operative procedure, and shunting, the incidence of perioperative stroke has decreased to 2 percent in some institutions. Immediate postoperative deficits may be due to embolization of the atheromatous debris during dissection, low flow while the carotid artery is clamped, or technical complications such as a raised intimal flap, resulting in vessel thrombosis.

With an acute stroke, the patency of the operated vessel must be promptly determined either by obtaining a noninvasive study or taking the patient directly back to surgery. If the artery is patent, heparinization is suggested. If the artery is not patent, thrombectomy is urgently performed. The artery is explored to locate any luminal irregularities that may have led to occlusion. On closure, patch angioplasty is sometimes used to widen the lumen of the artery if that was not done previously. Heparin may be added after the second operation.

BOX 14–3

Patient Education

PREOPERATIVE TEACHING

- Explain to patient that carotid artery disease is usually the result of atherosclerosis. Carotid endarterectomy is the surgical removal of atherosclerotic plaque from the artery, performed to prevent symptoms from occurring and to decrease the incidence of stroke. The surgeon will discuss potential neurologic deficits and cranial nerve injuries preoperatively with the patient and the family.
- Teach and discuss preoperative and postoperative routines with patient. Assess level of understanding, and reinforce teaching.
- Provide written material if available.

POSTOPERATIVE TEACHING

Activity

- Recovery from surgery varies from person to person. Return to normal activity at a gradual but regular pace using common sense. Move the neck as you would normally. No heavy lifting (greater than 10 lb) is allowed for 1 month after surgery.
- Restriction on sexual activity depends on the philosophy of the physician.

Bathing

- Instruct the patient that bathing or showering is acceptable on the second or third day after surgery if subcuticular sutures are used. Clean the incision with mild soap and water, and dry well. No special wound care is required unless otherwise indicated.

Risk Factor Reduction (see Chapter 10)

Risk factors are habits, traits, or conditions that may increase a person's likelihood of developing atherosclerosis. Review pertinent risk factors with the patient and family.

- Diet—Instruct patient on a low-fat, low-cholesterol diet unless specified. When appropriate, diet for modification of hyperlipidemia, hypertension, or diabetes should also be reviewed. American Heart Association guidelines specify that a total cholesterol level should be less than 200 mg/dl with low-density lipoprotein (LDL) of less than 100.
- Smoking—Explain to the patient that smoking accelerates atherosclerosis, increases blood pressure, and decreases heart rate. Encourage the patient to quit smoking.
- Hypertension—Instruct patient to resume preoperative antihypertensive medication, and emphasize importance of future blood pressure management.

Driving

- Inform patients that they may resume driving when they can move the neck as freely as they did before surgery. Instruct patients not to drive after taking narcotic pain medicine or sleeping pills.

Wound Care

- Inform patient that bruising, discoloration, and minimal swelling are not uncommon and will disappear. Inform patient that sutures are internal and do not need to be removed.
- Men may shave around the incision using an electric razor. Use of a bladed razor should be avoided until the swelling around the incision is gone.

Cranial Nerve Deficits

- Instruct patient regarding any postoperative cranial nerve deficits. Most symptoms will resolve in time.

Medical Follow-up/Indications for Physician Notification

- Instruct patient/significant other to inform physician of recurrent or new symptoms:
  Transient ischemic attack (TIA) or permanent (stroke)
  Motor or sensory deficits in extremities
  Speech impairments (difficulty expressing self or understanding spoken words)
  Visual deficits, especially loss of vision in one eye
  Sudden onset of swelling around the incision, increase in the size of the neck, or difficulty breathing
  Sudden severe headache
- Do not ignore any symptoms.
- Attend scheduled follow-up visits and duplex scan recommended by physician.

TABLE 14–1 Clinical Pathway for Same-Day Admission Carotid Endarterectomy

	OR Day; ICU/Floor	POD #1; Floor
Vital Signs/Parameters	VS/neurochecks q 1 hr I/O q 4 hr	VS/neurochecks q 4 hr I/O q 8 hr
IV and PO Drugs	Aspirin (recovery room) Antibiotic, pain med prn IV vasopressors prn IV; A-line prn	Aspirin q day Pain med prn Discontinue A-line IV line prn
Treatment	Observe for hematoma, respiratory distress q 1 hr Elevate HOB 30°	Observe for hematoma and respiratory distress Discontinue Foley catheter prn MD changes first dressing in AM Discharge home
Activity	Bed rest	OOB 2-3 times Ambulate as tolerated
Diet	NPO	Low fat, low cholesterol
Tests	ECG prn Labs prn ABGs prn O_2 prn CBC, SMA-7, PTT/PT prn	
Patient Education	Assess family level of understanding Discuss postop course with family	Discuss progress with pt and family Provide discharge teaching Offer risk reduction class and information

OR, Operating room; *ICU,* intensive care unit; *POD,* postoperative day; *VS,* vital signs; *q,* every; *I/O,* intake and output; *IV,* intravenous; *PO,* by mouth (oral); *D/C,* discontinue; *prn,* as needed; *A-line,* arterial line; *HOB,* head of bed; *MD,* physician; *ad lib,* freely; *OOB,* out of bed; *NPO,* nothing by mouth; *CBC,* complete blood count; *UA,* urinalysis; *ECG,* electrocardiogram; *MRA,* magnetic resonance angiography; *CT,* computed tomography; *T&S,* type and screen; *ABG,* arterial blood gas; *PTT/PT,* partial thromboplastin time/prothrombin time; *pt,* patient.

Deficits due to acute occlusion will often resolve when flow is restored. Deficits due to atheromatous embolization may or may not resolve.

Hypertension/Hypotension

Hypertension is a common problem, which can threaten the arterial anastomosis. Hypotension may also occur and predispose the patient to carotid artery thrombosis. Extremes in blood pressure may complicate any existing cardiac disease. Hypertension or hypotension should be treated if systolic blood pressure is greater than 180 mm Hg or less than 100 mm Hg with vasoactive infusions in an ICU setting.

Hyperperfusion Syndrome

While rare, hyperperfusion syndrome can occur, usually 2-3 days postoperatively, in patients who have preoperative high-grade stenosis, long-standing hypoperfusion, and chronic hypertension. This syndrome is caused by increased blood pressure in brain capillary beds distal to arterioles that have chronically lost the ability to autoregulate and vasoconstrict. Patients may experience severe unilateral headaches, seizures, and stroke.

Cranial Nerve Injuries

Some patients will experience sensory or motor deficits involving the cranial nerves or the greater auricular nerve, which may be misinterpreted as a stroke. The most frequent injuries are summarized in Table 14-2. These result from traction or inadvertent transection during the operation. The neuroanatomy of the neck is demonstrated in Figs. 14-14 and 14-15. Although most of these injuries resolve in time, patients undergoing staged bilateral endarterectomies may require laryngoscopy between the operations to identify any vocal cord paralysis. The spinal accessory, vagus, and sympathetic plexus can be disturbed during vertebral artery surgery.

Wound Complications/Respiratory Distress

Wound complications are infrequent after extracranial vascular reconstruction. Bleeding and wound hematomas should be aggressively managed because the airway may be compromised by tracheal compression. Cervical hematomas are usually the result of coughing or straining during extubation. Reoperation is performed to identify and correct a suture line bleed and to drain the hematoma. A small closed drain is used in these situations.

Restenosis

Patients and health care providers alike are often frustrated by recurrent carotid artery disease, which can occur at any time following CEA. Most recurrent lesions are caused by either of two factors: (1) myointimal hyperplasia, a collagenous proliferation of the medial layer of the arterial wall that appears to be more prevalent in women and usually is discovered within the first 3 postoperative years or, (2) secondary atherosclerosis occurring later in the follow-up period, which is more closely associated with smoking and hyperlipidemia.[29] The actual incidence and clinical implications of recurrent carotid stenosis are unclear. All patients undergoing CEA should be counseled to control risk factors. Management of recurrent disease requires an annual examination and ultrasonographic scanning. If the restenosis exceeds 50 percent or if the patient has symptoms, reoperation may be required.

Carotid Stenting

Recently, angioplasty with stenting has been used for the treatment of carotid artery stenosis. Indications for carotid stenting are fibromuscular dysplasia, recurrent stenosis, radiated neck, high bifurcation, and high surgical risk. The combined stroke and death rate for carotid stenting is between 5.9 and 11 percent.[30,31] Carotid stenting is an emerging technology (Fig. 14-16).[32-34] Early results of the SAPPHIRE (Stenting and Angioplasty with

TABLE 14–2 Summary of Nerve Injuries After Carotid Endarterectomy

Cranial Nerve	Postoperative Injury
Hypoglossal (XII)	Affects the ipsilateral tongue, difficulties with speech and mastication; patient will be hoarse and have difficulty attaining high-pitched phonation
Superior laryngeal vagus (X) branch	Minor swallowing problems and easily fatigued voice
Recurrent laryngeal–anterior vagus (X)	Vocal cord paralysis, hoarseness present, and inadequate gag reflex
Glossopharyngeal (IX)	Difficulty swallowing with ipsilateral Horner's syndrome (ptosis, exophthalmos, reduced sweating); a rare injury
Facial (VII)	Drooping of the corner of the lip on the ipsilateral side and inability to smile symmetrically
Spinal accessory (XI)	Limitations in neck, shoulder movement in terms of alignment and horizontal motion
Greater auricular	(A branch of brachial plexus rather than a cranial nerve) Paresthesias of the face and ear

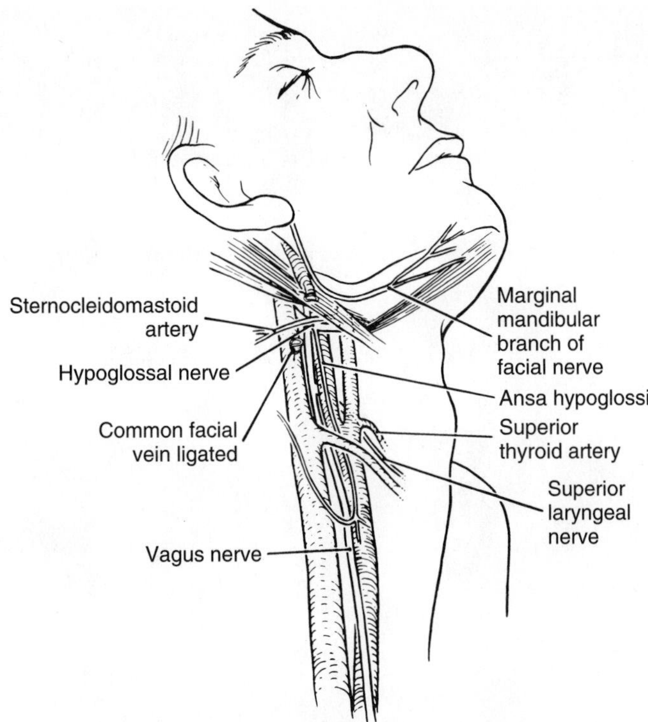

FIG. 14–14. Cranial nerves in relation to the carotid artery. (From Bergan JJ, Flinn WR, Yao JST: Cranial nerve injury in carotid surgery. In Bergan JJ, Yao JST, eds: *Cerebrovascular insufficiency,* New York, 1983, Grune & Stratton, p 454.)

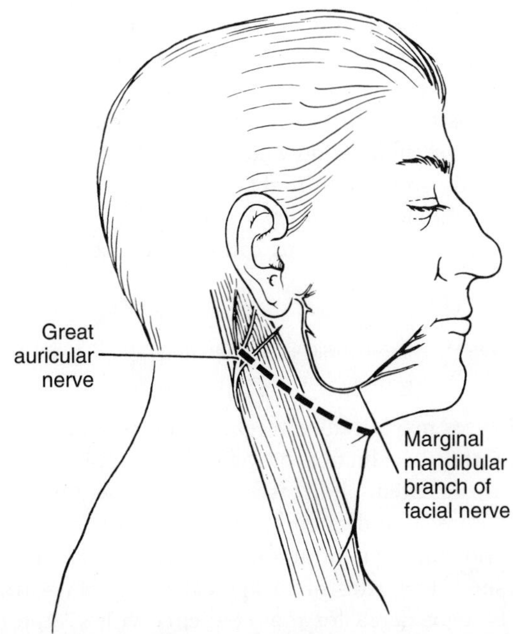

FIG. 14–15. Greater auricular and facial nerves in relation to the carotid artery. (From Bergan JJ, Flinn WR, Yao JST: Cranial nerve injury in carotid surgery. In Bergan JJ, Yao JST, eds: *Cerebrovascular insufficiency,* New York, 1983, Grune & Stratton, p 452.)

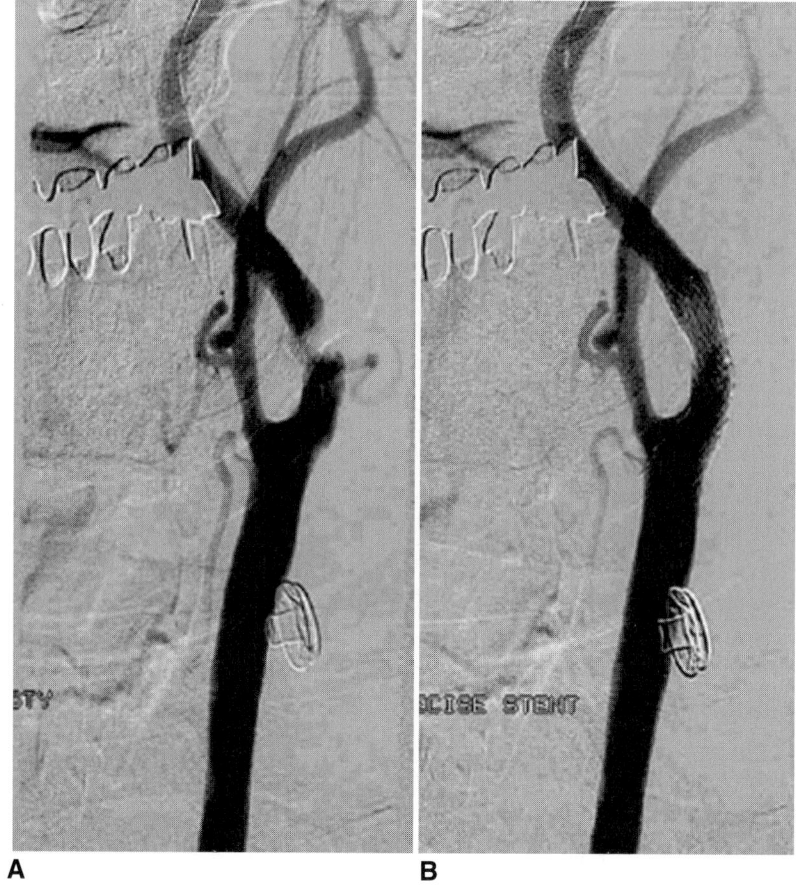

FIG. 14–16. Recurrent left internal carotid artery stenosis in a 76-year-old man. **A,** Before treatment. **B,** After percutaneous balloon angioplasty and stent placement.

Protection in Patients at High Risk for Endarterectomy) trial were recently presented, which demonstrated a decrease in perioperative morbidity in high-risk patients undergoing carotid artery stenting as compared to patients undergoing carotid endarterectomy.[35] The safety and efficacy of carotid stenting is being further studied in several other clinical trials including the CREST trial (Carotid Revascularization Endarterectomy Versus Stent Trial). The CREST trial is a FDA-approved study sponsored by the National Institute of Health (NIH) and the National Institute of Neurological Disorders and Stroke (NINDS). Cerebral protection devices used to prevent embolic events during carotid artery stenting are also currently being evaluated.[36,37]

CONCLUSION

Although a variety of diseases may produce cerebrovascular insufficiency, the most common cause is atherosclerosis. Careful evaluation of the patient by physical examination and noninvasive testing will define the extent of disease and direct planning for the appropriate treatment. Carotid endarterectomy is indicated for patients with moderate to severe stenosis, regardless of symptoms, and with no contraindications to surgery. The surgeon must be experienced and be able to show low rates of complications. Supra-aortic trunk and vertebral reconstructions should be considered for most patients with symptoms. These procedures can be carried out with low risk and great benefit to selected patients. In addition to post-procedure management of the patient, nurses are instrumental in providing education and support for lifestyle changes to reduce the risk of further disease.

REFERENCES

1. American Heart Association: *Heart & stroke encyclopedia: A to Z guide,* http://www.americanheart.org/presenter.jhtml?identifier=10000056, Dallas, 2002, The Association.
2. Sullivan ED, Herzter NR: Extracranial cerebrovascular arterial disease. In Young JR, Olin JW et al, eds: *Peripheral vascular disease*, ed 2, St Louis, 1996, Mosby, pp 288-304.
3. Moore WS: Fundamental consideration in cerebrovascular disease. In Rutherford RB, ed: *Vascular surgery,* Philadelphia, 1995, WB Saunders, pp 1456-1473.
4. Hass WK, Fields WS, North RR et al: Joint study of extracranial arterial occlusion. II. Arteriography, techniques, sites and complications, *JAMA* 203:961-968, 1968.
5. Carr SC, Cheanvechai V, Virmani R et al: Histology and clinical significance of the carotid atherosclerotic plaque: implications for endovascular treatment, *J Endovasc Surg* 4:321-325, 1997.
6. Lee NS, Jones HR: Extracranial cerebrovascular disease, *Cardiol Clin* 9:523-534, 1991.
7. Francfort JW, Smullens SN, Gallagher JF et al: Airway compromise after carotid surgery in patients with cervical irradiation, *J Cardiovasc Surg* 30:877-881, 1989.
8. Spittell JA, Spittell PC: Dissection of the aorta and other arteries. In Young JR et al, eds: *Peripheral vascular diseases,* St Louis, 1991, Mosby-Year Book, pp 321-329.
9. Green RM: Management of spontaneous dissection and fibromuscular dysplasia of the carotid artery. In Yao JST, Pearce WH, eds: *Arterial surgery: management of challenging problems,* Norwalk, Conn, 1996, Appleton & Lange, pp 127-139.
10. Calabrese LH, Clough JD: Systemic vasculitis. In Young JR, Olin JW et al, eds: *Peripheral vascular diseases*, ed 2, St Louis, 1996, Mosby, pp 380-406.
11. Hertzer NR, Beven EG, Young JR et al: Coronary artery disease in peripheral vascular patients: a classification of 1000 coronary angiograms and results of surgical management, *Ann Surg* 199:223-233, 1984.
12. Young JR: Physical examination. In Young JR, Olin JW et al, eds: *Peripheral vascular diseases*, ed 2, St Louis, 1996, Mosby, pp 18-32.
13. North American Symptomatic Carotid Endarterectomy Trial: Methods, patient characteristics, and progress, *Stroke* 22(6):711-720, 1991.
14. MRC European Carotid Surgery Trial: Interim results for symptomatic patients with severe (70-99%) or with mild (0-29%) carotid stenosis, European Carotid Surgery Trialists' Collaborative Group, *Lancet* 337(8752):1235-1243, 1991.
15. Barnett HJ, Taylor DW, Eliasziw M et al: Benefit of carotid endarterectomy in patients with symptomatic moderate or severe stenosis, *N Engl J Med* 339(20):1415-1425, 1998.
16. Hobson RW, Weiss DG, Fields WS et al: Efficacy of carotid endarterectomy for asymptomatic carotid stenosis, *N Engl J Med* 328:221-227, 1993.
17. Executive Committee for the Asymptomatic Carotid Atherosclerosis Study: Endarterectomy for asymptomatic carotid artery stenosis, *JAMA* 273(18):1421-1428, 1995.
18. Gent M, Blakely TA, Easton JD et al: The Canadian American Ticlopidine Study (CATS) in thromboembolic stroke, *Lancet* 1:1215-1220, 1989.
19. Callow AD: Carotid endarterectomy: ten-year follow up. In Yao JST, Pearce WH, eds: *Long-term results in vascular surgery,* Norwalk, Conn, 1993, Appleton & Lange, pp 61-68.
20. American College of Physicians: Indications for carotid endarterectomy, *Ann Intern Med* 111(8):675-677, 1989.
21. Berguer R, Morasch MD, Kline RA: A review of 100 consecutive reconstructions of the distal vertebral artery for embolic and hemodynamic disease, *J Vasc Surg* 27:852-859, 1998.
22. Berguer R, Flynn LM, Kline RA et al: Surgical reconstruction of the extracranial vertebral artery: management and outcome, *J Vasc Surg* 31:9-18, 2000.
23. Wilson PWF, Hoeg JM, D'Agostino RB et al: Cumulative effects of high cholesterol levels, high blood pressure, and cigarette smoking on carotid stenosis, *N Engl J Med* 337:516-522, 1997.
24. Biller J, Feinberg WM, Castaldo JE et al: Guidelines for carotid endarterectomy: a statement for healthcare professionals from a special writing group of the Stroke Council, American Heart Association, *Circulation* 97:501-509, 1998.
25. Christensen CR: Carotid endarterectomy clinical pathway: nursing perspective, *J Vasc Nurs* 15:1-7, 1997.
26. Morasch MD, Hodgett D, Burke K et al: Selective use of the intensive care unit following carotid endarterectomy, *Ann Vasc Surg* 9:229-234, 1995.
27. Amjad I, Paramo JC, Sendzischew H et al: Carotid endarterectomy critical pathway: application and benefits in a private teaching hospital, *Surg Rounds* 24(11):562-571, 2001.
28. Hirko MK, Morasch MD, Burke K et al: The changing face of carotid endarterectomy, *J Vasc Surg* 23:622-627, 1996.

29. Hertzer NR: Postoperative management and complications following carotid endarterectomy. In Rutherford RB, ed: *Vascular surgery*, ed 5, Philadelphia, 2000, WB Saunders, pp 1881-1906.
30. Wholey MH, Wholey MH, Jarmolowski CR et al: Endovascular stents for carotid artery occlusive disease, *J Endovasc Surg* 4:326-338, 1997.
31. Diethrich EB, Ndiaye M, Reid DB: Stenting in the carotid artery: initial experience in 110 patients, *J Endovasc Surg* 3:42-62, 1996.
32. d'Audiffret A, Desgranges P, Kobeiter H et al: Technical aspects and current results of carotid stenting, *J Vasc Surg* 33:1001-1007, 2001.
33. Diethrich EB: Endovascular repair for carotid lesions. In Pearce WH, Yao JST, eds: *Advances in vascular surgery,* Chicago, 2002, Precept Press, pp 127-141.
34. Hobson RW II, Lal BK: Carotid angioplasty and stenting for carotid restenosis after carotid endarterectomy. In Pearce WH, Yao JST, eds: *Advances in vascular surgery,* Chicago, 2002, Precept Press, pp 159-166.
35. SAPPHIRE Trial Investigators: Stenting and Angioplasty with Protection in Patients at High Risk for Endarterectomy (SAPPHIRE) trial. Presented at the American Heart Association Meeting, November, 2002, Chicago, IL.
36. Parodi JC, La Mura R, Ferreira LM et al: Initial evaluation of carotid angioplasty and stenting with three different cerebral protection devices, *J Vase Surg* 32:1127-1136, 2001.
37. Ohki T, Parodi J, Veith FJ et al: Efficacy of a proximal occlusion catheter with reversal of flow in the prevention of embolic events during carotid artery stenting: an experimental analysis, *J Vasc Surg* 33:504-509, 2001.

15

Upper-Extremity Problems

KAREN R. BRUNI

Upper-extremity ischemia is much less common than lower-extremity ischemia, due in part to the fact that arteries of the upper extremity are relatively spared from the atherosclerotic process. Extensive collateral pathways around the shoulder effectively compensate in most cases when major arterial obstruction threatens the upper extremities, making upper-extremity limb loss an unusual circumstance.

Although the upper extremities and hands are often taken for granted, humans depend tremendously on them to carry out the simple routines of life. For most persons, the prospect of amputation or disability of an upper extremity represents a considerably greater impairment than the loss of a lower extremity. For this reason, the diagnosis and treatment of upper-extremity problems presents a distinct challenge.

ANATOMY

Knowledge of upper extremity anatomy is essential to an understanding of factors responsible for arm ischemia and its treatment (Fig. 15-1). The subclavian artery originates from the brachiocephalic trunk on the right side and from the distal transverse aortic arch on the left and exits from the chest over the first rib on each side. At its junction with the first rib, the subclavian artery passes just behind the anterior scalene muscle, giving off the vertebral, internal mammary, and thyrocervical branches. Just beyond the anterior scalene muscle, the subclavian artery becomes the axillary artery, at which point close approximation with the axillary vein and brachial plexus occurs. The axillary artery then becomes the brachial artery and courses through the medial upper arm to just below the antecubital fossa, where it divides into the ulnar, radial, and interosseous arteries. These branches course deep to the flexor muscles of the forearm.

The radial artery (lateral) and the ulnar artery (medial) supply most of the hand circulation. Intercommunications at the palmar level are multiple, with one dorsal and two palmar arches (superficial and deep) providing a variety of inflow pathways to the digits. In most persons the superficial palmar arch is the dominant arterial circulation to the fingers, supplying common digital arteries that then branch into proper digital arteries on either side of the fingers. The distal circulation of the hand tends to be much more variable than that of the larger, proximal arteries of the upper extremity.

ETIOLOGY AND CLINICAL PRESENTATION

Unlike lower-extremity ischemia, in which the majority of patients suffer from atherosclerotic arterial occlusive disease, upper-extremity ischemia may have a wide variety of etiologic factors. An exhaustive listing is beyond the scope of this chapter. Box 15-1 summarizes the pathologic processes commonly responsible for upper-extremity arterial problems. The symptoms of upper-extremity arterial insufficiency vary considerably, depending on the level and acuteness of obstruction, the degree of collateral circulation, and the presence of vasospasm.

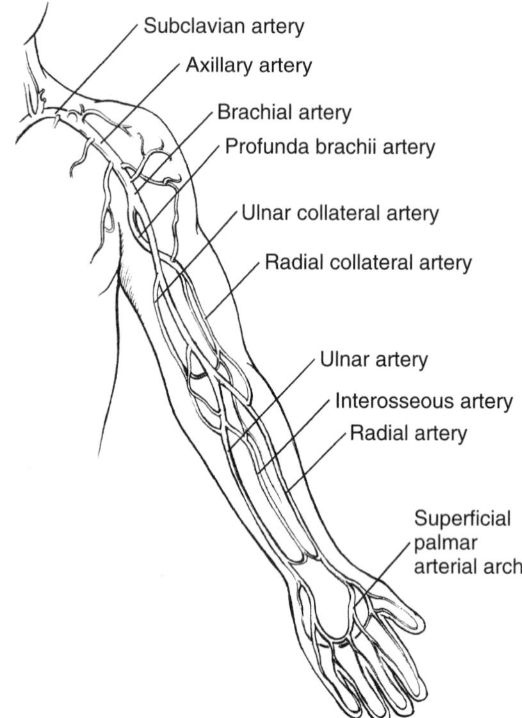

FIG. 15–1. Anatomy of the major arteries of the upper extremity. (Jillian O'Malley, Copyright 2002.)

Atherosclerosis

Although unusual, upper-extremity atherosclerosis is well recognized; the proximal left subclavian artery is involved twice as often as the right subclavian artery, with innominate artery involvement a distant third.[1,2] As with atherosclerosis elsewhere, the disease process is one of advancing age, with most patients being more than 50 years old. In chronic occlusion of major arteries, presenting symptoms may include forearm fatigue after exercise, pain at rest, gangrene, a cold hand, and loss of functional use of the hand.[3]

In cases of a left subclavian artery occlusion, a significant amount of blood may flow to the arm because of reversal of blood flow in the left vertebral artery (Fig. 15-2). The source

BOX 15–1

Etiology of Upper-Extremity Problem

- Atherosclerotic embolization
- Ischemic monomelic neuropathy
- Atherosclerosis
  - Generalized atherosclerosis
  - Subclavian steal syndrome
  - Atherosclerotic embolization
  - Atherosclerotic aneurysms
- Emboli
  - Cardiac source
  - Proximal arterial source
  - Inadvertent drug injections
  - Iatrogenic
- Trauma
  - Violent
  - Iatrogenic
  - Occupational
  - Frostbite
  - Irradiation
- Posttraumatic pain syndrome
- Immune arteritis
  - Polyarteritis
  - Hypersensitivity
  - Giant-cell
  - Buerger's disease
  - Thoracic outlet syndrome
- Hyperhidrosis

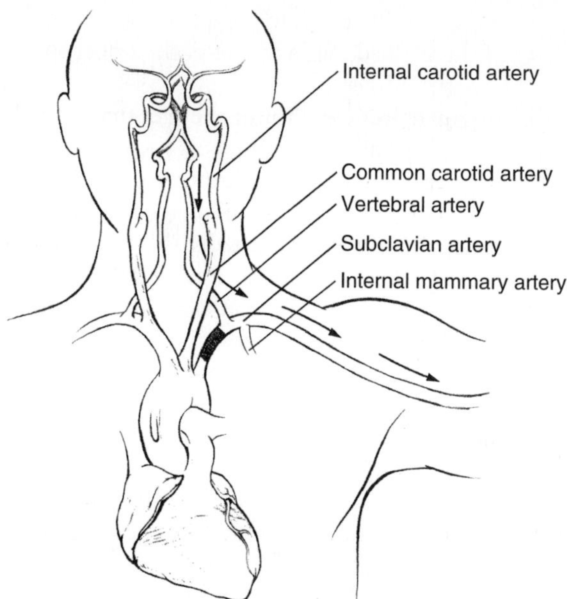

FIG. 15–2. Demonstration of "subclavian steal syndrome" with reversal of vertebral artery flow due to proximal subclavian artery occlusion. (Jillian O'Malley, Copyright 2002.)

of this flow is the basilar artery in the brain, which has received its circulation from the right vertebral artery or the carotid arteries via the circle of Willis. This forms the basis of the subclavian steal syndrome. It has been suggested that patients who complain of vertigo, dizziness, drop attacks, or visual disturbances suffer because the arm "steals" blood from the circulation intended for the posterior aspect of the brain. In fact, very few patients actually have these symptoms, despite reversed flow in the vertebral arteries. The current theory is that patients who present with cerebral symptoms have associated or coincidental stenosis of the carotid arteries.[4] Treatment of the carotid artery lesions usually relieves these symptoms.

It is also because of rather extensive collateral circulation from the vertebral arteries and around the shoulder that patients seldom develop symptoms of arm ischemia from proximal subclavian artery occlusive disease alone. Aneurysms of the upper-extremity arteries are uncommon. However, they may be associated with trauma, infections, or thoracic outlet syndrome.[5,6]

Embolism

Embolization to the upper extremity is a relatively common cause of acute arm ischemia, but only 10 percent of all embolic episodes involve the upper extremities.[7,8] These emboli may originate from proximal arterial lesions; however, most often they come from the heart (Box 15-2). In some patients, however, atherosclerotic lesions may be the source of distal embolization of atherosclerotic debris or small organized clots resulting in digital artery occlusion.[9] Diagnosis of microemboli may be difficult because presenting symptoms are often

BOX 15–2

Emboli From the Heart

Left ventricular mural thrombi after myocardial infarction
Left atrial thrombi in patients with atrial fibrillation
Cardiac tumors such as atrial myxoma
Debris from diseased cardiac valves
Thrombi that have developed on prosthetic valves

subtle. A blue finger may be present. Physical signs such as livedo reticularis, petechiae of the skin, splinter hemorrhage of the nailbed, or gangrene of the fingertips may be confused with other disorders.[3]

In general, emboli that originate from the heart are larger than emboli from proximal arterial sources and contain mainly thrombus (thromboembolism). Cardiac emboli, therefore, lodge primarily in the larger vessels of the upper extremity, involving the subclavian (10 percent), axillary (22 percent), and brachial arteries (64 percent).[10] Emboli that originate from proximal arterial sources (atheroembolism) are usually the result of platelet deposition and thrombus formation at points of atherosclerotic arterial damage. These emboli lodge more distally in the palmar arches or digital vessels and at times in the ulnar or radial arteries.[10,11] Mural thrombus that develops in a subclavian artery aneurysm may also embolize to the distal arm arteries. Inadvertent arterial injection of drugs of abuse, embolization during arterial catheterization procedures or arteriography, and embolization from indwelling arterial monitoring lines also may be seen.

Trauma

Traumatic injuries of the upper extremities stand out as a leading cause of upper-extremity ischemia. Penetrating injuries from knife wounds, lacerations, and gunshot wounds present a relatively straightforward mechanism for arterial injury. Blunt injuries to arterial structures may result from clavicular fractures, inferior shoulder dislocations, dislocations of the elbows, or humeral fractures. Prolonged use of crutches may result in continued trauma to the axillary artery with either arterial thrombosis or aneurysm formation.

Diagnostic and therapeutic procedures that require arterial puncture may lead to iatrogenic arterial injuries, including arterial thrombosis, hemorrhage, or distal embolization. Cardiac catheterization, commonly performed through the brachial artery (Sones technique), is often performed in patients with generalized atherosclerosis. The brachial artery may be difficult to repair after catheterization.[12] Puncture of the brachial or axillary arteries for arteriography likewise may be complicated by arterial thrombosis or hemorrhage. Bleeding into the axillary sheath may result in significant nerve compression and upper extremity dysfunction without the loss of distal pulses. Radial arterial lines for blood pressure monitoring and blood specimen withdrawals in critically ill patients likewise may result in arterial thrombosis and hand ischemia.

Increasing use of upper-extremity arteries and veins as access sites for chronic hemodialysis has resulted in a proportionate increase in iatrogenic hand ischemia. Several mechanisms may be at fault, including arterial injury at operation, distal embolization, pseudoaneurysm formation, or infection and mycotic aneurysm formation at anastomotic sites.[13]

Although many occupations lend themselves to an inordinate risk of blunt or penetrating trauma of the upper extremities, one particular mechanism for arterial damage and hand ischemia stands out. The "hypothenar hammer syndrome" (HHS) reported by Conn, Bergan, and Bell[5] in 1970 describes the association of ulnar artery injury with use of the heel of the palm to hammer, push, or twist objects. Ulnar artery thrombosis or aneurysm formation with distal embolization can then result in digital ischemia. Another mechanism described in association with digital ischemia has been the chronic use of vibratory tools. Unlike hypothenar hammer syndrome, in which intermittent severe blows are incurred, the vibratory tool syndrome results in arterial injury due to prolonged repetitive vibratory damage from pneumatic tools.[14] A recent study concludes that HHS occurs when persons with pre-existing palmar ulnar artery fibrodysplasia experience repetitive palmar trauma. This revised theory for the etiology of HHS explains why HHS does not develop in most patients with repetitive palmar trauma.[15]

Frostbite is the tissue injury that occurs as a result of overexposure to cold temperatures. The severity varies with the temperature and the duration of exposure, with most injuries occurring on exposure at temperatures between 0° C and 7° C for more than 7 hours. Increased humidity and wind velocity accelerate the withdrawal of heat from the body and may shorten the exposure time necessary to result in significant tissue damage. Although some acclimatization may occur, extremities previously injured from frostbite remain permanently susceptible to future cold injury because of an intensified vasoconstrictor response. Although direct freezing with cell membrane disruption may play a significant role in extremely low temperature frostbite injuries, many authorities believe that the mechanisms of vasoconstriction, decreased blood flow, arterial thrombosis, and ischemic necrosis are responsible in the majority of frostbite cases.[16]

Radiation therapy for various malignant processes can result in arterial injury.[2] Intimal thickening, cellular infiltration, and scarring result in arterial lesions very similar in appearance to those of atherosclerosis. Small-artery occlusion and large-artery stenosis may occur soon after irradiation or may develop gradually over many years. Irradiation of various cancers of the head, neck, breast, and lung most commonly results in subclavian artery lesions, while irradiation of soft-tissue tumors of the arm causes axillary or brachial artery damage. Another problem that may arise after irradiation is exposure of underlying arteries as a result of breakdown of overlying skin and subcutaneous tissue. Resultant arterial infection, desiccation, or disruption with blowout are complications that may arise because of inadequate coverage of underlying vascular structures.

Posttraumatic Pain Syndrome

Posttraumatic pain syndromes (causalgia, reflex sympathetic dystrophy) are intensely painful symptom complexes that are poorly understood and difficult to diagnose accurately. Posttraumatic pain may develop after peripheral nerve injury or irritation. Frequently, ischemia may be the inciting event. However, at times, the cause may be so insignificant as not to be readily apparent.

Three clinical stages of posttraumatic pain syndrome have been recognized. The acute stage is reversible, and the patient experiences burning, redness, swelling, sweating, and extreme tenderness to light tactile stimuli. After 2 months, symptoms may resolve spontaneously or patients may exhibit patchy areas of osteoporosis. In the dystrophic stage, symptoms progress to coolness, cyanosis, brawny edema, continuous pain, and diffuse osteoporosis. The atrophic phase is characterized by increasingly severe pain, even beyond the injured area, and accompanied by skin atrophy, muscle wasting, and trophic ulceration. Bones show advanced demineralization with joint contractures and ankylosis.

Patients who exhibit a majority of these symptoms are more likely to have an accurate diagnosis and are considered to have "major causalgia." Most patients, on the other hand, present with "minor" or "mimo" causalgia and complain of only some of these symptoms.

The differential diagnosis may include nerve entrapments, Raynaud's syndrome, arterial ischemia, and thoracic outlet syndrome. Response to sympathetic nerve block may help make the diagnosis. Patients with posttraumatic pain syndromes experience dramatic relief of pain with sympathetic nerve block, and this may be a useful predictor of the result of surgical sympathectomy.

Raynaud's Phenomenon

Raynaud's phenomenon occurs with episodic attacks of well-demarcated blanching (white finger) or bluish discoloration of one or more digits. The attacks are confined to the fingers and toes. The hands and feet are not involved. Vasospastic attacks occur on exposure to the cold or at times with emotional upset. During the attack, the digit becomes white and numb; the pallor may then be replaced by cyanosis due to slow blood flow, and finally the digit turns red during a hyperemic phase. During this phase, the patient may have throbbing pain.

Raynaud's phenomenon is termed primary (or idiopathic) when no underlying cause is present or secondary when it is caused by an underlying disease, drug, or inciting event. The precise classification of primary and secondary Raynaud's phenomenon is often difficult. Some authors prefer to use the term "Raynaud's syndrome" to characterize patients with episodic vasospastic disease of the hands. Raynaud's phenomenon must not be confused with Raynaud's disease, which is a primary disease without an underlying cause and is diagnosed after exclusion of all etiologic factors.[3]

Ischemic Monomelic Neuropathy

Ischemic monomelic neuropathy is a rare pain syndrome with a predilection for the upper extremity. It was originally described as a consequence of acute arterial compromise and now is more often seen in diabetic renal failure patients following upper-extremity dialysis graft insertion. The pathologic feature of multiple axon-loss mononeuropathies distally in the limb without muscle necrosis is diagnostic.[17,18]

The clinical presentation includes prominent sensory symptoms of numbness, dysesthesias, and burning causalgia-type pain with milder levels of motor weakness and loss of coordination in conjunction with acute ischemia. The pain is continuous, may persist for months, and rarely disappears completely even in the face of correction of the inciting ischemic event. The syndrome has no clinical, arterial, or neurologic predictors, and delay in diagnosis is common.

Immune Arteritis

Immune arteritis is a complex topic with many different categories and classifications (see Chapter 1). The specific term *arteritis* implies inflammation of the arterial wall with cellular infiltrates and eventual necrosis. The term does not imply the arterial involvement that is inevitable in the multitude of inflammatory processes with perivascular round-cell infiltrates. Immune arteritis is associated with intimal damage, scarring, and stenosis leading to arterial occlusions.[19] Most commonly, the small and medium-sized arteries are involved, although Takayasu's arteritis involves only the large aortic branch arteries.

Although an in-depth discussion is beyond the scope of this chapter, features that distinguish the types of arteritis will be briefly discussed. The polyarteritis nodosa group of diseases most commonly affects older patients, with male/female ratio of 2:1. Focal, transmural inflammation of the small and medium-sized arteries results in necrosis, arterial thrombosis, and formation of small aneurysms. The hepatic, renal, and mesenteric circulations are frequently involved. Although significant upper-extremity involvement is not common, Raynaud's phenomenon and upper-extremity symptoms may be the first clue to the underlying disease.

Hypersensitivity angiitis encompasses a broad group of problems affecting the small arteries. Characteristic arterial thickening, connective tissue swelling, and vascular occlusion occur with relatively little inflammatory reaction. Except for scleroderma, most of these conditions result from exposure to some antigen, with the formation of antigen/antibody immune complexes. At times, the inciting antigen is not known, but fragments of DNA, RNA, hepatitis B virus, or specific tumor antigens are commonly responsible.

Giant-cell arteritis is characterized by localized periarteritis with mononuclear and giant-cell infiltrates and disruption of elastic fibers of the arterial wall. Temporal arteritis or systemic giant-cell arteritis may involve any artery but most commonly involves the branches of the carotid arteries of older women. Takayasu's arteritis affects younger Asian women, with typical involvement of the aortic arch and its branches and, less frequently, involvement of the pulmonary artery.

Buerger's disease (thromboangiitis obliterans) represents a controversial clinical condition that is believed to represent a severe form of distal atherosclerotic arterial occlusive disease. Significant evidence, however, supports the belief that it does exist as a discrete pathologic entity.[9] The disease occurs predominantly in young men of Jewish familial descent who have a strong history of cigarette smoking. Transmural cellular infiltration of the small and medium-sized arteries results in fibrous obliteration of vascular lumen. Superficial thrombophlebitis and venous involvement are characteristic, involving the lower extremities more commonly than the upper extremities. Specific cellular immunity against antigens has been suggested as an etiologic factor.

Thoracic Outlet Syndrome

Thoracic outlet syndrome entails a complex of upper-extremity symptoms of the neurovascular bundle as it exits from the thoracic cage (Fig. 15-3). The disorder affects women more commonly than men and is usually seen in young and middle-aged adults.

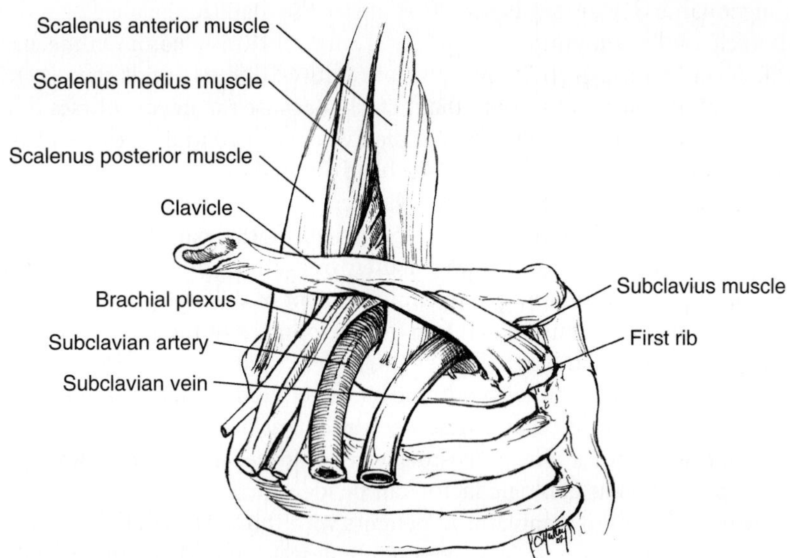

FIG. 15–3. Diagram of the right thoracic outlet demonstrating the relationship of the vein and artery and brachial plexus to the clavicle, first rib, and scalenus muscles. (Jillian O'Malley, Copyright 2002.)

The first rib forms the floor of the thoracic outlet, with the clavicle and the subclavius muscle forming the superior portion. Laterally, the scalenus medius muscle inserts inferiorly on the first rib and is in close proximity to the posterior aspect of the brachial plexus. The subclavian artery lies just anterior to the brachial plexus, so that the neurovascular bundle (brachial plexus and subclavian artery) lies between the scalenus medius and scalenus anticus muscle bundles. The scalenus anticus muscle inserts on the first rib between the subclavian artery and the subclavian vein and, with the subclavius muscle tendons, forms the medial border of the thoracic outlet by inserting on the first rib at its junction with the costal cartilage. Therefore, any affliction that impinges on this rather limited outlet may result in compression of the nerve, artery, or vein (Fig. 15-4). Neurologic symptoms due to brachial plexus compression predominate.

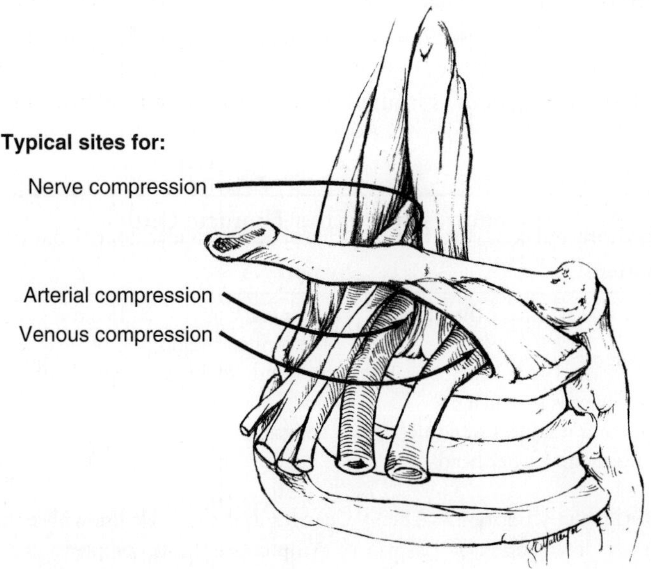

FIG. 15–4. Diagram of right thoracic outlet syndrome demonstrating artery, vein, and nerve compression. (Jillian O'Malley, Copyright 2002.)

Both congenital and acquired factors may upset this delicate balance of structures and result in thoracic outlet symptoms. A congenital cervical rib is a common mechanism. This may take the form of a complete bony rib or of multiple fibrous bands that stretch from an elongated cervical transverse process to the first rib. Because the nerve courses in close proximity to the posterior aspect of this brachial plexus, nerve irritation is caused by the scissor compression action of the cervical rib/fibrous band anomalies.

Trauma is frequently associated with the thoracic outlet syndrome. Callus formation due to a fractured clavicle or first rib may cause obvious outlet narrowing. Hyper-extension-flexion (whiplash) injuries may be followed acutely or even remotely by severe spasm of multiple cervical or upper back muscle groups. Involvement of the scalenus medius muscle may be responsible for the symptoms related to overdevelopment of the muscles of the neck and shoulder region that occurs in baseball pitchers, golfers, swimmers, and weight lifters.

In many patients, thoracic outlet syndrome has no obvious congenital or traumatic cause. Although it has been suggested that a shoulder girdle that lies exceptionally low in the thorax may be associated with a narrow costoclavicular space, this is not always the case. In many patients, no particular etiologic factor can be identified.

Pain is the most common complaint in patients with thoracic outlet syndrome. Although symptoms are quite subjective, patients commonly describe a dull, aching pain that radiates down the arm from the shoulder. At times, patients may experience sharp pains limited to specific muscle groups. Pain may involve the neck, shoulder, forearm, or hand, may be constant or intermittent, and may be related to specific physical activities such as lifting or working with the arms overhead. Numbness and paresthesia may accompany the pain. The ulnar nerve distribution is most commonly affected, with or without median nerve involvement. Radial nerve symptoms are infrequently seen. Although sensory symptoms predominate in the early stages, long-standing neurovascular compression frequently results in weakness of upper-extremity muscle groups; with time, muscle wasting may be seen.

Arterial complications that may result from thoracic outlet syndrome include thickening and fibrosis with early atherosclerotic changes and plaque formation because of continued arterial trauma. Poststenotic dilation and aneurysm formation may result. Complications include arterial thrombosis and distal embolization of thrombotic and atherosclerotic debris, whereas rupture is rarely seen. At times, hypertrophy of the anterior scalenus muscle in athletes may result in arterial compression during hyperabduction (Fig. 15-5). Table 15-1 describes the physical examination and symptoms of arterial compression of the thoracic outlet.

Effort Thrombosis of the Subclavian Vein (Paget-Schroetter Syndrome)

When compression of the subclavian vein occurs suddenly as the result of unusual physical movement of the arms, a person may develop acute damage of the subclavian vein at the thoracic outlet. The endothelium is injured, leading to immediate thrombosis of the vein at

TABLE 15–1 Arterial Compression of the Thoracic Outlet*

Physical Examination	Symptoms
The arm is abducted to 90° or over the head.	Numbness, tingling, and coldness of the hand; blanches the arm and hand; the pulse is lost by palpation and restored when the arm is dependent.
Adson maneuver—Patient is instructed to take a deep breath and hold it, extending the neck fully, turning his or her head toward the affected side.	Obliteration or decrease of the radial pulse suggests compression.
Costal clavicular test (military position)—The shoulders are drawn down and back.	Changes in the radial pulse with reduction of symptoms indicate compression.
Allen test—see Figure 4-3.	

*Involves numbness, tingling, and coldness of the hand.

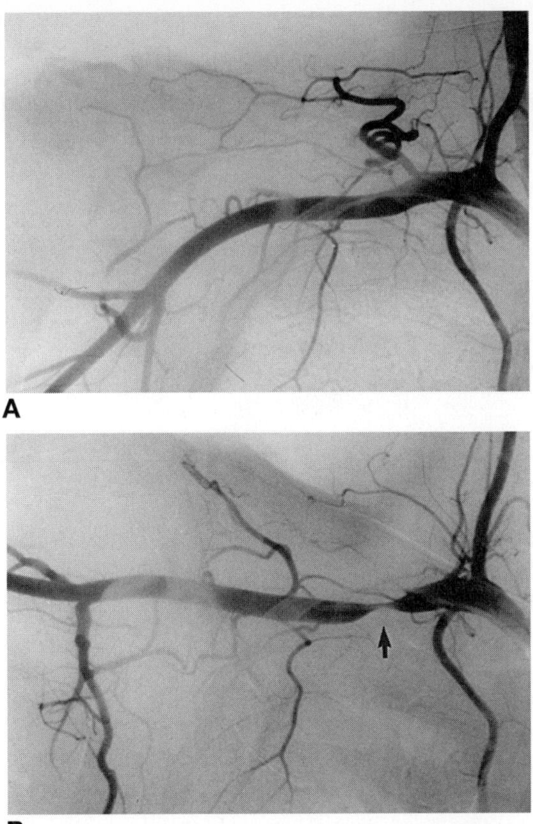

FIG. 15–5. Arteriogram of a professional baseball pitcher demonstrating **(A)** neutral position of subclavian artery and **(B)** compression of the subclavian artery *(arrow)* in the pitching position (hyperabduction). (From Yao JST: Occupational vascular problems. In Rutherford RB, ed: *Vascular surgery,* Philadelphia, 1989, WB Saunders, p 1203.)

that level and extending quickly toward the arm distally. This sequence of events is known as Paget-Schroetter syndrome, or effort thrombosis of the subclavian and axillary veins, and can occur without anatomic abnormalities. Causes of this syndrome include lifting a heavy weight with the arms down along the body, and a sudden pull of the arm to support the body weight during a fall or climbing. Baseball pitching, swimming, tennis, weight lifting, climbing, and other activities involving sudden movements with the arm may cause this syndrome. Young people are usually affected by this syndrome, because they frequently are physically active in sports.

Symptoms include a sudden sharp pain in the area of the subclavian region along the shoulder and into the arm. Within minutes, severe edema and congestion of the affected arm occur, with bluish discoloration of the arm and engorgement of the veins that extend from the shoulder level down to the fingers. It is important that the patient be treated immediately to prevent further extension of the thrombus into the arm, which can result in damage and fibrosis of the entire arm's venous network. Once this damage occurs, nothing can be done, leaving the patient permanently disabled.[20] Box 15-3 summarizes the recommended treatment for patients who present with this disorder.

Hyperhidrosis

Primary palmar hyperhidrosis is a condition marked by excessive perspiration beyond physiologic need and is reported to have an incidence of 0.6% to 1.0% in the Western population. The excessive sweating often begins in childhood and is primarily of the upper extremities but may involve the plantar surfaces of the hands and axillae as well. The symptoms range from occasional excessive sweating to constant wetness, chronic dermatitis, and fungal infections. Although the pathophysiology of the condition is uncertain, it is believed that the

BOX 15–3

Management of Paget-Schroetter Syndrome

DIAGNOSIS

Duplex ultrasound exam

Venogram—To determine extent of clot once diagnosis is established with ultrasonography

TREATMENT

Intravenous (catheter-directed) thrombolytic therapy

Possible percutaneous transluminal angioplasty (PTA) and/or venous stent placement

Systemic anticoagulation for 3 months

First-rib resection for residual compression

PTA for residual stenosis

overactivity of the sympathetic cholinergic fibers passing through the upper dorsal sympathetic ganglia at T2-T3 causes abnormal innervation of the eccrine glands responsible for sweat secretion, resulting in subsequent vasoconstriction and cooling of skin.

Hyperhidrosis is a peculiar condition in which sweating exceeds thermoregulatory needs. Sweat glands are anatomically normal but respond abnormally to certain stimuli such as anxiety and stress, chewing, or sudden temperature shifts. It is considered a benign condition; however, the psychologic, social embarrassment, and professional burden to those afflicted with hyperhidrosis can be disabling.

There are numerous conservative therapies used in the treatment of hyperhidrosis, including antiperspirants, tap water iontophoresis, botulinum toxin A, anticholinergic drugs, atropine-like medications, and psychotherapy. Most patients, however, seldom find permanent relief from conservative management.

HISTORY AND PHYSICAL EXAMINATION

In the majority of patients, the diagnosis is determined by careful history and physical examination. The identification of acute hand ischemia related to upper-extremity trauma, cardiac catheterization, or other arterial diagnostic or monitoring procedures is relatively straightforward. A history of renal failure requiring hemodialysis should include diagrams of previous arteriovenous fistulae or shunts. Previous infections, graft problems, and ischemic symptoms should be noted. When a history of previous cardiac valve prosthesis, cardiac arrhythmias (especially atrial fibrillation), or myocardial infarction is obtained, embolization is the likely cause. Intraarterial injection of drugs of abuse can be determined by history as well.

An occupational history may reveal repetitive trauma to the hand by either blunt (hypothenar hammer syndrome) or vibratory mechanisms, which can result in acute or chronic hand ischemia. Specific questions regarding athletic endeavors, training methods, or repetitive strenuous motions should be asked. Many cases of atherosclerotic upper-extremity arterial disease have a history of atherosclerotic problems elsewhere, most commonly coronary artery disease, cerebrovascular disease, or lower-extremity arterial occlusive disease. Documentation of tobacco use, sensitivity to cold, diabetes mellitus, familial diseases, medication history (especially vasoconstrictors, ergot alkaloids, dopamine), drug sensitivities, and previous operations or irradiation is of importance as well.

Physical examination of the upper extremity should begin with inspection. The presence of gangrene, muscular atrophy, swelling or edema, and discoloration, such as blanching, erythema, or cyanosis, should be documented. Microemboli produce characteristic punctate lesions on the fingertips that are associated with cyanosis (Fig. 15-6). Ischemic changes

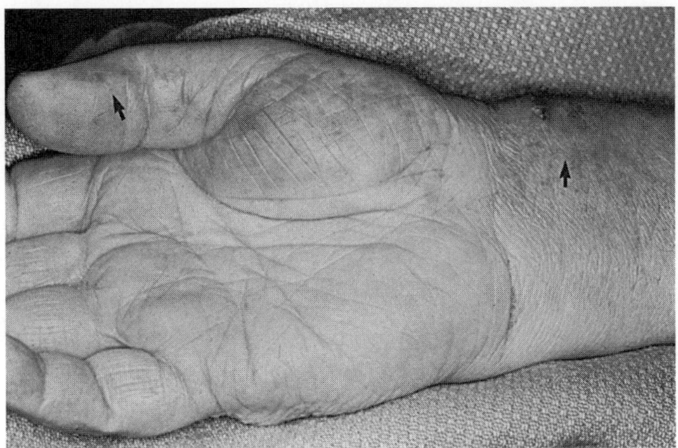

FIG. 15–6. Pseudoaneurysm of the radial artery *(right arrow)* due to arterial line trauma. Note the punctate lesions on the thenar eminence *(left arrow)* from distal microembolization.

secondary to scleroderma can often be identified because of the tight, shiny, atrophic skin characteristic of this systemic disorder.

Exposure to the cold may prompt the characteristic color changes associated with Raynaud's phenomenon. Symmetric blanching of the digits due to spastic closure of the small arterioles is followed by cyanotic mottling as cutaneous flow resumes sluggishly. This is followed by a hyperemic phase, with purplish rubor that remains for several minutes after rewarming.

In cases of trauma, careful description with drawings of upper-extremity wounds, puncture sites, and arm circumferences is vital. In some patients with acute arterial ischemia, increases in the pressure within the muscular compartments of the forearm may result in a tense, swollen, painful arm. Measurement of upper arm and forearm circumferences at initial assessment and at later examinations may be valuable.

Auscultation may reveal bruits at areas of arterial stenosis and should be performed over the subclavian, axillary, and brachial arteries in both neutral and hyperabducted arm positions. Pulses in the carotid, axillary, brachial, radial, and ulnar arteries should be palpated. The examination should include assessment of the pulse strength, an estimation of the character of the underlying artery (compliant vs. sclerotic), and a description of any aneurysm dilation or tortuosity. The disappearance of upper-extremity pulses during hyperabduction may provide a clue to the diagnosis of thoracic outlet syndrome.

The Adson maneuver is one method of demonstrating compression of the subclavian artery at the thoracic outlet. With the patient sitting erect, the radial pulse is located and continuously palpated while the patient inspires deeply and turns the head strongly to the affected side. The tension of the scalenus anticus muscle against the first rib results in compression of the subclavian artery in the narrow thoracic outlet. Although the Adson maneuver may be positive in a significant number of persons who have no evidence of upper-extremity ischemia, it may be important in patients with no obvious source of upper-extremity ischemia and lead to the diagnosis of a potentially curable lesion.

The Allen test is another maneuver that should be performed routinely to assess patency of the palmar arch. In this maneuver, the radial and ulnar arteries are compressed while the patient makes a fist to evacuate the blood from the hand. When the hand is open, the palm appears pale and mottled. In a patient with a normally patent palmar arch, release of either the radial or the ulnar artery results in prompt, even reactive hyperemia of the entire palm, with disappearance of the pallor and mottling. In the presence of radial artery occlusion, however, release of radial artery compression while occlusion of the ulnar artery is maintained does not relieve the pallor and mottling. Only on release of the ulnar artery compression does perfusion return to the hand. Likewise, with ulnar artery occlusion, color returns to the hand only after release of the radial artery, which is supplying the majority of perfusion to the hand (see Fig. 4-3).

Upper-extremity examination should be supplemented by a complete physical examination. Specific areas of interest include examination for signs of previous cerebrovascular accident, auscultation of the carotid arteries for bruits, complete cardiac evaluation, and a thorough investigation for aortoiliac or lower-extremity arterial disease. At times, systemic diseases responsible for upper-extremity ischemia result in signs or symptoms in the feet or lower extremities that are similar to those seen in the upper extremities.

DIAGNOSTIC EVALUATION

The diagnostic evaluation of patients with symptoms suggestive of upper-extremity arterial ischemia centers on establishment of the diagnosis and documentation of the location and degree of hemodynamically significant lesions. Noninvasive vascular testing (see Chapter 5) has become an important supplement to the clinical evaluation of patients with a variety of arterial and venous diseases but is especially applicable to upper-extremity arterial insufficiency. Although arteriography remains the definitive diagnostic tool, especially in patients who require operative intervention, it can now be used selectively on the basis of noninvasive hemodynamic test results.

Noninvasive Testing

The continuous-wave direction Doppler probe is the instrument most commonly used for upper-extremity arterial examinations. Flow velocity waveforms obtained by placement of the ultrasound probe over the subclavian, axillary, brachial, ulnar, radial, and digital arteries normally are triphasic. In the presence of significant proximal arterial stenosis, however, the arterial signal becomes damped and monophasic. Comparison with the opposite upper extremity is useful.

Patency of the palmar arterial arch can be determined by obtaining arterial waveforms at the midthenar and hypothenar regions in the hand. By alternately compressing the ulnar and radial arteries, the examiner can easily determine the vessel responsible for supplying the palmar arch and the one most responsible for the circulation of the hand. This is similar to the Allen test.

Arterial waveforms can also be obtained at the common digital vessel at the base of each finger and at the proper digital vessels along the shaft of each finger. Again, interpretation is dependent on comparison with more proximal waveforms and with the opposite extremity. The inability to detect any flow in an underlying artery with the directional Doppler probe is usually diagnostic of total occlusion of that particular artery.

In addition to the waveform analysis, the continuous-wave Doppler probe can be used to determine systolic blood pressures at different levels in the upper extremity. This is done by placing a regular blood pressure cuff on the upper arm and forearm and listening with the Doppler probe at the brachial, radial, and ulnar arteries, respectively. More distal blood pressure measurements are possible with the use of very small (2.5 cm) specialized blood pressure cuffs at the base of each finger. A reduction in the systolic blood pressure of more than 20 mm Hg is significant. For example, a reduction in the upper arm blood pressure when compared with the opposite extremity signifies innominate, subclavian, axillary, or proximal brachial arterial stenosis. A normal upper-arm blood pressure in conjunction with a reduction in the forearm blood pressure is diagnostic of distal brachial, radial, or ulnar arterial occlusive disease. Similarly, if the forearm blood pressure is normal, reduction in digital pressure implies occlusive disease distal to the major forearm arteries.

At times, in patients in whom arterial ischemia is suspected, various maneuvers may be extremely helpful in establishing the cause of upper-extremity symptoms. Patients with intermittent obstruction of the subclavian artery as a result of thoracic outlet syndrome may have an entirely normal upper-extremity arterial examination at rest. The exaggerated military position (with shoulders back and chest forward), hyperabduction of the arm, or the Adson maneuver (abduction and external rotation of the arm with the head turned first toward the arm, and then away) may result in damping of the brachial artery waveform and reduction in the upper-arm systolic blood pressure.

In patients with no evidence of proximal or digital arterial occlusion, a useful means of documenting vasospastic disorders is the digital temperature recovery time. In normal persons, the finger temperature returns to normal within 10-15 minutes after a 20-second submersion in an ice water bath. In patients with an abnormal vasospastic response to cold (Raynaud's phenomenon), finger skin temperatures return to normal much more slowly (recovery times exceeding 20-25 minutes). Bilaterally symmetric responses to cold submersion are characteristic of vasospasm. In patients with an asymmetric response, or those in whom only selected digits are affected, digital artery occlusive disease should be suspected.

As with ultrasound techniques elsewhere in the body, B-mode scanning and color flow imaging are especially useful in the diagnosis of arterial aneurysms. Atherosclerotic subclavian aneurysms, poststenotic subclavian dilatation, mycotic aneurysms, traumatic pseudoaneurysms, and even arteriovenous fistulae can be documented noninvasively.[21] Detection of small aneurysms or pseudoaneurysms, even at the palmar arch level, is possible as well (Fig. 15-7). In addition, occlusive lesions due to emboli, atherosclerotic plaque, or traumatic thrombosis at the axillary, brachial, and more distal arteries can be diagnosed with ultrasound imaging.[22]

Diagnostic Imaging

Arteriography continues to be the definitive test for the diagnosis of most arterial problems and is essential if operative intervention is to be considered. With the increasing use of noninvasive Doppler testing, however, arteriography plays a less prominent role in the evaluation of vasospastic disorders, especially when the extremity is not in jeopardy.

The transfemoral route, in which the Seldinger technique and catheters are used to selectively inject upper-extremity arteries, is the preferred method. Visualization of the aortic arch and proximal arch arteries is essential, and proximal arterial occlusive lesions, including subclavian and axillary aneurysms and ulcerative plaque, are easily identified. In assessing for thoracic outlet compression, hyperabduction maneuvers are used during arteriography. Proximal subclavian occlusion with subclavian steal and retrograde flow in the vertebral

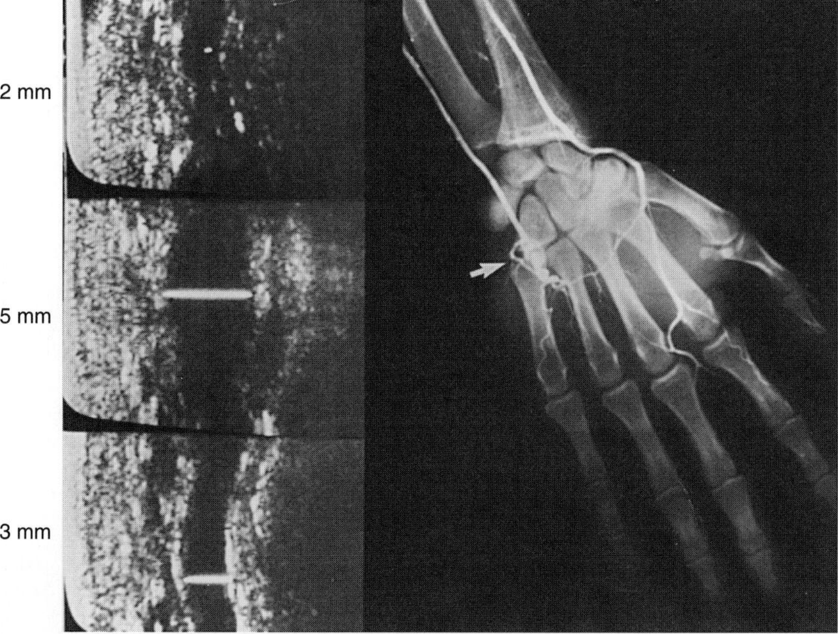

FIG. 15–7. B-mode ultrasound image of a 5-mm ulnar artery aneurysm *(left)*. The corresponding angiogram *(right)* demonstrates the aneurysm *(arrow)*.

artery is easily demonstrated arteriographically if delayed films are obtained. It is more difficult, however, to determine when angiographically detected "steal" is of clinical significance.

Arteritis of the aortic arch vessels usually causes solitary or multiple tapered stenosis without atherosclerotic plaques or ulcerations. Distinction between giant-cell arteritis and Takayasu's arteritis is difficult, however, on the basis of arteriography alone.

Atherosclerotic occlusions, embolic occlusions, traumatic lesions, and vasospasm usually are readily diagnosed by arteriography. In addition, variations in the normal arterial anatomy, which may be an important consideration at operation, and the degree of collateral circulation and distal runoff can be documented on arteriography.

Several techniques that have significantly improved the ability to visualize the small hand and digital arteries have been developed (Fig. 15-8). Warming of the hand and intraarterial injection of vasodilators, such as tolazoline hydrochloride (Priscoline) or papaverine, prevent vasospasm, which is often induced by high-pressure injection of contrast. In this way, the more distal arterial tree can usually be visualized and the vasospastic hypersensitivity characteristic of Raynaud's disease can be differentiated from vasospasm (Raynaud's phenomenon) that implies underlying arterial disease. In patients with underlying collagen vascular disease, arteriographic findings include the bilateral occurrence of distal lesions with no evidence of atherosclerosis. Typical smooth, tapering, string-like arteries or multiple segmental lesions may be seen. Collateral circulation is limited and often appears as winding "corkscrew" vessels. Routine and computerized digital subtraction techniques eliminate overlying bony shadows and significantly improve image quality as well.

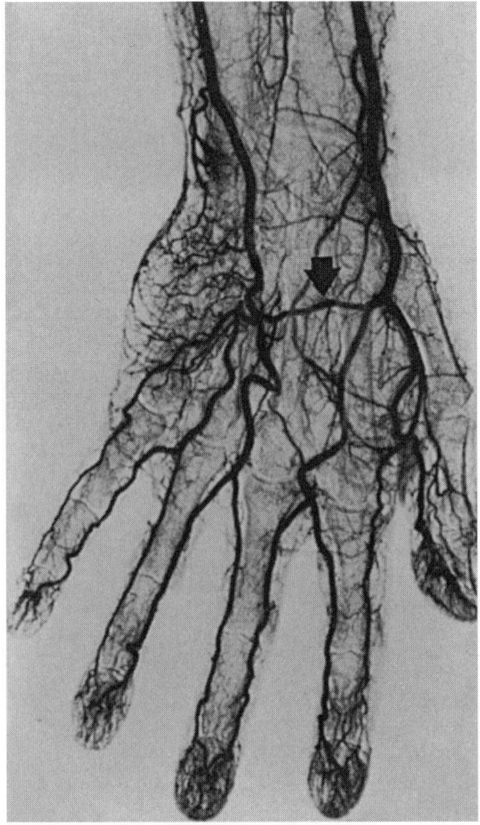

FIG. 15–8. Excellent visualization of digital arteries demonstrating a patent palmar arch *(arrow)*. (From Janevsky BK: Arteriography of the upper extremity: technique and essentials of interpretation. In Bergan JJ, Yao JST, eds: *Evaluation and treatment of upper and lower extremity circulatory disorders,* Orlando, Fla, 1984, Grune & Stratton, p 223.)

Refinements in computed tomography (CT) and magnetic resonance techniques have added new dimensions to diagnostic imaging for upper-extremity maladies. Cross-sectional display of vascular structures with magnetic resonance angiography (MRA), now available in most medical centers, may supplement arteriography or may offer a less invasive alternative. Technologic advances have come so rapidly that equipment and institutional experience vary widely, making comparisons of applicability difficult.

Spiral CT, electron beam CT, spin echo, and two-dimensional time-of-flight MRA imaging are just a few examples of the emerging vocabulary necessary to keep pace in this rapidly advancing field.[23] Although most operative decisions and transcatheter treatment options continue to be directed by conventional arteriography, the complicated anatomy of the thoracic outlet is displayed much more thoroughly by CT or magnetic resonance imaging (MRI). Fully three-dimensional vascular imaging is now possible, but the role of this exciting new information is yet to be determined.

Laboratory Evaluation

Routine hospital admission laboratory testing is usually not helpful in patients with upper-extremity arterial ischemia. In patients with atherosclerotic arterial occlusive disease, additional information is seldom provided by laboratory evaluation; however, appropriate testing for diabetes mellitus (fasting glucose, glucose tolerance test), hyperlipidemia (serum lipid profile), renal disease (creatinine, blood urea nitrogen, serum electrolytes, urinalysis), hypercalcemia (serum calcium, phosphorus, albumin, protein), or hypercoagulable states (see Chapter 9) may be extremely important.

Although careful inspection of the routine chest radiograph may identify a cervical rib that is causing thoracic outlet syndrome, cervical spine films may be necessary to adequately rule out this diagnosis. Electrocardiography may lead to the diagnosis of recent or remote myocardial infarction, atrial fibrillation, or other cardiac abnormalities, which might be responsible for upper-extremity embolization. More complete investigation would include 24-hour Holter monitoring, echocardiography, or transesophageal echocardiography.

Although a wide variety of serologic tests are available, they are not all useful in any individual patient. The sequence of workup for patients in whom a systemic cause of upper-extremity arterial insufficiency is suspected may vary depending on the clinical situation. Scleroderma (systemic sclerosis) and the CREST syndrome (calcinosis cutis, Raynaud's phenomenon, esophageal stricture, sclerodactyly, telangiectasis) may be suspected in patients with skin atrophy or calcinosis. Radiographs of the hands may reveal distal phalangeal tuft reabsorption or evidence of soft-tissue atrophy, and barium swallow may be diagnostic of an esophageal motility disorder. The immunologic abnormalities are less specific and include hypergammaglobulinemia, elevated serum rheumatoid factor, and antinuclear antibodies in 40-70 percent of cases.

Systemic lupus erythematosus is characterized by elevated anti-DNA antibodies, low levels of serum complement, and the presence of acute-phase reactants such as C-reactive protein and elevated fibrinogen and erythrocyte sedimentation rates. Mixed connective tissue disease, a variant of systemic lupus erythematosus, is often associated with Raynaud's phenomenon in the upper extremity. Circulating antinuclear antibodies directed against acidic nuclear proteins is the distinguishing feature of this systemic abnormality. In patients with suspected immune arteritis, the erythrocyte sedimentation rate is usually elevated; however, this test is nonspecific. At times, skin or temporal artery biopsies may be necessary before the diagnosis can be made. In patients with suspected thromboangiitis obliterans (Buerger's disease), precise diagnosis is possible only on microscopic evaluation of the involved small arteries and veins.

The detection of the abnormal serum protein cryoglobulin, which precipitates on exposure to cold, may provide a clue to excessive upper-extremity sensitivity to cold temperatures. Cryoglobulinemia may occur in an essential form or may be associated with abnormal protein production caused by other collagen vascular disorders, myeloma, lymphosarcoma, or macroglobulin anemia. In some cases, cold agglutination of red blood cells occurs when exposed to extremely cold temperatures.

TREATMENT

Methods of treatment of upper-extremity ischemia depend on the severity of ischemia, the cause, and at times, the potential for future problems.

Operative Treatment

Arterial bypass is the treatment for significant proximal arterial occlusive lesions, although endarterectomy of localized areas with vein patch angioplasty is an alternative. At the present time, bypass with prosthetic graft materials (usually polytetrafluoroethylene) is optimal because of appropriate size match and proven long-term patencies.[21] In cases of chronic arterial occlusion distal in the arm, arterial bypass has been shown to be an effective treatment (Fig.15-9). Reversed autogenous saphenous vein is the bypass graft material of choice. Arm revascularization for ischemia can be performed with reasonable mortality and morbidity rates.

Incisions commonly used for upper-extremity arterial surgery are depicted in Fig. 15-10. For the most part, intrathoracic procedures (aortic-subclavian artery bypass) have been replaced by extra-anatomic bypasses (axillary-axillary bypass, carotid-subclavian bypass [Fig. 15-11], carotid-axillary bypass) because hemodynamic improvement obtained is adequate and the complications of thoracotomy are avoided.[24] Management and potential complications following upper-extremity bypass are shown in Box 15-4.

Patients who have an acute arterial occlusion as a result of emboli or trauma are almost always considered for early operation. The treatment of embolic lesions is dependent on the severity of ischemia and the overall condition of the patient. Thromboembolectomy can at times be a fairly simple procedure in patients with acute occlusion of proximal large arteries with relatively little distal arterial thrombosis. An arteriotomy followed by removal of thrombotic debris with a balloon catheter suffices to restore distal circulation. More complicated

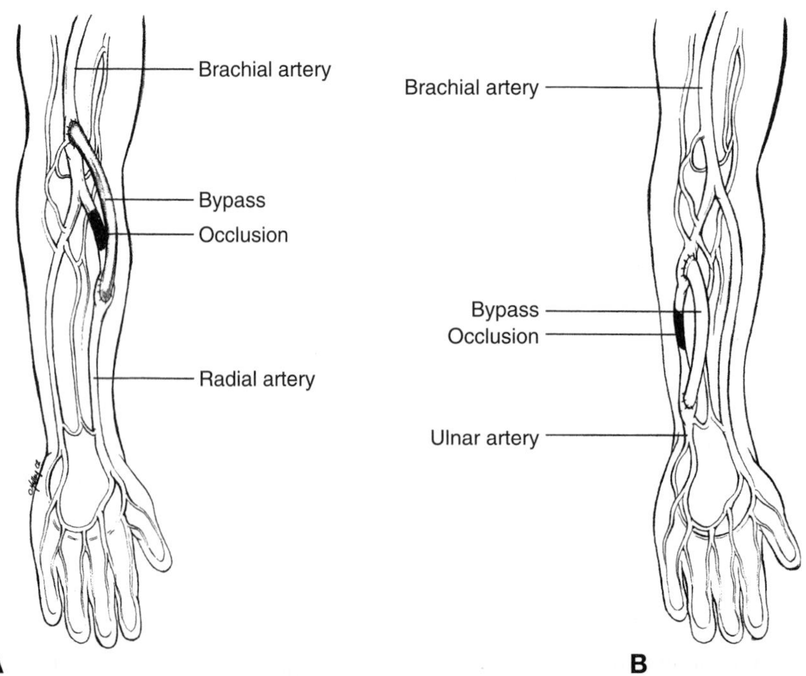

FIG. 15–9. A, Brachial-radial artery bypass. **B,** Ulnar artery bypass. (Jillian O'Malley, Copyright 2002.)

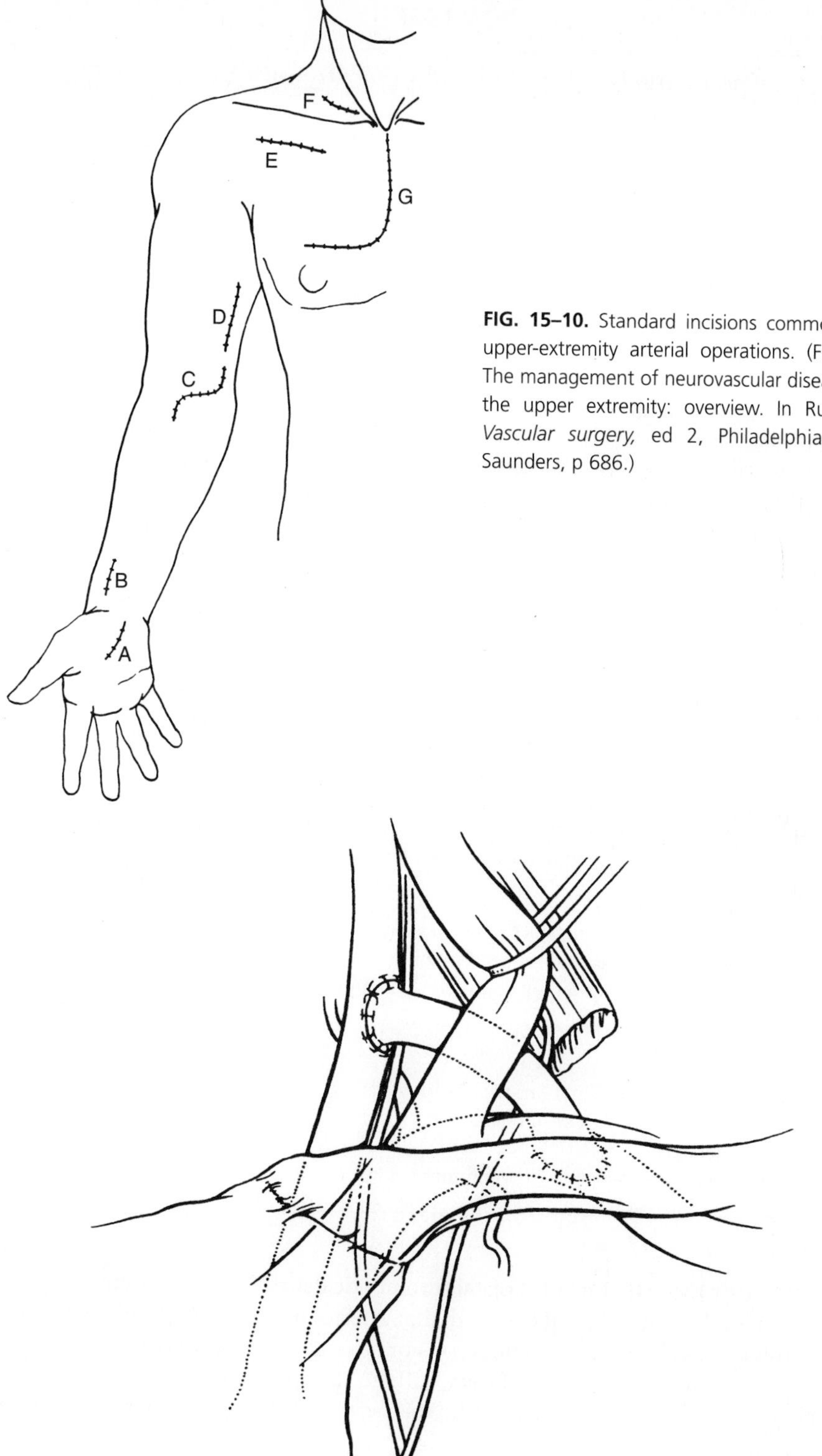

FIG. 15–10. Standard incisions commonly used for upper-extremity arterial operations. (From Roos D: The management of neurovascular diseases involving the upper extremity: overview. In Rutherford RB: *Vascular surgery,* ed 2, Philadelphia, 1977, WB Saunders, p 686.)

FIG. 15–11. Carotid-subclavian bypass tunneled under the jugular vein. (From Berguer R: Reconstruction of the supra-aortic trunks and vertebrobasilar system. In Moore WS, ed: *Vascular surgery: a comprehensive review,* Philadelphia, 1998, WB Saunders, p. 602. With permission)

BOX 15–4

Postoperative Care After Upper-Extremity Bypass

ISCHEMIA

Monitor pulses hourly by Doppler and palpation × 24 hours then q 4 hours.
Obtain forearem Doppler blood pressure (BP) q 2-4 hours × 24 hours then qd.
Assess motor and sensory function.
Monitor pain status of hands and fingers.
Check for warmth and capillary refill of extremity.

HEMATOMA/HEMORRHAGE

Monitor for swelling that may indicate hemorrhage and hematoma formation.
Observe for signs of shock, including increase in pulse, decrease in blood pressure, anxiety, restlessness, pallor, cyanosis, thirst, oliguria, clammy skin, venous collapse, and level of consciousness.
Monitor dressing/incision for excessive drainage.
Monitor for presence of false aneurysm, a pulsatile mass at the incision site.
Check laboratory values for signs of bleeding, e.g., hematocrit, hemoglobin, and notify physician if abnormal.

COMPARTMENT SYNDROME/MYOGLOBINURIA/METABOLIC COMPLICATIONS

Monitor for severe swelling of arm, which may be indicative of compartmental hypertension. Remove dressing when necessary to examine the incision site.
Assess arm and hand for motor and sensory function.
Elevate arm on pillow for mild swelling.
Observe for myoglobinuria (change in color of urine [reddish brown] and the presence of red blood cells secondary to the release of myoglobin due to muscle ischemia).
Monitor urine output and creatine level.
Monitor for hyperkalemia and acidosis due to increased concentration of lactic acid and potassium. Monitor creatine phosphokinase (CPK) levels.

IMPAIRED PHYSICAL MOBILITY

Assess reasons for immobility, the patient's range of motion, and ability to use extremity.
Encourage use of upper extremity and range of motion.
Request physical or occupational therapy consults when appropriate.
Encourage independence.

PAIN

Assess patient's pain level, type, duration, and location.
Provide comfort measures and means of distraction.
Medicate as per orders prn.
Evaluate the effectiveness of analgesic after administration.

situations, especially those that involve distal thrombotic debris, require systemic heparinization to discourage additional thrombosis of digital arteries in association with vasospasm.

In patients with subclavian artery aneurysms or arterial injury secondary to thoracic outlet syndrome, resection of the diseased artery with an interposition graft is accompanied by resection of the first rib when indicated. In this way, the thoracic outlet compression is relieved in addition to removal of the arterial abnormality. The pros and cons of treatment in patients with symptomatic thoracic outlet syndrome without obvious arterial damage are quite variable and beyond the scope of this chapter. Division of hypertrophied scalenus anticus muscles (scalenotomy or scalenectomy) in highly developed athletes may provide relief of symptoms secondary to intermittent arterial compression.

Aneurysms of the subclavian artery are treated to prevent distal embolization and thrombosis of the aneurysm. In patients with aneurysm formation in the distal arteries of the forearm or hand from occupational trauma (Fig. 15-12), resection with an interposition graft is

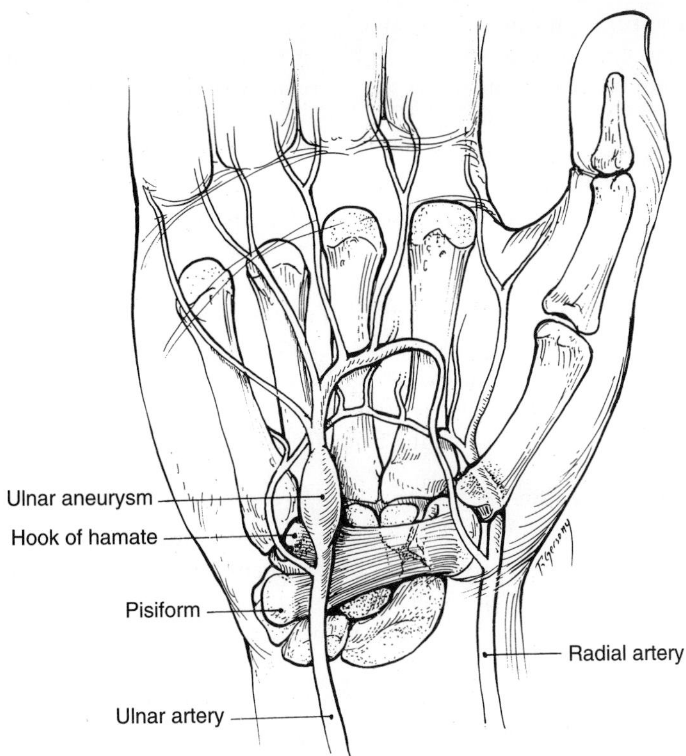

FIG. 15-12. Posttraumatic ulnar artery aneurysm in the typical anatomic position adjacent to the hamate bone and distal to the deep palmar artery. (From Dalman RL: Upper extremity arterial bypass distal to the wrist, *Ann Vasc Surg* 11:551, 1997.)

indicated. In patients with infected or mycotic aneurysms, resection with ligation of the proximal and distal vessels is performed, if collateral circulation is adequate to maintain viability of the distal extremity. At times, extra-anatomic bypass with reversed saphenous vein through uninvolved tissues is necessary.

With many iatrogenic or laceration injuries, minimal debridement with primary repair of the injured artery will suffice. Traumatic lacerations or arterial intimal injuries, however trivial, should be promptly repaired, because these may take the form of chronic thrombosis, arteriovenous fistulae, or pseudoaneurysms.[25] Vein-patch angioplasty may be necessary to avoid narrowing of the arterial lumen. In patients with blunt injuries and contaminated penetrating injuries or gunshot wounds, excision of devitalized tissue is necessary; although end-to-end arterial anastomoses are at times possible, an interposition graft of reversed saphenous vein is often required. In cases of high-velocity gunshot wounds, injuries to the accompanying nerves are responsible for the majority of functional disability postoperatively (see Chapter 22).

In the past, removal of the sympathetic ganglia (sympathectomy) was a popular treatment for a variety of upper-extremity maladies, including severe ischemia, when direct arterial repair and bypass were not possible. The theoretic benefits of sympathectomy are based on the fact that the sympathetic chain innervates arterial vasoconstrictor fibers as well as eccrine (sweat) glands. Sympathectomy removes these potential vasoconstrictors and eliminates the stimulus for sweat production. Unfortunately, the diseased atherosclerotic peripheral arteries are minimally influenced by this fine sympathetic innervation, and lasting improved perfusion is not usually seen. Some practitioners continue to use it as a last resort in selected patients with ischemic ulceration or gangrene. Short-term relief of pain, decreased tissue loss, and improved wound healing may be seen. Patients with Raynaud's syndrome in the absence of digital arterial occlusion seldom benefit from this treatment.

Posttraumatic pain syndromes (causalgia or reflex sympathetic dystrophy) may respond favorably to sympathectomy in severe cases. Best results are achieved if sympathectomy is performed before the development of fixed pain patterns or atrophic skin changes.[26] Treatment may also include physical therapy, analgesia, and stellate ganglion nerve blocks prior to sympathectomy.

Several surgical approaches, including supraclavicular, axillary, transthoracic, and cervical, are available. Surgical complications of sympathectomy are included in Box 15-5. Endoscopic and percutaneous sympathectomy are newly developed alternatives that may offer lower complication rates, but the benefit is not yet proven.[27]

Thoracoscopic sympathectomy is primarily performed for the treatment of palmar hyperhidrosis. By resecting the sympathetic chain and ganglia in the upper thoracic region (T2-T3), blood flow is increased through the cutaneous arteriovenous fistula and sweating is decreased in the ipsilateral hand. This technique has had impressive technical and patient satisfaction rates, with success rates ranging from 71 percent to 100 percent.[28]

Interventional Techniques

Thrombolytic therapy, percutaneous angioplasty, and intravascular stents and stented grafts may be used as an alternative means of treatment for thrombotic and occlusive arterial lesions. Although reports of upper-extremity transcatheter treatment experiences are limited, the results are good and parallel the broader experience in lower-extremity disease.[29]

Thrombolysis may play a role both as primary treatment and as an adjunct to surgical treatment, such as bypass or thromboembolectomy. Transcatheter approaches allow access to the upper-extremity vessels through remote routes, thus limiting direct arterial trauma and providing a means of regional delivery of thrombolytic agents. Lysis of even well-organized thrombus in larger arteries may be used, and recanalization of smaller peripheral vessels may restore flow when thromboembolectomy might not have been technically feasible. Alternatively, lysis of obscuring luminal thrombus may reveal underlying causative arterial lesions and help direct definitive treatment.[30]

Thrombolytic therapy is limited at times by the potential for serious hemorrhage either at the catheter insertion site or at remote areas. Other limitations include the relative inability of the forearm fascial compartments to expand, increasing the possibility of compartmental hypertension, and the tendency of the upper-extremity arteries to vasospasm.

Suboptimal results following arterial dilation can often be improved by the placement of an intraarterial stent. Residual stenosis due to arterial recoil, subintimal dissection, and at times, even arterial rupture can be treated successfully by stent placement.

Use of stents as primary treatment of arteriovenous fistulae or arterial lacerations secondary to subclavian trauma is inviting because direct operative repair in this area is technically challenging. Longer segments of arterial disease not amenable to dilation alone are now being treated with prosthetic grafts secured intramurally by stents. Early success in patients

BOX 15–5

Complications of Surgical Sympathectomy

- Horner's syndrome
- Postsympathetic neuralgia
- Atelectasis
- Pleural effusion
- Pneumonia
- Pneumothorax
- Winged scapula
- Hemothorax
- Subcutaneous emphysema
- Sweating in the trunk or lower extremities
- Intercostal neuralgia

with aorto-ilio-femoral disease suggests that stented grafts may be a popular option in the future, but it is difficult to predict that this modality will fulfill a similar role in upper-extremity arterial disease.[31,32]

Medical Treatment

The medical management of patients with upper-extremity ischemia is extremely variable and can be broken down into three main areas: (1) treatment of vasospasm, (2) protection from further injury, and (3) treatment of systemic diseases.

Because vasospasm is commonly a reaction to exogenous stimuli, simple removal of the stimulus is often effective. Keeping the upper extremity warm with gloves, cotton batting, avoidance of cold stimuli, or a warm water bath is an effective method of preventing cold-induced vasospasm.

Medical management of vasospasm is not uniformly effective; however, oral administration of guanethidine or calcium channel blockers such as nifedipine has shown some promise. Short-term relief may be provided in some cases by the intravenous or intraarterial administration of arterial smooth muscle relaxants (vasodilatory agents: papaverine, reserpine, Priscoline).

Protection of the upper extremity from obvious or subtle injury includes the avoidance of continued occupational trauma. Avoidance of hyperabduction of the upper extremity is important to avoid compression of the subclavian artery at the thoracic outlet.

Although there are a variety of specific medical treatments for the multitude of underlying systemic conditions that may be associated with upper-extremity ischemia, their discussion is beyond the scope of this chapter. In general, anticoagulation, regional sympathetic blockade, and administration of vasodilators, both systemically and locally, have shown no convincing proof of efficacy.[6] In the treatment of giant-cell arteritis, early initiation of steroid therapy is of proven value and often results in the restoration of upper-extremity pulses. In Takayasu's arteritis, steroids are less beneficial.

Systemic anticoagulation with heparin is indicated in patients with acute upper-extremity ischemia caused by embolization. In most instances, chronic anticoagulation should be continued with warfarin (Coumadin) in an attempt to decrease the risk of re-embolization of thrombotic material from proximal sources. Low-molecular-weight heparin products are now available as an alternative method of long-term outpatient anticoagulation.

NURSING INTERVENTION

Nursing care may have a significant impact on the outcome of treatment in patients with upper-extremity ischemia, who may have a systemic disorder responsible for or in conjunction with their upper-extremity problem. An overall nursing plan is vital.

In general, an ischemic upper extremity should not be elevated or dependent but should be kept at the level of the heart. The arms should be protected from further injury by avoidance of areas of increased pressure for any prolonged period of time. Constrictive circumferential dressings and tourniquets should be avoided, and any cast materials should be inspected for tightness on a regular basis. The forearm should be assessed for excessive swelling or tightness that might be a sign of compartmental hypertension. Routine physical examination with circulatory, motor, and sensory function is of critical importance.

Postoperative Monitoring

Patients who have had arterial repairs, upper-extremity bypass, or diagnostic or therapeutic interventions require postoperative monitoring to assure successful outcome. Box 15-4 discusses the postoperative care after upper-extremity bypass.

Although mild swelling in the upper extremity often accompanies revascularization in both acute and chronic ischemia, severe swelling is abnormal and may indicate hemorrhage and hematoma formation or compartmental hypertension. Hematomas may compress the brachial plexus or axillary nerve, and the resulting nerve damage may be permanent if decompression is not perform promptly. Hemorrhage may also take the form of frank bleeding from the wound, and in these instances, prompt exploration is often indicated. Any evidence of acutely intensified postoperative pain, upper-extremity swelling, or hemorrhage should be brought to the immediate attention of the surgeon. Mild swelling may be relieved by elevation of the arm. Nonconstricting elastic bandages may prove useful, and a sling may provide added support during ambulation.

Revascularization of acutely ischemic muscular tissue may result in systemic elevations in serum creatine phosphokinase, potassium, and myoglobin levels. This may result in excretion of these by-products in the urine (myoglobinuria), causing dark urine and possible renal dysfunction. The patient's potassium, urine output, and creatinine levels should be monitored closely.

Wound Care

Operative incisions for upper-extremity arterial surgery can be covered with dry gauze for 1-2 days postoperatively. Ischemic ulcerations or gangrenous areas on the hands or fingers are managed with gentle cleansing, conservative debridement, and dressings. Tape on the skin should be avoided. At times, wet to dry dressings will hasten debridement of slightly dirty wounds. Traumatic wounds of the upper extremity need to be kept very clean. Dressing changes should be preformed with an aseptic technique. Sharp debridement frequently plays a role in the ultimate healing process. Excessive moisture between the fingers can be prevented by lightly bandaging the hand with dry gauze between the fingers. Any bandages on the upper extremity should allow easy access for frequent physical examination of the digits and the radial and ulnar pulses. Avoid reinforcing dressings with excessive bandaging. A variety of newly developed gel dressings and enzymatic debriding agents are useful adjuncts for lesser amounts of tissue necrosis.

Patient Education

The nurse plays a vital role in the patient education process, with regard to both in-hospital care and posthospitalization management (Box 15-6). Patients welcome additional information about the disease process responsible for their upper-extremity problems, as well as information regarding the operation performed. Diagrams of upper-extremity anatomy and the specific procedures performed on individual patients are extremely useful.

Patients should be informed about their activity level postoperatively. Exercises of gradually increasing duration and intensity can be coordinated through the occupational and physical therapy departments. The patient and the family should be educated about dressing changes and wound management, allowing them to acquire the skills necessary to perform them independently. Patients usually need counseling concerning medications that will be required after their discharge from the hospital.

BOX 15–6

Patient Education

Provide diagrams of upper-extremity anatomy and surgical procedure.
Coordinate range-of-motion exercise with occupational and physical therapy.
Bathe 4-5 days after surgery.
Cover incisions for 1-2 days with a dry sterile dressing; if no drainage, leave open to air. Otherwise, all draining incisions should be covered.
Provide anticoagulation education when indicated (see Chapter 8).

SUMMARY

Although uncommon, arterial ischemia and other upper-extremity problems may be the cause of significant morbidity and disability. Recognition of the multitude of causes requires a careful, systematic approach to achieve an accurate diagnosis and ultimately to provide the appropriate treatment. Nurses play a vital role in the care of patients with upper extremity disease.

REFERENCES

1. Ehrenfeld WK, Rapp JH: Direct revascularization for occlusion of the trunks of the aortic arch, *J Vasc Surg* 2:228-230, 1985.
2. Machleder HI: Vascular disease of the upper extremity and the thoracic outlet syndrome. In Moore WS, ed: *Vascular surgery: a comprehensive review,* Philadelphia, 1998, WB Saunders, pp 613-625.
3. Yao JT: Upper extremity ischemia. In Dean RH, Yao JST, Brewster DC et al: *Current diagnosis and treatment in vascular surgery,* 1995, Appleton & Lange, pp 153-159.
4. Walker PM, Paley D, Harris KA, et al: What determines the symptoms associated with subclavian artery occlusive disease? *J Vasc Surg* 2:154-157, 1985.
5. Conn J, Bergan JJ, Bell JL: Hypothenar hammer syndrome: post traumatic digital ischemia, *Surgery* 68:1122-1128, 1970.
6. Miller CM, Sanginiolo P, Schanyer H et al: Infected false aneurysms of the subclavian artery: a complication in drug addicts, *J Vasc Surg* 1:684-688, 1984.
7. Banis JC, Rich N, Whelan TJ: Ischemia of the upper extremity due to noncardiac emboli, *Am J Surg* 134:131-139, 1997.
8. Ahmed AM, Eduards JM, Porter JM: Nonatherosclerotic vascular disease. In Moore WS, ed: *Vascular surgery: a comprehensive review,* Philadelphia, 1998, WB Saunders, pp 111-145.
9. Taylor LM, Bauer GM, Porter JM: Finger gangrene caused by small artery occlusive disease, *Ann Surg* 193:453-461, 1981.
10. Gross WS, Flanigan DP, Kraft RD et al: Chronic upper extremity arterial insufficiency: etiology, manifestations and operative management, *Arch Surg* 113:419-422, 1978.
11. Dietrich EB, Koopot R, Kinard SA et al: Treatment of microemboli of the upper extremity. *Surg Gynecol Obstet* 148:584-587, 1979.
12. Finkelmeier WR: Iatrogenic arterial injuries resulting from invasive procedures, *J Vasc Nurs* 9:12-17, 1991.
13. Valji K, Hye RJ, Roberts AC et al: Hand ischemia in patients with hemodialysis access grafts: angiographic diagnosis and treatment, *Radiology* 196:696-700, 1995.
14. Bartel P, Blackburn D, Peterson L et al: The value of noninvasive tests in occupational trauma of the hands and fingers, *Bruit* 8:15-18, 1984.
15. Ferris BL, Taylor LM Jr, Oyama K et al; Hypothenar hammer syndrome: proposed etiology, *J Vasc Surg* 31(1 Pt 1):104-113, 2000.
16. Porter JM, Snider RL, Bardana EJ et al: The diagnosis and treatment of Raynaud's phenomenon, *Surgery* 88:11-23, 1975.
17. Wilbourn AJ, Furlan AJ, Hulley W et al: Ischemic monomelic neuropathy, *Neurology* 3:447-451, 1983.
18. Hye RJ, Wolf YG: Ischemic monomelic neuropathy: an under-recognized complication of hemodialysis access, *Ann Vasc Surg* 8:578-582, 1994.
19. Fauci AS, Haynes BF, Katz P: The spectrum of vasculitis, *Ann Intern Med* 206:521-528, 1978.
20. Molina JE: Compression syndromes of the thoracic outlet. In Hiatt WR, Hirsch AT, Regensteiner J: *Peripheral arterial disease,* 2001, CRC Press, pp 417-420.
21. Brewster DC, Moncure AC, Darling RC et al: Innominate artery lesions: problems encountered and lessons learned, *J Vasc Surg* 2:99-112, 1985.
22. Payne KM, Blackburn DR, Peterson LK et al: B-mode imaging of the arteries of the hand and upper extremity, *Bruit* 10:168-174, 1986.
23. Esposito MD, Arrington JA, Blackshear MN et al: Thoracic outlet syndrome in a throwing athlete diagnosed with MRI and MRA, *J Magn Reson Imaging* 7:598-599, 1997.
24. Moore WS: Extra-anatomic bypass for revascularization of occlusive lesions involving the branches of the aortic arch, *J Vasc Surg* 2:230-232, 1985.
25. Hardin WD, O'Connell RC, Adinolfi MF et al: Traumatic arterial injuries of the upper extremity: determinants of disability, *Am J Surg* 150:266-270, 1985.
26. May J, Harris JP: Upper extremity sympathectomy: a comparison of the supraclavicular and axillary approaches. In Bergan JJ, Yao JST, eds: *Evaluation and treatment of upper and lower extremity circulatory disorders,* Orlando, Fla, 1985, Grune & Stratton, pp 69-85.

27. Malone PS, Cameron AEP, Rennie JA: Endoscopic thoracic sympathectomy in the treatment of upper limb hyperhidrosis, *Ann R Coll Surg Engl* 69:93-94, 1986.
28. Ro MK, Cantor RM, Lange KL et al: Palmar hyperhidrosis: evidence of genetic transmission, *J Vasc Surg* 33:1-5, 2001.
29. Bonn J, Soulen MC: Thrombolysis and angioplasty in upper extremity arterial disease. In Strandness DE, Van Breda A, eds: *Vascular diseases: surgical and interventional therapy,* New York, 1995, Churchill Livingstone, pp 539-555.
30. Wheatley MJ, Marx MV: The use of intraarterial urokinase in the management of hand ischemia secondary to palmar and digital artery occlusion, *Ann Plast Surg* 37:356-363, 1996.
31. Martinez R, Rodriguez-Lopez J, Torruella L et al: Stenting for occlusion of the subclavian arteries: technical aspects and followup results, *Tex Heart Inst J* 24:23-27, 1997.
32. Kumar K, Dorros G, Bates MC et al: Primary stent deployment in occlusive subclavian artery disease, *Cathet Cardiovasc Diagn* 34:281-285, 1995.

16

Renovascular Hypertension and Renal Artery Occlusive Disease

KIM MULKAY □ MARSHALL E. BENJAMIN

Renovascular hypertension (RVH) is the clinical manifestation that results from the restriction of blood flow to the kidney. Most commonly, it is the result of an occlusive lesion in the renal artery, secondary to atheroemboli, fibromuscular dysplasia, or from the more common atherosclerotic plaque. Renovascular hypertension tends to be a relatively severe form, accounting for approximately 33 percent of patients with severe hypertension.

It appears that severe hypertension at the two extremes of life carries the highest probability of being renovascular in origin. Dean et al[1] have shown that the majority of children admitted for hypertension were found to have occlusive disease of the renal arteries as the cause. After childhood, the age group that is next most likely to have RVH is the elderly. RVH is present in 7-10 percent of relatively healthy elderly Americans and in approximately 33 percent of patients over age 60 who are admitted for evaluation of hypertension.[1]

Any lesion that impedes blood flow in the renal artery can lead to RVH. The majority of lesions are located at the origin or orifice of the artery and represent "spillover" or extension of aortic disease into the renal artery (Fig. 16-1). Therefore, most of these patients are elderly, frequently with other manifestations of atherosclerosis.

Fibromuscular dysplastic lesions account for approximately 25 percent of all causes of RVH and represent an array of histologic patterns. The cause is not known. These lesions are usually classified by the layer of the artery wall most predominately involved: intimal dysplasia, medial dysplasia, medial hyperplasia, and perimedial dysplasia. Medial dysplasia is the most common, representing 85 percent of the cases. It is encountered almost exclusively in women, most commonly 50-60 years of age. On arteriographic evaluation, medial dysplasia most frequently appears as a "string of beads" (Fig. 16-2).

The coexistence of renal artery stenosis and hypertension does not establish a causal relationship. Many normotensive patients, especially those over the age of 50 years, have renal artery stenosis.

With respect to the prevalence of RVH, it is inappropriate to view all hypertensive patients in the same way. Rather, the probability of finding a renovascular cause correlates with the severity of the hypertension. Thus, the search for the disease should be directed to the subset of patients with the more severe degree of hypertension.

Because the prevalence of RVH in the entire hypertensive population is small, much effort has focused on finding demographic or physical clues that might help discriminate between RVH and essential hypertension. The most frequently cited among these are the recent onset of hypertension, young age, lack of family history of hypertension, and the presence of an abdominal bruit. The most complete study comparing the clinical characteristics of patients with RVH and those with essential hypertension was the Cooperative Study of Renovascular Hypertension.[2] In that study, the prevalence of certain clinical characteristics in 339 patients with essential hypertension was compared with their prevalence in 175 patients with RVH. The conclusion of the study was that no clinical characteristic had sufficient discriminative value to be used to exclude patients from

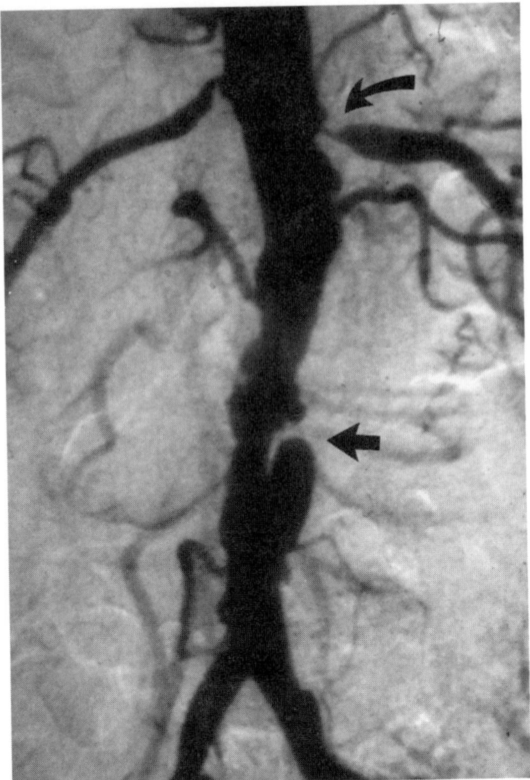

FIG. 16–1. Typical arteriogram of a patient with severe aortic disease *(straight arrow)*, as well as bilateral renal artery stenosis *(curved arrow)*.

further diagnostic investigation for RVH. Therefore, one should base the decision for diagnostic study on the severity of hypertension. The more severe the hypertension, the greater the probability that it is from a renal cause. With this in mind, one should consider evaluating all patients with a diastolic blood pressure above 115 mm Hg for a correctable origin of hypertension.

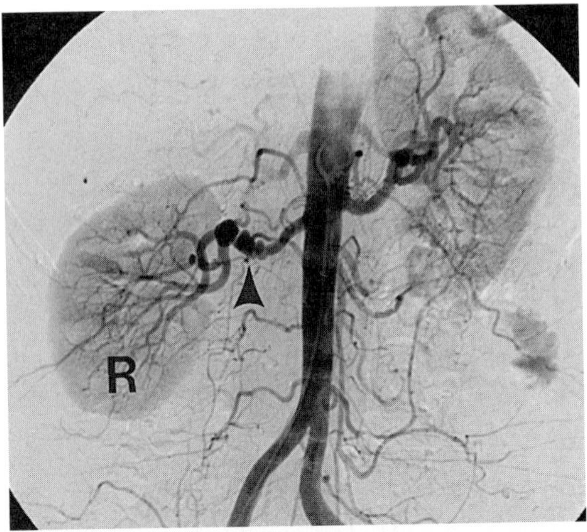

FIG. 16–2. Arteriogram showing right renal artery fibromuscular dysplasia. Note the "string of beads" appearance *(arrow)* and also note ptosis, or downward displacement, of the right kidney (*R*).

PATHOPHYSIOLOGY

Harry Goldblatt provided more support for the concept that a renal hormonal mechanism could induce hypertension. By the late 1920s and early 1930s, the association between hypertension and renal artery disease was increasingly recognized, but not proven. What was not agreed on was the order of occurrence. Did hypertension cause arteriolar sclerosis, or did primary arteriolar sclerosis produce the hypertension? Goldblatt reasoned arteriolar nephrosclerosis was the equivalent of millions of tiny vascular clamps limiting inflow into the glomerulus. Published in 1934, his observation that hypertension developed after a clamp was placed on the renal artery of dogs confirmed his suspicions: arteriolar nephrosclerosis produced hypertension. What he did not expect to find was the dissipation of hypertension that occurred when he subsequently removed the occluding clamp. These events made up the beginning of our current understanding of RVH.

In 1939, cooperative studies in the laboratories of Page in the United States and Braun-Menendez in Argentina led to the characterization of renin as a proteolytic enzyme and the discovery of a rapidly acting, potent pressor by-product. This was followed by the structural characterization of angiotensin I, angiotensin-converting enzyme, and angiotensin II by Skeggs and Lentz in the 1950s. Cook localized renin production to the juxtaglomerular apparatus by the end of that decade while the rapid conversion of angiotensin I to angiotensin II during its passage through the lungs was demonstrated by Ng and Vane in the late 1960s.[3]

The renin-angiotensin system is responsible for the hypertensive response seen with renal artery disease (Fig. 16-3). The physiologic effect of the renin-angiotensin system influences renal, cardiovascular, neural, adrenal, and microcirculatory function.

These 60 years of laboratory investigation led to an initial understanding of renovascular hypertension and the development of new methods of medical and surgical intervention. Clinical application of these discoveries has significantly improved diagnostic capabilities and has significantly lengthened or saved many patients lives.

DIAGNOSTIC EVALUATION

The most important screening tests for patients presenting with hypertension are the medical history, physical examination, and routine blood studies (Box 16-1). From this simple approach, selected patients can be identified for more complex screening tests to confirm renal artery occlusive disease. Currently, the most popular screening tests are renal duplex sonography (RDS) (Fig. 16-4) and isotope renography before and after captopril ingestion or exercise. Unfortunately, a large number of the medical community still evaluate patients for RVH only when medications are not tolerated and hypertension remains severe and uncontrolled.

General evaluation of all hypertensive patients is outlined in Box 16-1. Electrocardiography is important to gauge the extent of secondary myocardial hypertrophy or associated ischemic heart disease. Estimation of renal function is necessary. A rough gauge of excretory impairment can be obtained simply by measuring the serum creatinine. When an impairment is present, a 24-hour creatinine clearance measurement may be indicated. Finally, assessment of the urinary 17-hydroxy-corticosteroid, 17-ketosteroid, and vanillylmandelic acid (VMA) levels will effectively identify the rare patient with a pheochromocytoma or a functioning adrenal cortical tumor. These latter studies are performed only when some part of the medical history or initial assessment increases the suspicion of their presence.

Special studies are required to establish the functional significance of renal artery lesions. Many studies have come and gone over the years; however, experience has shown that properly performed renal vein renin assays can predict that a good blood pressure response can be expected following successful renal artery bypass operation in over 95 percent of cases.[4] This involves obtaining a venous blood sample from both renal veins and vena cava. If a

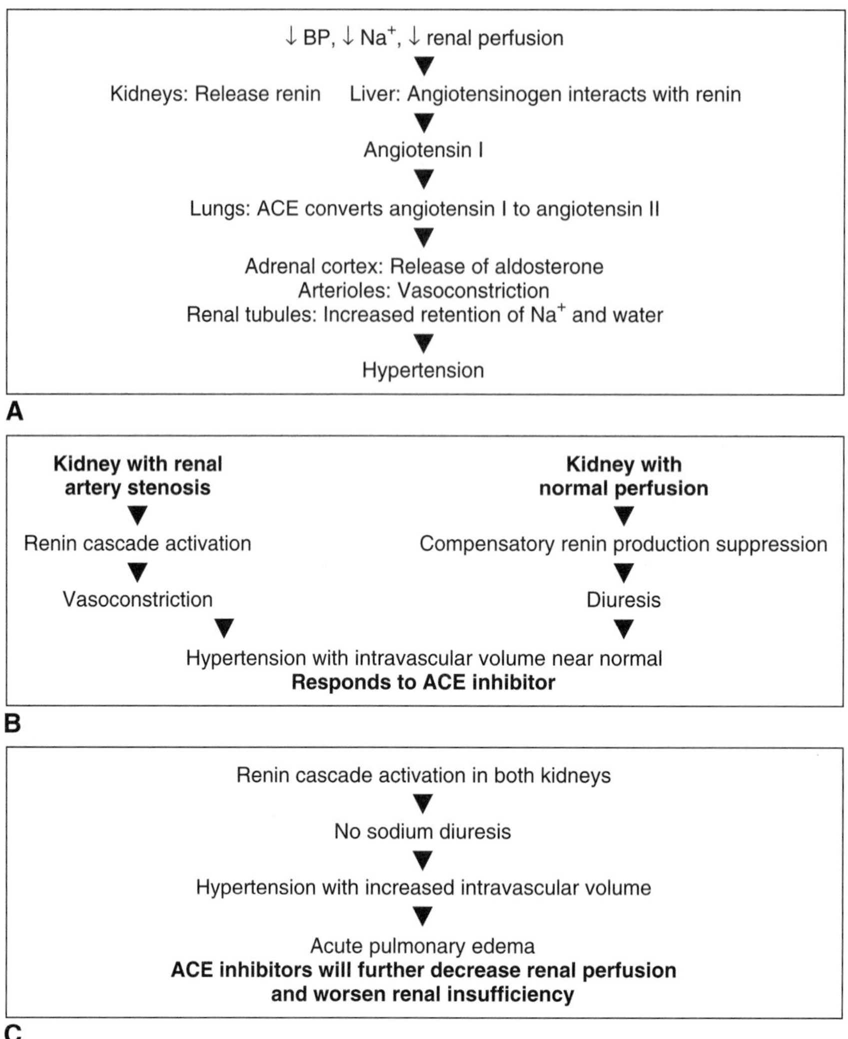

FIG. 16–3. Renin-angiotensin-aldosterone cascade. **A,** Physiologic mechanisms. **B,** Unilateral renal artery stenosis. **C,** Bilateral renal artery stenosis. *BP,* Blood pressure; *Na^+,* sodium; *ACE,* angiotensin-converting enzyme.

kidney is producing increased renin, secondary to activation of the renin-angiotensin system (i.e., from a renal artery lesion), then these elevated levels should be seen in the appropriate renal vein sample when compared to the inferior vena cava (IVC).

Isotope renography continues to be proposed as a valuable screening test, yet the methods employed are being modified continuously with the hope of improving the sensitivity and specificity. The most common version consists of renal scans performed before and after exercise or captopril infusion.[5] With these methods, a test is interpreted as positive when there is augmentation of derangements in renal perfusion following exercise or captopril infusion. Although these methods have improved the specificity of isotope renography, their reliance on activation of the renin-angiotensin system leads to an unacceptable incidence of false-negative results, especially in patients with renal dysfunction (elevated creatinine).

The screening test of choice is RDS. This examination provides both anatomic and physiologic information about the renal artery. The information obtained includes an image of the vascular anatomy, as well as the hemodynamics of the renal parenchyma and its blood flow. Similarly, vascular images using magnetic resonance imaging (MRI) may hold great promise (Fig. 16-5). Current expense, lack of widespread availability, and limitations of patient selection criteria prevent the use of this application as a widespread screening tool.

BOX 16–1

General Evaluation of Patients With Hypertension

HISTORY AND PHYSICAL EXAMINATION

- Complete blood count (CBC), electrolytes, blood urea nitrogen (BUN), creatinine, glucose, urinalysis, urine culture, serum potassium (three times)
- Electrocardiogram and chest x-ray
- Analysis of 24-hour urine collection for creatinine clearance, electrolytes, catecholamines, vanillylmandelic acid, and 17-hydroxy-corticosteroids and 17-ketosteroids (if indicated)
- Creatinine clearance
- Renal duplex sonography

RDS has been proposed by several investigators as a useful screening test with which candidates for arteriography can be identified. The group at Wake Forest University have reported their extensive experience with RDS and evaluated its sensitivity and specificity for identification of renovascular occlusive disease. When single renal arteries are present, RDS has approximately a 93 percent sensitivity, 98 percent specificity, and an overall accuracy of

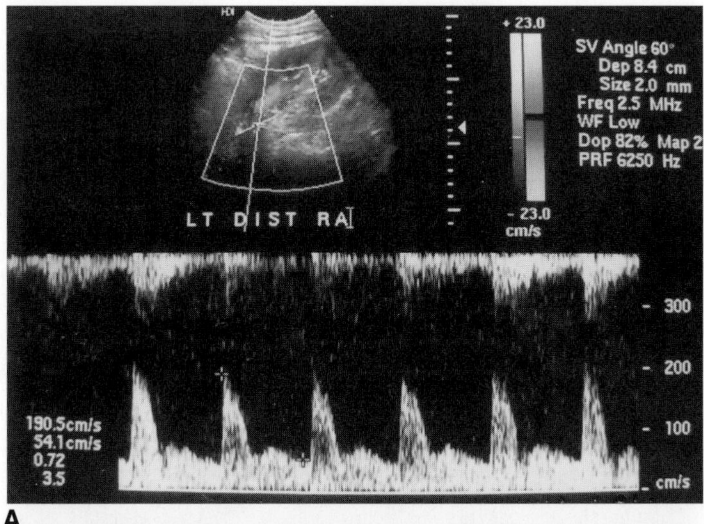

A

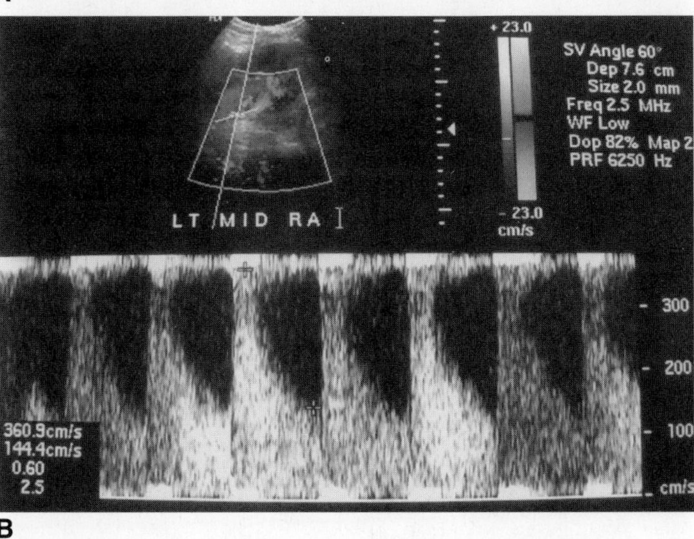

B

FIG. 16–4. A, Normal renal artery duplex ultrasound. **B,** Renal artery duplex ultrasound, showing critical (>60 percent) renal artery stenosis.

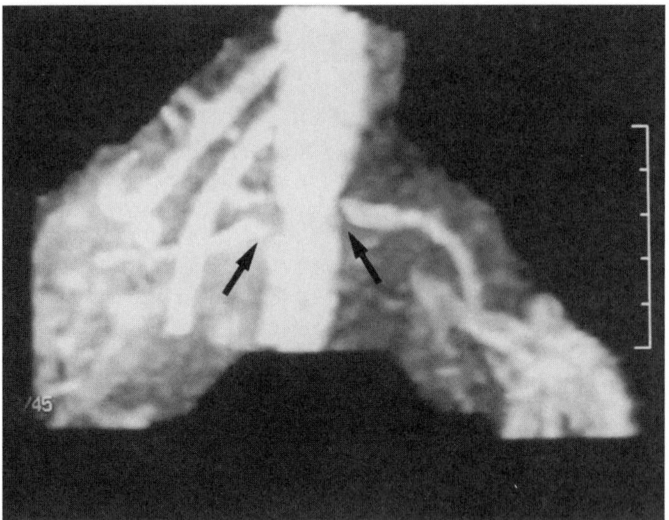

FIG. 16–5. Magnetic resonance angiography (MRA) showing bilateral renal artery stenosis (>60 percent) (*arrows*).

96 percent.[6] Thus, RDS can be a valuable screening test in the search for correctable renovascular disease causing global renal ischemia and secondary renal insufficiency (ischemic nephropathy).

Because the accuracy of RDS is limited in its identification of accessory or branch vessels, arteriography is performed when this situation is suspected or when severe hypertension occurs in pediatric-age patients.

The more invasive, intraarterial digital subtraction angiography is used to further evaluate the renal arteries in cases of a positive screening study (see Fig. 16-1). Frequently, multiple oblique and selective renal injections are necessary for adequate assessment of the renal vasculature and juxta-renal aorta (Fig. 16-6). The fact that arteriography in patients with severe renal insufficiency, especially those with concomitant diabetes mellitus, can aggravate renal failure is widely recognized and must be considered. In this setting, CO_2 angiography (Fig. 16-7) or magnetic resonance angiography may provide adequate information. Nevertheless, some imaging study of the renal artery and kidney is mandatory prior to revascularization.

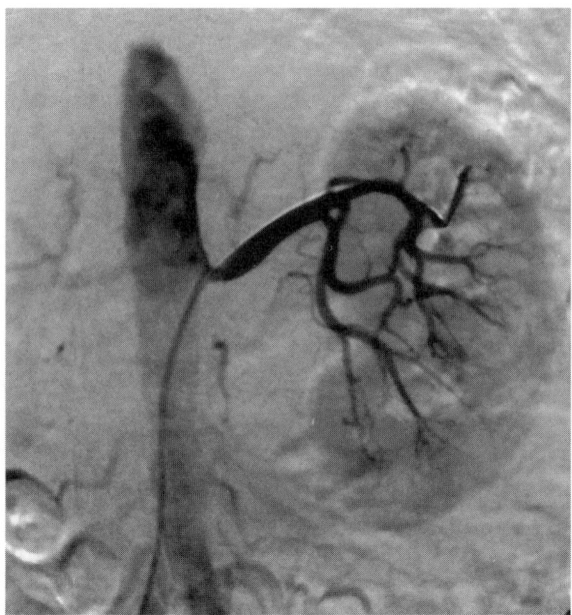

FIG. 16–6. Selective left renal arteriogram.

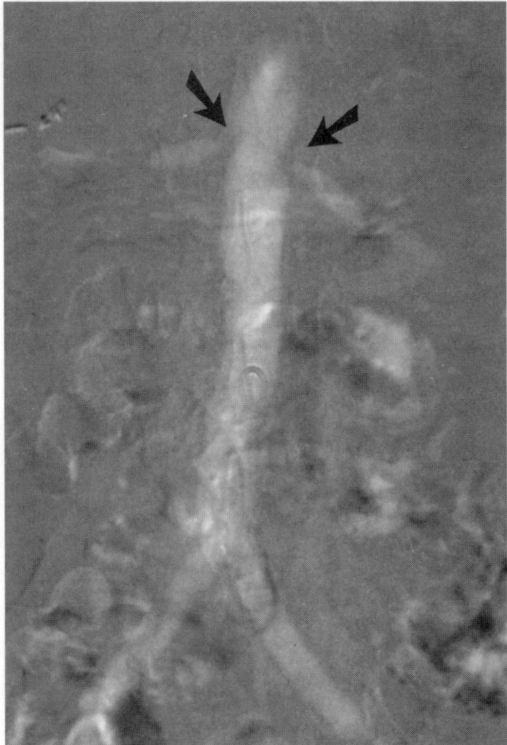

FIG. 16–7. CO_2 angiogram demonstrating bilateral renal artery stenosis (*arrows*).

CURRENT INDICATIONS FOR INTERVENTION

Indications for correction of occlusive lesions of the renal arteries have continued to evolve, yet remain controversial. Significant renal disease found at the time of an aortic reconstruction has led to an empiric and liberal approach to simultaneous renal revascularization in many centers, yet the exercise of clinical judgment in the application of a selective approach to such combined procedures is more appropriate. A prerequisite for considering simultaneous renal revascularization is the presence of hypertension. If the patient is normotensive, then operation, for the most part, should be limited to the aortic procedure. If unilateral renal artery stenosis is found in a hypertensive patient, then simultaneous renal revascularization should be considered.

When a patient has bilateral renal artery stenoses and hypertension, the decision to correct the renovascular disease simultaneously with correction of the aortic disease is based on the severity of both the hypertension and the renovascular lesions. When the two renal artery lesions are not similarly severe, but instead, there is severe disease on one side and only mild or moderate disease on the contralateral side, then the patient is treated as if only a unilateral lesion exists. If both lesions are only moderately severe (65-80 percent stenosis), then renal revascularization is undertaken only if the hypertension is severe. In contrast, if the lesions are both severe (>80 percent stenosis) and the patient has drug-dependent hypertension, then bilateral simultaneous renal revascularization is undertaken.

Our results in 133 patients who underwent combined aortorenal revascularization (simultaneous aortic and renal repair) over an 8.5-year period demonstrated perioperative mortality was higher in the combined aortorenal revascularization group (5.3 percent) than in patients undergoing isolated aortic (0.74 percent) or isolated renal (1.65 percent) repair. However, statistical significance was only reached when compared to the isolated aortic group.[6]

One of the most controversial indications for intervention is the prophylactic management of all anatomically severe lesions without regard to their functional significance, that is, even in the absence of hypertension. The typical viewpoint held by most vascular surgeons has remained rather conservative and is outlined below.

Most surgeons find no justification for prophylactic renal artery surgery, either as an independent surgical procedure or as an additional procedure performed in conjunction with infrarenal aortic surgery. More specifically, a lesion that may be found incidentally, in the absence of hypertension, for the most part should be left alone. A unilateral lesion in the presence of severe or difficult-to-control hypertension despite multiple medications should be considered for intervention.

THERAPEUTIC OPTIONS

Therapeutic options for the treatment of RVH must be carefully evaluated for each patient. Appropriate forms of therapy consist of drug therapy, percutaneous transluminal angioplasty (PTA) and renal stents, or operative management.

Percutaneous Transluminal Angioplasty and Renal Stents

The wide use of PTA has made selective application for its use appropriate in patients with uncontrolled hypertension and fibromuscular dysplasia. It is now considered the treatment of choice for patients with renovascular hypertension and fibromuscular dysplasia, as well as nonostial atherosclerotic lesions. In this regard, PTA of nonostial atherosclerotic lesions has an immediate success rate of 72-82 percent, as compared to 60-62 percent success rate for PTA of ostial atherosclerotic renal-artery stenosis.[7] PTA of medial fibrodysplastic lesions in the main renal artery yields an 82-100 percent success rate; these results are comparable to the results of surgery if carried out by surgeons experienced in this technique.[8] In contrast, the use of PTA for the treatment of congenital lesions, fibrodysplastic lesions involving renal artery branches, and ostial atherosclerotic lesions is associated with inferior results and increased risk of complications.

The idea of stenting the renal artery (Fig. 16-8) was first introduced in the United States in 1988 as part of a multicenter trial, with 263 patients entered into the trial.[9] During this

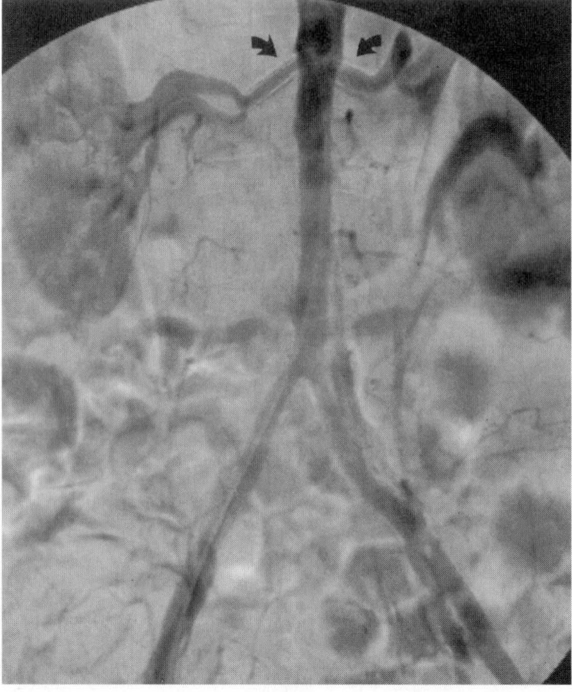

FIG. 16–8. Arteriogram showing bilateral renal artery stents (*arrows*).

same period, the Palmaz and Wall stents were being used in Europe. Currently, no stent has been approved for renal artery use in the United States. The most common indications for renal artery stenting include (1) elastic recoil of the vessel immediately after angioplasty, (2) dissection after angioplasty, and (3) restenosis after angioplasty. Improvement or cure in hypertension was seen in only 61 percent at 1 year in this multicenter trial, and angiographic restenosis occurred in 32.7 percent of patients in follow up of less than 1 year.[9]

These multicenter results have not been overly impressive when compared to contemporary surgical results (see below), and for this reason, we believe that renal artery bypass surgery remains the initial treatment of choice for select good-risk patients.

These studies have shown that when the intervention was for the treatment of hypertension alone, a beneficial result was achieved in approximately 60 percent of those treated with PTA and stent versus approximately 90 percent for those treated surgically. When the intervention was for ischemic nephropathy, the differences were even more dramatic. PTA and stent yielded a beneficial response in approximately 13 percent of patients versus 60 percent treated surgically.[9] Thus, at our center, we believe that when treating RVH, the beneficial hypertensive response between percutaneous and operative therapy is small. If the patient has ischemic nephropathy, however, the optimal outcome is with surgical revascularization even considering the magnitude of the operation.

Given the high recurrence rate of PTA and stenting, approximately 30 percent at 1 year, repeat PTA and stent is not rare and carries a higher risk.[9] Additionally, if unsuccessful, a subsequent surgical intervention is limited and more difficult.

Techniques for Renal Revascularization

When possible, it is preferable to delay surgical revascularization for at least 24 hours after arteriography. In addition, since approximately one third of these patients will have a contractive blood volume due to chronic diuretic therapy or the disease itself, overnight intravenous hydration is of critical importance prior to revascularization. Failure to correct this deficit may lead to operative hypotension and further insult on an already compromised kidney. A pulmonary artery catheter to monitor myocardial performance and fluid balance, as well as a radial artery catheter to monitor blood pressure, are standard and typically continued for the first 48 hours after operation. Mannitol (12.5 mg) is administered intravenously approximately 10 minutes before renal artery cross-clamping, and heparin (100-200 units/kg) is given intravenously.

Aortorenal Bypass

Aortorenal bypass is customarily performed with either autogenous saphenous vein and rarely, autogenous hypogastric artery or some type of synthetic prosthesis.[6] When a synthetic prosthesis is preferred, polytetrafluoroethylene (PTFE) has proven to be technically superior to Dacron with regard to the ease of handling and suturing to the small renal vessels. The use of synthetic grafts is limited to instances of proximal atherosclerotic lesions where the distal renal artery is relatively large (>4 mm in diameter). In most circumstances, autogenous saphenous vein is preferred for renal artery bypass, regardless of whether the etiology is atherosclerotic or fibromuscular dysplasia, even when the repair extends to the branch level.[6]

When an end-to-side renal artery bypass is employed (Fig. 16-9, *A*, *B*, and *C*), the distal anastomosis is performed first. Since this is generally the most difficult anastomosis, it is easier if the graft is completely mobile. The aortic anastomosis is then performed. The aorta is cross-clamped below the renal arteries, and a portion of aortic wall is excised.

In contrast to the end-to-side bypass technique, when performing an end-to-end renal artery bypass, the proximal aortic anastomosis is constructed first. With completion of the proximal anastomosis, the native renal artery is ligated proximally and transected (Fig. 16-9, *A*, *B*, and *D*). The renal artery and graft are then spatulated, and the anastomosis completed with 6/0 monofilament suture. This technique minimizes renal ischemia time.

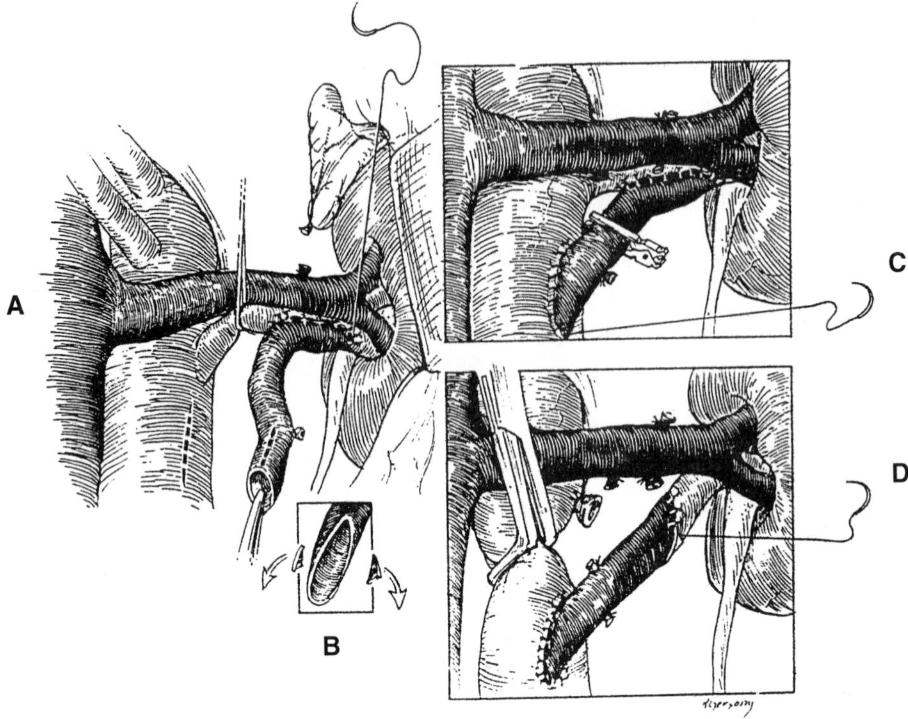

FIG. 16–9. Diagram of renal artery bypass showing **(A)** exposure and distal anastomosis, **(B)** vein spatulation, and **(C)** end-to-side and **(D)** end-to-end configurations. (With permission from Benjamin ME, Dean RH: Techniques in renal artery reconstruction, part I, *Ann Vasc Surg* 10:306-314, 1996.)

Renal Artery Thromboendarterectomy

TRANSRENAL TECHNIQUE (TRANSVERSE AORTOTOMY). In some cases of bilateral atherosclerotic disease of renal artery origin, simultaneous bilateral endarterectomy may be the most appropriate method of revascularization. The preference in most instances is a transverse or transrenal incision (Fig. 16-10, A, B, C). This arteriotomy is carried out across the aorta and along the renal artery to a point beyond the stenosis. With this technique, the distal intima can be inspected directly. Following completion of the endarterectomy, the arteriotomy is usually closed with a Dacron or PTFE patch angioplasty to ensure that the newly repaired renal artery is left widely patent (Fig. 16-11). Intraoperative duplex sonography is used to verify a flawless technical result (Fig. 16-12).

Renal Artery Reimplantation

Frequently, the renal artery is redundant after it has been dissected from the retroperitoneal tissue. When the disease is limited to the origin, and the artery sufficiently redundant, the renal artery can be transected, spatulated, and reimplanted into the aorta slightly inferior to its native location. This is especially advantageous in children, thereby eliminating the need for a graft (Fig. 16-13).

Ex Vivo Renal Revascularization

Disease affecting the renal hilar vessels requires a more extensive exposure through Gerota's fascia, the fascia directly covering the kidney, and usually an ex vivo reconstruction. The usual etiologies for this pattern of disease include fibromuscular dysplasia, renal artery aneurysm, or dissection. The preferred approach for complex branch renal artery disease requiring ex vivo revascularization without autotransplantation is an extended subcostal incision, carried to the posterior axillary line.[6] A midline xiphoid to pubis incision is reserved for revascularizations where combined aortic reconstruction is planned. The ureter is always mobilized, but left

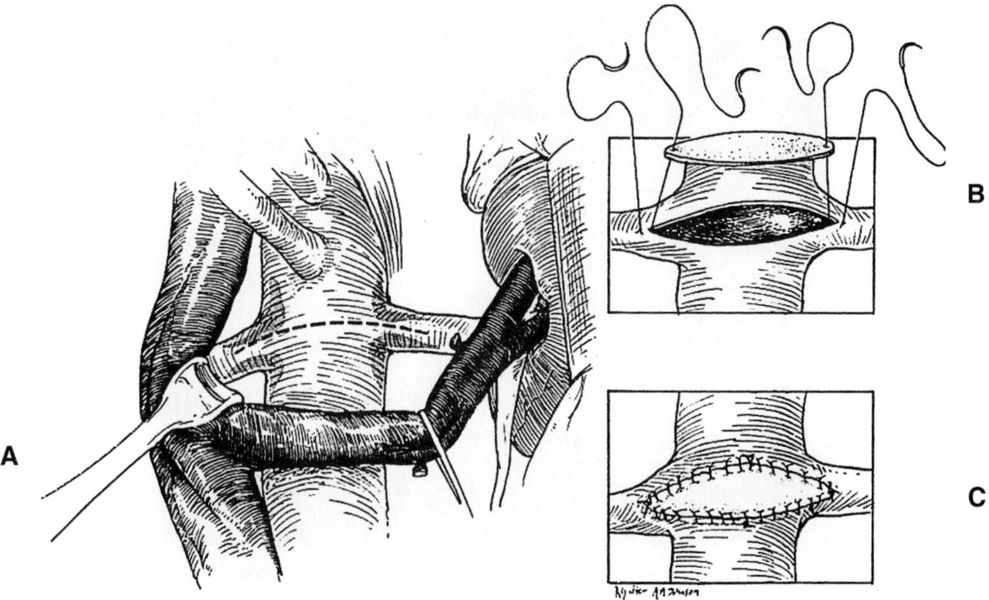

FIG. 16–10. Diagram of transrenal endarterectomy. **A,** General exposure and transrenal aortotomy. **B,** Patch angioplasty following endarterectomy. **C,** Completed patch closure. (With permission from Benjamin ME, Dean RH: Techniques in renal artery reconstruction, part I, *Ann Vasc Surg* 10:306-314, 1996.)

intact with a silastic sling placed around it to prevent collateral perfusion, inadvertent rewarming, or continued blood loss through the ureter. Before the renal vein is transected, a large vascular clamp is positioned to partially occlude the vena cava where the renal vein enters the cava. A small ellipse of the vena cava wall is excised with the renal vein, as the vessels are divided. The kidney is mobilized, placed on the abdominal wall, and perfused with a renal preservation solution. Chilled "transplant" solution (500 ml) is flushed through the kidney immediately, and, after each anastomosis is completed, an additional 150-200 ml of solution

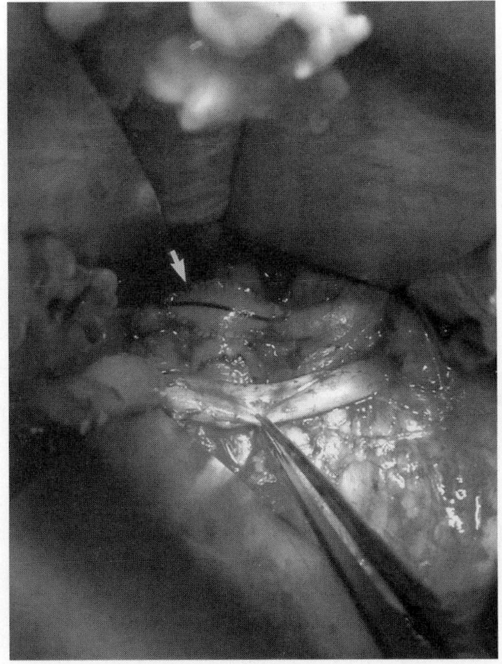

FIG. 16–11. Intraoperative photograph of transrenal endarterectomy with Dacron patch closure (*arrow*).

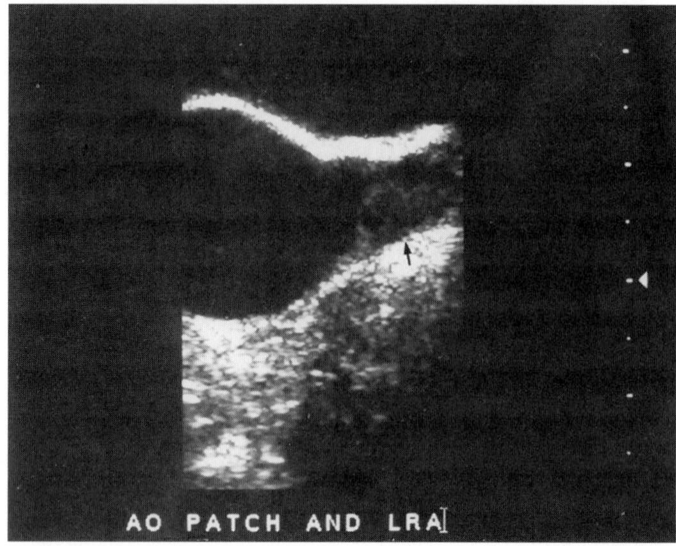

FIG. 16–12. Intraoperative duplex ultrasound of the same patient as in Fig. 16-11.

are infused (Fig. 16-14). It provides excellent protection during the relatively short period (2-3 hours) required for the ex vivo dissection and reconstruction, although surface hypothermia is employed. A constant drip of chilled saline solution can maintain renal core temperatures of 10°C to 15°C throughout the period of reconstruction. With completion of the arterial anastomoses, the kidney is placed back in its native bed and the ellipse of vena cava is reattached to its original position with the running monofilament suture. The renal artery graft is then attached to the aorta in a standard end-to-side fashion. Finally, the envelope of Gerota's fascia is reattached to secure the kidney in its original position. A branched segment of the greater saphenous vein is the commonly employed bypass conduit.

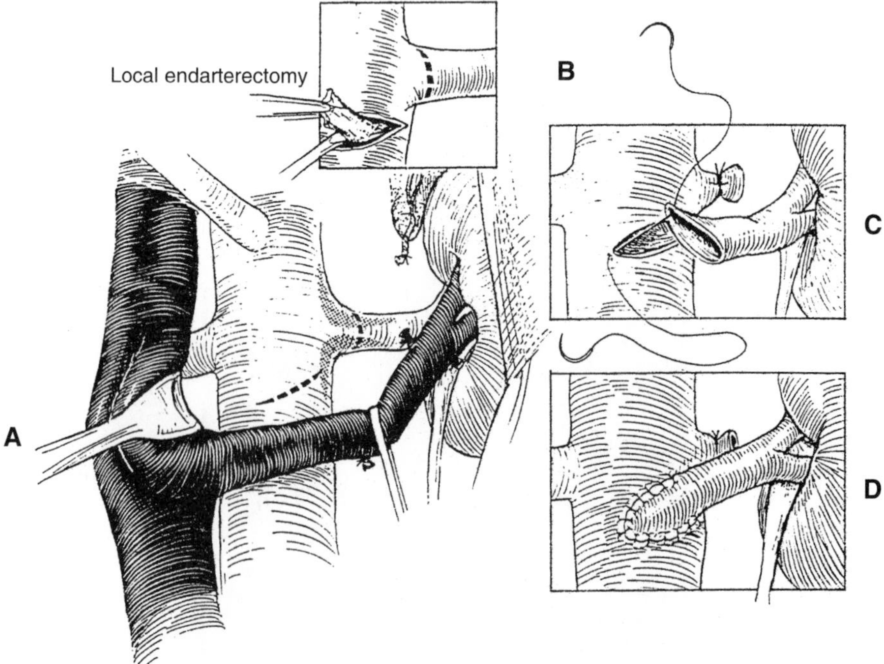

FIG. 16–13. Diagram of renal artery reimplantation. **A,** General exposure. **B,** Local aorta endarterectomy at proximal anastomosis. **C,** Ligation of left renal artery and proximal anastomosis. **D,** Completed reimplantation. (With permission from Benjamin ME, Dean RH: Techniques in renal artery reconstruction, part I, *Ann Vasc Surg* 10:306-314, 1996.)

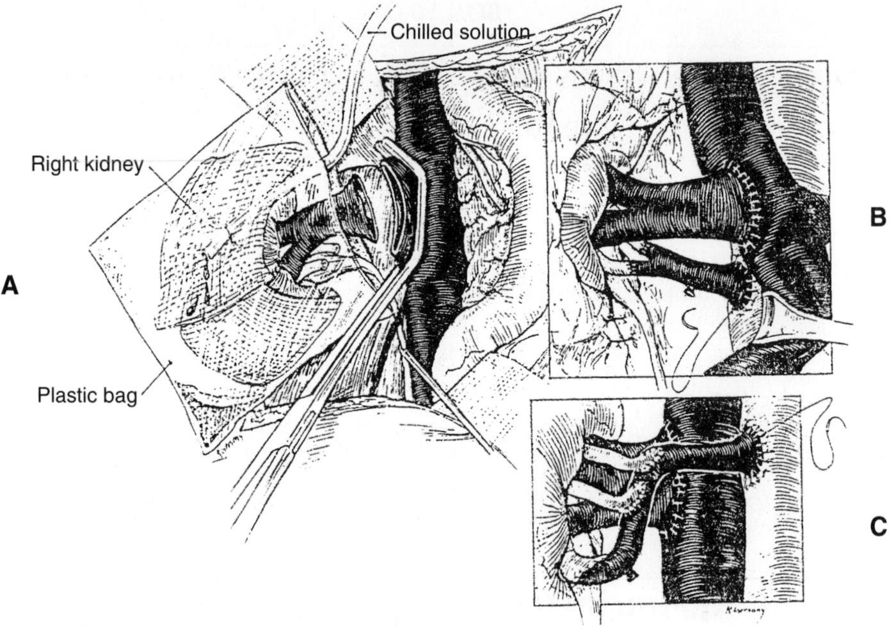

FIG. 16–14. Diagram of the ex-vivo type of renal artery repair. **A,** Intraoperative set-up. **B,** Bifurcated saphenous vein interposition graft for arterial reconstruction. **C,** Various arterial configurations for arterial reconstruction. (With permission from Benjamin ME, Dean RH: Techniques in renal artery reconstruction, part II, *Ann Vasc Surg* 10:409-414, 1996.)

Nephrectomy

Nephrectomy is usually limited to the minority of patients with renovascular hypertension in whom the kidney responsible for the hypertension has nonreconstructable vascular disease or minimal residual excretory function. In these situations, nephrectomy can allow for improved control of the blood pressure with minimal effect on overall excretory function. In all other circumstances, when some measure of excretory renal function exists, we believe that exploration and attempted revascularization is far better than nephrectomy.[6]

Effect of Surgery on Hypertension

Most of the controversy surrounding the role of operative treatment of RVH relates to the risk of operation, unacceptable frequency of technical failures, and a low rate of favorable blood pressure response to operation. The literature adequately documents the fact that poorly performed operations in poorly selected patients will result in a less favorable blood pressure response. Current results of operative intervention in centers experienced in the management of RVH, however, underscore the predictability of success. Most of these centers have found a beneficial hypertension response in approximately 90 percent of patients with atherosclerotic renal disease.[10] For patients with nonatherosclerotic disease (i.e., fibromuscular dysplasia), a higher beneficial hypertension response is typically seen.

NURSING CARE

Close attention must be paid to patients having undergone renal artery bypass surgery or angioplasty and stenting. Strict monitoring of blood pressure, intake and output, and response to any antihypertensive medications should be documented. Renal function is followed with serial blood urea nitrogen (BUN) and creatinine levels, and patency of the renal arteries is assessed by RDS. Patient education at all levels, including explanation of and preparation for diagnostic testing, intervention, and follow-up care, is important (Box 16-2).

BOX 16–2

Nursing Management of Patients With Renovascular Hypertension

PATIENT EDUCATION RELATED TO:
- Diagnostic testing: renal duplex sonography, magnetic resonance imaging, angiography
- Renal artery angioplasty and stenting
- Renal artery bypass surgery

POSTOPERATIVE MONITORING
- Blood pressure, including medication and response
- Intake and output
- Blood urea nitrogen (BUN) and creatinine levels

FOLLOW-UP CARE
- Surveillance renal artery duplex scans
- BUN and creatinine as indicated

ISCHEMIC NEPHROPATHY

As the preceding section has shown, renovascular hypertension, when properly recognized, diagnosed, and treated, can carry an excellent prognosis. Historically, diagnostic and therapeutic strategies have focused on restoring adequate renal blood flow to alleviate hypertension secondary to stimulation of the renin-angiotensin system. More recently, however, decreased excretory function (i.e., renal failure), also resulting from inadequate renal blood flow, has been recognized and cited as an indication for renal revascularization.[11] The term given to decreased renal excretory function in an ischemic kidney has been *ischemic nephropathy*. In this section, we will briefly review the diagnosis and treatment of this disease entity.

Ischemic nephropathy may be present in up to 24 percent of patients 50 years of age or older who have chronic or progressive renal failure.[7] Once patients become dialysis dependent from ischemic renovascular disease, their prognosis is extremely poor. In a study evaluating mortality in dialysis-dependent patients, Mailloux et al[12] found end-stage renal disease (ESRD) from a renovascular cause to have the highest associated mortality from all causes of ESRD. In that subset of patients, the median survival was 27 months and the 5-year survival rate following dialysis initiation was 12 percent. This equates to a death rate in excess of 20 percent per year.

Diagnosis and Treatment

The recent onset of renal insufficiency in a hypertensive patient in the atherosclerotic age group warrants evaluation for possible ischemic nephropathy. Accordingly, at our center, using RDS, we currently screen all patients over 50 years of age with new onset of renal insufficiency (creatinine >2.0 mg/dl) and concomitant hypertension of any magnitude. A positive RDS study warrants further imaging (i.e., angiography, CO_2 angiography, or MRI/MRA) to plan operative strategy in suitable candidates. Our conviction is that the risk associated with medical management and eventual dialysis are significant and justify an aggressive attitude toward evaluation and intervention in these patients.

With regard to excretory renal function and prevention of ischemic renal failure, operative intervention with renal artery bypass surgery is directed at improvement in renal function with improvement or cure of concomitant renovascular hypertension.[13] Response to renal revascularization can be segregated into an immediate impact of revascularization on the glomerular filtration rate (GFR) and the effect of improved perfusion on the subsequent rate of decline in GFR over a prolonged follow-up period. The coupling of these effects results in prolongation of the dialysis-free interval by immediately increasing GFR and retarding subsequent disease progression from a new level of critical excretory renal function. As mentioned in the previous section, most studies have demonstrated that a beneficial functional response can be achieved with surgery in approximately two thirds of patients.[14] The rapidity of decline in a patient's renal function is important in assessing the retrievability of renal function. A rapid deterioration in renal function warrants diagnostic evaluation to rule out a correctable renovascular etiology. These patients may have salvageable and/or retrievable renal function, which obviates the need for dialysis. In fact, studies have shown that nearly 80 percent of those patients newly placed on dialysis, and considered permanently dialysis dependent, can be permanently removed from dialysis.[14]

CONCLUSION

Much progress has been made in the diagnosis, treatment, and ultimate outcome for patients with RVH. What is now needed is additional education of primary care providers to include renal duplex sonography in their evaluation of hypertensive patients when initial history, physical, and routine blood studies indicate.

Data continues to be collected concerning indications for intervention and therapeutic options for treatment of RVH. It is the expectation that along with further experience will come more definitive criteria for both intervention and treatment type.

What is certain, however, is the beneficial response of RVH patients to treatment performed by an experienced team. As is true for so many potentially fatal diseases, early detection and treatment of RVH are key to long-term patient survival. As is also true, it is the responsibility not only of providers, but of patients as well, to become educated in appropriate lifestyle habits to promote health and prevent disease. These include proper diet and exercise, routine medical visits with a primary care provider and screening for age- and gender-appropriate diseases, and smoking or substance abuse cessation. It should be our goal as nurses to provide this education in all feasible patient encounters.

REFERENCES

1. Dean RH, Keyser JE, Dupont WD et al: Aortic and renal vascular disease, *Ann Surg* 200:336-344, 1984.
2. Simon N, Franklin SS, Bleifer KH et al: Clinical characteristics of renovascular hypertension, *JAMA* 220:1209, 1972.
3 Tobian L: Relationship of juxtaglomerular apparatus to renin and angiotensin, *Circulation* 25:189, 1962.
4. Vaughn ED, Buhler FR, Larach JH et al: Renovascular hypertension: renin measurements to indicate hypersecretion and contralateral suppression, estimate renal plasma flow, and score for surgical curability, *Am J Med* 55:402, 1973.
5. Meier GH, Sumpio B, Black HR et al: Captopril renal scintigraphy: an advance in the detection and treatment of renovascular hypertension, *J Vasc Surg* 11:770-777, 1990.
6. Dean RH, Benjamin ME, Hansen KJ: Surgical management of renovascular hypertension, *Cur Probl Surg* 34:3:209-316, 1997.
7. Safian RD, Textor SC: Renal artery stenosis, *N Engl J Med* 344(6):431-441, 2001.
8. Hansen KJ: Renovascular hypertension: an overview. In Rutherford RB, ed: *Vascular surgery*, ed 5, Philadelphia, 2000, WB Saunders, pp 1593-1600.
9. Rees CR: *Renovascular interventions*. Twenty-first Annual Meeting of the Society of Cardiovascular and Interventional Radiology, Seattle, March 1996, pp 311-314.
10. Hansen KJ, Starr SM, Sands RE et al: Contemporary surgical management of renovascular disease, *J Vasc Surg* 16:319-331, 1992.
11. Scobie JE, Maher ER, Hamilton G et al. Atherosclerotic renovascular disease causing renal impairment: a case for treatment, *Clin Nephrol* 31:119, 1989.
12. Mailloux LU, Bellucci AG, Mossey RT et al: Predictors of survival in patients undergoing dialysis, *Am J Med* 84:855, 1988.
13. Dean RH, Krueger TC, Whiteneck JM et al. Operative management of renovascular hypertension: results after 15-23 years follow-up, *J Vasc Surg* 1:234, 1984.
14. Hansen KJ, Thomason RB, Craven TE et al: Surgical management of dialysis-dependent ischemic nephropathy, *J Vasc Surg* 21:197-211, 1995.

17

Mesenteric Ischemia

KELLI J. STOTT □ B. TIMOTHY BAXTER

Mesenteric ischemia remains one of the most difficult diagnostic challenges in contemporary vascular surgery. Although recognized as early as the fifteenth century, successful revascularization of ischemic bowel did not occur until the 1950s.[1] Basic scientific investigation has led to dramatic progress in our understanding of the mediators of injury following experimental gut ischemia and reperfusion, including important effects on distant organs. Unfortunately, this progress has not yet had a meaningful impact on patient outcome as the mortality of mesenteric ischemia with infarction remains in excess of 60%.[2] While comorbid disease contributes to this high mortality rate, timely diagnosis relative to the onset of ischemia is the most critical factor in patient outcome. The delay is often caused by failure to consider mesenteric ischemia in the differential diagnosis or reluctance to order mesenteric arteriography once the diagnosis is considered. Recognizing and establishing the diagnosis of intestinal ischemia requires the input of an entire health care team, a team that is well versed in the clinical features of this rare but deadly problem.

ANATOMY AND PATHOPHYSIOLOGY

Localized ischemia and infarction play an important role in the pathophysiology of a wide array of surgical problems, including appendicitis, strangulation associated with herniation, and segmental ischemic colitis. Rather than discuss these focal processes, this chapter will address four specific entities that affect blood flow in the major arteries or veins of the intestine (Table 17-1). Atherosclerotic stenosis, arterial and venous thrombosis, and embolization can all cause mesenteric ischemia. Understanding the arterial anatomy of the gut provides the basis for understanding differences in the clinical presentation of acute, subacute, and chronic intestinal ischemia.

The embryologic foregut, midgut, and hindgut derive their arterial supply from the celiac artery, the superior mesenteric artery (SMA), and the inferior mesenteric artery (IMA), respectively.[3] These three major arteries arise from the abdominal aorta (Fig.17-1). Additionally, branches of the internal iliac artery supply the distal colon. The celiac artery is the first major branch of the abdominal aorta arising from the anterior surface at the level of the twelfth thoracic or first lumbar vertebra. It supplies the stomach, duodenum, liver, pancreas, and spleen. Approximately 1.5 cm below the celiac axis, the SMA originates. It supplies the remainder of the small bowel from the ligament of Treitz, the ascending and transverse colon, and the pancreas. The IMA, which begins midway between the renal arteries and the aortic bifurcation, is the blood supply to the descending and sigmoid colon. The hypogastric arteries or internal iliac arteries supply the rectum as well as the remainder of the pelvis. All of these vessels divide and anastomose with each other to form a rich vascular network. The major collateral between the celiac artery and the SMA is the anterior pancreaticoduodenal arcade. The meandering mesenteric artery is the important central collateral between the SMA and IMA. The middle and superior hemorrhoidal arteries form an anastomosis between the IMA and hypogastric arteries.

TABLE 17–1 Four Entities That Affect Intestinal Blood Flow

Type of Ischemia	Cause
Chronic mesenteric	Atherosclerosis and thrombosis
Acute mesenteric	Embolus
Nonocclusive mesenteric ischemia	Low cardiac output
Mesenteric vein thrombosis	Hypercoagulability

The importance of these collaterals cannot be overestimated since gradual occlusion of all three of the vessels has been reported without infarction.[4] Conversely, acute occlusion of a single artery, as might occur from cardiac embolization, can result in rapid segmental infarction.[2,5] Because of the remarkable ability of the gut to develop compensatory collateral blood flow, ischemia from chronic occlusive disease represents the end stage of progressive occlusion of all major arteries to the gut.[4] Decreased gut perfusion from low cardiac output can cause intestinal infarction.[6-8] Venous outflow occlusion from mesenteric vein thrombosis causes venous hypertension followed by compromised arterial inflow and, finally, infarction.[9,10]

The basic insult of compromised gut blood flow occurs when the critical threshold of oxygen for cellular viability is not met. The cells of the mucosa are highly active metabolically and are, therefore, exquisitely sensitive to ischemia. The mucosal cells at the tip of the villi are the first to be lost. These early changes affecting the villi may be seen microscopically within 10 minutes of total ischemia.[11] The acute ischemic insult is usually associated with intense peristalsis, which is manifest clinically as vomiting, diarrhea, or both. Inflammatory cells, necrotic debris, fibrin, and bacteria accumulate at the mucosal surface. With progression, ulcers begin to form on the lumenal surface. Fortunately, some degree of collateral blood flow is usually present to attenuate the injury and slow the progression. If flow is not restored, the lamina propria breaks down.[11] Loss of this barrier is a critical

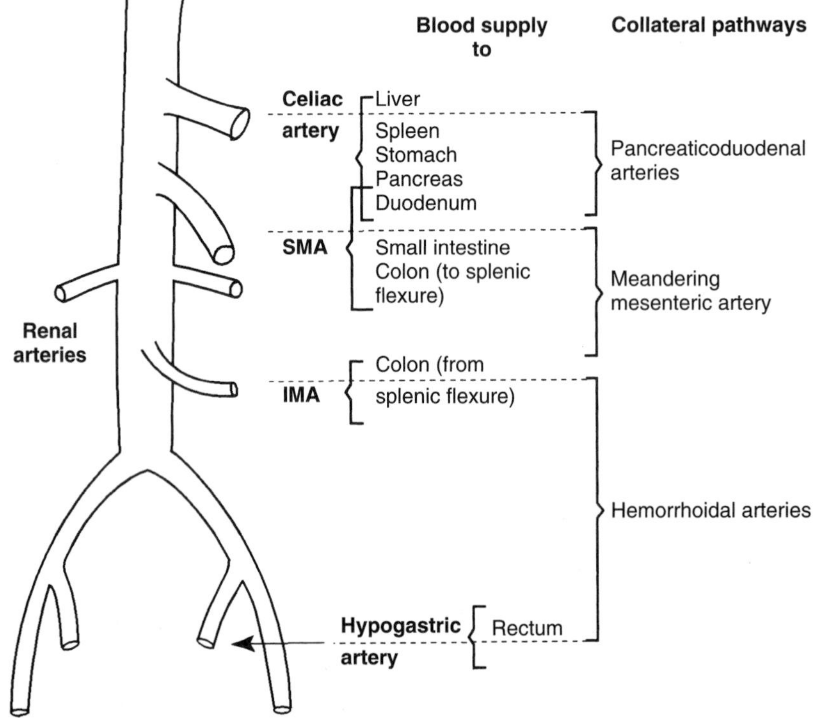

FIG. 17–1. The intraabdominal aorta perfuses the gastrointestinal tract through the celiac artery, the superior mesenteric artery (SMA), the inferior mesenteric artery (IMA), and the hypogastric arteries. The organs perfused by each artery are shown as are the collateral pathways between major arteries.

event, allowing egress of fluid and ingress of bacteria. These fluid shifts may lead to significant intravascular volume depletion. The signs of sepsis, including leukocytosis, fever, hypotension, and altered mental status, may appear at this point. Typically, pain is severe but poorly localized within the abdomen until transmural injury causes inflammation of the parietal peritoneum.

There are multiple other local and systemic physiologic responses that arise and contribute to the clinical picture.[3,12] Autonomic, humoral, and local factors all affect the eventual outcome of the intestine. Autonomic factors, including alpha- and beta-adrenergic stimuli, cause an initial brief period of vasodilation followed by sustained vasoconstriction. The humoral factors, angiotensin II and vasopressin, exacerbate local vasoconstriction. The ischemic process causes both local and systemic activation of the immune system. Activated neutrophils may initiate remote organ injury in the lungs or liver.[13] These destructive processes may be greatly amplified following reperfusion of the ischemic bowel.[14] Ongoing experimental work will help to identify pharmacologic approaches that, in the future, may attenuate the inflammatory cascade and reduce morbidity and mortality associated with ischemia and revascularization.

CLINICAL MANIFESTATIONS

The key to prevention of transmural infarction is early diagnosis. This can only be accomplished if a high index of suspicion is maintained in a patient who fits the "clinical criteria" outlined below. While these signs and symptoms may be quite nonspecific, when considered with the patient's history and comorbid problems, they are often highly suggestive of the correct diagnosis.

Acute Intestinal Ischemia

Acute ischemia may occur in association with acute embolic occlusion of a mesenteric vessel, as the final thrombotic event in patients with chronic mesenteric ischemia, or from shock (hypovolemic or cardiogenic). Of these three, acute embolic occlusion is most readily recognized because of the sudden and dramatic onset of symptoms.[2,5] It begins with severe, acute abdominal pain and may be followed by prompt emptying of the gastrointestinal tract, either by vomiting or diarrhea or both. The intense pain is caused by vigorous intestinal contractions, and bowel sounds are usually increased at this stage. Since the patient will often be writhing in pain, it is surprising to find the abdomen soft and minimally tender on physical examination. Abdominal distention is not a consistent feature. A history of previous emboli, cardiac arrhythmias, or poor ventricular function lends further support to the diagnosis.

Thrombosis of the last patent mesenteric artery in a patient with progressive atherosclerotic occlusive disease will be more insidious than acute embolic occlusion.[2,5] The more subtle presentation may result because patients are debilitated from malnutrition or because they have long suffered from vague abdominal pain. Weight loss is an essential feature of this process, while chronic postprandial abdominal pain is less consistent. Many of these patients develop a subconscious fear of eating that they fail to recognize. In the presence of unexplained weight loss, mesenteric angiography is a critical diagnostic study. Unfortunately, the study is often delayed because the diagnosis of mesenteric ischemia is not considered. Many of these patients will have other gastrointestinal pathology such as gastritis or diverticulosis that may obscure the underlying ischemia.

The clinical presentation associated with nonocclusive mesenteric ischemia is a subacute process and a diagnostic dilemma because of the underlying medical condition of the patient.[7,8] The signs and symptoms of bowel ischemia usually arise during the course of treatment for some other life-threatening condition. A careful review of the records will identify a period of hypotension, often requiring pharmacologic support, during the previous 72 hours. These patients are often obtunded, and there is a significant delay in recognizing the intestinal ischemia until signs of more advanced ischemic changes or infarction (leukocytosis, abdominal distention, and acidosis) are present.

Chronic Intestinal Ischemia

Although the initial clinical features of chronic mesenteric ischemia are vague, with time, a pattern of signs and symptoms will emerge.[4] Weight loss is invariable and must be present to consider the diagnosis. This is associated with "food fear," avoidance of food because of the associated pain. Abdominal pain occurs within minutes of eating and is initially only associated with large meals. The patient makes adjustments by eating smaller amounts more often as the atherosclerosis progresses. Eventually these smaller meals are associated with pain, and caloric intake is no longer adequate; weight loss begins. Diarrhea is often present during this time, presumably related to malabsorption. Other complications of atherosclerosis such as cerebral, coronary, or lower extremity ischemia and vascular reconstruction usually precede the development of mesenteric ischemia.

Mesenteric Vein Thrombosis

Mesenteric vein thrombosis is a distinct entity that can also cause intestinal infarction.[9,15] Any extensive infectious process within the mesenteric venous drainage such as appendicitis or diverticulitis can cause thrombosis. It is also seen as a manifestation of hypercoagulability. This may occur in patients with a history of venous thrombosis and defined abnormalities such as a deficiency in antithrombin III, protein C, or protein S. Hypercoagulability associated with cancer can also cause mesenteric vein thrombosis.

Mesenteric vein thrombosis results in increased venous pressures. This will interfere with capillary flow, and tissue damage results. When this is associated with infarction and peritonitis, the mortality rate is high. Mesenteric vein thrombosis can have a relatively benign course with mild abdominal pain and flu-like symptoms in some patients.[15]

DIAGNOSIS

With suspected acute ischemia, urgent and aggressive diagnostic measures should be undertaken. Unfortunately, laboratory and noninvasive radiologic procedures are not diagnostic in the early, reversible phase of the process. Development of a rapid and reliable diagnostic marker has been elusive despite active investigation. Again, however, a pattern of diagnostic findings may help to exclude other more common diagnoses and lead to definitive angiographic assessment.

Laboratory Tests

A serum marker specific for intestinal ischemia has long been sought. This is especially difficult because the liver acts as a filter between mesenteric venous drainage and systemic venous drainage. Leukocytosis is present in 75% of patients but is, obviously, nonspecific. Metabolic acidosis is a late sign associated with infarction. The BB isoform of creatine kinase is abundant in smooth muscle cells. There are conflicting reports of its sensitivity in gut ischemia.[16] While smooth muscle cells are also rich in phosphate, and elevated serum levels may occur with mesenteric infarction, it is not clear this is a sensitive marker of ischemia.[16] Peritoneal lavage can be performed in patients with suspected ischemia, and animal studies suggest that an elevation in peritoneal leukocytes and phosphate occurs with gut ischemia. This has not been evaluated in clinical trials. D-lactate is a product of bacterial fermentation not produced in mammalian tissues.[17] Although animal studies suggested it might be a good marker for early ischemia, it has been disappointing in identifying ischemic bowel in clinical trials.

Noninvasive Radiologic Tests

In the past decade, duplex ultrasonography has emerged as a valuable tool in the diagnosis of chronic mesenteric ischemia.[18-20] In the hands of a skilled technician, it can accurately detect both stenosis and occlusion in both the celiac artery and SMA. Gaseous distention and pain limit the utility of duplex in the setting of acute ischemia. Keen et al have suggested that these limitations might be overcome by using endoscopic transgastric ultrasonography.[21]

Technological advances in computed tomography (CT) scanning have led to a resurgence of interest in this modality.[22,23] It is invaluable as a tool to exclude other more common causes of abdominal pain. More rapid spiral scanning with timed contrast infusion may allow assessment of bowel perfusion. Bowel wall thickening, intestinal pneumatosis, or portal vein gas are late findings associated with advanced ischemia or infarction. Contrast CT scan is the definitive diagnostic study for mesenteric vein thrombosis, and the frequent use of CT for unexplained abdominal pain may well account for the recently reported decline in mortality from this entity.[2]

Arteriography

Despite the technologic advances in noninvasive diagnosis of other disease processes, mesenteric angiography remains the single best diagnostic study for bowel ischemia of arterial etiology.[5] Since mesenteric ischemia caused by thrombotic occlusion, embolus, and nonocclusive mesenteric ischemia have distinct angiographic features, the underlying process can also be identified (Fig. 17-2). Chronic occlusive disease is ostial and is best seen on lateral views of the aorta. Emboli usually lodge more distally in the superior mesenteric artery. Nonocclusive mesenteric ischemia is associated with narrowing and spasm in the peripheral arcades of the bowel with little filling of mesenteric branches. Besides the diagnostic value of mesenteric angiograph in nonocclusive mesenteric ischemia, catheters can be left in place for selective infusion of vasodilators to help reverse local spasm.[7] Furthermore, mesenteric angioplasty (discussed below) can also be performed at the same setting. Since angiography is the definitive diagnostic study, clinicians should have a low threshold for obtaining mesenteric angiography when the diagnosis is even remotely considered.

TREATMENT

The goal of treatment of mesenteric ischemia is to restore normal bowel function. The patient's overall age and medical condition and the extent of bowel infarction must be considered in choosing the best treatment. Options include local infusion of vasodilators, revascularization by angioplasty or open surgical procedure, and in some unusual cases where infarction is extensive, observation and supportive therapy alone (Table 17-2).

Whether surgery is anticipated or not, the initial treatment for patients with suspected bowel ischemia is the same: (1) correct intravascular volume loss, (2) optimize cardiac function and mesenteric flow, (3) limit the existing thrombotic or embolic process, and (4) correct electrolyte and acid/base abnormalities. These measures will limit bowel infarction and begin to address the adverse systemic effects of the ischemic process.

Medical Management and Resuscitation

Fluid shifts with bowel ischemia can be dramatic. For this reason, all patients should have a bladder catheter and central venous line to help continuously assess volume status. If blood pressure is labile, an arterial line should be placed. When there are questions about cardiac function, a pulmonary artery catheter can be very helpful. Because of coexistent cardiac disease, hypotension should not always be equated with hypovolemia. Knowledge of the central venous pressure or pulmonary artery pressure is essential in making the important distinction between cardiogenic and hypovolemic shock.

Saline solutions or plasma may be used to correct the fluid loss. Dextran may also be used and may be of further benefit because of its antiplatelet properties. Regardless of the solution used, a central venous or pulmonary artery catheter is necessary to carefully monitor volume replacement.

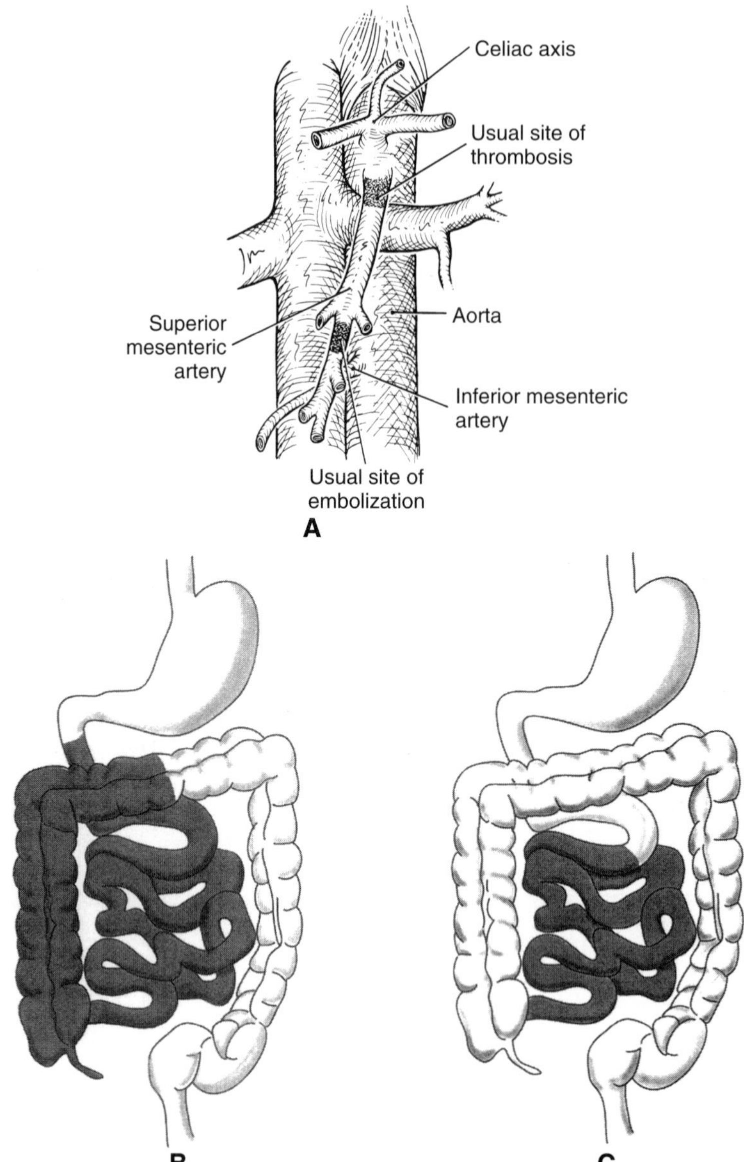

FIG. 17–2. The usual site of mesenteric artery thrombosis is at the origin of the vessel **(A),** resulting in the pattern of ischemia shown in **B.** Embolic occlusion of the superior mesenteric artery (SMA) **(A)** typically occurs distal to the origin of the middle colic artery, sparing the transverse colon as shown in **C.** (**A** from Bergan JJ: Operative procedures in acute mesenteric infarction. In Bergan JJ, Yao JST, eds: *Operative techniques in vascular surgery,* New York, Grune & Stratton, 1980, p 106. Reprinted with permission.)

TABLE 17–2 Treatment Options for Mesenteric Ischemia

Type of Ischemia	Treatment
Chronic occlusive mesenteric ischemia	Bypass, endarterectomy, or angioplasty
Acute embolus to superior mesenteric artery (SMA)	Embolectomy
Nonocclusive mesenteric ischemia	Circulatory support, local vasodilators
Mesenteric vein thrombosis	Anticoagulation

During resuscitation, other measures should be directed at improving mesenteric arterial flow. This is best achieved by optimizing cardiac function. Dobutamine may be particularly useful in improving function and selectively improving mesenteric blood flow. Catheters are left in the SMA after arteriography when nonocclusive mesenteric ischemia is diagnosed.[7] Intraarterial papaverine hydrochloride provides a local vasodilating effect, correcting intestinal ischemia and promoting maximum bowel viability. Papaverine is diluted to a concentration whereby 1 mg/ml can be infused at a rate of 30-60 mg/hr. The infusion continues for one or more 24-hour periods, often with repeat arteriography at the end of each 24-hour period.[15] During this time, the patient must be continually assessed for bowel infarction and peritonitis.

Patients who present after embolization from a cardiac source are at significant risk of recurrent embolization. This risk is dramatically reduced by intravenous heparin infusion. In thrombotic occlusive disease, heparin prevents propagation of newly formed thrombus. Thus, anticoagulant therapy is initiated with heparin sodium while the patient is carefully monitored for any increase in intestinal bleeding due to bowel infarction and mucosal injury. Long-term warfarin therapy is considered along with the risk of this treatment.

When bowel infarction is suspected on clinical grounds, an antibiotic that covers gram-negative and anaerobic organisms should be given. Arterial blood gas values will indicate the need for sodium bicarbonate therapy to correct the acidosis found with bowel infarction.

Nonoperative treatment has a place in the management of nonorganic intestinal ischemia, and angioplasty has been used to treat chronic mesenteric occlusive disease. Surgery, however, remains the most definitive technique for revascularization. When there are obvious physical and radiographic signs of extensive infarction in a severely debilitated and elderly patient, it may be reasonable in consultation with the family to provide only supportive treatment. After initial diagnosis and resuscitation, open surgery or laparoscopy offers the only opportunity to assess bowel viability, resect dead bowel, and treat the underlying vascular problem.

Angioplasty

In those suffering from chronic mesenteric ischemia, nonoperative approaches have also been used in the last 10-15 years. Angioplasty has been used successfully in the coronary and peripheral circulation. The objective of angioplasty is to dilate hemodynamically significant stenosis (greater than 50%) in the celiac or superior mesenteric artery.[24] Most authors are reporting initial success rates of greater than 80%. As may occur with angioplasty in other arteries, restenosis is a problem occurring at a rate of 33% within 10 months.[24] Whether primary stenting will improve short-term restenosis rates is unclear. Another benefit of angioplasty is that it may be diagnostic in that an immediate improvement in pain confirms the diagnosis of mesenteric ischemia. Because of the superior durability, surgical revascularization remains the best treatment for chronic mesenteric ischemia.

Surgical Treatment

Surgery continues to have a central role in the management of mesenteric ischemia for two reasons. The first is that surgical revascularization provides the best long-term outlook for the patient.[25] Second, laparotomy may be required to determine the extent of the ischemic process and resect nonviable intestine. In acute embolic occlusion, embolectomy of the superior mesenteric artery using a balloon catheter can usually restore adequate flow (Fig.17-3). During surgery, the bowel is carefully examined to determine the need for any resection. If the majority of bowel appears ischemic but is not infarcted, a second operation (second look) is performed to observe the condition of the bowel 24 hours after revascularization and to determine whether bowel resection is necessary.[5]

Acute thrombotic occlusion or chronic mesenteric artery occlusion can be treated with bypass or endarterectomy. The former is more common and can be done with either saphenous vein or prosthetic material (Fig. 17-4). Because all of the arteries will be involved to some degree, a bypass to both the celiac and superior mesenteric arteries provides some

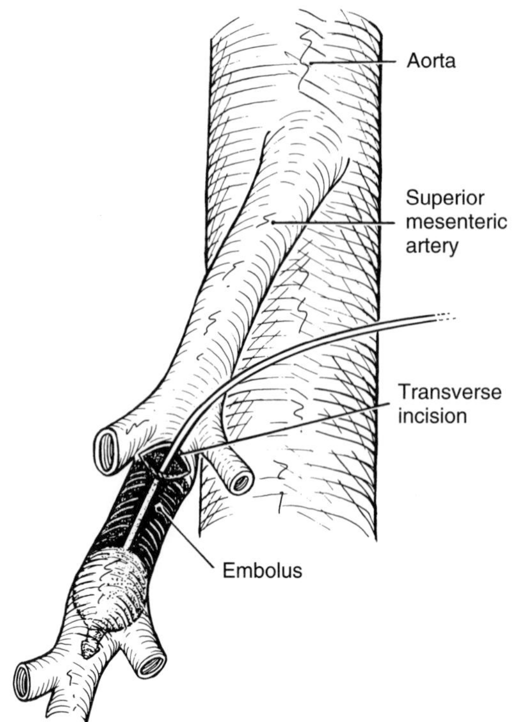

FIG. 17–3. Embolectomy of the superior mesenteric artery by means of a Fogarty catheter. (From Bergan JJ: Operative procedures in acute mesenteric infarction. In Bergan JJ, Yao JST, eds: *Operative techniques in vascular surgery,* New York, Grune & Stratton, 1980, p 106. Reprinted with permission).

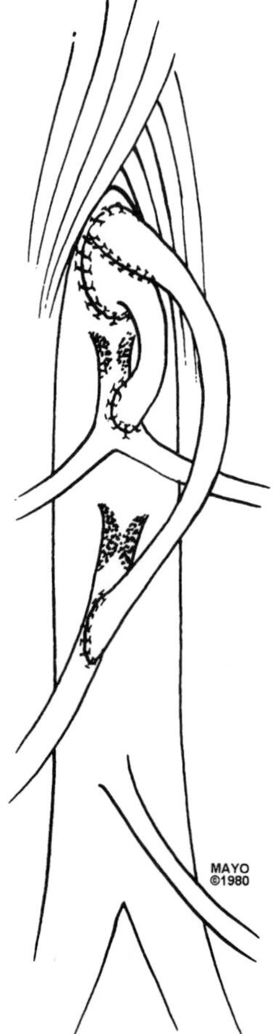

FIG. 17–4. Antegrade aortomesenteric bypass reconstructing the celiac axis and superior mesenteric artery. (From Lipski DL, Ernst CB: Visceral ischemic syndromes. In Moore WS, ed: *Vascular surgery,* ed 5, Philadelphia, 1998, WB Saunders, p 547. By permission of Mayo Foundation and WB Saunders.)

insurance if one of the grafts eventually fails.[25,26] The comparative mortality rates for embolic and thombotic causes of intestinal ischemia are shown in Table 17-3.

NURSING POSTOPERATIVE CARE

The postoperative phase requires vigilant observation and skilled nursing care including (1) observation for signs of recurrent ischemia, (2) correction of fluid and electrolyte losses, (3) correction of metabolic acidosis, and (4) monitoring of gastrointestinal function.

The patient must be constantly assessed for signs of intestinal ischemia secondary to recurrent mesenteric embolization or thrombosis of the graft or endarterectomy site. Key symptoms are abdominal pain similar to the preoperative pain and not related to the incision site, an elevated white blood cell count, and gut emptying (diarrhea or vomiting).

Fluid and electrolyte management may be challenging. Hypotension may occur, as the preoperative fluid losses are now aggravated by additional fluid loss during surgery and activation of the inflammatory cascade. Blood pressure measurements and vital signs must, therefore, be carefully monitored.

The patient's cardiac status is a factor to consider during this fluid replacement therapy. If there is compromised cardiac function, frequent central venous or pulmonary artery pressure readings help in attaining a balance between hypovolemia and cardiac overload. Some medications used to improve cardiac function (including digitoxin) may cause vasoconstriction of the abdominal viscera; these drugs may have to be limited or discontinued during this time. Exact intake and output records are important in fluid management as well as in assessment of renal function.

Pulmonary complications such as pneumonia can be reduced with aggressive measures. Many patients with vascular disease are cigarette smokers with chronic obstructive pulmonary disorders. Vigorous pulmonary care should be started on admission to the intensive care unit. Arterial blood gas analysis provides helpful information regarding oxygen exchange (Po_2) and ventilation (CO_2). Metabolic acidosis occurs after revascularization, as a result of the release of agents from ischemic tissue.

A nasogastric tube will provide gastric decompression. Time for return of bowel function may be prolonged. When normal bowel sounds have returned, a liquid diet can be resumed. A period of malabsorption presumably related to recovery of the mucosa has been reported and may last for several weeks.

TABLE 17–3 Comparative Mortality Rates for Embolic and Thombotic Causes of Intestinal Ischemia

Author	Year	Arterial Embolism % Deaths	Arterial Thrombosis % Deaths	Venous Thrombosis % Deaths	Overall Mortality
Ottinger, Austen[27]	1967	76	95	80	83%
Smith, Patterson[28]	1976	86	90	100	90%
Kairaluoma, Karkola, Heikkinen et al[29]	1977	91	90	—	91%
Hertzer, Beven, Humphries[30]	1978	57	100	—	67%
Sachs, Morton, Schwartz[31]	1982	64	100	36	68%
Bergan, McCarthy, Flinn et al[32]	1987	83	75	—	79%
Klempnauer, Grothues, Bektas et al[33]	1997	76	81	37	62%
Endean, Barnes, Kwolek et al[2]	2000	59	62	13	48%

To prevent the complications associated with bed rest, activity should be encouraged as soon as tolerated. Pneumatic compression stocking and subcutaneous heparin should be used for deep vein thrombos (DVT) prophylaxis. With improvement the patient may be transferred to the floor and discharged when ambulatory with adequate oral intake.

Patient Education

When the patient has stabilized and is recovering comfortably, patient education should be initiated. Mesenteric occlusion is usually due to atherosclerosis, so patient education should focus on the following: (1) identification of risk factors such as smoking, high cholesterol, hypertension, diabetes, and lack of exercise, and (2) methods to control these risk factors through diet instruction, smoking-cessation classes, exercise therapy, and control of blood pressure. In patients with chronic ischemia and its attendant weight loss or resection of a substantial length of small bowel, nutrition will also be an important issue. The patient's weight should be monitored after discharge as parenteral or enteral support may be needed. After hospital discharge, nursing referral can be made for the teaching to be reinforced by the physician's office nurse, a visiting nurse, or a vascular rehabilitation program.

CONCLUSION

Few challenges in vascular nursing are greater than that of caring for the patient with mesenteric ischemia. Any member of the health care team who recognizes the constellation of signs and symptoms associated with mesenteric ischemia should suggest it be included in the differential diagnosis. Simply considering the diagnosis may help to expedite the evaluation and confirm a diagnosis of mesenteric ischemia. Perioperatively, patients with mesenteric ischemia are extremely challenging because of a combination of sepsis, activation of the inflammatory cascade, and underlying cardiovascular disease. Providing optimal patient care requires knowledge of these processes. Nursing care before and after surgery will have a critical impact on overall patient outcome.

Often the immediate need for prompt lifesaving interventions allows time for only a brief nursing assessment focused on the patient's physical status. However, emotional and educational support are also important for both the patient and family dealing with a life-threatening illness. Continued support, combined with skillful assessment and technical expertise, is required of any nurse facing the clinical challenge of mesenteric ischemia.

REFERENCES

1. Boley SJ, Brandt LJ, Sammartano RJ: History of mesenteric ischemia, *Surg Clin North Am* 77(2):275-278, 1997.
2. Endean ED, Barnes SL, Kwolek CJ et al: Surgical management of thrombotic acute intestinal ischemia, *Ann Surg* 233(6):801-808, 2001.
3. Rosenblum JD, Boyle CM, Schwartz LB: The mesenteric circulation: anatomy and physiology, *Surg Clin North Am* 77(2):289-306, 1997.
4. Baxter BT, Pearce WH: Diagnosis and surgical management of chronic mesenteric ischemia. In Strandness E, Van Berda A, eds: *Vascular diseases: surgical and interventional therapy,* New York, 1996, Churchill, pp 795-702.
5. McKinsey JF, Gewertz BL: Acute mesenteric ischemia, *Surg Clin North Am* 77(2):307-318, 1997.
6. Howard TJ, Plaskon LA, Wiebke EA et al: Nonocclusive mesenteric ischemia remains a diagnostic dilemma, *Am J Surg* 171(4):405-408, 1996.
7. Bassiouny HS: Nonocclusive mesenteric ischemia, *Surg Clin North Am* 77(2):319-326, 1997.
8. Lock G, Scholmerich J: Non-occlusive mesenteric ischemia, *Hepatogastroenterology* 42(3):234-239, 1995.
9. Rhee RY, Gloviczki P: Mesenteric venous thrombosis, *Surg Clin North Am* 77(2):327-338, 1997.
10. Crespo I, Murphy J, Wong RK: Superior mesenteric venous thrombosis masquerading as Crohn's disease, *Am J Gastroenterol* 89(1):116-118, 1994.
11. Pearce WH, Bergan JJ: Acute intestinal ischemia. In Rutherford RB, ed: *Vascular surgery,* ed 3, Philadelphia, 1989, WB Saunders, pp 1086-1096.

12. Patel A, Kaleya RN, Sammartano RJ: Pathophysiology of mesenteric ischemia, *Surg Clin North Am* 72(1):31-41, 1992.
13. Kim FJ, Moore EE, Moore FA et al: Reperfused gut elaborates PAF that chemoattracts and primes neutrophils, *J Surg Res* 58(6):636-640, 1995.
14. Koike K, Moore EE, Moore FA et al: Gut phospholipase A2 mediates neutrophil priming and lung injury after mesenteric ischemia-reperfusion, *Am J Physiol* 268(3 pt 1):397-403, 1995.
15. Abdu RA, Zakhour BJ, Dallis DJ: Mesenteric venous thrombosis—1911-1984, *Surgery* 101:383-388, 1987.
16. Kurland B, Brandt LJ, Delany HM: Diagnostic tests for intestinal ischemia, *Surg Clin North Am* 72(1):85-105, 1992.
17. Murray MJ, Gonze MD, Nowak LR et al: Serum D(−)– lactate levels as an aid to diagnosing acute intestinal ischemia, *Am J Surg* 167(6):575-578, 1994.
18. Bowersox JC, Zwolak RM, Walsh DB et al: Duplex ultrasonography in the diagnosis of celiac and mesenteric artery occlusive disease, *J Vasc Surg* 14:780-786, 1991.
19. Jager K, Bollinger A, Valli C et al: Measurement of mesenteric blood flow by duplex scanning, *J Vasc Surg* 3:462-469, 1986.
20. Roobottom CA, Dubbins PA: Significant disease of the celiac and superior mesenteric arteries in asymptomatic patients: predictive value of Doppler sonography, *AJR Am J Roentgenol* 161(5):985-988, 1993.
21. Keen RR, Yao JS, Astleford P et al: Feasibility of transgastric ultrasonography of the abdominal aorta, *J Vasc Surg* 24(5):834-842, 1996.
22. Taourel PG, Deneuville M, Pradel JA et al: Acute mesenteric ischemia: diagnosis with contrast-enhanced CT, *Radiology* 199(3):632-636, 1996.
23. Klein HM, Lensing R, Klosterhalfen B et al: Diagnostic imaging of mesenteric infarction, *Radiology* 197(1):79-82, 1995.
24. Hackworth CA, Leef JA: Percutaneous transluminal mesenteric angioplasty, *Surg Clin North Am* 77(2):371-380, 1997.
25. Derrow A, Seeger JM, Douglas DA et al: The outcome in the United States after thoracoabdominal aortic aneurysm repair, renal artery bypass, and mesenteric revascularization, *J Vasc Surg* 34(1):54-61, 2001.
26. Kasirajan K, O'Hara PJ, Gray BH et al: Chronic mesenteric ischemia: open surgery versus percutaneous angioplasty and stenting, *J Vasc Surg* 33(1):63-71, 2001.
27. Ottinger LW, Austen WG: A study of 136 patients with mesenteric infarction, *Surg Gynecol Obstet* 24(2):251-261, 1967.
28. Smith JS, Patterson LT: Acute mesenteric infarction, *Am Surg* 42:562-567, 1976.
29. Kairaluoma MI, Karkola P, Heikkinen D et al: Mesenteric infarction, *Am J Surg* 133(2):188-193, 1977.
30. Hertzer NR, Beven EG, Humphries AW: Acute intestinal ischemia, *Am Surg* 44(11):744-749, 1978.
31. Sachs SM, Morton JH, Schwartz SI: Acute mesenteric ischemia, *Surgery* 92(4):646-653. 1982.
32. Bergan JJ, McCarthy WJ 3rd, Flinn WR et al: Nontraumatic mesenteric vascular emergencies, *J Vasc Surg* 5(6):903-909, 1987.
33. Klempnauer J, Grothues F, Bektas H et al: Acute mesenteric ischemia following cardiac surgery, *J Cardiovasc Surg* 38(6):639-643, 1997.

PART FOUR

VENOUS DISEASES

18

Venous Thromboembolic Disease

M. EILEEN WALSH □ KAREN L. RICE

Venous thromboembolic disease (VTE), which includes deep vein thrombosis (DVT) and pulmonary embolism (PE), represents the third most common cardiovascular disorder, affecting over 2 million Americans each year.[1,2] For many years, it was initially thought that only a small fraction of DVTs progressed to PE. However, we now know that PE occurs in approximately 80 percent of patients with proximal DVT, 46 percent with calf DVT, and 10 percent with superficial venous thrombosis.[3] Although the exact incidence of venous thrombosis is not known, it is estimated that more than 200,000 Americans are hospitalized each year for first-time VTE, with approximately 25 percent dying within 7 days of symptom onset. In addition, about 22 percent of all patients with VTE will die because of insufficient time to initiate appropriate intervention for PE.[4,5] Despite a heightened awareness about VTE, the annual incidence of PE is estimated at 69 per 100,000 patients, with a mortality rate of up to 30 percent if untreated. In addition, more than 400,000 cases of PE occurring each year in the United States are never diagnosed.[6]

A recent review of hospitalized patients in Minnesota over a 10-year period reported a more than 100-fold increase in the incidence of VTE when compared to community-dwelling residents. Surprisingly, the incidence rate of VTE in this latter study exhibited little change over the 10-year period despite increased awareness and advances in diagnosis, prophylaxis, and treatment.[7] Although these statistics suggest little progress has been made in addressing this potentially lethal health care problem, it is reasonable to speculate that despite the major advances made to date, problems related to early diagnosis, treatment, and prophylaxis still exist.[8,9]

A wide variety of medical conditions, as well as surgical and interventional procedures, place many patients at increased risk for the development of VTE. In addition, many hypercoagulable states, including those influenced by pharmacologic agents, continue to further complicate the problem. Although VTE most commonly develops in the chronically ill, in patients with spinal cord disorders, and in surgical patients, it can occur even in the healthy person with no obvious cause.[5] Because of the impact of prophylaxis, along with early diagnosis and treatment, all fields of nursing play a key role in significantly reducing the morbidity and mortality associated with VTE.

This chapter focuses on the etiology, prophylaxis, clinical manifestations, diagnostic evaluation, treatment, and nursing management of VTE. Refer to Chapter 2 for a review of anatomy and physiology of the venous system.

VENOUS THROMBOSIS

Venous thrombosis is an obstruction of a vein in which the thrombus is composed mainly of erythrocytes in a fibrin mesh with few platelets and is therefore known as a red thrombus (Fig. 18-1). In 1846, Virchow identified three factors as the most important initiators of venous thrombosis: stasis of venous blood flow, damage to the endothelial lining of the vein wall, and changes in the coagulation mechanisms of the blood.[4]

Venous stasis is a state in which blood remains in contact with the venous wall for a prolonged time. It is probably the most important predisposing factor. Because forward movement

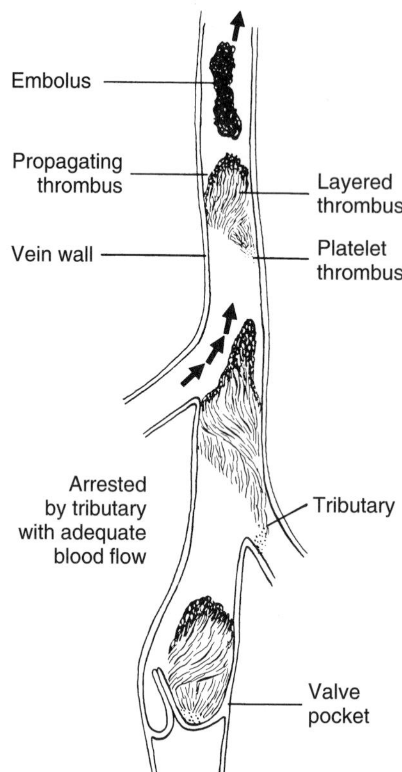

FIG. 18–1. Development of deep vein thrombosis and embolus. (From *Critical Care Nursing Quarterly*, Vol 8, No 2, p 82 with permission of Aspen Publishers, 1985.)

depends on the action of the voluntary muscles and adequacy of the venous valves, venous stasis can occur when muscles are inactive or when the valves are incompetent.[4,10] In an immobilized limb, forward venous flow is completely abolished unless the limb is elevated above the level of the heart.

The normal venous endothelium is an intact, smooth, single layer of nonthrombogenic cells containing various substances to prevent platelet adhesion and clot formation.[6,11] Local venous trauma, however, can result in alteration of this epithelial lining, reducing the intrinsic capacity of the vessel to inhibit thrombus formation. Local platelet aggregation and fibrin entrapment of red blood cells, white blood cells, and additional platelets also occur, resulting in thrombus formation.[4,10]

Changes in the coagulation mechanism of the blood can result from hematologic disorders included in Table 18-1. For example, antithrombin III, a circulating anticoagulant, inactivates thrombin and other clotting factors. Therefore, an antithrombin III deficiency allows thrombin and other clotting factors to proliferate, increasing the risk of thrombus formation.

Etiology

Virchow's triad is still supported today as the primary theory responsible for thrombus formation. Table 18-1 outlines major risk factors for VTE.[4,11] It is important to emphasize that the presence of multiple risk factors has a multiplicative effect rather than an additive effect on the overall risk for VTE. Although Table 18-1 addresses risk factors in general, several factors are especially noteworthy and thus are discussed in more detail in the text.

Age

Advanced age (>60 years) is commonly accepted as a risk factor for VTE. The geriatric patient is at increased risk, in part, due to increased comorbidity and age-related alterations in drug pharmacokinetics. Based on reports from the World Health Organization and other countries,

TABLE 18–1 Risk Factors for Venous Thrombosis

Acquired	Mixed	Inherited
Prior history of venous thromboembolic disease	Vitamin B_6 deficiency	Protein C deficiency
Major comorbid chronic illness (congestive heart failure, myocardial infarction, stroke with paralysis)	Vitamin B_{12} deficiency	Protein S deficiency
Surgical procedure (i.e., abdomen, pelvis, lower-extremity orthopedic)	Folate deficiency	Factor V Leiden
Transvenous cannulation (i.e., central line, pacemaker)	Hyperhomocysteinemia	Prothrombin mutation
Femoral fracture	High factor VIII levels	Antithrombin III deficiency
Tibial fracture	Non-O blood groups	Dysfibrinogenemia
Spinal cord injury	High von Willebrand factor	
Major head trauma	High fibrinogen levels	
Long air flights		
Antiphospholipid syndrome		
Trauma with immobilization		
Advancing age		
Hypertension		
Malignancy		
Immobility (i.e., hospitalization, nursing home residence)		
Currently on oral contraceptive		
Pregnancy		
Puerperium		
Myeloproliferative disorders		
Polycythemia vera		
Heparin-induced thrombocytopenia		
Smoking		
Obesity		

Modified from Kim V, Spandorfer J: Epidemiology of venous thromboembolic disease, *Emerg Med Clin North Am* 19(4):840, 2001.

there appears to be a linear increase in the prevalence of PE up to age 65 followed by a more rapid acceleration.[12,13] The probability of VTE has been estimated to rise from 0.5 percent at age 50 to 10.7 percent by the age of 80 years.[14] Short-term in-hospital mortality rates for this high-risk population have been reported at rates of 3 percent for DVT and 21 percent for PE. Additionally, 1-year mortality rates also remained high with an incidence of 39 percent and 21 percent, respectively.[15]

Invasive Procedures

Surgical and interventional procedures, as well as other invasive interventions, have long been established as risk factors for VTE. It has been theorized that trauma to major vessels during these invasive procedures, prolonged immobilization, and anesthetic agents all play a contributory role. The Sixth American College of Chest Physicians (ACCP) Consensus Conference (2000) has recommended that prophylaxis should be guided by risk stratification based on the type of surgical procedure. Table 18-2 provides an overview of the levels of risk associated with VTE when no thromboprophylaxis is used.[16]

Although surgical procedures in general place patients at an increased risk for VTE, major trauma, orthopedic procedures, and abdominal surgery (gastrointestinal and genitourinary) are associated with the highest risk. Orthopedic procedures in particular pose a significant risk for VTE, not only during the immediate postoperative period but for several months following. The prevalence of DVT at 7-14 days postoperatively for total hip arthroplasty, total

TABLE 18–2 Levels of Thrombotic Risk in Surgical Patients Without Prophylaxis

Level of Risk	Calf DVT (%)	Proximal DVT (%)	Clinical PE (%)	Fatal PE (%)
LOW RISK				
Minor surgery in patients <40 years without additional risk factors	2	0.4	0.2	0.002
MODERATE RISK				
Minor surgery with additional risk factors Nonmajor surgery in patients 40-60 years without additional risk factors Major surgery in patients >40 years without additional risk factors	10-20	2-4	1-2	0.1-0.4
HIGH RISK				
Nonmajor surgery in patients >60 years without additional risk factors Nonmajor surgery in patients <60 years with additional risk factors Major surgery in patients >40 years without additional risk factors Major surgery in patients <40 years with additional risk factors	20-40	4-8	2-4	0.4-1.0
HIGHEST RISK				
Major surgery in patients >40 years plus prior VTE, cancer, or hypercoagulable state Hip or knee arthroplasty Hip fracture Hip fracture surgery Major trauma Spinal cord injury	40-80	10-20	4-10	0.2-5

DVT, Deep vein thrombosis; *PE,* pulmonary embolism; *VTE,* venous thromboembolic disease.

knee arthroplasty, and hip fracture surgery is reported in the range of 50-60 percent, with rates of proximal DVT at 25 percent, 15-20 percent, and 30 percent, respectively. In addition, it has been documented that up to 2 percent of patients receiving pharmacologic prophylaxis still develop PE.[16]

The increasing use of central venous cannulation for both diagnostic (i.e., right heart catheterization) and therapeutic procedures (i.e., pacemaker wires, central line infusion) is responsible for an increasing trend in upper extremity–related VTE. It has been reported that upper-extremity DVT is associated with a 5-10 percent incidence of PE. However, peripheral ports are associated with a significantly higher incidence of DVT (11.4 percent) when compared to chest ports (4.8 percent).[17] In addition, subclavian catheters are the most common cause of catheter-related upper-extremity VTE, primarily because of fibrin sleeve formation. The clinical significance of fibrin sleeve formation lies in the risk of thrombi being detached and embolized at the time of catheter removal.[18]

Medical Illnesses

Similar to major surgery, both acute hospitalization and nursing home confinement pose a substantial risk for VTE. These patient groups are felt to be vulnerable to VTE because of restricted mobility and the specific illness itself. Several nonmalignant medical illnesses are associated with an increased risk for VTE. These include myocardial infarction, stroke, congestive heart failure (New York Heart Association Functional Level III or IV), respiratory insufficiency, spinal cord injury, septic shock, and nephrotic syndrome.[5,9]

Although restricted physical activity plays a key role in the increased incidence of VTE in the chronically ill, mechanisms such as pulmonary vasoconstriction (i.e., hypoxia, congestive heart failure, respiratory insufficiency), the stimulation of thrombogenic factors (i.e., spinal cord injury, myocardial infarction), and the excretion of anticoagulant proteins such as antithrombin III (i.e., nephrotic syndrome) also contribute to the overall risk.[4] In an investigation of 911 community residents, Heit et al reported that almost one third of all VTE cases occur in recently hospitalized patients within 12 days from hospital discharge.[5]

Travel

It is generally accepted that travel is associated with an increased risk of VTE. It is believed that an increase in venous stasis is created by the high pressures exerted on the posterior calves from the edge of an individual's seat with prolonged sitting. The resultant decrease in venous blood flow is also associated with a gradual increase in hematocrit and concomitant rise in plasma protein concentration. Ferrari et al reported that 24.5 percent of patients with VTE had a journey longer than 4 hours, opposed to 7.5 percent of those in the control group.[19] Although all methods of prolonged travel place individuals at increased risk for VTE, air travel has been particularly scrutinized and is thus believed to pose a higher risk when compared to other modes of travel.[4,20] This theory is attributed to the associated hemoconcentration that results from decreased urine output and increased urine osmolality that is unique to air travel. In addition, a decrease in spontaneous endothelial fibrinolysis is associated with the fall in ambient oxygen concentration, which occurs in flight.[4]

Recurrent Venous Thromboembolism

A history of VTE remains a strong risk factor for a new event. Empiric data support that the risk for recurrent VTE is highest immediately after hospitalization for treatment and gradually declines, reaching a plateau at about 3 years. The risk of recurrent VTE is reported to be highest during the first 6 to 12 months after the initial thrombotic event but never falls to zero. Although a history of VTE alone poses a significant risk, the addition of malignancy or a hypercoagulable state increases the risk of recurrence even higher.[4] Of particular interest is that those who developed VTE associated with surgery, trauma, fracture, pregnancy, postpartum, or hormone therapy demonstrated a lower incidence of recurrent thrombosis when compared with those in whom the etiology was due to other circumstances.[21]

Pregnancy and Postpartum

Although the true incidence of VTE in pregnancy is unknown, there is strong clinical evidence to support that there is an increased incidence when compared to those who are not pregnant. The risk of VTE is higher following cesarean section, particularly in emergency cases, when compared to vaginal delivery. During pregnancy, alterations in several clotting factors occur that contribute to the risk of thrombosis and may persist for up to 2 weeks following delivery. These alterations include relative increases in procoagulants such as fibrinogen, factor VII, factor X, and factor VIII, and relative decreases in protein S. Incidence may be higher during the third trimester due to the mechanical obstruction of the iliac veins by the fetus and the maximal procoagulant effects associated with this final phase. Because of the compressive effects on the left iliac vein by the right iliac artery where they cross, approximately 90 percent of DVTs associated with pregnancy occur in the left leg. Therefore, a greater proportion of DVT during pregnancy involve the iliofemoral veins, where embolization is more likely to occur.[22,23] Table 18-3 stratifies the risk of VTE associated with pregnancy.[9]

During the postpartum period, the risk for VTE is threefold to fivefold higher than during pregnancy. It is estimated that 2.3 to 6.1 per 1000 women giving birth will develop DVT during the puerperium. This increased risk of VTE is because the puerperium is shorter than pregnancy.[24]

Malignancy

The incidence of VTE in patients with cancer is reported to range from 16.5 to 32 percent.[4] The increase in thrombogenicity associated with malignancy is thought to be related to the production of certain procoagulants by neoplastic cells. In many instances, the diagnosis of idiopathic VTE is followed by the identification of a malignancy.[4] Although multiple studies support the increased risk of VTE in cancer, there is variability in the association with specific types. In the past, lung cancer was responsible for about 25 percent of associated VTE, followed by malignancies involving the pancreas, stomach, colon, prostate, ovary, breast, and kidney.[4,25] However, more recently, Levitan et al identified that the highest rates of VTE occurred in carcinomas involving the kidney, stomach, pancreas, brain, and lymphoma; the lowest rates involved carcinomas of the head/neck, bladder, breast, esophagus, uterus, and cervix.[26] Strong associations have also been reported to occur with carcinomas of the ovary and non-Hodgkin's lymphoma. In addition, malignancy is also associated with a significantly higher rate of recurrent VTE.[4]

Inherited Hypercoagulable States

Although inherited hypercoagulable states are responsible for only a small percentage of VTE, they do pose a significant risk if present. Table 18-1 lists inherited disorders that commonly

TABLE 18–3 Pregnancy and the Risk for Venous Thrombosis

Risk Stratification	Patient Characteristics
Low	Family history of deep vein thrombosis (DVT)
	Protein C or S deficiency
	Heterozygous factor V Leiden
Moderate	Homozygous factor V Leiden
	History of single DVT and thrombophilia
	History of recurrent spontaneous abortion
	History of severe pre-eclampsia/HELLP syndrome* and thrombophilia
High	Acute VTE in current pregnancy
	Prosthetic heart valve
	Antithrombin III deficiency
	History of prior thrombosis on anticoagulants
	History of complex thrombophilic defects

*HELLP syndrome is hemodialysis, elevated liver enzymes, low platelet count.

cause coagulopathies. In patients with inherited disorders, approximately one half of those with VTE will demonstrate an increased risk from additional risk factors, such as surgery, pregnancy, or the use of oral contraceptives. In this same high-risk group of patients, approximately 50 percent with a single DVT will develop reoccurrence without lifelong anticoagulation.[4,27] Thrombotic disorders are reviewed in greater detail in Chapter 9.

Medications

The thrombogenicity of oral contraceptives and hormone replacement therapy have been known for many years. Although the impact of second- and third-generation oral contraceptives containing levonorgestrel on the incidence of VTE continues to be debated, there has been a substantial decline since the reduction of estrogen content. However, it has been hypothesized that the thrombogenicity associated with oral contraceptives is mediated only in part by the effects of estrogen on the hemostatic system. Some have proposed the role of an immunologic response to estrogen, which causes secondary deficiencies in protein S, hence, mediating thrombosis. In addition, others report that progesterone also plays a role in the pathogenesis of thrombosis. Of noteworthy significance is that the highest risk for VTE occurs during the first year of use.[28] The relative low incidence of VTE in young females has created speculation that patients who develop VTE while using oral contraceptives could have an underlying coagulopathy, such as factor V Leiden. In such instances, the activated protein C resistance and the metabolic derangements of the clotting cascade caused by oral contraceptives act synergistically to enhance each other's effects.[4,29]

The relative risk of VTE associated with hormone replacement therapy is reported to be comparable to that conferred by oral contraceptives, despite a significantly lower amount of estrogen. Although empiric data addressing this issue are limited, careful risk-benefit analysis on an individual basis is warranted, especially in those with a prior history of VTE or malignancy.[4] More recent reports support an increased risk for VTE, which is associated with postmenopausal estrogen replacement, especially during the first year of therapy.[30,31]

Chemotherapeutic agents have also been associated with an increased incidence of VTE because of drug-induced hypercoagulation. In addition, chemotherapeutic agents and other caustic infusates have been associated with superficial thrombophlebitis.

VENOUS THROMBOEMBOLISM PROPHYLAXIS

The primary reason for thromboprophylaxis is based on the high prevalence of VTE among hospitalized patients and its associated potential mortality. Since both DVT and PE produce few specific symptoms, and the first manifestation may be fatal, thromboprophylaxis becomes as important as the actual treatment. Prevention is the most effective weapon against the morbidities of postthrombotic syndrome, pulmonary hypertension, and PE. Therefore, patients at risk for VTE should be identified and thromboprophylaxis implemented. Since this is not a simple task, a combination of pharmacologic agents and adjunctive prevention strategies are used to optimize patient benefit while minimizing the risk for serious complications. Recommendations by the Sixth ACCP Consensus Conference on Antithrombotic Therapy (2000) provide guidelines for thromboprophylaxis in medical, surgical, and pregnant patients (Table 18-4).[16,22] However, clinicians need to be cognizant of the need for thromboprophylaxis in those patients in whom circumstances may not be clearly delineated in consensus guidelines.

Pharmacologic Measures

Pharmacologic thromboprophylaxis consists of the use of antithrombotic agents that inhibit blood coagulation and interrupt the progression of the thrombotic process. Effective antithrombotic regimens include low-dose heparin (LDH), low-molecular-weight heparin (LMWH), and warfarin. Table 18-5 outlines the Sixth ACCP Consensus Conference's recommendations for antithrombotic agents in preventing VTE.[16,22]

TABLE 18–4 Guidelines for Thromboprophylaxis in the Surgical Patient

Level of Risk*	Prevention Strategies
Low risk	No specific measures
Moderate risk	Aggressive mobilization Low-dose unfractionated heparin (LDUH) q12h or low-molecular-weight heparin (LMWH) or external pneumatic compression Compression stockings
High risk	LDUH q8h or LMWH or compression stockings or external pneumatic compression
Highest risk	LMWH or oral anticoagulants Compression stockings or external pneumatic compression

*Refer to Table 18-2 for stratification of preoperative risk for thrombosis.

Low-Dose Unfractionated Heparin

Unfractionated heparin acts rapidly following both subcutaneous and intravenous administration. It has a short half-life and exerts its antithrombotic effect by binding with antithrombin III, accelerating its ability to inhibit clotting factors IX, X, and II. Unfractionated heparin administered at a low dose has been shown to be both safe and effective for VTE prophylaxis in moderate-risk general surgery patients. However, it has been less successful in surgical procedures involving the lower extremity. Unfractionated heparin may be poorly absorbed when administered by the subcutaneous route and thus may result in an unpredictable anticoagulant response.[32]

In those patients with contraindications to LMWH or warfarin, unfractionated heparin may be considered the best option. In these circumstances, a fixed-dose or adjusted-dose heparin may be administered. However, it is important to note that the adjusted-dose heparin has a greater VTE risk reduction when compared to a fixed dose of 5000 U heparin subcutaneously every 12 hours. The adjusted heparin dose is determined by monitoring the activated partial thromboplastin time (APTT). Alterations in the dose are made with the intent of keeping the APTT in the range of 31.5 to 36 seconds.

Major disadvantages associated with unfractionated heparin include bleeding, postoperative wound hematoma, the risk of heparin-induced thrombocytopenia, and thrombosis. Patients receiving unfractionated heparin should also have screening of stool for occult blood as well as regular monitoring of the platelet count.

Low-Molecular-Weight Heparin

LMWH is a classification of heparin commonly used for VTE prophylaxis. LMWH is derived from heparin by either chemical or enzymatic depolymerization. Its mechanism of action is due to the inhibition of factor Xa and IIa activity that results in less bleeding when compared with other types of heparin.[32]

The major advantages of LMWH are subcutaneous route of administration and relatively consistent anticoagulant response. Thus, LMWH produces a sustained stable anticoagulant effect, which eliminates the need for laboratory monitoring of coagulation in most instances. However, in certain clinical situations, such as renal failure or morbid obesity, determining the therapeutic dose of LMWH may be guided by laboratory assay. Although the chromogenic anti-Xa assay has been recommended by the College of American Pathologists, minimal therapeutic levels have not been established definitively. Dose determination is guided by the premise that anti-Xa levels are inversely related to thrombus propagation.[32]

Despite a lower incidence of heparin-induced thrombocytopenia (HIT) with LMWH as compared to unfractionated heparin, periodic laboratory monitoring of the platelet count is recommended. In addition, stools should be screened for occult blood since some risk for bleeding is present with all anticoagulants.

Current LMWH agents approved by the Food and Drug Administration (FDA) are enoxaparin (Lovenox), ardeparin (Normiflo), dalteparin (Fragmin), and danaparoid (Orgaran); however, other agents are currently under investigation or in use in other areas of the world.[16,32] These agents, indications, and dosages are outlined in Table 18-5.

The major disadvantages of using LMWH include expense and appropriate administration following patient discharge. It is important to note that the incidence of bleeding complications with LMWH has been reported to be higher than those associated with warfarin.[32] In addition, an increased incidence of spinal/epidural hematomas has been associated with neuraxial anesthesia and LMWH. Regardless of the specific LMWH agent used, patient compliance and safety play an important role in optimizing clinical outcomes. Box 18-1 provides an overview of several important concepts that should be included in patient education.

TABLE 18–5 Antithrombotic Agents and Dosing Regimens for VTE Prophylaxis

Pharmacologic Agent	Description
Low-dose unfractionated heparin	Heparin 5000 U SC q8-12h starting 1-2h preop
Adjusted-dose heparin	Heparin SC q8h starting with approximately 3500 U SC and adjusted by + 500 U SC; dose to maintain a mid-high normal value
Low-molecular-weight heparin	**Medical conditions**
	Dalteparin 2500 U SC once daily
	Danaparoid 750 U SC q12h
	Enoxaparin 40 mg SC once daily
	General surgery, moderate risk
	Dalteparin 2500 U SC 1-2h preop and once daily postop
	Enoxaparin 20 mg SC 1-2h preop and once daily postop
	Nadroparin 2850 U SC 2-4h preop and once daily postop
	Tinzaparin 3500 U SC preop and once daily postop
	General surgery, high risk
	Dalteparin 5000 U SC 8-12h preop and once daily postop
	Danaparoid 750 U SC 1-4h preop and q12h postop
	Enoxaparin 40 mg SC 1-2h preop and once daily postop
	Enoxaparin 30 mg SC q12h starting 8-12h postop
	Orthopedic surgery
	Dalteparin 5000 U SC 8-12h preop and once daily starting 12-24h postop
	Dalteparin 2500 U SC 6-8h postop then 5000 U once daily
	Danaparoid 750 U SC 1-4h preop and q12h postop
	Enoxaparin 30 mg SC q12h starting 12-24h postop
	Enoxaparin 40 mg SC once daily starting 10-12h preop
	Nadroparin 38 U/kg SC q12h preop, 12h postop, and once daily on postop days 1-3, then increase to 57 U/kg once daily
	Tinzaparin 75 U/kg SC once daily starting 12-24h postop
	Tinzaparin 4500 U SC 12h preop and once daily postop
	Major trauma
	Enoxaparin 30 mg SC q12h starting 12-36h post-injury if hemostatically stable
	Acute spinal cord injury
	Enoxaparin 30 mg SC q12h
Perioperative warfarin	Start daily dosing regimen with 5-10 mg the day of or day after surgery; adjust the dose for a target INR of 2.5 (range of 2-3)

Modified from Deitelzweig SB: Management and prevention of venous thromboembolism including surgery and the pregnant state, *Ochsner J* 4:23–29, 2002.

VTE, Venous thromboembolic disease; *SC,* subcutaneously; *INR,* international normalized ratio.

BOX 18–1

Patient Teaching Guidelines for Anticoagulation Therapy

PRESCRIBED DRUG__________
NAME__________
GENERAL ACTION__________
DOSAGE__________
SIDE EFFECTS__________

- **Contraindications to anticoagulation therapy**
  Active major bleed
  Thrombocytopenia
  Hypersensitivity to heparin or pork products
- **Signs of unusual bleeding**
  Bleeding gums
  Nosebleeds
  Excessive bruising
  Blood in urine or stool
  When to report to health care professional
- **Drug administration guidelines**
  Give at same time each day.
  Do not stop taking unless advised by health care professional.
  If injection is missed, take as soon as possible but do not double the dose (alter timing of next injection dose).
- **Drugs administered by injection**
  Inject into abdominal subcutaneous tissue at least 2 inches from navel.
  Rotate injection sites to avoid irritating the skin.
  Discard used needle in appropriate dispenser (not in trash).
- **Drug administered orally (warfarin)**
  Maintain a log of dosage, lab values, and dosage adjustments.
  Monitor dietary intake of dark green and yellow vegetables, which are sources of vitamin K that counteract anticoagulant effects.
- **Substances that may have anticoagulant effects unless authorized**
  Aspirin
  Certain vitamins, nutritional, and herbal agents (i.e., vitamin E, green tea, nutritional shakes)
  Limit alcohol intake.
  Consult health care professional if at increased risk of bleeding.
  Complete blood tests as ordered by health care professional (i.e., INR, platelet count).
  Carry an emergency identification bracelet or card listing drug name, dosage, health care professional name, and phone number.

INR, International normalized ratio.

Warfarin

Oral anticoagulants, such as warfarin, inhibit vitamin K–dependent clotting factors II, VII, IX, X, and proteins C and S.[33] When low-intensity warfarin (5-10 mg) is administered the night prior to surgery, therapeutic anticoagulation is usually achieved on the third postoperative day.[33,34] This dosing method was instituted to prevent delays in warfarin's anticoagulant effect, yet avoid the excess bleeding associated with full anticoagulation during surgery. The dosage of warfarin is adjusted daily to maintain the international normalized ratio (INR) in the range of 2 to 3.

Major advantages of warfarin are its low cost and route of oral administration. Disadvantages include the length of time to achieve therapeutic effect (a window of 36 to 72 hours), potential bleeding complications, and dose adjustments that depend on daily laboratory monitoring of the INR. Patient teaching guidelines are included in Box 18-1.

BOX 18–2

Nursing Management: Venous Thromboembolism Prophylaxis
• **Identify patients at increased risk for DVT:** Refer to Tables 18-1 and 18-2 • **Monitor for early signs and symptoms associated with DVT by assessing extremities at least every shift, being vigilant for:** Unilateral or bilateral edema Pain that is atypical for operative procedure Generalized tenderness Venous distention • **Promote venous return:** Maintain fluid balance. Use stool softener. Perform passive and active ROM exercises. Encourage early ambulation. • **Apply graduated compression stockings:** Assess for appropriate application at least every shift. Look for circumferential constriction. Remove twice daily for 60 minutes; inspect skin. Inspect heels for redness and soreness. Apply skin emollient prn. • **Use intermittent pneumatic compression:** Assess for appropriate extremity/foot sleeve application and pump function at least every shift. Ensure bladder of sleeve is positioned over calf muscle. Inspect skin and soft tissue under sleeve at least every shift.

DVT, Deep vein thrombosis; *ROM,* range of motion.

Adjunctive Prevention Strategies

Adjunctive prevention strategies include external pneumatic compression pumps, use of compression stockings, leg elevation, and early mobilization. These strategies are beneficial as either primary prophylaxis or as an adjunct combined with pharmacologic measures.[35] However, successful prophylaxis using these adjunctive strategies depends on both consistency and accuracy in appropriate use. Nursing management associated with DVT prophylaxis is outlined in Box 18-2.

External Pneumatic Compression

External pneumatic compression (EPC) of the thigh and/or calf, or plantar venous plexus decreases the incidence of DVT by augmenting the calf muscle pumps in evacuating the sinuses of blood and reducing venous stasis by stimulating endogenous fibrinolytic activity. Some investigators report that even unilateral application results in benefit to both extremities as this triggers systemic fibrinolytic activity.[36]

A synthetic sleeve or boot encircles the extremity and provides alternating periods of compression to the calf alone, the calf and thigh, or the foot. EPC devices are available in single-chamber and multichamber types, providing intermittent or sequential pressure at predetermined time periods. The single-chamber device produces uniform compression of the calves at predetermined time periods, whereas the more frequently used multichamber device produces graded sequential or intermittent compression. Figs. 18-2 and 18-3 illustrate the extremity and pedal pump systems.

Factors such as patient comfort, site accessibility, staff familiarity, and cost all play a role in the selection of pump type. Comparisons of efficacy in preventing DVT between these diverse pump systems are varied. In general, using the pump on the patient is more important in preventing VTE than the type of pneumatic compression device.[37,38]

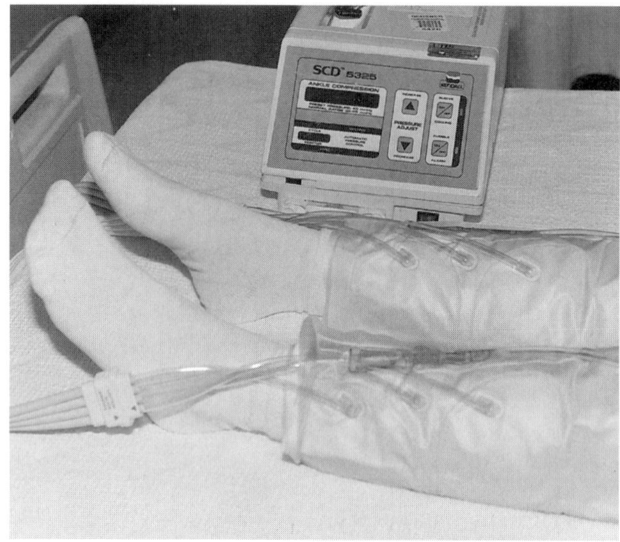

FIG. 18–2. Segmental compression pump with sleeves on lower extremities.

Complications, although extremely rare, may include skin blisters and sensations of warmth/heat. Oftentimes, graduated compression stockings are used simultaneously to protect the skin and increase venous return.

Compression Stockings

Compression stockings are useful adjuncts in the prevention of VTE by promoting venous return from the lower extremities.[16,39] These stockings are made of various materials, such as natural rubber and synthetics, including latex. They are available in a variety of colors, lengths (calf to thigh high), and ranges of compression with the greatest pressure at the ankle (Fig. 18-4). Most are available as ready-made products. Normal resting venous pressures are 18 mm Hg at the ankle to 8 mm Hg at the upper thigh. Therefore, hospital compression stockings are generally calibrated to 20 mm Hg for DVT prophylaxis in the recumbent patient. Patients with pre-existing venous disease may have higher resting pressures that would require additional compression for appropriate prophylaxis. Despite the availability of different lengths, knee-high stockings are more effective in the prevention of DVT; they are less expensive and easier to apply.

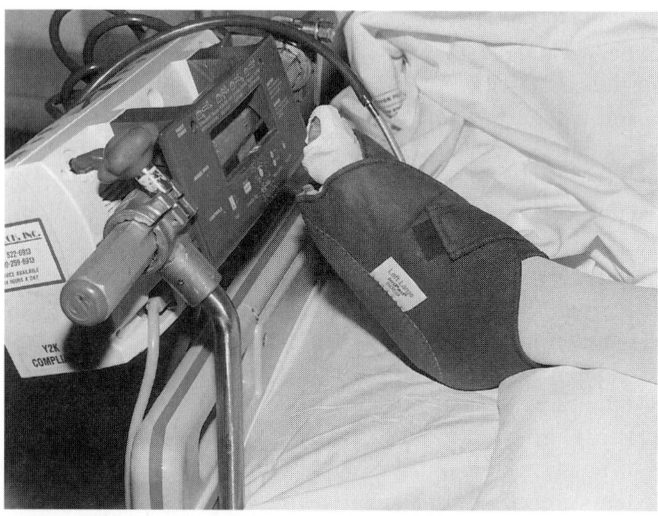

FIG. 18–3. Plantar compression device.

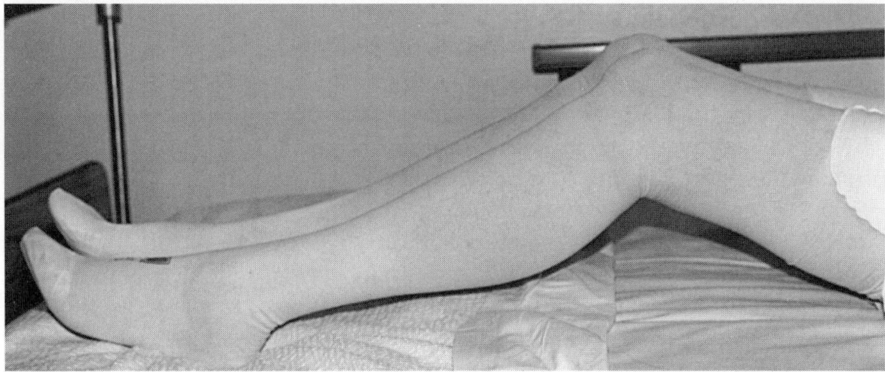

FIG. 18–4. Thigh-high compression stockings.

As with compression pumps, the effectiveness of stockings in DVT prophylaxis is dependent upon appropriate fit and use. To fit a patient, the circumference and length of each extremity must be accurately measured according to manufacturer's instructions. An appropriate fit is important to prevent the stocking from rolling down, forming a rubber-band–like constrictive effect. Patients should be taught the proper use and care of compression stockings (see Box 18-2).

Leg Elevation and Early Mobilization

Leg elevation is an important adjunct in DVT prophylaxis. However, its effectiveness is dependent on the angle of elevation. To reduce leg edema, the angle of elevation should be 10° to 20° above the level of the heart in the nonambulatory patient. All patients should be ambulating as soon as their condition permits.[16,39] Once ambulation has begun, the patient should be encouraged to avoid prolonged standing and sitting without leg elevation. Walking and other types of physical activity using the calf muscles should be encouraged on a regular basis.

VENOUS THROMBOEMBOLIC EVENTS

Venous thromboembolic disease may be manifested as a variety of clinical pictures. Although some patients may appear to be asymptomatic, closer analysis of signs and symptoms usually reveals clues to establishing a diagnosis. This section will provide an overview of superficial thrombophlebitis, deep vein thrombosis, and pulmonary embolism.

Superficial Thrombophlebitis

Superficial thrombophlebitis, estimated to affect 125,000 individuals within the United States, results from both thrombosis and inflammation within a superficial vein.[40] In the lower extremity, the greater or lesser saphenous veins are most often involved. Superficial thrombophlebitis is more commonly seen in women during pregnancy.[4,15] There is also an increased incidence within the postoperative period and in patients with varicose veins. In the upper extremity, superficial thrombophlebitis is seen in the arm and subclavian veins. Superficial thrombophlebitis is typically associated with a precipitating factor such as trauma, infection, venous stasis, vasculitis, cancer, and/or hypercoagulable state. The specific types of superficial thrombophlebitis are discussed below.

Traumatic superficial thrombophlebitis is the most common type. Trauma to the vein results from a direct injury or an iatrogenic event, such as intraluminal cannulation of a vessel and the administration of intravenous therapy, including chemotherapeutic agents, hypertonic solutions (e.g., potassium chloride), specific pharmacologic agents (e.g., benzodiazepines, barbiturates), and radiographic contrast.[4]

Infectious/suppurative thrombophlebitis is a relatively rare but potentially fatal disorder. An infectious process usually develops at the site of a cannulated vein. *Staphylococcus epidermidis, Staphylococcus aureus,* and many types of *Candida* are common pathogens. As these microorganisms proliferate, pus accumulates and an abscess forms.[40] This can progress to microorganism seeding in the blood, leading to septicemia and sometimes endocarditis, particularly in those patients with prosthetic heart valves or valvular heart disease.

Superficial thrombophlebitis associated with varicose veins is more likely to develop secondary to trauma and adjacent to venous stasis ulcers. Typically, the greater or lesser saphenous veins are painful, erythematous, and swollen. This type of superficial thrombophlebitis is more common in older patients with long-standing venous insufficiency.

Migratory thrombophlebitis refers to the presence of multiple superficial venous thromboses. Migratory thrombophlebitis frequently occurs in patients with an underlying carcinoma, particularly those with pancreatic cancer. This type of thrombophlebitis also develops in patients with a hypercoagulable problem or an underlying pathology, such as vasculitis.[40]

Clinical Manifestations

Superficial thrombophlebitis is easily recognized on physical examination. The area is erythematous, swollen, and painful along the course of the affected superficial vein. The area is warm and often has a red linear streak. A firm, subcutaneous tender cord may be palpable (see Fig. 4-14). With recent trauma or intravenous cannulation, ecchymosis may be present.

Infectious/suppurative thrombophlebitis, however, is not as easily recognized on physical examination. Most often there are no local signs of thrombophlebitis. The presence of a high-grade fever may indicate suppurative thrombophlebitis. In some cases, septic pulmonary emboli are the first indication of its presence.

Diagnostic Evaluation

Superficial thrombophlebitis is typically diagnosed on the basis of the physical exam alone. An elevated white blood cell count and/or positive blood cultures may be present. In the lower extremity, a venous duplex ultrasound may be indicated to identify the extent of the thrombus into the saphenofemoral junction or the deep femoral system.

Treatment and Nursing Management

Several strategies directed at the prevention of superficial thrombophlebitis are outlined in Box 18-3. However, when prophylaxis fails, treatment of superficial thrombophlebitis is based on the type and extent of the disease process. Superficial thrombophlebitis can last for a few days or a few weeks. With traumatic superficial thrombophlebitis, any indwelling catheter should be immediately removed.[18] The affected extremity should be elevated to promote venous return and reduce swelling. The application of local moist heat for 20-30 minutes several times a day frequently alleviates pain and reduces inflammation. Compression stockings or an elastic bandage may provide comfort in lower-extremity thrombophlebitis once inflammation begins to resolve.

Nonsteroidal anti-inflammatory drugs, such as ibuprofen, may be administered to relieve symptoms. Aspirin may be given to provide an antithrombotic effect. Other pharmacologic agents, such as antibiotics and corticosteroids, are usually not indicated in noncomplicated situations. However, suppurative thrombophlebitis requires surgical excision of the affected vein and its tributaries. In addition, specific antibiotic therapy is administered on the basis of the culture results.[18]

If the thrombus extends into the proximal greater saphenous vein or to the saphenofemoral junction, more aggressive management is indicated to prevent propagation of the clot into the deep venous system. In this instance, either systemic anticoagulation or surgical ligation proximal to the thrombosis is indicated.[40] The choice of treatment is generally dictated by the overall health status of the patient. Patients at risk of hemorrhagic complications or pregnant women are best treated without anticoagulation using surgical ligation of the affected vein under local anesthesia with conscious sedation if necessary.

BOX 18–3

Nursing Management: Superficial Thrombophlebitis Prophylaxis

Use strict aseptic technique during venous cannulation, intravenous dressing changes, and intravenous therapy.
Assess intravenous sites every 4-8 hours for signs of thrombophlebitis.
Check temperature every 4-8 hours.
Change intravenous tubing every 24-48 hours.
Change intravenous catheter sites every 72-96 hours.
Adhere to dilution requirements of intravenous medications.
Use large veins only for potentially irritating solutions.
Secure indwelling venous catheters.
Pad bed rails of disoriented patients.
Use arm/leg restraints with extreme caution.
Avoid using the lower extremity for venous access.
Insert peripherally inserted central catheter (PICC) line for long-term access.
Use a central venous line for select patients.

Deep Vein Thrombosis

DVT is an acute, potentially life-threatening condition that may necessitate hospitalization. DVT, more common in the veins of the lower extremity, develops in the deep veins of the calf muscles or, less frequently, in the proximal deep veins of the lower extremity. DVT limited to the calf veins is generally associated with a low risk of PE. If untreated, 20 percent of calf vein thromboses will propagate into the proximal venous system (Fig. 18-5), increasing the risk of fatal PE to 10 percent.[16] Recent reports suggest that most DVT that develop, despite prophylaxis, will resolve without causing localizing symptoms. However, many of these asymptomatic DVTs have been associated with the late development of PE and postphlebitic syndrome.[41]

Clinical Manifestations

Patients with DVT may be asymptomatic or symptomatic. Signs and symptoms of DVT vary, depending on the size of the thrombus, location, if the lumen is partially or totally

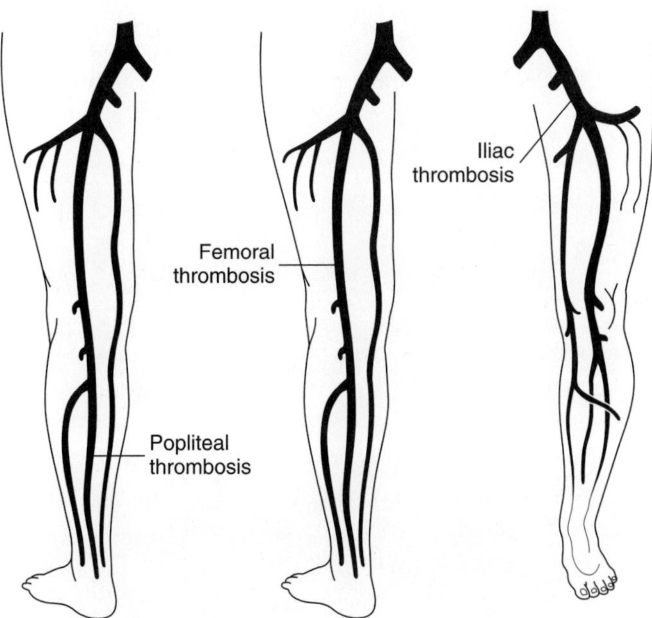

FIG. 18–5. Common patterns of deep vein thrombosis. (From Belcaro G, Nicolaides AN, Veller M: *Venous disorders: a manual of diagnosis and treatment*, Philadelphia, 1995, WB Saunders.)

obstructed, and adequacy of collateral circulation. Hence, physical findings may be absent in cases of partial obstruction or when collateral channels reconstitute flow around a complete obstruction. Classic symptoms of DVT include sudden onset of unilateral swelling of the extremity, pain, and possible tenderness (Fig. 18-6). Table 18-6 describes common signs and symptoms associated with calf, femoral, and iliofemoral thrombosis. However, these symptoms can also be related to disorders such as superficial thrombophlebitis, cellulitis, ruptured muscle or tendon, muscle strain, internal derangement of the knee, ruptured popliteal cyst (Baker's cyst), cutaneous vasculitis, or lymphedema.[10] A ruptured Baker's cyst frequently produces a clinical syndrome of calf pain that mimics DVT (pseudothrombophlebitis). The presence of calf pain on dorsiflexion of the foot, Homan's sign, is not a reliable predictor since it is not consistently found in patients with DVT.[3,4,10]

In the presence of DVT, collateral venous channels develop in an effort to reconstitute venous flow around the obstruction.[4,10] This process may precipitate clues to establishing a diagnosis of DVT such as visible dilation of superficial veins adjacent to the obstruction (Fig. 18-7). For example, venous collaterals are often visible through the skin over the shoulder and infraclavicular area in axillary or subclavian vein thrombosis, and over the groin and lower abdomen in patients with iliofemoral venous thrombosis. In addition, the inflammatory response involving the superficial venous system may be significant enough to exhibit increased local warmth and erythema of the involved extremity.[10]

While most extremities affected by acute DVT appear near normal, obstruction of the iliofemoral veins commonly manifests obvious clinical signs and symptoms. Advanced forms of iliofemoral venous thrombosis include phlegmasia alba dolens and phlegmasia cerulea dolens. Phlegmasia alba dolens, also known as "milk leg," was first described in postpartum patients. The affected limb is characterized by diffuse swelling, pallor, and moderate pain. This is caused by a severe perivenous inflammatory reaction extending to the periarterial sympathetic nerve fibers, producing arterial spasm or compression.[11] Clinical manifestations in combination with tenderness over the common femoral vein and visible collaterals in the groin is generally diagnostic of iliofemoral venous thrombosis.

Phlegmasia cerulea dolens is commonly seen in advanced stages of some cancers. The iliac, common femoral, superficial femoral, popliteal, tibial, and greater saphenous veins and

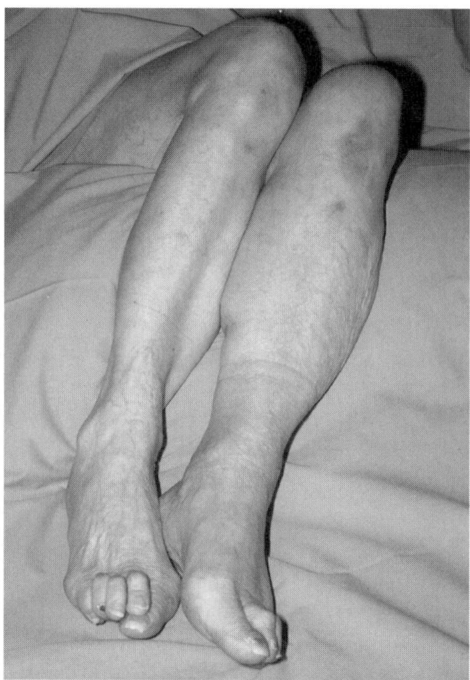

FIG. 18–6. Patient with unilateral leg swelling indicative of deep vein thrombosis.

TABLE 18–6 Common Signs and Symptoms Associated With Deep Vein Thrombosis

Site	Signs and Symptoms
Calf thrombosis	Calf tenderness Distal swelling (slight to absent) of affected extremity
Femoral thrombosis	Tenderness and pain in distal thigh and popliteal regions Swelling more prominent than with calf vein thrombosis alone Swelling may extend to level of knee
Iliofemoral thrombosis	Massive swelling in affected extremity Tenderness and pain involving entire extremity
Upper-extremity thrombosis	Swelling of affected extremity Dilated superficial veins Tenderness and pain Impaired mobility of extremity

their tributaries may all be involved. This extensive process results in almost total occlusion of venous outflow, with increased pressure contributing to arterial inflow obstruction. Pedal pulses may be reduced or absent, and compartment pressures are likely to be elevated. Multiple petechiae are common and may progress to hemorrhagic bullae. Patients typically have sudden onset of deep pain, massive edema, and cyanosis of the extremity. Hypotension and hemoconcentration, which result from entrapment of blood in the leg and massive fluid loss into the interstitium, may further compound the thrombotic cycle. If untreated, gangrene is likely to develop. The mortality rate is high, especially in the presence of venous gangrene. Survivors frequently require amputation of the involved limb.

Diagnostic Evaluation

Physical examination is only accurate for DVT in 30 percent of cases; therefore, it serves to increase clinical suspicion for those at risk rather than eliminate the possibility of VTE.[3] Wells et al developed a clinical model to guide the diagnostic approach in patients suspected of having DVT.[42] The clinical model categorizes patients as high, moderate, or low probability of having DVT, which is based on the presence of clinical features (nine-item checklist) commonly associated with DVT and identification of alternative diagnosis. Box 18-4 outlines both the pretest and DVT risk classification.[41,42] This model is reported to be accurate

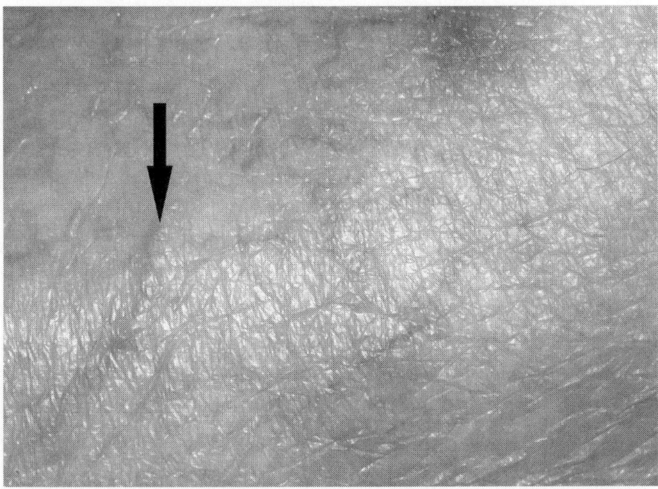

FIG. 18–7. Collateral veins (*arrow*) adjacent to deep vein thrombosis involving the popliteal and superficial femoral veins.

BOX 18–4

Predicting Probability of Deep Vein Thrombosis Using a Clinical Model

PRETEST*
Active cancer (treatment ongoing, within prior 6 months, or palliative)
Paralysis, paresis, or recent plaster immobilization of the lower extremities
Recent confinement to bed >3 days or major surgery within 4 weeks
Swelling of thigh and calf
Localized tenderness along the distribution of the deep vein system
Calf swelling 3 cm > symptom-free side (measured 10 cm below tibial tuberosity)
Dilated superficial veins (nonvaricose) in symptomatic extremity
Pitting edema in symptomatic leg
Alternative diagnosis as likely as or more likely than deep vein thrombosis (DVT)

DVT RISK CLASSIFICATION
High probability
>3 points
Moderate probability
1-2 points
Low probability
0 points

*One point is given for each positive finding in the pretest, and 2 points are subtracted if an alternative diagnosis as likely as DVT is identified.

in predicting whether a diagnosis of DVT will actually be found. Patients categorized as high probability were accurately diagnosed with DVT in 85 percent of the cases. Patients designated as moderate pretest probability had DVT diagnosed 30 percent of the time. In those patients identified as low probability, only 5 percent of patients were diagnosed with DVT.[41]

As previously stated, clinical manifestations alone are not reliable in establishing a diagnosis of DVT. Therefore, additional diagnostic techniques must be incorporated in order to facilitate a comprehensive evaluation of the patient. Diagnostic modalities identified to be reliable in diagnosing VTE include color flow duplex ultrasound imaging, the D-dimer test, ascending phlebography, computerized tomography venography, and magnetic resonance venography.

COLOR FLOW DUPLEX ULTRASOUND IMAGING. Color flow duplex ultrasound imaging (CFDI) allows rapid and clear visualization of thrombi (Figs. 18-8 and 18-9), including identification of unstable or floating thrombi, which may cause emboli (see Chapter 5). Full diagnostic components of the examination include Doppler spectral analysis, color flow Doppler imaging, transducer compression, and high resolution B-mode imaging. CFDI is reported to have a 95 percent sensitivity and 98 percent specificity for compression ultrasound.[42] Occasionally false positives result from proximal obstructions caused by extrinsic masses or venous distention secondary to congestive heart failure. Technical difficulty attributed to obesity or edema has also been associated with false negatives. Despite a few pitfalls, CFDI is currently the mainstay of DVT diagnosis and has essentially replaced indirect physiologic diagnostic modalities.

D-DIMER TEST. Patients with VTE usually have elevated D-dimer levels because D-dimer is released into the circulation when cross-linked fibrin is degraded by plasmin. Therefore, a normal level is valuable in ruling out DVT. However, because D-dimer is generated in the presence of thrombus, it may also be positive in those who have undergone recent surgery, sustained minor trauma, or in the presence of an active inflammatory process. Dryjski and co-workers reported that when D-dimer and pretest probability were utilized to establish a diagnosis of DVT, there was a 100 percent sensitivity, 100 percent negative predictive value, and a specificity of 25 percent.[43,44] The four basic methods capable of measuring D-dimer

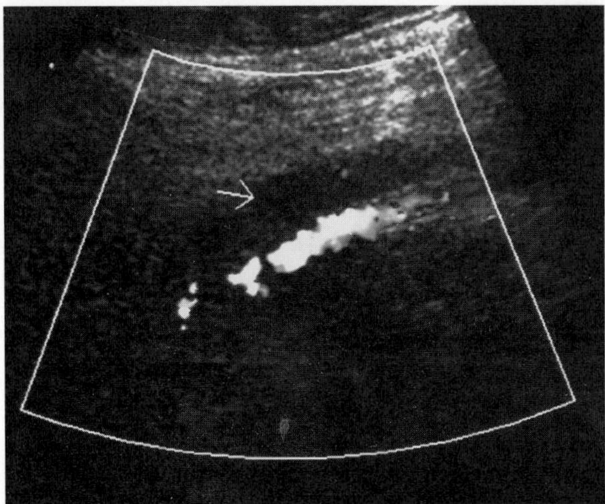

FIG. 18–8. Acute vein thrombosis vein (*arrow*) with expanded hypoechoic vein with no flow seen on color flow Doppler imaging. (Reprinted from Olsan AD, Matthew CC, Sullivan MA: Pulmonary thromboembolic disease: a new role for computed tomography, *The Ochsner Journal,* Vol 4, No. 1, p 16 with permission, 2002.)

concentration include latex agglutination, microplate enzyme-linked immunosorbent assay (ELISA), membrane ELISA, and whole blood agglutination. The ELISA determinations are the best methods for D-dimer analysis; however, they are time consuming and not practical for clinical use. The whole blood agglutination assay has been found to be the most advantageous method; it requires only a drop of whole blood, and results are available in just a few minutes.[43]

ASCENDING PHLEBOGRAPHY. Prior to the development of sophisticated ultrasonography available today, venography was considered the gold standard for the diagnosis of DVT. Ascending venography is performed by the injection of a radio-contrast agent into a superficial vein on the dorsum of the foot. The contrast material mixes with the blood and flows proximally. Radiographic images of the leg and pelvis show the calf, popliteal, and femoral veins, which drain into the external iliac vein. A thrombus is diagnosed by the presence of an intraluminal filling defect, flow diversion, abrupt termination of contrast visibility, and failure to opacify segments or the entire deep venous system. Venography accurately identifies 90 percent of thrombi.[6,8,45] In addition, a negative venogram excludes the presence of lower-extremity thrombosis. The small veins and sinuses of the calf, however, may be difficult to visualize, and deep femoral vein opacification in the presence of DVT is identified in only 50 percent of patients.[10,11] Other limitations of venography include increased cost and increased risk of lower-extremity thrombophlebitis associated with an invasive procedure (see Chapter 6).

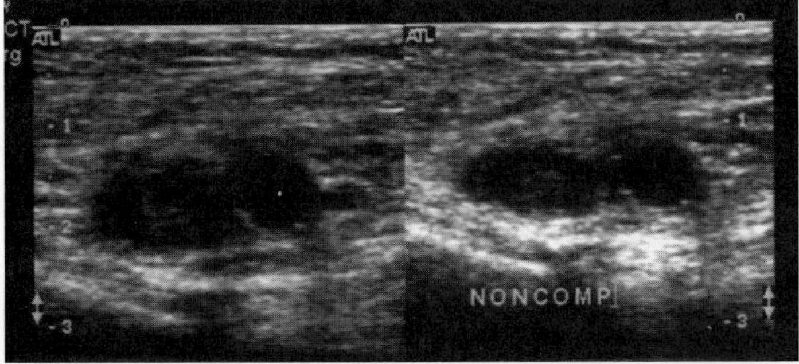

FIG. 18–9. Transverse gray scale images of the common femoral vessels with acute deep vein thrombosis. The image on the left is without compression, and the image on the right demonstrates the noncompressible vein and adjacent artery. (Reprinted from Olsan AD, Matthew CC, Sullivan MA: Pulmonary thromboembolic disease: a new role for computed tomography, *The Ochsner Journal,* Vol 4, No. 1, p 16 with permission, 2002.)

COMPUTED TOMOGRAPHY VENOGRAPHY. The diagnostic capability of computed tomography venography (CTV) in the diagnosis of DVT may equal ultrasound and in some instances actually be superior (Fig. 18-10). Loud et al[46] recently reported a 97 percent sensitivity and 100 percent specificity for the detection of femoropopliteal DVT by computed tomography venography when compared to venous sonography. This alternative to ultrasound may be particularly beneficial in selective cases, such as in the morbidly obese or when pelvic or abdominal thrombosis is suspected.

MAGNETIC RESONANCE VENOGRAPHY. Magnetic resonance venography has also demonstrated excellent sensitivity for the diagnosis of proximal DVT. However, availability, cost, contraindication with metallic implants, and claustrophobia limit its application. When more traditional diagnostic studies are inadequate, particularly in patients with pelvic and vena caval thrombosis, magnetic resonance venography provides an alternative.[46,47]

DIAGNOSTIC STRATEGIES. Although CFDI using compression is the current study of choice for the diagnosis of DVT, recent investigations suggest that pretest probability and D-dimer testing may be sufficient alone to exclude the diagnosis.[43,48] Table 18-7 describes proposed diagnostic strategies in evaluating patients for DVT.

A negative D-dimer test provides good assurance that the patient does not have DVT. However, a positive D-dimer assay in the presence of a negative CFDI necessitates further evaluation with computed tomography venography, magnetic resonance venography, or ascending phlebography as described above. Both CTV and magnetic resonance venography have demonstrated excellent sensitivity for the diagnosis of proximal venous thrombosis in comparison to ascending phlebography. The true value of CTV and magnetic resonance venography is likely to be in the obese patient or when the diagnosis of pelvic and vena caval thrombosis is suspected, for which traditional phlebography is inadequate.[43,47]

Other components of the diagnostic evaluation include blood testing to detect coagulopathies. A coagulation profile should be completed, including measurement of APTT, prothrombin time (PT), INR, circulating fibrin, monomer complexes, fibrinopeptide A, serum fibrin degradation products, proteins C and S, and antithrombin III levels. Chapter 9 discusses these coagulation measurements in more detail.

Treatment and Nursing Management

Treatment interventions are based on the location of the thrombus. The goals of treatment are to prevent propagation of the clot, prevent the development of new thrombi, prevent pulmonary emboli, and limit venous valvular damage. The nursing management of the patient closely reflects the implementation of the treatment interventions, which include bed rest, leg elevation, compression stockings, and administration of antithrombotic agents.[9,35]

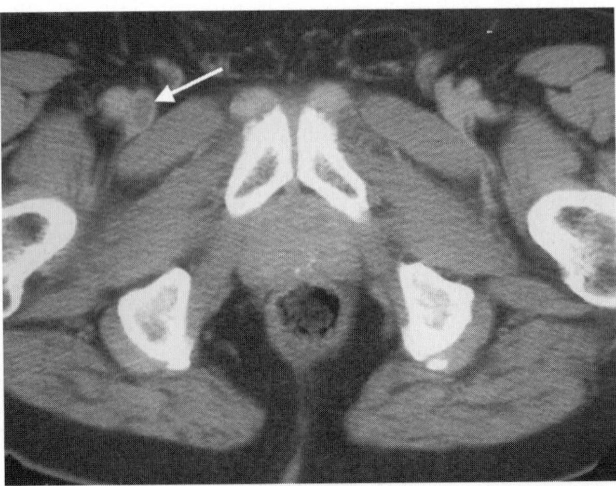

FIG. 18–10. Computed tomography venogram demonstrating acute deep vein thrombus (*arrow*) in the right common femoral vein. (Reprinted from Olsan AD, Matthew CC, Sullivan MA: Pulmonary thromboembolic disease: a new role for computed tomography, *The Ochsner Journal,* Vol 4, No. 1, p 16 with permission, 2002.)

TABLE 18–7 Applying the Pretest Probability Clinical Model to the Diagnostic Evaluation of DVT

Patient Category	Proposed Diagnostic Strategy
High-risk probability	Direct duplex ultrasound imaging with compression
Low-risk and moderate-risk patients with positive D-dimer	D-dimer and duplex ultrasound imaging with compression
Low-risk and moderate-risk patients with negative D-dimer	D-dimer

Modified from Wells PS, Ginsberg JS, Anderson DR et al: Use of a clinical model for safe management of patients with suspected pulmonary embolism, *Ann Intern Med* 129:997–1005, 1998.
DVT, Deep vein thrombosis.

If thrombosis is suspected, the patient should be kept on bed rest until examined by the physician. The calf and thigh should be measured at specific points, such as 10 cm above the upper edge of the patella, 10 cm below the tibial crest, and 20 cm below the tibial crest. Any changes from the baseline measurements should be promptly reported to the physician.

BED REST. Bed rest is usually recommended for approximately 4-5 days until the thrombus is stable and has adhered to the intraluminal wall. Progressive ambulation can be started after this period. This length of time varies with physician preference; some patients are currently being treated as outpatients.

LEG ELEVATION. The affected extremity should be elevated at least 10-20 degrees above the level of the heart to enhance venous return and reduce swelling. Elevation of the foot of the bed is permitted if the head of the bed remains flat, because this will prevent inguinal congestion. Pillows may be used to elevate the affected extremity; they should support the entire length of the leg to prevent compression of the popliteal space. If the thrombosis is located in the upper extremity, the arm can be elevated with a stockinette attached to an intravenous pole. Once ambulation has begun, the patient should be encouraged to avoid prolonged standing and sitting without leg elevation. If the patient has significant edema, ambulation should be restricted.

COMPRESSION STOCKINGS. A compression garment, such as stockings or an elastic bandage, should be worn at all times. Compression promotes venous return and decreases leg swelling. Initially, 4-inch elastic bandages are applied snugly, with consistent tension from the toes to just below the knee with edges overlapped. If an iliofemoral venous thrombosis is present, a 6-inch elastic bandage may be applied above the knee. Once the edema has subsided, the patient should be measured for graded compression stockings (or an upper-extremity sleeve). To fit the stocking correctly, the nurse should measure the largest calf and ankle circumference and the leg length from bottom of heel to bend of knee. Pressure at the ankle should be at least 30-40 mm Hg to counteract the high venous pressure; pressure should decrease proximally. Knee-high stockings are more effective in the treatment of DVT, whereas thigh-high stockings are more effective in the treatment of proximal vein DVT (see Fig. 18-4).

PHARMACOLOGIC MEASURES. In general, pharmacologic measures consist of anticoagulation with heparin or LMWH, followed by long-term oral anticoagulation with warfarin.[49] However, in recent years the benefits of treating extensive DVT with thrombolytic therapy have been identified. While anticoagulation is essentially prophylaxis because these medications do not actively dissolve thrombus, thrombolytic agents potentially prevent PE and decrease the incidence of postphlebitic syndrome.[50] Guidelines for the duration of anticoagulation therapy are included in Table 18-8.

Unfractionated Heparin. Heparin therapy is initiated after baseline laboratory determinants of APTT, PT with INR, and platelet count are drawn. If a DVT is suspected based on the clinical history and examination, either a fixed-dose bolus of heparin (5000 U) or weight-based dosing (80 U/kg) is initially administered intravenously. It is then followed by a heparin drip to maintain the APTT ratio between 1.5 and 2.5 times the control. The majority of patients

TABLE 18–8 Recommended Duration of Anticoagulation

Duration of Therapy	Characteristics
3 to 6 months	First event with time-limited or reversible risk factor (e.g., trauma, immobilization, surgery, estrogen use)
>6 months	Idiopathic venous thromboembolic event First-time event
12 months to lifetime	First-time event with (one of the following) Cancer, until resolved Antithrombin deficiency Anticardiolipin antibody Recurrent event, idiopathic or thrombophilia

initially require 1000-2000 U/hr or 18 U/kg/hr to achieve adequate anticoagulation. It is generally accepted that adequate anticoagulation must be maintained in order to achieve an effective antithrombotic effect. Therefore, body weight–based dosing of intravenous heparin provides a guided approach to maintaining therapeutic anticoagulation. Table 18-9 outlines dosing guidelines and associated APTT monitoring for weight-based dosing of heparin.[49]

Heparin should be continued for 5-10 days, the usual time the body needs to dissolve the clot completely. Oral anticoagulation should be overlapped with heparin. For iliofemoral thrombosis, a longer period of heparin therapy may be considered. Currently, the accepted approach is to begin heparin and oral anticoagulation together at the time of diagnosis and discontinue the heparin between the fourth and seventh day of therapy. Heparin therapy is generally discontinued when the INR is >2, while oral anticoagulation is continued for approximately 3 months. Clinical trials have also demonstrated the effectiveness of subcutaneous heparin and LMWH as treatment for DVT. For subcutaneous treatment of DVT with unfractionated heparin, 250 U/kg every 12 hours is recommended.[49]

HIT is a well-recognized complication of heparin occurring in up to 10 percent patients.[50] Heparin-induced antiplatelet antibodies cause platelet aggregation, leading to thrombocytopenia. The nurse should carefully monitor the platelet count and notify the physician if it is less than 100,000/mm^3 or 40 percent below pretreatment level.[50] This platelet aggregation may activate the clotting mechanism and result in arterial thromboembolism and extension or recurrence of existing venous thromboembolism, as well as skin slough and wound hematoma.[50] Mild asymptomatic elevation of liver enzymes in some patients occurs between days 5 and 10 of heparin therapy. These elevations have been associated with either normalization during treatment or following treatment cessation without untoward long-term effects.

Low-Molecular-Weight Heparin. There is a growing trend in the use of LMWH, as a replacement for unfractionated heparin, in the treatment of DVT. As previously discussed,

TABLE 18–9 Guidelines for Weight-Dosing Heparin

APTT parameter	Dose Change (U/kg/hr)	Instructions	Next APTT
<35	+4	Rebolus with 80 U/kg	6 hours
35-45	+2	Rebolus with 40 U/kg	6 hours
46-70	0	0	6 hours
71-90	−2	0	6 hours
>90	−3	Stop infusion for 1 hour	6 hours

APTT, Activated partial thromboplastin time.

the benefit of using LMWH includes no laboratory monitoring unless the treatment period exceeds 7 days. Similar to the use of unfractionated heparin, oral anticoagulation therapy should overlap LWMH administration in order to maintain therapeutic levels of anticoagulation. In addition, LMWH may be efficaciously administered at home; therefore, there is the possibility of early discharge or initial treatment as an outpatient. Factors to be considered in identifying appropriate patients for early discharge or outpatient therapy include stable condition, low bleeding risk, absence of severe renal insufficiency, and the presence of a practical system for the administration and surveillance of treatment/complications.[49,50]

Warfarin. Oral anticoagulation with warfarin should begin simultaneously with initiation of intravenous heparin or LWMH anticoagulation. Because warfarin has a very short half-life, there is a period of hypercoagulability that occurs during the first few days of treatment. Heparin should not be discontinued until therapeutic INR values of 2-3 are maintained.[33,49]

Oral anticoagulation is generally continued for 3-6 months to prevent recurrent thrombosis in patients with proximal vein thrombosis and symptomatic calf vein thrombosis.[33,49] Oral anticoagulation is maintained indefinitely in patients with recurrent venous thrombosis, antithrombin III deficiency, protein C deficiency, protein S deficiency, and malignant neoplasm.[49] An anticoagulation flow sheet is a useful tool to document laboratory results and to calculate heparin and warfarin dosages. The nurse should monitor the patient for signs of Coumadin necrosis (see Chapter 8).

Thrombolytic Therapy. Thrombolytic agents, such as streptokinase, urokinase, and recombinant tissue plasminogen activators (rt-PA, such as Alteplase and Reteplase), have all been reported as effective in dissolving existing thrombi. Although the best results generally occur when treatment is begun during the first 24 hours of the thrombotic event, benefit has been associated with catheter-directed thrombolysis in instances of DVT up to 10 days old.[51,52] Still others report that there is no convincing evidence to support that catheter-directed thrombolysis is superior to infusion through a peripheral vein.[49]

Thrombolytic agents impair coagulation by increasing fibrinolytic activity through the conversion of circulating plasminogen to plasmin. Streptokinase, urokinase, and rt-PA are currently the only agents approved for clinical use in VTE. While reteplase is not currently approved for VTE, this agent shows promise for rapid venous thrombolysis. Heparin should be infused concurrently with rt-PA, but not with streptokinase or urokinase because of the associated increased risk for bleeding complications. Because of the significant risk of hemorrhage, particularly intracranial bleeding, thrombolytic therapy is usually reserved for individuals in which the benefit outweighs the risk, such as younger patients with massive iliofemoral thrombosis.[49]

While the patient is anticoagulated or receiving thrombolytic therapy, the nurse should watch for any signs of bleeding (see Chapter 8). If the patient is receiving thrombolytic therapy, the nurse should alert the physician to a fibrinogen level that is less than 100 mg/dl.

Special Considerations

Calf Vein Thrombosis

The treatment of calf vein thrombosis remains controversial. Isolated calf vein thrombosis usually does not cause major sequelae and does not place the patient at high risk for pulmonary embolism. However, calf vein thrombi can embolize and propagate proximally to the large deep veins of the thigh. Current studies support the need to treat calf vein thrombosis, which includes the popliteal fossa, with 3 months of anticoagulant therapy.[49] If untreated with anticoagulants, the patient should be monitored with venous duplex ultrasound until the high-risk period has passed and the patient returns to full ambulation.

Femoral Popliteal Venous Thrombosis

Venous thrombosis of the superficial femoral and popliteal veins is the most common type of thrombosis requiring treatment. Anticoagulation is the standard form of therapy. Thrombolysis may be useful in appropriate candidates. Once clot lysis is achieved, the patient should be converted to intravenous heparin followed by long-term anticoagulation (see Chapter 6).

Iliofemoral Venous Thrombosis

Iliofemoral venous thrombosis may not be common, but the devastating sequelae pose more than an increased risk of PE.[41,49] Approximately 95 percent of patients with iliofemoral thrombosis treated with anticoagulation alone exhibit severely compromised muscle function and valvular incompentency at 5 years following treatment, despite improved venous outflow.[53,54] Surgical thrombectomy with the creation of an arteriovenous fistula is reported to have a long-term patency rate of approximately 80 percent; many patients rethrombose due to incomplete thrombectomy.[55,56] However, this procedure is rarely performed in the United States. While systemic lytic therapy has been associated with a fourfold increase in lysis of venous thrombi, the incidence of PE has not been significantly impacted in this high-risk group. More recently, positive strides have been made in using catheter-directed lytic therapy with angioplasty and stenting of residual stenosis (Fig. 18-11, *A* and *B*). Empiric data support lysis with stenting as a more effective method of treating iliofemoral vein thrombosis when compared to conventional therapy.[54,57]

Pulmonary Embolism

As previously stated, PE is the third leading cause of death from cardiovascular disease, exceeded only by atherosclerotic heart disease and stroke.[8,9,13,68] It is hypothesized that more than 200,000 deaths occur each year due to PE, which exceeds the combined death rate of acquired immunodeficiency syndrome (AIDS), motor vehicle accidents, and breast cancer.[9] Despite improvements in medical diagnosis and treatment, the actual number of clinically diagnosed cases is significantly less than the true incidence.[4,13,14,42] PE may be the most common preventable cause of death throughout the world.[9,12,13]

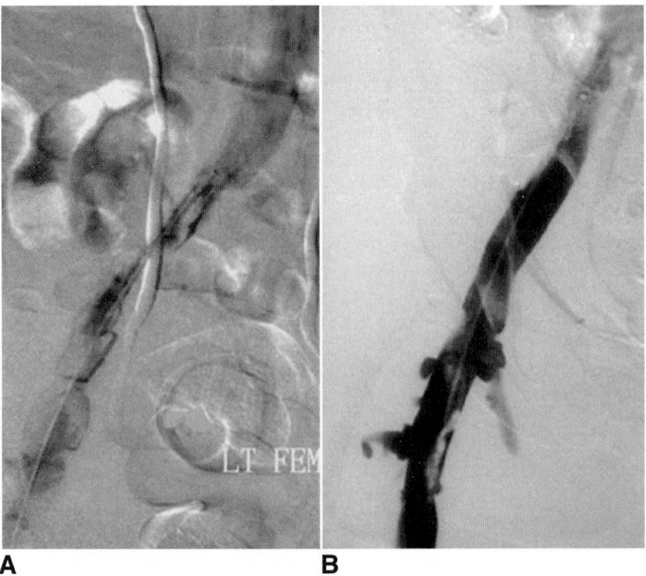

FIG. 18–11. A. Selective venography of left iliac vein thrombosis with partial restoration of flow following catheter-directed thrombolysis. **B,** Restoration of left iliac venous flow following stent placement. (Reprinted from Subramanian R, White CJ: Mechanical interventions and thrombolytic therapy in venous thrombosis and pulmonary embolism, *The Ochsner Journal,* Vol 4, No. 1, p 33 with permission, 2002.)

PE occurs in any clinical setting; it is rarely seen in young healthy patients, whereas the elderly, immobilized, or trauma patients have the highest incidence.[5,6] An increased risk has also been identified during pregnancy and in the puerperium.[4,5,7,15] Other factors that increase the risk of pulmonary embolism include all types of heart disease, low cardiac output, surgical procedures, the use of oral contraceptives, and having blood group A.[41,48]

PE is a direct consequence of DVT. More than 90 percent are due to thrombus formation in the deep veins of the legs.[4,11] The incidence of PE increases with more proximal DVT.[42,44] The iliac and femoral veins, because of their large size, are the source of most PE. The upper extremity and the pelvic veins are less common sites. Superficial leg veins generally do not cause pulmonary embolus unless the thrombosis propagates into the larger veins of the deep system. Tumor embolization of the lungs and cardiac tumors involving the right atrium and ventricle may also cause PE, but the incidence is rare.

Clinical Manifestations

The clinical manifestations of PE are directly related to the magnitude of the pulmonary circulatory obstruction caused by migration of a blood clot.[3,9] Many times symptoms are nonspecific and similar to those of other cardiopulmonary diseases. Symptoms of dyspnea and chest pain have been identified as the most common symptoms of patients with documented PE.[4] However, any abrupt or unexplained episode of hypotension, chest pain, or respiratory distress should be considered suspicious of pulmonary embolism (Box 18-5). Research studies support that PE, as a sudden cause of death identified at autopsy, is suspected in only about 30 percent of this population.[4]

Auscultation of the heart may reveal an accentuated pulmonic second sound (tricuspid regurgitation murmur). Findings may differ between patients with the severity varying from transient dyspnea to acute right heart failure and cardiopulmonary arrest. Acute cor pulmonale with abrupt onset of cardiovascular collapse, syncope, and sudden death is generally associated with massive pulmonary embolism. Small PE in the pulmonary parenchyma of a relatively healthy patient may be asymptomatic. Yet the same size PE may cause distressing symptoms in a patient with severe cardiopulmonary disease.[9,42]

Diagnostic Evaluation

Diagnostic evaluation of patients suspected of a PE may include easily obtained bedside studies, such as pulse oximetry, arterial blood gases, electrocardiogram, and chest x-ray.

ARTERIAL BLOOD GASES. Arterial blood gases are normal in approximately 10 percent of patients with PE; however, hypoxemia and primary respiratory alkalosis are common.[58-60] In patients with PE, a low arterial Po_2 is highly suspicious especially when the chest x-ray does not reveal any obvious pulmonary cause for the hypoxia.

ELECTROCARDIOGRAM. The electrocardiogram (ECG) is useful primarily to identify myocardial infarction, arrhythmias, or other cardiac causes of the patient's symptoms; however,

BOX 18–5

Most Frequent Clinical Manifestations of Pulmonary Embolism

Dyspnea	Increased pulmonic second sound
Chest pain	Cough
Sudden-onset dyspnea	Decreased breath sounds
Tachypnea	Palpitations
Tachycardia	Distended neck veins
Diaphoresis	

in the presence of PE, it may show a pattern of right heart strain. Although most electrocardiograms are normal in patients with PE, changes may include nonspecific ST-T changes.[59]

CHEST X-RAY. Because the clinical manifestations of PE may mimic other types of pulmonary pathology, a baseline chest x-ray should be obtained. The initial chest x-ray may not demonstrate abnormal findings on the basis of PE, but rather changes in radiodensity associated with other pulmonary disease processes.[59] Congestion is not usually present during the early phase of PE. Later, however, wedge-shaped or triangular defects in the pleural surface may be seen, which are indicative of pulmonary infarct. A pleural effusion may also develop if the pleura becomes inflamed.

VENTILATION/PERFUSION LUNG SCAN. A ventilation/perfusion (V/Q) scan assesses airflow patterns and circulation of the lungs. The perfusion scan demonstrates the distribution of pulmonary artery blood flow and underperfused areas in the lung. The perfusion component of the scan involves intravenous injection of albumin labeled with technetium (^{99m}Tc) or iodine (^{133}I) and should exhibit a radiolucent area of underperfusion. However, preexisting lung disease, such as atelectasis, pneumothorax, emphysema, and chronic pulmonary disease, or neoplasm may demonstrate a defect that produces a false-positive result.[58,61] Hence, the perfusion scan must be interpreted in conjunction with a recent chest x-ray and the patient's clinical status. A normal perfusion scan essentially excludes PE, but an abnormal test may be due to several other causes as described above.

Xenon-133 ventilation, the ventilation component of a V/Q scan, increases the utility of establishing a diagnosis of PE. It increases the sensitivity of identifying underperfused and underventilated areas by collecting information regarding the distribution of inhaled gas. PE typically causes perfusion defects in an area of normal ventilation. However, ventilation defects are often found in the presence of perfusion defects. Therefore, a positive study produces a mismatch between the ventilation and perfusion components of the scan, whereas an inconclusive scan generally warrants further workup to establish a diagnosis.[59]

The V/Q scan may be repeated 1-3 days after the initial scan if a PE remains suspect. Noninvasive modalities, such as venous duplex/color duplex ultrasound, may be used to assess DVT presence and rule out PE to pursue other differential diagnoses including pneumonia, acute myocardial infarction, dissecting aortic aneurysm, pneumothorax, and pericarditis.[59,62]

PULMONARY ANGIOGRAPHY. Pulmonary angiography remains the gold standard for establishing a diagnosis of PE.[59,63] A positive angiogram, via right heart catheterization, demonstrates an internal filling defect in the pulmonary arteries (Figs. 18-12 and 18-13, *A*). Although angiography can clearly demonstrate PE, several factors limit its clinical use. Because it is an invasive procedure that requires injection of contrast material, it is associated with some risk, especially in patients with severe pulmonary hypertension, right-sided heart failure, or respiratory failure.[63] However, sophisticated radiologic equipment and technical expertise are not available in all hospitals, and, if available, the test may not be provided on nights or weekends. Because of these limitations and the high cost, pulmonary angiography is inappropriate for screening and routine use in establishing the diagnosis of PE.

ECHOCARDIOGRAPHY. Echocardiography, including transesophageal echocardiography, provides valuable data to evaluate cardiac function in patients with PE. Although echocardiography cannot visualize most of the pulmonary arterial circulation, it is very useful in evaluating the presence of acute cor pulmonale. More than 50 percent of pulmonary arterial obstructions, pulmonary arterial hypertension, and distention of the right ventricle are due to PE.[13] Thus, echocardiography serves as a useful tool to quantitate the degree of right ventricular distention due to high pressures, which occur with PE. Because the size of ventricular distention can be measured accurately with echocardiography, the effectiveness of fibrinolytic agents can be evaluated during or following thrombolytic therapy.

SPIRAL COMPUTED TOMOGRAPHY. Although pulmonary angiography is unsurpassed at detecting subsegmental pulmonary emboli, spiral computed tomography (CT) may be superior in visualizing clot within the central or segmental pulmonary arteries. Spiral CT is expected to assume an increasingly valuable role in evaluating patients suspected of PE, particularly in the emergency setting.[64]

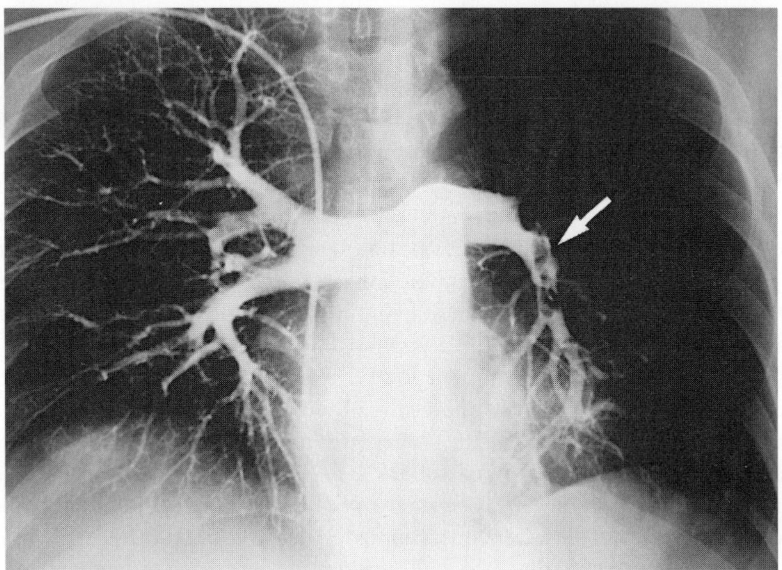

FIG. 18–12. Pulmonary angiogram of filling defect (*arrow*) in pulmonary artery with absence of flow in left pulmonary artery branches. Sudden cut-off of left pulmonary artery branches is demonstrated. (Reprinted from *Critical Care Nursing Quarterly,* Vol 8, No. 2, p 84 with permission of Aspen Publishers, Inc., 1985.)

Treatment

Successful management of PE requires prompt, accurate diagnosis and proper treatment. When PE is suspected, initial treatment is directed toward stabilizing the patient with supportive therapy and initiating antithrombotic therapy.

SUPPORTIVE THERAPY. Supportive measures to improve clinical symptoms should be implemented as soon as possible. The head of the bed should be elevated higher than 30° to enable the patient to breathe easier and minimize dyspnea. If the patient is in shock, care

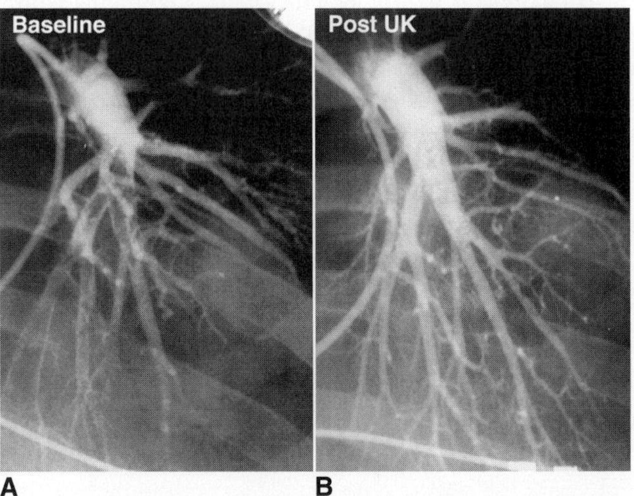

FIG. 18–13. A, Selective angiogram of left pulmonary artery exhibiting filling defects and restricted flow involving the branches of the left pulmonary artery due to pulmonary embolism. **B,** Selective angiogram of left pulmonary artery exhibiting resolution of filling defects with restoration of flow in the left pulmonary artery and its branches following catheter-directed delivery of urokinase. (Reprinted from Subramanian R, White CJ: Mechanical interventions and thrombolytic therapy in venous thrombosis and pulmonary embolism, *The Ochsner Journal,* Vol 4, No. 1, p 32 with permission, 2002.)

should be taken to monitor blood pressure carefully and avoid cerebral hypoperfusion.[58] Oxygen should be administered by nasal cannula, face mask, or both. In patients with respiratory distress, endotracheal intubation and mechanical ventilation may be required. However, these supportive measures may not be effective alone because the major cause of hypoxia is lack of perfusion of the pulmonary parenchyma.

Small doses of intravenous opiates (e.g. 1-2 mg of morphine) may help the patient's discomfort and apprehension, along with reduction of systemic afterload. Larger doses of narcotics should be used cautiously as they may cause respiratory depression. Intravenous access should also be established as soon as possible for rapid delivery of appropriate medications. In addition, intravenous fluid intake should be monitored closely because of the risk of exacerbation of right ventricular dysfunction.

HEPARIN. The cornerstone of treatment for PE is intravenous heparin.[49] Maintenance of therapeutic anticoagulation values usually results in improved outcomes. In treating acute PE, APTT values must be closely monitored, particularly after the first 48 hours, to avoid over-anticoagulation. As previously described for DVT, a continuous heparin infusion should be titrated to maintain the APTT at 1.5-2.5 times the patient's baseline.[49] An initial bolus of 5000-10,000 U of heparin should be given intravenously, followed by 1000-2000 U/hr thereafter, depending on the laboratory results. Of equal importance is ensuring the patient's level of anticoagulation does not fall into a low range, placing him or her at an increased risk of recurrent and sometimes fatal PE. Initially, the patient may require high doses of heparin, especially with major PE; however, the dose can usually be decreased after the first 24-48 hours. The most common mistake that occurs is to give too little heparin initially when the heparin requirement is high, and too much heparin later, when the heparin requirement is generally low.

WARFARIN. Oral anticoagulation with warfarin is generally initiated during heparin administration. However, heparin should not be discontinued until therapeutic anticoagulation with warfarin has been obtained.[33,49] Heparin is frequently continued for about 7-10 days. Therefore, administration of a continuous heparin infusion concomitantly with warfarin for 2-3 days is not uncommon.[49]

The starting dose of warfarin is usually 10 mg daily for the first 2 days, however, lower doses may be used initially in specific high-risk populations such as the elderly. Thereafter, the daily maintenance dose is adjusted to yield an INR of 2-3. Oral anticoagulation should be continued for at least 3 months, and sometimes indefinitely.[32,49]

THROMBOLYTIC THERAPY. A few thrombolytic agents, streptokinase, urokinase, and rt-PA (alteplase and reteplase), are approved by the FDA for treatment of massive pulmonary embolus.[49] Indications for thrombolytic therapy include the presence of a large clot, profound refractory hypoxemia, or significant hemodynamic compromise. Although the risks associated with thrombolytic therapy may result in a negative outcome, failure to lyse the clot generally leads to pulmonary hypertension and end-stage heart disease. Therefore, early lysis of the thrombus may be lifesaving in situations in which the patient may not survive long enough for spontaneous dissolution to occur.

Thrombolytic therapy is induced into the main pulmonary artery through the catheter used for the pulmonary arteriogram (Fig. 18-13, *A* and *B*). This technique enables pulmonary arteriography to be repeated at specific intervals to assess the arteriographic effect of the infusion.

Streptokinase. Streptokinase was the first thrombolytic agent employed for treatment of pulmonary embolism and is relatively inexpensive. However, streptokinase does not lyse as rapidly as urokinase and rt-PA, and it is more likely to be associated with hypersensitivity.[49] Because of the efficacy of urokinase and rt-PA, and the risk of anaphylaxis, streptokinase is rarely used today.

Urokinase. Urokinase has been used effectively for lysis of pulmonary embolism. Its ability to lyse clots rapidly is superior in comparison to streptokinase but not as rapid as rt-PA in reconstituting venous flow.[48] The treatment guidelines for administration of urokinase are an initial loading dose of 4400 IU/kg over 10 minutes, then 4400 IU/kg/hr infused over 12-24 hours.

Recombinant Tissue Plasminogen Activator. Research comparing the efficacy of rt-PA to urokinase in massive PE reports that rt-PA (such as alteplase and reteplase) is more efficacious.

rt-PA dissolves the obstructive embolus more rapidly and completely than urokinase.[49] In addition, administration can be completed in a shorter time frame than other agents. The treatment guideline for administration of alteplase is 100 mg as a continuous intravenous infusion over 2 hours. More recently, other thrombolytic agents have become available using recombinant DNA technology, but because of differences in molecular structure, dosing and administration differ between agents.

Precautions. The most serious bleeding complication associated with thrombolytic agents is intracranial bleeding, occurring in approximately 1 percent of the patients.[49] A retroperitoneal hemorrhage can also be life-threatening. None of these thrombolytic regimens uses concomitant heparin therapy in the early stage of PE because of the increased risk of bleeding. A thorough assessment of the patient's risk factors for hemorrhage and avoidance of unnecessary venipunctures may limit bleeding complications.

VENA CAVA INTERRUPTION. Most patients with DVT with or without PE can be successfully treated with heparin. In specific situations, however, heparin cannot be used, and interruption of the vena cava is necessary to prevent recurrent PE and potentially fatal PE.[65] Filters function by intercepting emboli traveling to the pulmonary vasculature. There are several vena caval filters available, including the stainless steel Greenfield filter (Fig. 18-14), nitinol filter, "bird's nest" filter (Fig. 18-15, *A* and *B*), Venatech filter, titanium Greenfield filter, and the TrapEase (Fig. 18-16).[51] In recent years, vena caval filters have become smaller in size and may be introduced percutaneously. Filters are inserted through the femoral vein and placed in the vena cava inferior to the renal veins to avoid obstruction of blood flow from the kidneys. Complications after filter placement include recurrent pulmonary emboli, venous insufficiency, air embolism, and improper placement or migration of the device.

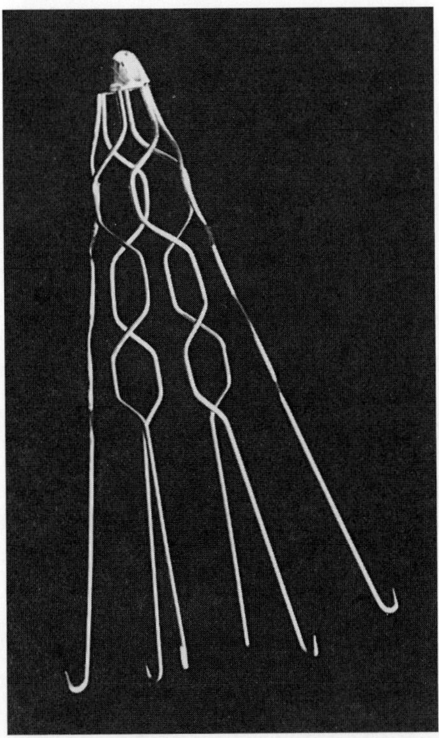

FIG. 18–14. Greenfield stainless steel vena cava filter. (Reprinted from McCarthy WJ, Fahey VA, Bergan JJ et al: The veins and venous disease. In James EC, Corry RJ, Perry JF, eds: *Principles of basic surgical practice*, Philadelphia, 1987, Hanley & Belfus, p 461 with permission.)

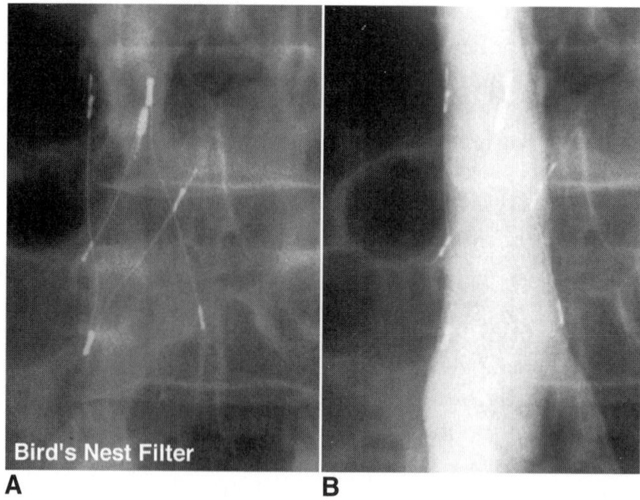

FIG. 18–15. A, Fluoroscopic image of a bird's nest filter in the inferior vena cava **B**, Vena cavagram confirmation of flow across the bird's nest filter in the inferior vena cava. (Reprinted from Subramanian R, White CJ: Mechanical interventions and thrombolytic therapy in venous thrombosis and pulmonary embolism, *The Ochsner Journal*, Vol 4, No. 1, p 34 with permission, 2002.)

PULMONARY EMBOLECTOMY. Pulmonary embolectomy is rarely indicated since thrombolytic therapy and vena caval filters have become available.[51] However, when a patient with an acute PE presents with a terminal comorbidity or is not a candidate for thrombolytic agents, emergency pulmonary embolectomy should be considered. Yet most patients with massive PE who are candidates for pulmonary embolectomy either die before being transported to the operating room or become hemodynamically stable, no longer requiring embolectomy .

Nursing Management. Initial evaluation of the patient with suspected PE should include assessment of the respiratory and cardiovascular systems and vital signs. Initial stabilization of the patient with oxygen therapy, continuous pulse oximetry, arterial blood gas analysis, cardiac monitoring, and intravenous access is critical to the survival of the patient. The head of the bed should be raised to facilitate breathing and promote comfort. Medications should be administered to relieve pain, manage blood pressure changes, treat cardiac dysrhythmia, and reduce fluid overload. Further nursing management is dependent upon the patient's condition.

In summary, nurses play a key role in not only the treatment, but the prevention and detection of venous thromboembolism, including superficial thrombophlebitis. Knowledge of appropriate prevention strategies and an awareness of the signs and symptoms of VTE and its life-threatening sequelae are paramount in the management of patients, particularly those at high risk. With prompt recognition of risk factors and signs and symptoms associated with VTE, the incidence and potentially life-threatening complications will be reduced.

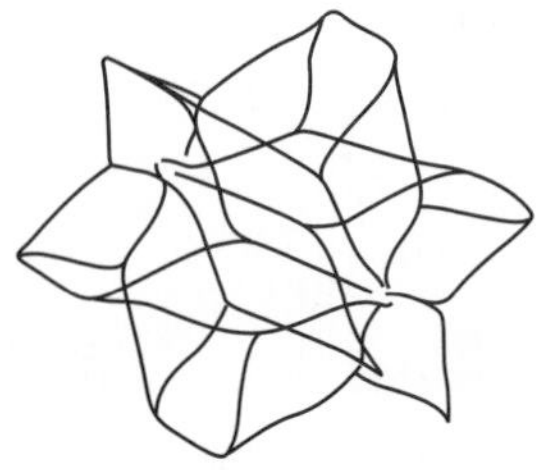

FIG. 18–16. TrapEase vena cava filter. (Reprinted from *Filter Guide* from the Cordis Corporation with permission, 2001.)

REFERENCES

1. Hirsh J, Hoak J: Management of deep vein thrombosis and pulmonary embolism: a statement for healthcare professionals, *Circulation* 93:2212-2245, 1996.
2. Jaff MR: Venous thromboembolic disease, *Ochsner J* 4:6-8, 2002.
3. Kennedy D, Setnik G, Li J: Physical examination findings in deep venous thrombosis, *Emerg Med Clin North Am* 19:869-876, 2001.
4. Kim V, Spandorfer J: Epidemiology of venous thromboembolic disease, *Emerg Med Clin North Am* 19:839-859, 2001.
5. Heit JA, Silverstein MD, Mohr DN et al: Risk factors for deep vein thrombosis and pulmonary embolism: a population-based case-control study, *Arch Intern Med* 160:809-815, 2000.
6. Weiner SG, Burstein JL: Nonspecific tests for pulmonary embolism, *Emerg Med Clin North Am* 19:943-955, 2001.
7. Heit JA, Melton J, Lohse CM et al: Incidence of venous thromboembolism in hospitalized patients vs community residents, *Mayo Clin Proc* 76:1102-1110, 2001.
8. Hyers TM: Venous thromboembolism, *Am J Respir Crit Care Med* 159:1-14, 1999.
9. Deitelzweig SB: Management and prevention of venous thromboembolism including surgery and the pregnant state, *Ochsner J* 4:23-29, 2002.
10. Meissner MH, Strandness DE: Pathophysiology and natural history of acute deep venous thrombosis. In Rutherford RB, ed: *Vascular surgery*, ed 5, Philadelphia, 2000, WB Saunders, pp 1920-1937.
11. DeWet CJ, Pearl RG: Postoperative thrombotic complications: venous thromboembolism—deep-vein thrombosis and pulmonary embolism, *Anesthesiol Clin North Am* 17:895-922, 1999.
12. Ferrari E, Baodouy M, Cerboni P et al: Clinical epidemiology of venous thromboembolic disease: results of a French multicentre registry, *Eur Heart J* 18:685-691, 1997.
13. Silverstein MD, Heif HA, Mohr DN et al: Trends in the incidence of deep vein thrombosis and pulmonary embolism: a 25-year population based study, *Arch Intern Med* 158:585-593, 1998.
14. Hansson P, Welin L, Tibblin G et al: Deep vein thrombosis and pulmonary embolism in the general population: "The Study of Men Born in 1913," *Arch Intern Med* 157:1665-1670, 1997.
15. Farrell SE: Special situations: pediatric, pregnant, and geriatric patients, *Emerg Med Clin North Am* 19:1013-1023, 2001.
16. Geerts WH, Heit JA, Clagett GP et al: Prevention of venous thromboembolism, *Chest* 119:132S-175S, 2001.
17. Kuriakose P, Colon-Otero G, Paz-Fumagalli R: Risk of deep venous thrombosis associated with chest versus arm central venous subcutaneous port catheters: a 5-year single-institution retrospective study, *J Vasc Interv Radiol* 13:179-184, 2002.
18. Volturo GA, Repeta RJ: Non-lower extremity deep vein thrombosis, *Emerg Med Clin North Am* 19:877-893, 2001.
19. Ferrari E, Chevallier T, Chapelier A et al: Travel as a risk factor for venous thromboembolic disease: a case-control study, *Chest* 115:440-444, 1999.
20. Giangrande PL: Air travel and thrombosis, *Int J Clin Pract* 55:690-693, 2001.
21. Heit JA, Mohr DN, Siverstein MD et al: Predictors of recurrence after deep vein thrombosis and pulmonary embolism: a population-based cohort study, *Arch Intern Med* 160:761-768, 2000.
22. Ginsberg JS, Greer I, Hirsh J: Use of antithrombotic agents during pregnancy, *Chest* 119:122S-131S, 2001.
23. James KV, Lohr JM, Deshmukh RM et al: Venous thrombotic complications of pregnancy, *Cardiovasc Surg* 4:777-782, 1996.
24. Rosendaal FR: Risk factors for venous thrombosis: prevalence, risk, and interaction, *Semin Hematol* 34:171-187, 1997.
25. Rickler FR, Edwards RL: Activation of blood coagulation in cancer: Trousseau's syndrome revisited, *Blood* 62:14-31, 1983.
26. Levitan N, Dowlati A, Remick SC et al: Rates of initial and recurrent thromboembolic disease among patients with malignancy versus those without malignancy: risk analysis using Medicare claims data, *Medicine* 78:285-291, 1999.
27. Alving B: Update on recognition and management of patients with acquired or inherited hypercoagulability, *Compr Ther* 24:302-309, 1998.
28. Rosendaal FR, Helmerhorst FM, Vandenbroucke JP: Female hormones and thrombosis, *Arterioscler Thromb Vasc Biol* 22:201-210, 2002.
29. Rosing J, Tans G: Effects of oral contraceptives on hemostasis and thrombosis, *Am J Obstet Gynecol* 180:S375-382, 1999.
30. Miller J, Chan BKS, Nelson HD: Postmenopausal estrogen replacement and risk for venous thromboembolism: a systematic review and meta-analysis for the U.S. Preventive Services Task Force, *Ann Intern Med* 136:680-690, 2002.

31. Writing Group for the Women's Health Initiative Investigators: Risks and benefits of estrogen plus progestin in healthy postmenopausal women: principal results from the Women's Health Initiative randomized control trial, *JAMA* 288:321-333, 2002.
32. Hirsh J, Warkentin TE, Shaughnessy SG et al: Heparin and low-molecular-weight heparin: mechanisms of action, pharmacokinetics, dosing, monitoring, efficacy, and safety, *Chest* 119:64S-94S, 2001.
33. Hirsh J, Dalen JE, Anderson DR et al: Oral anticoagulants: mechanism of action, clinical effectiveness, and optimal therapeutic range, *Chest* 119:8S-21S, 2001.
34. Ansell J, Hirsh J, Dalen J et al: Managing oral anticoagulants therapy, *Chest* 119:22S-38S, 2001.
35. Aquila AM: Deep venous thrombosis, *J Cardiovasc Nurs* 15:25-44, 2001.
36. Comerata AJ, Chouhan V, Harada RN et al: The fibrinolytic effects of intermittent pneumatic compression: mechanism of enhanced fibrinolysis, *Ann Surg* 226:306-314, 1997.
37. Anglen JO, Goss K, Edwards J et al: Foot pump prophylaxis for deep venous thrombosis: the rate of effective usage in trauma patients, *Am J Orthop* 27:580-582, 1998.
38. Vanek VW: Meta-analysis of effectiveness of intermittent pneumatic compression devices with a comparison of thigh-high to knee-high sleeves, *Am Surg* 64:1050-1058, 1998.
39. Launius BK, Graham BD: Understanding and preventing deep vein thrombosis and pulmonary embolism, *AACN Clin Issues Nurs* 9(1):91-99, 1998.
40. Ascher E, Hingorani A: Superficial thrombophlebitis. In Gloviczki P, Yao JST, eds: *Handbook of venous disorders,* ed 2, London, 2001, Arnold, pp 179-183.
41. Haas S: Deep vein thrombosis: beyond the operating table, *Orthopedics* 23:S629-632, 2000.
42. Wells PS, Ginsberg JS, Anderson DR et al: Use of a clinical model for safe management of patients with suspected pulmonary embolism, *Ann Intern Med* 129:997-1005, 1998.
43. Dryjski M, O'Brien-Irr MS, Harris LM et al: Evaluation of a screening protocol to exclude the diagnosis of deep venous thrombosis among emergency department patients, *J Vasc Surg* 34:1010-1015, 2001.
44. DiVittorio R, Bluth EI, Sullivan MA: Deep vein thrombosis: diagnosis of a common clinical problem, *Ochsner J* 4:14-17, 2002.
45. Davis JD: Prevention, diagnosis, and treatment of venous thromboembolic complications of gynecologic surgery, *Am J Obstet Gynecol* 184:759-775, 2001.
46. Loud PA, Katz DS, Bruce DA et al: Deep vein thrombosis with suspected pulmonary embolism: detection with combined CT venography and pulmonary angiography, *Radiology* 219:498-502, 2001.
47. Fraser DGW, Moody AR, Morgan PS et al: Diagnosis of lower-limb deep venous thrombosis: a prospective blinded study of magnetic resonance direct thrombus imaging, *Ann Intern Med* 136:89-98, 2002.
48. Kearon C, Ginsberg JS, Douketis J et al: Management of suspected deep venous thrombosis in outpatients by using clinical assessment and D-dimer testing, *Ann Intern Med* 135:108-111, 2001.
49. Hyers TM, Angelli G, Hull RD et al: Antithrombotic therapy for venous thromboembolic disease, *Chest* 119:176S-193S, 2001.
50. Brown KR, Towne JB: Hypercoagulable states in venous disease. In Gloviczki P, Yao JST, eds: *Handbook of venous disorders,* ed 2, London, 2001, Arnold, pp 84-93.
51. Subramanian R, White CJ: Mechanical interventions and thrombolytic therapy in venous thrombosis and pulmonary embolism, *Ochsner J* 4:30-36, 2002.
52. Mewissen MW, Seabrook GR, Meissner MH et al: Catheter-directed thrombolysis for lower extremity deep venous thrombosis: report of a national multicenter registry, *Radiology* 211:39-49, 1999.
53. Mohr DN, Silverstein MD, Heit JA et al: The venous stasis syndrome after deep venous thrombosis or pulmonary embolism: a population-based study, *Mayo Clin Proc* 75:1249-1256, 2000.
54. AbuRahma AF, Perkins SE, Wulu JT et al: Iliofemoral deep vein thrombosis: conventional therapy versus lysis and percutaneous transluminal angioplasty and stenting, *Ann Surg* 233:752-760, 2001.
55. Juhan MC, Alimi YS, Barthelemy PJ et al: Late results of iliofemoral venous thrombectomy, *J Vasc Surg* 25:417-422, 1997.
56. Roh B, Park K, Kim E et al: Prognostic value of CT before thrombolytic therapy in iliofemoral deep venous thrombosis, *J Vasc Interv Radiol* 13:71-76, 2002.
57. Raju S, Owen S, Neglen P: The clinical impact of iliac venous stents in the management of chronic venous insufficiency, *J Vasc Surg* 35:8-15, 2002.
58. Wheeler HB, Anderson FA: Pulmonary embolism. In Gloviczki P, Yao JST, eds: *Handbook of venous disorders,* ed 2, London, 2001, Arnold, pp 215-223.
59. McFadden PM, Ochsner, JL: A history of the diagnosis and treatment of venous thrombosis and pulmonary embolism, *Ochsner J* 4:9-13, 2002.
60. Kirksey KM, Holt-Ashley M, Goodroad BK: Easy method for interpreting the results of arterial blood gas analysis, *Crit Care Nurse* 21:49-54, 2001.
61. Epley D: Pulmonary emboli risk reduction, *J Vasc Nurs* 18(2):61-68, 2000.

62. Wells PS, Anderson DR, Rodger M et al: Excluding pulmonary embolism at the bedside without diagnostic imaging: management of patients with suspected pulmonary embolism presenting to the emergency department by using a simple clinical model and D-dimer, *Ann Intern Med* 135:98-107, 2001.
63. Stein PD, Athanasoulis C, Alavi A et al: Complications and validity of pulmonary angiography in acute pulmonary embolism, *Circulation* 85:462-468, 1992.
64. Holbert JM, Costello P, Federle MP: Role of spiral computed tomography in the diagnosis of pulmonary embolism in the emergency department, *Ann Emerg Med* 33:520-528, 1999.
65. Greenfield LJ, Proctor MC: Indications and techniques of inferior vena cava interruption. In Gloviczki P, Yao JST, eds: *Handbook of venous disorders,* ed 2, London, 2001, Arnold, pp 235-243.

19

Chronic Venous Disease

KIMBERLY A. KERR □ WILLIAM C. WATSON □ MICHAEL C. DALSING

Chronic venous disease is a common malady that affects all age groups. Findings range from small spider telangiectasias and varicose veins to disabling venous claudication and venous ulcers. The mainstay of therapy remains nonsurgical, but advanced surgical therapy is being reconsidered more aggressively in recent decades. This chapter discusses the pathophysiology, diagnosis, and treatment of chronic venous disease.

NORMAL ANATOMY AND PHYSIOLOGY

To understand venous disease, a working knowledge of the lower-extremity venous system is imperative. There are three basic components of the lower extremity venous system: deep veins, communicating (or perforating) veins, and superficial veins (Fig. 19-1, *A*). The deep system is composed of the iliac, the common, superficial, and profunda femoral veins, in addition to the popliteal and tibial veins. The greater and lesser saphenous veins compose the superficial system, which lies in the subcutaneous tissue. The communicating veins create the various connections between the superficial and deep systems. The deep veins are located below the investing fascia, travel adjacent to similarly named arteries, and are generally surrounded by muscle. Communicating veins pierce the fascia to connect the deep and superficial systems (Fig. 19-1, *B*).

Key to understanding the etiology of venous disease is the concept of the calf muscles as a pump, the "peripheral heart" (Fig. 19-2, *A* and *B*). The lower extremity, pelvic, abdominal, and chest central veins carry blood back to the cardiac chambers, while the venous valves act as one-way stopcocks to prevent the reflux of blood into the lower leg after peripheral pump contraction or when a person assumes an upright position. In this analogy, the deep veins within the gastrocnemius and soleus muscles correspond to the left ventricle. As the calf muscles contract with exercise, the deep venous system is compressed, and blood is propelled or pumped toward the heart. Deep within the muscle pump, pressures can rise to 300 mm Hg.[1] As pressure rises in the deep system, the valves in the communicating veins close, preventing both the backflow of blood into the superficial venous system and the transmission of these high pressures from the deep venous system to the superficial system. Blood is also moved toward the heart in the superficial veins because of compression of the fascia against the skin, even though these pressures may peak at lower levels (100-150 mm Hg).[1] Valves in the proximal or more cephalad superficial and deep veins open in response to the calf pump to allow blood to move toward the heart. As the pumping action ceases, blood is prevented from refluxing into the leg by the closure of the valves within the deep and superficial veins. Arterial flow begins to fill the venous system during rest. As the venous system fills, the valves in the foot, distal leg, and perforating system open to allow blood to enter the deep veins within the calf muscle pump.[2]

Normal pressures in a patient's leg can be measured by inserting an intravenous catheter into a vein of the foot. The catheter is connected to a pressure transducer and chart recorder. With the patient lying down, normal venous pressure is approximately 15 mm Hg, but may be zero with mild leg elevation. When the patient stands, gravity exerts its influence in the

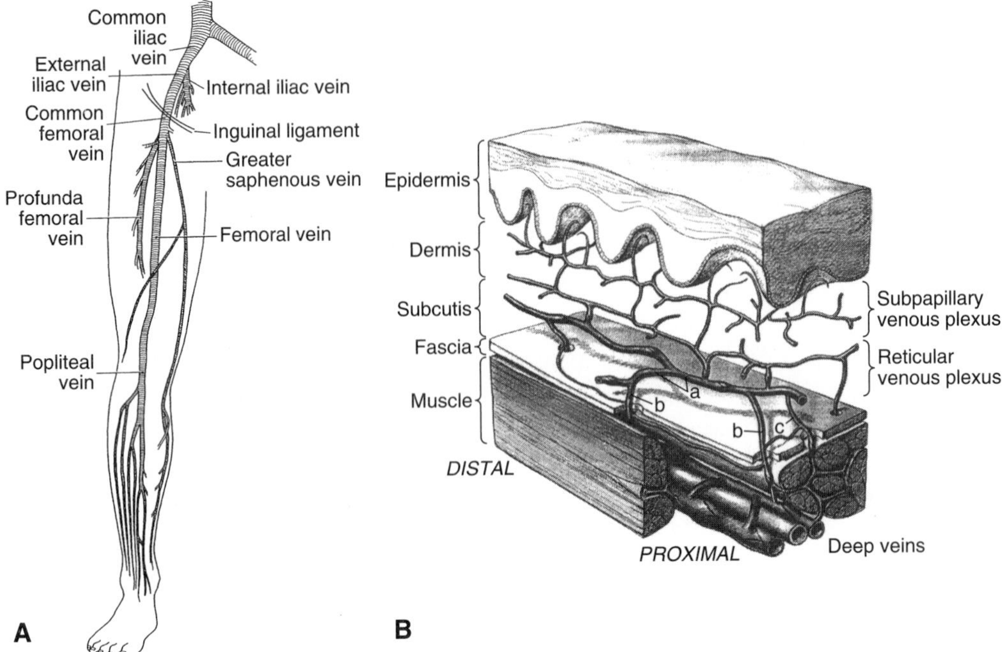

FIG. 19–1. A, Anatomic drawing of lower extremity venous system. **B,** Anatomic drawing of connections between the lower extremity deep and superficial venous system. Capillaries of dermal papillae are drained by subpapillary venous plexus, which joins the reticular venous plexus. Superficial veins *(a)* drain dermal veins and empty into deep axial veins through direct perforating veins *(b)*. Muscular venous sinuses may fill from superficial veins through indirect perforating veins *(c)* and are drained into the deep axial veins. (**A** reprinted with permission from Dalsing M: Venous valvular insufficiency: pathophysiology and treatment options. In Society of Cardiovascular and Interventional Radiology: *Venous interventions, syllabus V: venous interventions,* Fairfax, VA, 1995, p 225. **B** redrawn with permission from Ballard JL, Bergan JJ, eds: *Chronic venous insufficiency: diagnosis and treatment,* London, 2000, Springer-Verlag, p 26.)

form of hydrostatic pressure. Because the arteries and veins run in parallel, this pressure is exerted equally in both systems. When relaxed, the veins are flat and nondistended. However, as they begin to fill with blood, they become elliptical before proceeding to the circular shape of a fully distended vein. Once the veins become filled to capacity and have assumed a cylindrical shape, any increase in volume will dramatically increase pressure.[1] Prior to full vein diameter expansion, large volume changes can occur without dramatic changes in pressure (veins are very compliant until full expansion).

Ambulatory venous pressure measurements are a physiologic study designed to assess venous function in an active patient. A baseline erect pressure is obtained. This baseline pressure is the pressure exerted on the lower leg as reflected by the venous catheter measurement of a column of blood from the heart to the lower-extremity venous system. This pressure is generally 90 mm Hg or higher and is influenced by the height of the patient in addition to other less influential factors. The time it takes to achieve a steady-state pressure after rising from a supine position is called the venous filling time (VFT). The patient then is instructed to perform 10 tiptoe maneuvers at a rate of 1 per second, and the resultant drop in recorded pressure is labeled the ambulatory venous pressure (AVP). After this exercise, the patient remains still until the pressure returns to baseline. The time it takes to return to the baseline erect pressure from the AVP is called the venous refilling time (VRT). If the AVP is greater than 30 mm Hg, the sequelae of venous disease (ulceration) increases by 10-15 percent for each 10 mm Hg increase in AVP because exercise and valvular disease are ineffective in decreasing lower leg venous pressures when standing.[3] The VRT reflects the closure of

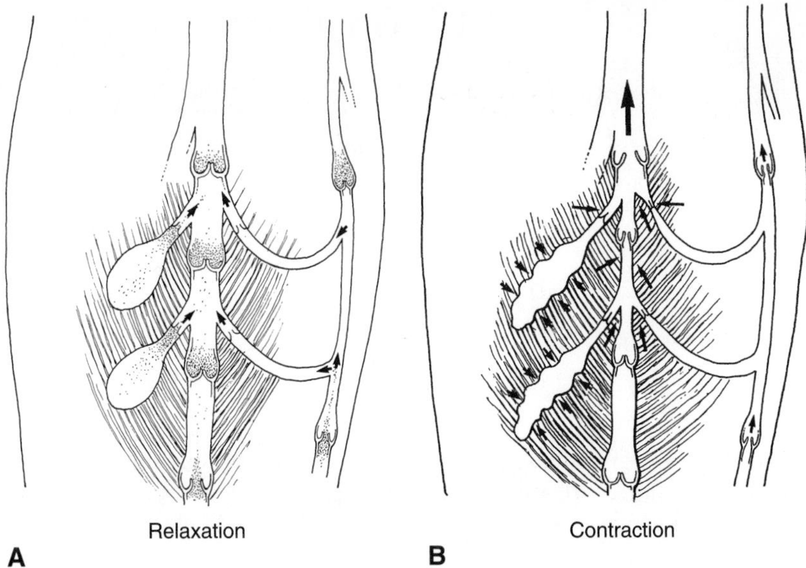

FIG. 19–2. A, Veins within the calf muscle pump during relaxation. Note the filling of the deep veins from the perforating veins and lower leg with proper deep venous valve closure in the standing patient. **B,** Veins within the calf muscle pump during muscle contraction with ejection of blood toward the heart. Note the proper closure of the valves of the communicating veins in a nondiseased venous system. (Reprinted with permission from Dalsing M: Venous valvular insufficiency: pathophysiology and treatment options. In Society of Cardiovascular and Interventional Radiology: *Venous interventions, syllabus V: venous interventions,* Fairfax, VA, 1995, p 225.)

venous valves to prevent blood from refluxing down the leg following exercise. If the VRT is greater than 20 seconds, the venous valvular system is intact and adequately prevents retrograde flow of blood in the veins. If the VRT is less than 20 seconds, overall valvular reflux throughout the lower leg is present.[3]

PATHOPHYSIOLOGY AND ETIOLOGY

Chronic venous disease occurs when there is failure of one or more of the components of a normal venous system. Three pathophysiologic states have been defined: venous obstruction, venous valvular insufficiency, and calf muscle pump malfunction.[4]

Elevated pressures within the venous system result from increased resistance to outflow due to venous obstruction. If the deep system is primarily involved, the increased pressure is eventually transmitted to the communicating system, which then gradually causes communicating vein valve dysfunction. With failure of the communicating vein valves, increased volume and venous hypertension are communicated to the superficial venous system and to the skin and subcutaneous tissues. Primary causes of obstruction are very uncommon and are the result of intrinsic or extrinsic factors (Box 19-1),[1] whereas secondary venous outflow obstruction is often the result of venous thrombosis. Venous thrombosis is by far the most common cause of venous obstruction in the United States population.

Extrinsic causes of venous obstruction in the lower limb include compression of iliac and pelvic veins by tumor, retroperitoneal fibrosis, or infection. Iliac vein compression syndrome occurs most commonly on the left side. The left iliac vein is compressed between the right common iliac artery and the lumbar vertebrae, also known as May-Thurner syndrome.[5,6] The femoral vein can be compressed by a herniation of fat through a femoral hernia defect and by soft tissue tumors limited to the thigh. Aneurysms of the common femoral, superficial femoral, or the deep femoral arteries can compress the thin elastic wall of the femoral vein. Popliteal masses (a popliteal artery aneurysm or Baker's cyst) can compress the popliteal vein and cause obstruction at this distal level.[1]

BOX 19–1

Etiology of Lower Limb Venous Obstruction

INTRINSIC
Aplasia (absence of veins)
Tumors (e.g., venous leiomyomata)
Intraluminal webs

EXTRINSIC
Tumor compression
Retroperitoneal fibrosis
Infection
Femoral hernia
Arterial aneurysms
Popliteal masses (e.g., Baker's cyst)
May-Thurner syndrome

Internal sources of outflow obstruction other than deep venous thrombus are even less common. Vein wall abnormalities such as the absence of the vein (aplasia) or tumors of the vein wall (leiomyomata) have been described.[1] A somewhat less obscure source of obstruction results from intraluminal webs.[7]

Valvular insufficiency may involve one or more of the three venous systems in the lower leg. This incompetence, congenital or acquired, allows for the transmission of high venous pressures to the lower leg on standing, which is not adequately relieved by exercise. The superficial system is involved in 60 percent of cases, while the deep system is involved 40 percent of the time.[8] Primary valvular insufficiency encompasses a variety of processes. The obvious is congenital absence of valves, a rare cause.[9] Venous valve prolapse, observed as floppy valve cusps, is also seen. These floppy valves can be seen in the very common hereditary varicose veins of the superficial venous system, but they are also observed in the deep and perforating systems. Alternatively, the problem may be dilation of the vein diameter, resulting in malapproximation of the valve cusps.[10] Approximately 50-60 percent of deep valvular dysfunction is a result of deep venous thrombosis (DVT), whereas the other 40-50 percent appears to be of a primary etiology.[11] Incomplete or nonexistent recanalization of the vein following DVT can damage the delicate bicuspid leaflets of the venous valves. Even with complete thrombus reabsorption, scarring can result in damage of these delicate structures. Prolonged exposure to high venous pressures will eventually cause the vein to dilate, preventing the valve cusps from meeting appropriately due to valve ring dilation.[1,12] Such high pressures can result from an abnormal artery to venous connection (arteriovenous fistula) or from prior proximal valve damage as a result of trauma, DVT, or other cause with resultant pressure on and subsequent failure of even more distal valves, not affected directly by the original insult. Lower leg venous hypertension is the ultimate result.

Varicose veins are one of the most common sequelae of chronic venous disease. Ten to thirty-five percent of the adult population is afflicted with superficial varicosities (Table 19-1).[13] There are two types of varicose veins—primary and secondary. Primary, or simple, varicose veins (Fig. 19-3) result from superficial vein incompetence. They are often familial in origin and have no underlying etiology. Secondary varicose veins are the result of previous vein pathology. Many of the risk factors for chronic venous insufficiency and varicosities are well established, while others are a bit more controversial (Box 19-2).[1,8] Individuals who are employed in jobs

TABLE 19–1 Prevalence of Lower Extremity Varicosities

Age	Female	Male
20-29	8%	1%
40-49	41%	24%
60-69	72%	43%

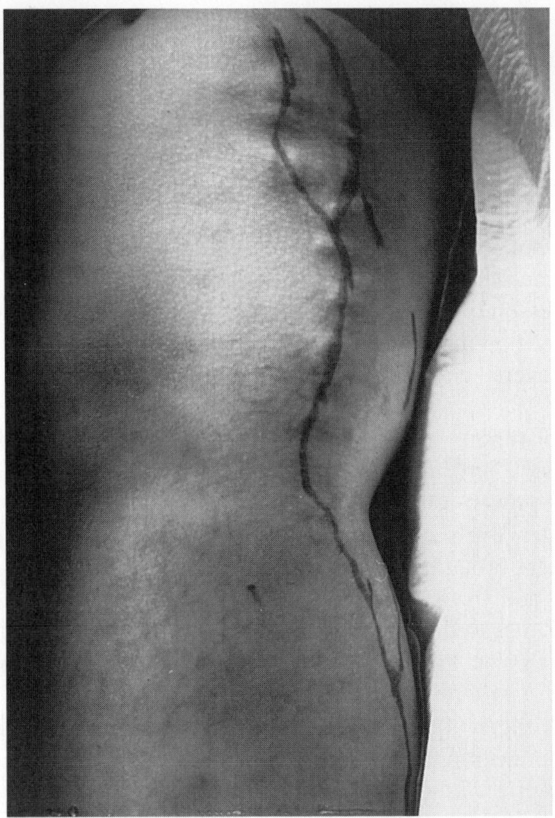

FIG. 19–3. Varicose veins on the thigh associated with greater saphenous vein insufficiency. These veins have been marked with permanent ink in preparation for surgery. (Reprinted with permission from Dalsing M: Venous valvular insufficiency: pathophysiology and treatment options. In Society of Cardiovascular and Interventional Radiology: *Venous interventions, syllabus V: venous interventions,* Fairfax, VA, 1995, p 225.)

that require prolonged periods of standing (as opposed to intermittent or constant periods of walking) are at an increased risk. Also patients with known hypercoagulable states and those afflicted with the sequelae of DVT have been identified as a portion of the chronic venous insufficiency population. Estrogen has been cited as a factor in varicose vein formation because of its effect on smooth muscle dilation.

Finally, there can be failure of the calf muscle pump either isolated or in combination with one or the other previously described venous disease states. Returning to the cardiac analogy, calf muscle pump failure is similar to congestive heart failure. The pump eventually is unable to generate the force necessary to eject a satisfactory volume of blood from the leg. The

BOX 19–2

Causes of Chronic Venous Insufficiency

ESTABLISHED	SUGGESTED
Age	Race
Sex	Geography
Genetic predisposition	Body mass
Hormonal influences	Dietary habits
History of deep vein thrombosis (DVT)/thrombophlebitis	Tight undergarments
Thrombophilia (hypercoagulable state)	Toilet posture
Lifestyle (e.g., standing occupation)	Cigarette smoking
	Lack of exercise

reasons for this are varied. Elderly patients with physiologic muscle wasting may not have the physical muscle strength sufficient to pump the blood out of the leg. This is also true for patients with muscle wasting diseases such as paraplegia, those with trauma injury, or bedridden patients (disuse).[1] Similarly, pathologic conditions that result in muscle fibrosis (e.g., muscular dystrophy, multiple sclerosis) will destroy the calf muscle pump. Acute or chronic thrombus in the deep veins within the gastrocnemius and soleus muscles can prevent blood from entering the pump itself, resulting in a deficient ejection volume. If outflow is obstructed for any reason, the excessive afterload causes dilation of the pump chambers (the veins within the calf muscle). Eventually the perforating vein valves are made incompetent from the excessive pressure placed on them with each pump contraction. The pressures generated by the calf muscle pump are then transmitted to the superficial venous system and surrounding tissue. The overall effect is venous stasis and venous hypertension within the lower extremity.

The final effects of venous stasis and hypertension are the skin changes associated with chronic venous disease. There are theories proposed to explain these changes, but they have yet to be definitively proven. Originally, venous stasis was thought to cause hypoxia as a result of the low oxygen levels associated with excessive venous blood pooling in the lower extremity. This was later brought into question by direct physiologic measurements. Several years later, the fibrin cuff theory became popular. This theory suggests that, as a result of venous hypertension, increased plasma proteins and cells were lost through the capillary wall into the surrounding tissues. Fibrinogen was a major component of these extravasated proteins. The fibrinogen was converted to fibrin by local enzymes, and fibrin buildup was believed to hamper oxygen diffusion through the tissues, resulting in tissue hypoxia.[14] However, fibrin has not been proven to be detrimental to the diffusing capacity of oxygen in many cases. Most recently, white blood cell trapping and activation have been postulated as a cause for observed skin changes. Patients with chronic venous disease were found to have "trapped" monocytes within the tissues affected by venous hypertension.[15] The activation of these monocytes could cause an inflammatory reaction, the normal function of white blood cells. This inflammatory reaction could then be responsible for some of the skin changes observed. Macrophages appear to be present no matter the acuity of the venous disease, while T-lymphocytes may be more prominent in early disease and mast cells more prominent in the latter stages.[16] This finding suggests a shift over time from an autoimmune response (eczematous skin) to a dermal fibrosis (hardened and damaged skin and soft tissue leading to ulcer formation and a chronic nonhealing wound). The theory that dermal fibrosis and poor healing is the ultimate fate of prolonged venous hypertension is supported by the upregulation of TGF-β1 (leading to dermal fibroblast collagen production and unabated fibrosis), phenotypically senescent fibroblasts (unable to provide for a stable wound), and increased matrix metalloproteinases (excessive proteolysis) in patients with advanced clinical class 4-6 venous disease.[16] This is an area of active investigation sure to become better defined in the near future.

CLINICAL SIGNS AND SYMPTOMS

Venous disease can present in a variety of ways (Box 19-3). Spider veins, also known as telangiectasias, often accompany varicose veins. These appear as fine blue-red branchings just under the surface of the skin. The greatest complaint is their unsightly appearance. However, each spider vein is often accompanied by a larger pathologically dilated vein located deeper in the subcutaneous tissue.[17]

Varicose veins of a hereditary nature will usually appear during the second decade of life. If there is an inciting event, such as thrombosis or trauma, the varicosities generally appear within several years as a natural progression of the disease. These veins appear as blue, dilated, tortuous, and palpable protrusions beneath the skin. They may be isolated or bunched into clusters in the general distribution of the greater or lesser saphenous veins and

BOX 19–3

Signs and Symptoms of Chronic Venous Disease

SIGNS
Telangiectases (spider veins)
Varicose veins
Edema
Hyperpigmentation
Lipodermatosclerosis
Venous ulcers

SYMPTOMS
Complaints of swelling
Heaviness
Pain with standing
Nocturnal calf muscle cramps
Aching
Leg tiredness
Itching
Venous claudication

their branches. Symptoms can range from a dull ache and itching to edema, cramping, and eventually skin damage. Tiredness, heaviness, and pain of and within the lower leg are commonly reported. The presence of varicose veins and related symptoms can be due to a variety of disease processes, and careful evaluation is required to determine the exact cause. The pain from varicosities should not be so severe as to warrant the use of narcotic medications; if it is, another source for the pain should be sought.

Even without obvious varicosities, venous disease can result in pain, edema, cutaneous hyperpigmentation (Fig. 19-4, *A*), stasis dermatitis or eczema (Fig. 19-4, *A*), and finally venous ulcers (Fig. 19-4, *B* and *C*).[18,19] These changes usually occur just above and around the medial malleolus, the location known as the "gaiter" area. The largest number of perforating veins per area exists in the medial calf. If their associated valves become incompetent or proximal obstruction exists, the high pressures generated by the calf muscle pump can be transmitted to the surface veins and the respective cutaneous capillary beds, resulting in tremendously high venous pressures and skin changes.[1] Similarly, if venous insufficiency and/or a malfunctioning calf pump are the underlying pathologic processes, the high intravenous pressures generated while standing cannot be relieved by exercise. High pressures generated while standing, and not relieved by normal physiologic processes, are most severe in the most dependent areas of the leg, the "gaiter" area.

One of the most severe pain syndromes associated with venous disease is termed venous claudication. Fortunately, this is a rare condition. The characteristics of this condition were described by Cockett and Thomas[5] and consist of leg pain with exercise, iliac vein obstruction, and venous hypertension, especially with exercise. Further investigation by Killewich et al[20] prompted the addition of cyanosis, sensations of increased swelling, and increased prominence of superficial veins to this symptom complex. These investigators also differentiated the pain of venous claudication from the pain of arterial insufficiency by noting a relief of symptoms with 15-20 minutes of rest in combination with elevation of the extremities in the former as opposed to pain relief with cessation of activity and the dangling of the legs in the latter.[20] Nonetheless, there are a wide range of presentations. Some patients are able to function in their everyday routine, while others are so debilitated that amputation has been requested.[5] The patients plagued with the most severe disease often have associated deep system incompetence in addition to an obstructive component. This also may be accompanied by superficial and/or communicating vein incompetence. The signs and symptoms of obstruction are related to both the level of the obstruction and the number and size of collaterals. This was best demonstrated by Labropoulus et al[21] in their study of venous obstruction. More proximal obstruction is associated with worse symptoms due to the decreased potential for adequate collateral formation.

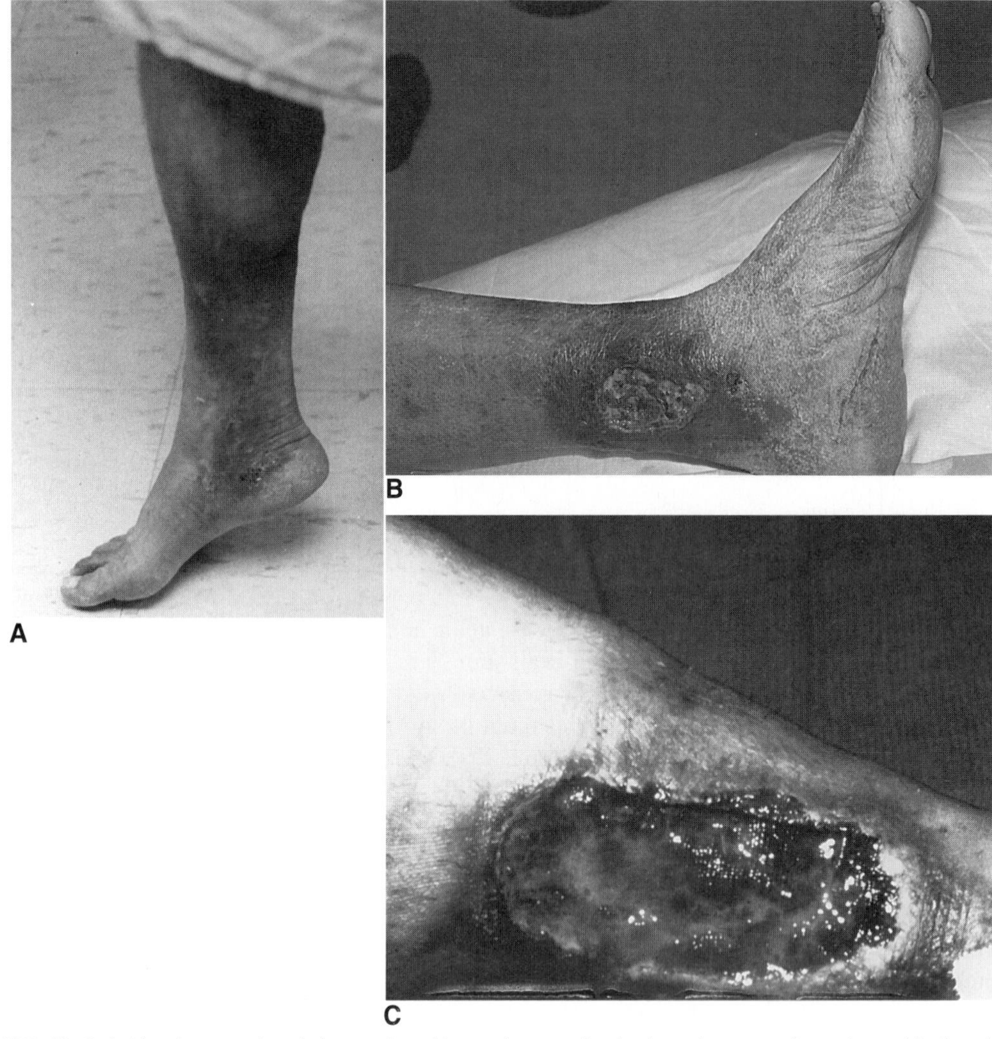

FIG. 19–4. A, Lipodermatosclerosis (eczema) and hyperpigmentation in the gaiter area of a patient with chronic venous disease. **B** and **C,** Venous ulcers of the lower extremity in patients with chronic venous disease demonstrating the wide variance in size and depth of such ulcers. (**B** from McCarthy WJ, Fahey VA, Bergan JJ, et al: The veins and venous disease. In James EC, Corry RJ, Perry JF, eds: *Principals of basic surgical practice,* Philadelphia, 1987, Hanley & Belfus, p 463.)

DIAGNOSTIC EVALUATION

The diagnosis of potential vein pathology begins with a thorough history and physical examination. A family history of venous disease (varicose veins), past episodes of venous thromboses, and a discussion of symptoms as related to dependency and/or exercise is very important. The leg swelling and pain are generally noted with standing and relieved by elevation and are the two most common complaints in chronic venous disease.[1,8,18] The presence of varicose veins confirms venous pathology as at least one component of the patient's problems. Chronic venous disease stigmata such as hyperpigmentation or venous ulcers are also significant signs of the disease often noted at a later stage in the pathologic process.

The Clinical Class-Etiology-Anatomic-Pathophysiologic (CEAP) classification system was created to standardize the description of chronic venous disease and to better define our ability to compare patients being studied around the country (Box 19-4).[22] It is applied clinically to help direct diagnostic testing and treatment options. The CEAP classification is further augmented by another assessment tool, the Venous Clinical Severity Score (VCSS), which is used to measure the success of treatment regimens. It is based on clinical parameters, including

BOX 19–4

CEAP Classification

CLINICAL CLASS (C)

Class 0: No visible or palpable signs of venous disease
Class 1: Telangiectases or reticular veins
Class 2: Varicose veins
Class 3: Edema
Class 4: Skin changes of venous disease (e.g., pigmentation, eczema, lipodermatosclerosis)
Class 5: Skin changes as above with healed ulceration
Class 6: Skin changes as above with active ulceration

ETIOLOGY (E)

Congenital (Ec)
Primary (Ep)—with undetermined cause
Secondary (Es)—with known cause
- Postthrombotic
- Posttraumatic
- Other

ANATOMY (A)

Superficial veins (AS), segments 1-6
- Telangiectases/reticular veins

Greater saphenous (GSV)
- Above the knee
- Below the knee

Lesser saphenous (LSV)
- Nonsaphenous

Deep veins (AD), segments 7-16
- Inferior vena cava iliac
  - Common
  - Internal
  - External
- Pelvic—gonadal, broad ligament, other femoral
  - Common
  - Deep
  - Superficial
- Popliteal
- Crural—anterior tibial, posterior tibial, peroneal
- Muscular

Perforating veins (Ap)
- Thigh
- Calf

PATHOPHYSIOLOGY (P)

Reflux (Pr)
Obstruction (Po)
Reflux and obstruction (Pr,o)

pain, varicose veins, edema, pigmentation, induration, inflammation, number of active ulcers, duration of active ulceration, size of the largest current ulceration, and compressive therapy. These parameters are graded on a scale of 0-3, for a total possible score of 30 (Table 19-2).[23] A patient's score is calculated on initial evaluation and on each visit after therapy is initiated. Comparing the scores over time allows for a quantifiable measure of therapy outcome.

Ambulatory venous pressure measurements are a direct measurement of venous hemodynamics and aid in the diagnosis of venous insufficiency but are not routinely obtained in the initial evaluation of patients with suspected venous disease. In the diseased state, the veins not only fill from arterial inflow but also from the reflux of blood down the veins. Blood pressure cuffs placed above and below the knee as well as at the ankle can be sequentially inflated to compress the greater saphenous vein, the lesser saphenous vein, and essentially all superficial and perforator veins affecting the ankle area; then VRT measurements can be repeated. If the VRT is still less than 20 seconds, the deep system may be a major component of the venous reflux present. With the various cuffs inflated, if the VRT is converted to normal, the problem resides within one or the other superficial or perforating venous systems. The arm-foot pressure differential as developed by Raju[24] is a quantitative measurement for venous obstruction. Venous cannulas are placed in both the hand and the foot. Simultaneously, pressures are measured in the hand and in the foot while the patient is lying down and again after a 3-minute thigh cuff occlusion that induces vasodilation upon cuff deflation. A normal reading after this reactive hyperemia is an arm-foot differential of less than 6 mm Hg with a resting pressure of less than 4 mm Hg. Venous obstruction is considered present when a pressure difference ranging from 6 to 20 mm Hg is detected with the exception of a normal pressure difference in the

TABLE 19–2 Vascular Severity Scoring

Parameter	Absent=0	Mild=1	Moderate=2	Severe=3
Pain	None	Occasional, no activity restriction, no analgesics	Daily, moderate activity limitation, occasional analgesics	Daily, severely limiting activities, regular analgesics
Varicose veins*	None	Few, scattered: branch VVs	Multiple: GS VV confined to calf or thigh	Extensive: thigh and calf, or GS and LS
Venous edema†	None	Evening ankle edema only	Afternoon edema, above ankle	Morning edema above ankle, requiring activity change, elevation
Skin pigmentation‡	None or focal (tan)	Diffuse, but limited in area and old (brown)	Diffuse over most of gaiter area or recent (purple)	Wider distribution and recent (purple)
Inflammation	None	Mild cellulitis, limited to marginal area around ulcer	Moderate cellulitis, involves most of gaiter area	Severe cellulitis, above gaiter or significant venous eczema
Induration	None	Focal, <5 cm, circummalleolar	Medial or lateral < lower third of leg	Entire lower third of leg or more
Number of active ulcers	None	1	2	>2
Active ulceration, duration	None	<3 months	>3 months <1 year	Not healed, >1 year
Active ulcer, size§	None	<2 cm diameter	2-6 cm diameter	>6 cm diameter
Compressive therapy	Not used, not compliant	Intermittent use of stockings	Wears elastic stockings most days	Full compliance (stockings and elevation)

VV, Varicose vein; *GS,* greater saphenous; *LS,* lesser saphenous.
*Varicose veins must be >4 mm in diameter
†Origin is venous and a regular finding, daily.
‡Focal pigmentation over VV does not qualify.
§Largest dimension/diameter of largest ulcer.

face of an abnormal resting pressure, in which case the patient has a fully decompensated venous system.[24] Although this invasive method was once the only technique capable of investigating the venous system, duplex scanning and air plethysmographic techniques are the primary anatomic and functional tests of choice in current medical practice.[25]

Plethysmography is an indirect method of assessing the venous system and of diagnosing obstruction, valve incompetence, or calf muscle pump dysfunction.[26] There are several plethysmographic methods, and all detect changes in blood volume. Obstruction can be determined by evaluating venous capacitance and the rate of venous outflow using impedance plethysmography. With impedance plethysmography, changes in volume are detected as changes in electrical resistance. Patients lie on a table, and bilateral thigh cuffs are placed to provide for venous occlusion while electrodes placed on the lower leg measure changes in volume (resistance). A baseline reading is obtained prior to cuff inflation, and then the cuffs are inflated to approximately 50 mm Hg to result in occlusion of venous outflow. Once the volume measurement stabilizes, a reading is taken and the cuffs are rapidly deflated. The time it takes to return to baseline is noted. Venous capacitance is then determined by subtracting the baseline from the volume plateau. Results are compared to a standard set of normal values.[26] If values lie outside the normal reading, venous obstruction is one component of the patient's venous disease. Previously used alone as a method of determining the presence of acute deep venous thrombosis, duplex evaluation has supplemented it in this role.

Light reflex rheography, similar to methods of plethysmography, can quantitate the VRT in patients with venous valvular incompetence. A small photoelectrode is placed on the patient's ankle. The time for venous refill is measured after 10 plantarflexion/dorsiflexion maneuvers. Normal refill is greater than 20 seconds, whereas reflux is considered to be present if the VRT is less than 20 seconds.[26] Changes in blood volume are detected as changes in light absorption and reflection. With the use of tourniquets, a rough estimation of the localization of reflux (superficial, perforator, deep) is possible much like the method described for intravenous pressure measurement.

Calf muscle pump function, venous insufficiency, and some estimation of venous obstruction can be evaluated by air plethysmography. A plastic cylinder filled with air is fitted over the calf. This cylinder is connected to a chart recorder, and changes in leg volume are detected by increases in pressure within the cylinder. After a baseline reading is taken, patients exercise by ankle dorsiflexion or heel raises to stimulate the calf muscle pump to empty the calf veins. The ejection fraction, the amount of blood propelled cephalad with a single muscle contraction, is determined. After a series of ankle flexions, the volume remaining in the leg is measured and is referred to as the residual volume. The residual volume is equivalent to the lowest ambulatory venous pressure obtained during exercise. These values can be compared with normal studies to determine the presence and the type of the patient's venous disease.[26] Abnormal resting and residual volumes suggest an abnormal muscle pump. To detect outflow obstruction a tourniquet is placed at the thigh and inflated to 80 mm Hg to increase the volume to a new level. Upon rapid deflation of the tourniquet, the venous outflow is recorded at 1 second and calculated as a percent of the total venous volume. The greater saphenous vein is then occluded at the knee, and the outflow is measured at 1 second. Varying degrees of obstruction are suggested by decreasing percentages of the outflow volume.[26] The venous volume refilling time after exercise can be used to characterize venous reflux problems. Because plethysmographic methods cannot provide an anatomic depiction of the venous system, many institutions will combine this type of study with ultrasonographic techniques to provide a complete venous evaluation.

Ultrasonographic techniques are a direct but noninvasive evaluation of the venous vascular system. A continuous-wave (CW) Doppler uses sound waves generated by a crystal in the Doppler head that are directed into the body to evaluate the underlying veins. By determining the shift in sound frequency as the sound wave hits flowing blood, one can determine blood flow velocity and other flow parameters. The drawback to a CW Doppler examination is the inability to be sure which vein is being evaluated because of the possible presence of duplicated veins or large collateral veins. Also, the existence of reflux, but not its severity, can be determined.

CW Doppler examination has been replaced by duplex scanning, currently the most popular and versatile noninvasive venous evaluation, which uses B-mode imaging to overcome the limitations of a CW Doppler study (Fig. 19-5). This procedure is able to identify specific venous structures and thereby eliminate the confusion involved with continuous-wave scanning. B-mode imaging uses sound waves to create a picture of the structure being examined. Long segments of vein can be analyzed with this method for easier evaluation of obstruction. In combination with color flow analysis, this method of ultrasonography gives anatomic detail that can be useful for planning surgical procedures. Venous obstruction appears as a segment of vein where there is loss of flow signal. Chronic obstruction can be differentiated from acute thrombosis. Acute thrombosis causes venous distention because the intraluminal clot has bulk and the vein is inflamed. Chronic occlusion causes fibrosis of the vein so that it is smaller than the normal caliber. Calcifications may be present in a chronic thrombus.[27] One can see recanalization of veins in chronic venous disease as well. All these findings can be seen in any of the venous structures imaged. With the use of venous compression maneuvers, incompetence of the venous valves can be observed (see Fig. 19-5). A reflux time of

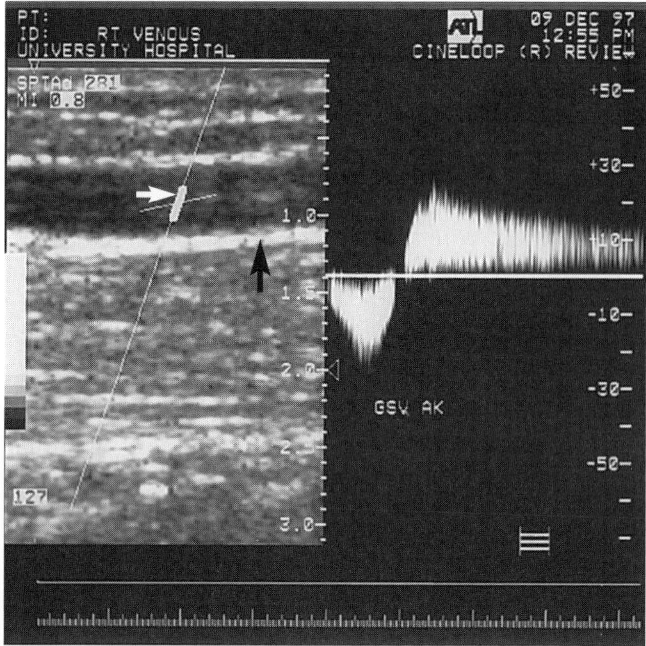

FIG. 19–5. B-mode Doppler study of a vein images the actual venous anatomy *(black arrow)*. The spectral histogram shows the venous wave pattern at the location indicated by the white bar on the B-mode image *(white arrow)*. This image shows venous valvular insufficiency as demonstrated by the antegrade flow with calf compression and prolonged reverse flow with release of compression.

more than 1.0 second is considered abnormal with routine distal compression maneuvers.[27] As a result of the very precise visualization capable with duplex scanning, evaluation of the vein valves can even be performed in some instances (Fig. 19-6, *A* and *B*). Of note, incompetent communicating veins can be seen on duplex scanning. When duplex imaging is used in combination with plethysmographic methods, a quantitative and qualitative assessment of the venous system can be achieved with surprising anatomic detail.

Ascending venography has the same purpose in the venous system as arteriography has for arterial disease. It provides a road map for anticipated surgical procedures. Placing an intravenous catheter into a foot vein and injecting contrast dye allows filling of the venous system. Occasionally during evaluation, the deep system does not fill with contrast dye. This may indicate DVT (Fig. 19-7). However, the placement of tourniquets at the ankle and thigh may help force the contrast agent into the deep system rather than passing only through the superficial veins. The deep veins may be damaged from previous disease rather than from acute thrombosis, and the contrast may have preferentially flowed into the superficial veins prior to the use of tourniquets.

Descending venography is used to detect valvular incompetence and is generally only obtained when surgical intervention is planned. This study is performed by entering another vein in the body (i.e., brachial or contralateral femoral vein) and advancing a catheter to the common femoral vein. This study is then performed in two stages.[28] The initial stage injects contrast material when the patient is at rest and in a semi-erect position with the weight of the patient on the opposite leg. The contrast material is heavier than blood and gently refluxes down the leg, outlining any valves that may be present (Fig. 19-8, *A*). The second part of the procedure is performed by injection of contrast dye while the patient performs a Valsalva maneuver. Competent valves will prevent reflux of blood down the leg (Fig. 19-8, *B*), whereas incompetence allows reflux of blood into the distal leg. Reflux is considered pathologic if blood reaches the calf veins in the second stage of the study. The presence or absence of structurally intact valves has surgical implications. The risks of venography include skin necrosis with extravasation of contrast dye, renal failure from the contrast dye,

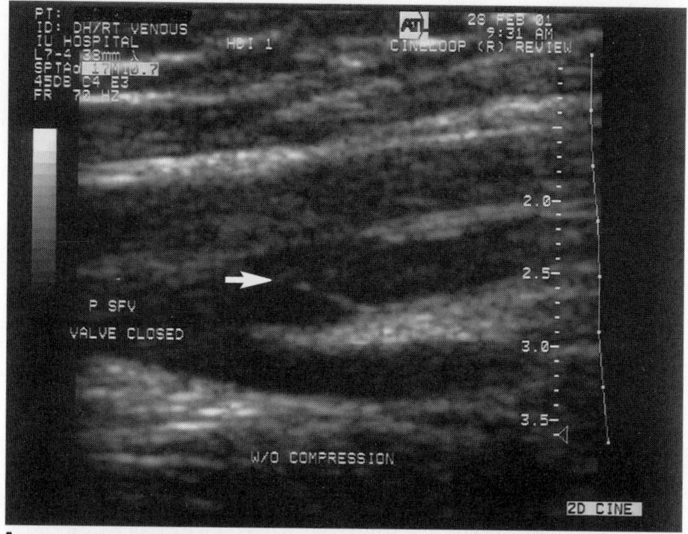

A

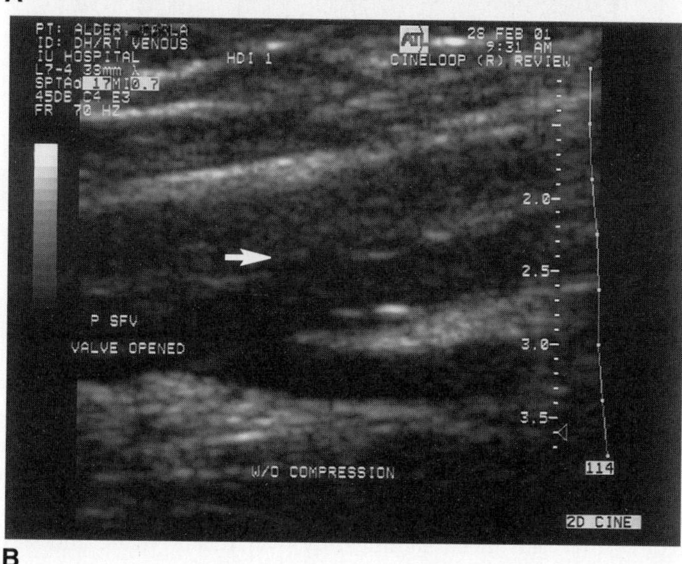

B

FIG. 19–6. Doppler study image of venous valve with **(A)** cusps closed *(arrow)* and **(B)** the valve cusps open to permit flow *(arrow)*.

thrombophlebitis, pulmonary embolus, and allergic reaction to the contrast agent, to mention some of the more common or life-threatening problems.[29]

TREATMENT OPTIONS AND RESULTS

Conservative Medical Therapy

Despite all the advances in modern medicine and in surgical technique, the mainstay of therapy for chronic venous disease has remained unchanged. The goals are to treat symptoms and restore as much normal physiologic function to the diseased limb as possible. Often these therapies are uncomfortable and difficult to perform during normal living. The full cooperation of the patient is required for these therapies to be successful. These measures include wearing high-quality compressive stockings (graded 30-40 mm Hg at the ankle), elevating the legs when possible during the day, avoiding prolonged periods of standing or sitting, elevating the foot of the bed 4-6 inches while sleeping, and applying bandages to ulcerations.[30,31] Appropriate education is required to perform these tasks well.

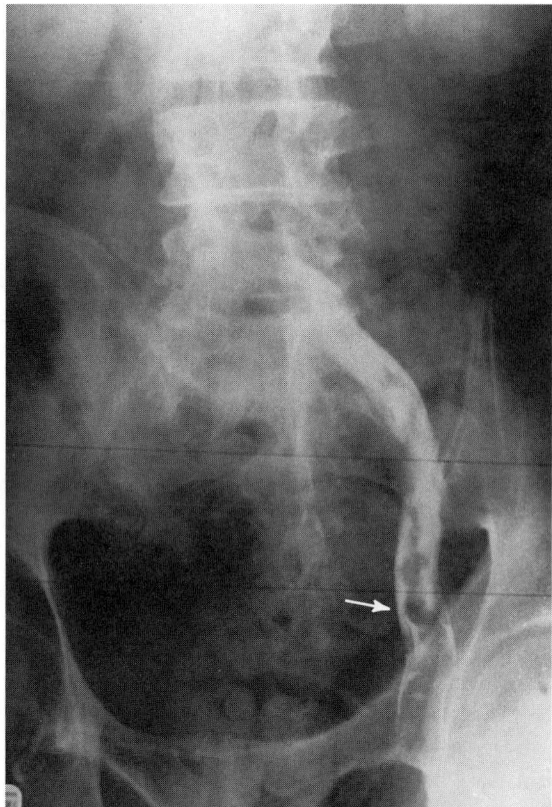

FIG. 19–7. Venogram demonstrating deep venous thrombosis of the left common iliac vein. The lumen of the vein is only partially occluded, and the thrombus is apparent as areas of the vein are not filled with white contrast material *(arrow)*.

Numerous types of compression garments have been developed. These garments range from elastic bandage wraps and compressive stockings to firm relatively inelastic wraps that provide graduated compression from the distal ankle to the proximal portion of the leg. Historically, compression stockings have been associated with poor patient compliance. However, their design has advanced significantly over recent years, and stockings are now available in various colors, styles, lengths, and degrees of compression.

Sclerotherapy

In the event that conservative measures are unsuccessful, surgery may be considered. Sclerotherapy (needle injection of caustic solutions directly into superficial veins) has been advocated for the treatment of small varicosities that remain after saphenous vein stripping, small individual varicosities, and telangiectasias in the thigh and around the knee. In general, it appears appropriate for patients without major superficial, perforator, or deep venous disease, although some would disagree. The most common sclerosing agents, sodium tetradecyl sulfate and hypertonic saline, can be caustic. These chemicals act by damaging the endothelium of the vein, inducing inflammation and scarring, and resulting in collapse of the vessel lumen.[32] These procedures are generally performed in an outpatient setting. Common complaints include burning, stinging, and itching or muscle spasm upon injection. If there is extravasation of the agent, fat or skin necrosis, ulcerations, and/or hyperpigmentation of the surrounding skin may result. The posttreatment veins are often a brown color as opposed to the blue-red pretreatment color. Other potential complications of sclerotherapy (Box 19-5) include allergic reactions to the sclerosing agent and toxicity if too many veins are treated at one sitting.[32] Therefore, a limited amount of sclerosing agent is typically injected during a single setting. Although the

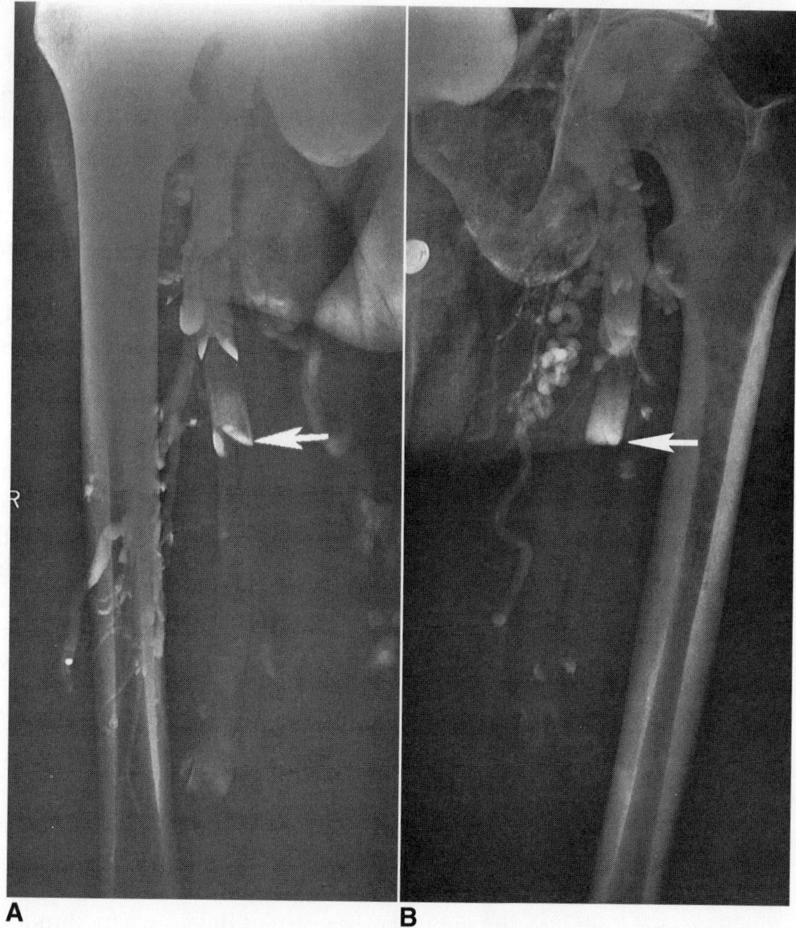

FIG. 19–8. Descending venogram with and without Valsalva maneuver. **A,** A picture of the presence of valves in the superficial femoral vein on quiet standing (see *arrow* showing valve). **B,** One of the proximal venous valves is competent (*arrow*) as the patient performs a Valsalva maneuver.

immediate postsurgical results are very satisfactory to most patients, the procedure often must be repeated if the larger diseased veins underlying each telangiectasia or small varicosity are not eliminated. Major venous insufficiency, if present, must be surgically managed to prevent recurrence following sclerotherapy.[32,33]

BOX 19–5

Complications of Sclerotherapy

ALLERGIC REACTION
Minor itching
Swelling of the lips and tongue
Bronchospasm
Skin blotching
Cardiovascular collapse

TOXICITY
Thirst
Shivering
Headache
Chest pain
Epigastric pain

TREATMENT FOR THESE COMPLICATIONS
Antihistamines
Hydration
Epinephrine
Oxygen
Limit volume of agent injected

Iliac Stenting and Venous Bypass

If less invasive measures fail, more aggressive surgical procedures are available for obstructive venous disease. The procedures include iliac vein stenting, cross-femoral venous bypass, saphenofemoral bypass, and inferior vena cava reconstruction, which have all been used in appropriate situations to decompress or bypass appropriate segments of the venous system.

In recent reports, endovascular stenting of iliac vein stenosis (placing a metallic endoskeleton within the vein via a percutaneous route) has improved the symptoms of venous occlusive disease, including edema and pain.[34,35] To ensure success after any venous reconstruction, it is imperative that the proper patient be selected. Direct venous measurements are required to determine the hemodynamic consequence of any obstruction or stenosis. This is usually done by measuring the pressure gradient across a stenosis or by performing an arm-foot pressure comparison. Some authors do not believe, however, that even these pressure measurements are sufficiently sensitive to determine who is a potential candidate for percutaneous interventions.[36]

The open surgical procedures use either native saphenous vein or polytetrafluoroethylene (PTFE) graft material as the conduit to bypass a nondiseased distal vein to a disease-free proximal vein. Vena caval reconstructions have been performed and often use PTFE grafts as the material of choice to allow a proper size match. Preoperatively, venous pressure studies are obtained to document venous hypertension that would be amenable to vena caval bypass.[18] Iliac vein decompression is utilized in the instance of extrinsic compression by an overlying right iliac artery (May-Thurner syndrome). If the iliac vein is severely stenosed or occluded, cross-femoral venous bypass can be performed, but the procedure of choice is direct repair of the involved segment of iliac vein or balloon angioplasty with stenting. Balloon angioplasty with stenting of the vein is becoming more popular as advances in endovascular surgery improve the success of this method of treatment.[34-37]

The indications for cross-femoral venous bypass include persistent unilateral iliac or common femoral venous occlusion in young patients, patients with subacute onset of progressive leg swelling due to extrinsic compression not amenable to direct surgical cure, and patients with threatened limb loss due to phlegmasia cerulea dolens where thrombectomy or thrombolysis has failed. If compression of the vein is due to a neoplastic growth, patient survival should be considered prior to aggressive surgical intervention. The cross-femoral venous bypass (femoral vein to femoral vein bypass graft) is performed by passing a chosen graft material through a suprapubic subcutaneous tunnel. The saphenous vein or prosthetic graft is then connected to each disease-free femoral vein by an end-to-side technique. The key to the success of this surgery is graft diameter. If the native vein is less than 4.5 mm in diameter, better success may be achieved with an 10-mm diameter PTFE graft.[18] An arteriovenous fistula can be created to increase flow and to improve graft patency in the immediate postoperative period. The fistula serves to increase blood flow across the anastomosis, thereby decreasing the early chances of occlusion. This fistula can then be ligated in 1-3 months.

Indications for a saphenopopliteal bypass are isolated femoral and/or popliteal vein occlusion, the common femoral and iliocaval system must be patent, a nonvaricosed saphenous vein must exist, and femoral phlebitis must be inactive for 1 year. In addition, conservative therapy to relieve chronic venous disease symptoms must have failed, and abnormal venous pressures of the diseased leg must be present. These distal to proximal venous bypasses use autogenous vein as the conduit of choice, and bypasses extend from distal to proximal nondiseased segments.[18]

Vein Stripping

In the face of superficial venous insufficiency, stripping of superficial varicosities can be employed. This operation should not be performed if deep venous obstruction is a significant component of the patient's problems because the superficial veins may be the only outflow tract for venous blood. However, it can be considered in cases of combined deep and superficial insufficiency.[38] Vein stripping includes ligation of the greater saphenous vein at the saphenofemoral junction in the groin followed by removal of the vein to the knee. If the below-knee saphenous vein is incompetent based upon preoperative diagnostic studies, it may also be excised. Preoperatively, with the patient standing to fully dilate the veins, the varicosities are marked with a permanent marker (see Fig. 19-3) for later operative visualization. Incisions are made to define the proximal (groin incision) and distal (ankle or calf incision) extent of the incompetent greater saphenous vein. The saphenofemoral junction is dissected in the groin, and all of the branches are ligated. By placing the patient in reverse Trendelenburg's position, the venous system is collapsed during stripper introduction and later vein extraction. A thin, flexible wire (the vein stripper) is placed in the lumen of the saphenous vein (Fig. 19-9, *A*) and advanced towards the groin. A third incision approximately 6 cm below the knee is made if the lower calf saphenous vein is to be stripped, and the original stripper is advanced to this incision. A second stripper is placed from the ankle to the knee incision. The wire is then secured proximally to the greater saphenous vein at the saphenofemoral junction. The saphenous vein is ligated flush with the common femoral vein and then transected (Fig. 19-9, *B*). The vein stripping device is then briskly pulled in a caudad direction, from groin to calf, thereby pulling the vein out of the leg. The distal end

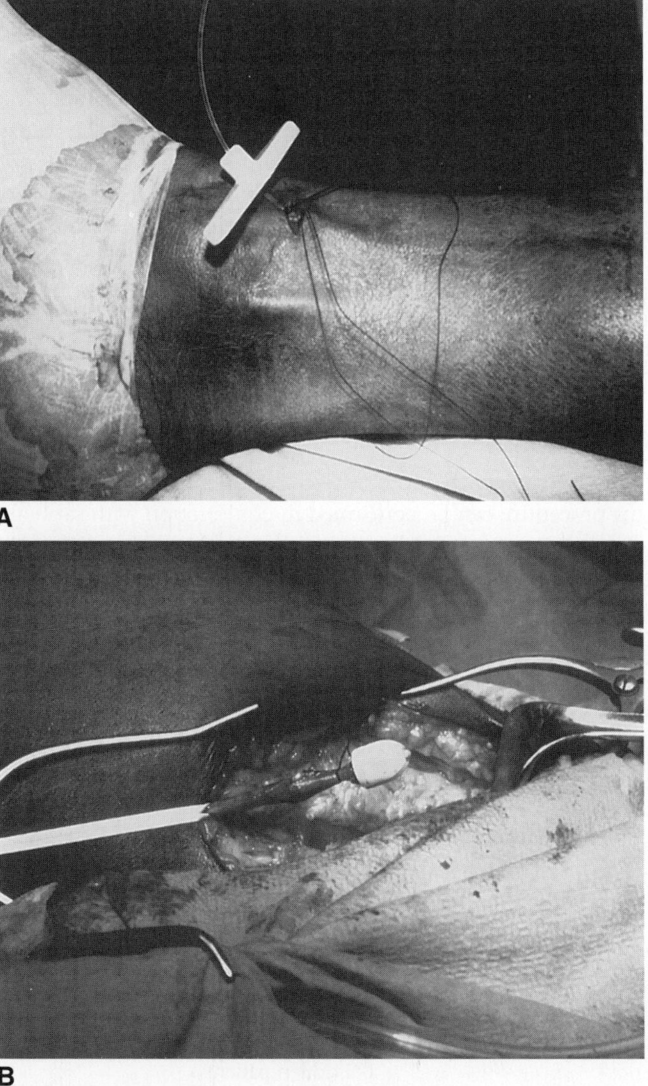

FIG. 19–9. A, A vein stripper device inserted at the ankle incision with a handle in place to aid in extracting the vein. **B,** A vein stripper device protruding from the greater saphenous vein at the saphenofemoral junction with cap placed prior to vein removal.

of the saphenous vein is removed in a similar fashion through the ankle and knee incision when appropriate.

Another method of removing the greater saphenous vein from the venous circulation is to thermally heat the inside (Closure technique).[39] A heating catheter is placed percutaneously inside the vein; once the catheter is activated, the vein is obliterated. After either approach to removing the greater saphenous vein for the venous circulation is accomplished, small incisions are made over the preoperatively marked branch varicosities. The veins are grasped and removed in long segments with a hemostat or another small instrument. Alternatively, a subcutaneous light-assisted powered phlebectomy has been suggested for removal of long lengths of branch varicosities via minimal incisions.[40] A long lighted probe with a powered suction and cutting tool is advanced along the trace of the branch varices to allow removal of long lengths.

Once all varicosities are excised, compressive stockings or elastic bandages are applied in the immediate postoperative period to prevent hematoma formation. Patients are discharged on the day of surgery and encouraged to ambulate aggressively but are told to avoid prolonged periods of standing or heavy lifting for 1-3 weeks. The operative compression stockings are typically removed the following day and then reapplied generally to the below-knee area in a graded pressure fashion to further decrease the risk of hematoma formation. It is difficult to obtain above-knee wrapping with any precision.

There are both temporary and absolute contraindications to performing a vein stripping procedure (Box 19-6). Complications of vein stripping are rare but include wound infection, DVT, nerve damage, and hematoma formation, to mention the most prominent.[41-43] Saphenous nerve injury can result in an area of numbness on the lateral foot.[13] Among properly selected patients undergoing a vein stripping procedure, recurrent saphenous varicosities will be noted in less than 15 percent of cases.[41] The lesser saphenous vein can be stripped if needed with similar results. Complications from this procedure are typically rare but include bleeding and hematoma formation, sural nerve damage, DVT, and wound infection.[44] A complication unique to the Closure procedure is thermal damage to adjacent structures that may include nerve and/or skin but appears to be mitigated by injecting a significant volume of local anesthetic around the vein.[39]

Perforator Vein Ligation

Ligation of perforating veins can be an effective treatment for patients with perforating vein incompetence. This procedure can be performed in conjunction with saphenous vein removal. Perforating vein ligation is performed by an open procedure with direct visualization of the offending veins or with minimally invasive endoscopic instruments. A Linton type of procedure utilizes an incision along the medial or posterior aspect of the leg and the creation of subfascial flaps.[45] The perforating veins are directly ligated. If a skin ulcer is present, this can be debrided simultaneously. If a large amount of soft tissue is affected, including the fascial layers, a skin graft can be placed to speed healing once the diseased tissues are removed.[45]

BOX 19–6

Contraindications to Vein Stripping

TEMPORARY	ABSOLUTE
Recent deep thrombophlebitis	Significant arterial disease
Weeping ulcers	Chronic lymphedema
Active cellulitis	Noncorrectable systemic disease
Uncontrolled metabolic disease (e.g., diabetes)	Advanced age
Pregnancy	Bedridden patient
Anemia	

Alternately, an endoscopic technique can be used.[46] The knee is slightly flexed, and two small (10-15 mm) incisions are made on the medial aspect of the lower leg near the knee and proximal to areas of induration and inflammation. Subfascial dissection is performed using blunt balloon and sharp dissection. Some surgeons place a tourniquet on the upper leg to prevent carbon dioxide (CO_2) embolus to the lungs just prior to subfascial insufflation of CO_2, which is used to improve visualization during the procedure. Other surgeons feel this step is not necessary because the venous system is better visualized with blood within the perforator veins and the risk of embolism is minimal. Under direct enhanced vision with a video camera, the perforating veins are ligated with metal clips and then divided. Some physicians have utilized mediastinoscopes through which a long clip applier can be advanced, obviating the need for a second incision. Once all of the vessels have been ligated, the instruments are removed and the incisions closed.

Elastic bandages are placed on the lower extremities, and the patients are allowed to ambulate the same day. Many surgeons mark the perforating veins preoperatively with duplex scanning to ensure that all offending veins are identified at the time of surgery. The most current follow-up of patients undergoing this method of perforator vein ligation is promising. Patients were shown to have decreased symptoms from their venous incompetence and were found to have near 90% ulcer healing rates at 2 years.[47]

Venous Ulcer Management

The goals of venous ulcer therapy are twofold: to heal the ulcer and to prevent its recurrence. As with all chronic venous disease, elevation and compression to control edema are paramount to therapy. Compression has been proven to be a vital part of venous ulcer therapy with several potential benefits (Box 19-7). The Unna paste boot (Fig. 19-10) is a dressing composed of gauze moistened with zinc oxide and calamine lotion containing glycerin.[31] The gauze is wrapped circumferentially to the affected limb and, when dry, it provides equal compression to the damaged skin. Care must be taken not to compromise the arterial circulation by applying the boot too tightly. A compressive bandage is placed over the boot to provide even more support. The boot is changed from a few times a week to once every 2 weeks, depending upon the amount of ulcer drainage. Its use must be discontinued if signs of infection develop such as erythema, purulent drainage, warmth, or pain.

Newer wound care products provide a substitute to the Unna boot and are aimed at providing a warm, moist, and clean environment for ulcer healing. Multilayer dressings (e.g., Profore, Dyna-Flex) provide compression and absorbency to protect the ulcer bed and surrounding skin from the wound fluid, which can impede wound healing.[31] Most of these dressings have one absorbent layer and one to three layers of elastomeric fibers, which provide compression. This group of dressings allow for weekly changes in most cases. Ulcers that have more copious amounts of drainage require more frequent dressing changes or the use of a hydrocolloid dressing. Such hydrocolloid and hydrogel dressings (e.g., AlgiDerm or AlgiSite Sorbsan) are able to absorb many times their weight in wound fluid. Therefore, these dressings can stay in place longer while maintaining a drier environment for the ulcer and surrounding tissues.

BOX 19–7

Effects of Compression Therapy

Enhances calf muscle pump function
Closes incompetent superficial veins and diverts flow into competent veins
Augments lymphatic flow
Reduces edema that separates skin from capillaries
Makes incompetent valves work by decreasing the diameter between the leaflets of valves in varicose veins

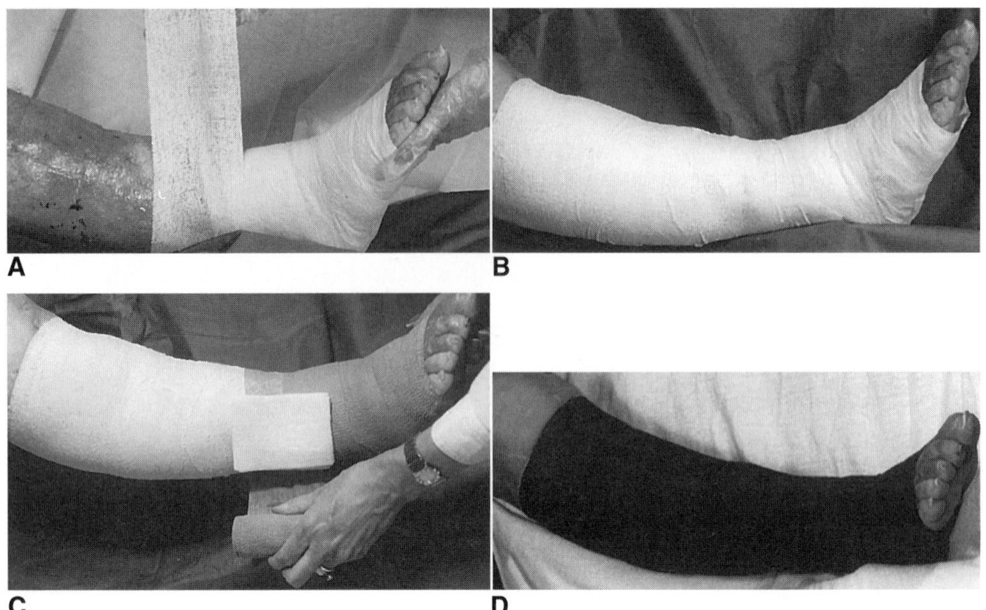

FIG. 19–10. Placement of an Unna boot. **A,** Venous ulcers are first wrapped with gauze or a medicated dressing. **B,** Lower leg completely wrapped with gauze. **C,** An extra dressing is placed over the site of the venous ulcer. **D,** An elastic bandage is placed around the entire lower extremity for uniform circumferential compression.

For the unresponsive or recurrent venous ulcers, skin grafting is an adjunctive option to control the underlying venous disease. These lesions can be extensive, and skin grafting allows for coverage of raw surfaces, thereby potentially speeding the healing process. Once the ulcer has a clean base of granulation tissue, a split-thickness skin graft can be applied. There are reports on improved healing with skin grafting for chronic venous ulceration,[48] but there are risks associated with the graft harvest site as well as the lack of potential cure. Skin grafting should only be considered if healing of the ulcer has not occurred with diligent conservative management.

An allogenic cultured bilayer skin equivalent (Apligraf) is being used for the treatment of venous stasis ulcers. Cultured skin consists of a layer of bovine collagen matrix, which has living human dermal fibroblasts, and an outer layer of living human keratinocytes. Its advantages over autogenous skin include application in an outpatient setting without the need for anesthesia, and there are no donor site risks. In trials, it has been shown to decrease the time to ulcer closure and increase the overall number of ulcers that are healed.[49] It can also be used as a preamble to skin grafting in some cases of extensive ulceration.

Venous Valve Repair or Replacement

Valve repair and reconstruction can be performed for primary deep venous valvular incompetence. Valve operations are generally performed only for end-stage disease symptoms, but in some circumstances surgery is performed for lifestyle-limiting disease. These operations attempt to restore one or more functional valves in the affected lower extremity.

A variety of open and direct valve cusp repair techniques have been described.[50,51] When undamaged valves exist within the vein, the affected vein is incised at the level of an anatomically preserved but nonfunctional valve and fine suture is used to tighten and reinforce the valve (Fig. 19-11). Angioscopy can be used to direct the valvuloplasty repair while avoiding the need to open the vein itself. With this procedure, the scope is placed through a side branch of the vein and is advanced until the incompetent valve is in view. One or more fine Prolene sutures are used to tighten the valve cusps. There have also been methods of valve repair described that do not require opening of the vein in any way but are applicable only in select patients.[50,51] These procedures are not without risks, however. Wound hematoma, infection, lymphatic leaks, thrombosis of the repaired vein, and recurrent reflux have all been reported.[51-54] The open

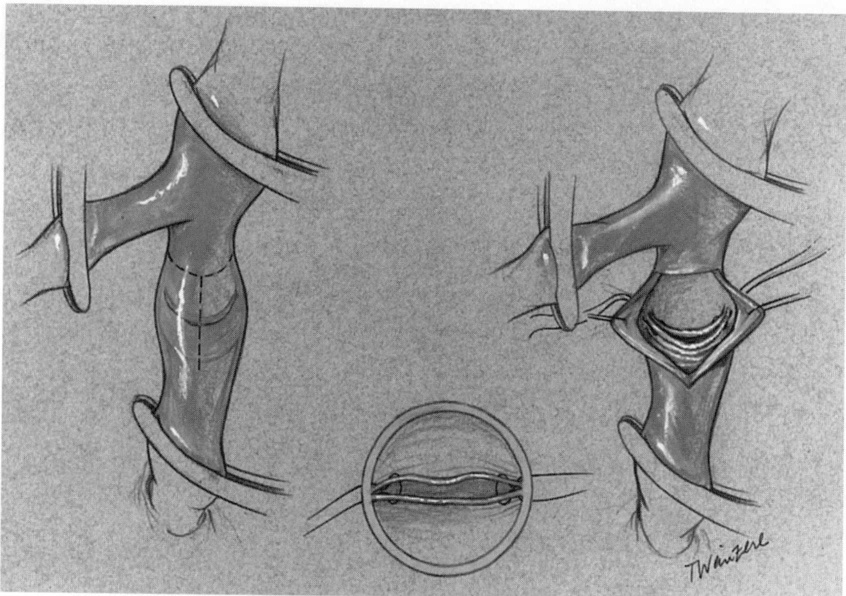

FIG. 19–11. An artist's depiction of a venous valve repair in a patient with primary venous valvular incompetency. The vein has been opened, and sutures are placed to tighten the valve for proper functioning.

vein technique has been studied more extensively than any other technique and has had very reasonable success ranging from 60-70 percent at 5-year follow-up.[51-54]

Finally, the use of a transposition procedure or venous valve transplantation has been attempted in patients with complete damage of the valves that are not amenable to repair. The transposition of valves requires the presence of a competent valve in some part of the lower-extremity venous system that can be used to provide reflux protection for the incompetent system. The incompetent venous system (often the superficial femoral vein) is ligated proximally, and the distal vein is sewn in a position below the available competent valve. This procedure is applicable in only 2-3 percent of potential patient candidates.[55]

Venous valve transplantation requires finding a competent valve in the upper extremity (or one that can be made competent) or opposite lower extremity saphenous system and then transplanting it into the incompetent lower leg venous system (Fig. 19-12). The valve must be transplanted below all pathologic reflux to be effective. The upper-extremity valve is usually obtained from the axillary venous system. The major obstacle to this technique has been the absence of a functional upper-extremity valve (40 percent of cases) or incompetence of the transplanted valve over time.[53,55,56] Clinically, however, approximately 60 percent of patients severely disabled prior to surgery have clinical improvement for more than 5 years with this approach.[54] There are currently investigations into valve substitutes that might provide an option for patients lacking an appropriate upper-extremity venous valve for transplantation.[57] There are also ongoing studies to determine if this approach is clinically feasible.[58] There is some indication that cryopreserved valves are prone to fibrosis. In addition, there are experimental and clinical trials to determine if percutaneously placed stents with valves could eventually be a treatment option.[59,60] Long-term results are lacking.

NURSING IMPLICATIONS

Varicose Veins

Patient education should include an explanation of the function of the veins and valves. The patient should be taught the cause of varicose veins as well as preventive measures and should be further informed about recommended treatment as discussed below.

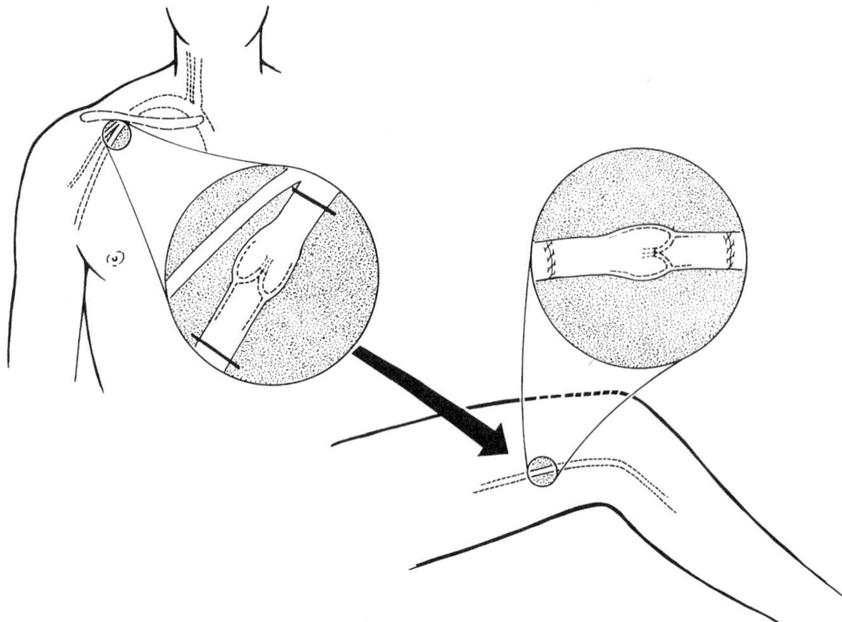

FIG. 19–12. The transplantation of a venous valve from the upper arm to the lower leg provides for reflux protection to the lower leg in a patient who otherwise has no competent valves in the lower leg.

Injection Therapy

A complete health history, including a list of current medications, drug allergies, and hypersensitivities, is obtained from the patient. The patient is advised to avoid platelet-inhibiting drugs for 1 week before treatment. Patients with known cardiac valvular disease should be treated with oral antibiotics.

The procedure and possible adverse effects should be fully explained to the patient. The patient should be told that multiple bruises from injections will appear 2-3 days after treatment and that the legs will look worse before they look better. The patient should be warned of the potential adverse effects, including pain during injection, hyperpigmentation, multiple superficial thrombi, ulceration, nodular fibroses, and blush-mat effects. A consent form should be obtained. Posttreatment instructions should be provided to the patient on discharge as follows:

ACTIVITY. Limit vigorous activities such as aerobics, racquet sports, biking, or running for 72 hours. Walking briskly for 30 minutes after treatment is recommended and is thought to enhance the effect of sclerosing agents injected into the veins. It may also decrease the risk of deep venous thrombosis.

ELASTIC STOCKINGS. Ankle-to-thigh compression dressings should be worn for 72 hours to 3 weeks, depending on the physician's discretion. Prescription compression stockings or elastic wrap bandages may be used. If elastic wrap bandages are used, care must be taken to rewrap as necessary to maintain firm compression. The patient should be taught to wrap the elastic bandage, beginning at the foot and ending at the thigh. The pressure applied should be more at the foot/ankle and decrease slightly as one applies the bandage up the leg and thigh.

BATHING. The initial compression dressing may be removed so that the patient can bathe only at a designated time to be determined by the physician. This time may vary from 24 hours to 3 days after injection. It must be reapplied promptly after bathing for best results.

SKIN CARE. Bruising near areas of injection is expected and is usually resolved within 2 weeks. Small, firm, tender, greenish blue nodular areas may also result after sclerotherapy. These are areas of superficial thrombosis and are easily evacuated when the skin is pierced with a large-bore needle and the thrombus is expressed. If untreated, the thrombus will eventually be reabsorbed but will often leave a brownish discoloration of the skin, which may persist for up to 1 year or longer. If the skin is damaged sufficiently, a superficial ulcer may develop that is treated with antibiotic ointments, bandages, and time. The skin will essentially heal, but a scar may remain.

Vein Stripping or Perforator Ligation Operation

Preoperative teaching should include an explanation of the function of the veins and valves, information regarding causes of varicose veins, preoperative and postoperative routines, and potential discoloration, bruising, leg swelling, scarring and discomfort after surgery. The patient should be made aware of possible nerve injury, and the operative consent should reflect this discussion. Operating room nurses should discuss with the surgeon any special equipment that may be needed.

POSTOPERATIVE CARE. Vital signs should be checked regularly. The nurse should monitor the patient for potential hemorrhage by checking leg dressings for excessive drainage. If bleeding is excessive, direct pressure should be applied over the wound, the leg should be elevated, and the surgeon should be notified. If bleeding is minimal, proper elastic support will control it. It is important to ascertain that the bandage is not applied so tightly as to compromise the circulation.

Elastic bandages are applied to the affected leg to decrease hematoma formation and prevent postoperative edema secondary to disruption of perivenous lymphatic vessels that accompany the venous trunks in the lower extremity. When one considers that nearly all lymphatic trunks from the lower extremities are grouped around the greater saphenous vein, it is surprising that edema is a rare complication.

Pedal pulses and sensory and motor function of the affected extremity should be checked every 2 hours for the first 8 hours. When the leg is in a dependent position, the patient should wear elastic support below the knee for 1-2 weeks. Leg swelling reduction can also be accomplished by raising the foot of the bed or by using a foam rubber block. Ambulation should be encouraged as soon as possible after surgery.

Venous Reconstruction or Venous Valvular Transplant Operations

An explanation of the procedure should be provided to the patient. Patients should be instructed that they will need to be up walking with support hose on that night or next day. They may have some swelling in the legs as well and will be required to elevate the legs (above the heart) as much as possible.

Patients must be monitored carefully in the postoperative period for the development of surgical complications. These complications include hematoma formation, incisional bleeding, and swelling of the leg more than anticipated. Adequate compression that does not compromise the circulation will solve these problems, but if this measure is unsuccessful, the physician must be notified. Also, if an arteriovenous fistula was performed for patients undergoing venous bypass procedures, distal pulse checks must be performed to ensure adequate distal circulation. Again, any change in the pulses necessitates physician notification. Because these are major surgical procedures, routine postoperative monitoring, including respiratory, cardiac, and vital signs, must be carefully documented, and results not within standard parameters conveyed to the physician.

Venous Ulceration

Success in healing a venous ulcer can be achieved only if the patient is a ready and willing participant in the plan of care. The patient needs to be educated about venous disease in order to make necessary adjustments in lifestyle to minimize the effects of the disease. Because the underlying problem in patients with venous ulceration is venous hypertension, nursing care is directed at reducing this high pressure. Efforts to accomplish this involve emphasizing the importance of bed rest, leg elevation, and external elastic support.

A complete assessment of the lower extremities should be performed at each visit, and any abnormalities or changes from baseline should be noted. Pedal pulses and motor/sensory function should be assessed. Thorough documentation of ulcer characteristics should be made at each dressing change to evaluate effectiveness of treatment. Ulcer characteristics to note include size, condition of granulation tissue, color, odor, consistency and amount of drainage, and condition of the limb (i.e., swelling, redness, warmth, and amount and character of pain). Signs of infection at any time or unsatisfactory progress in ulcer healing within 2-3 weeks of treatment necessitate re-evaluation of the patient's treatment regimen. Concurrent medical problems (such as congestive heart failure, lymphedema, malnutrition, and diabetes) must be controlled to afford optimal healing. Providing patients with the guidelines listed in Box 19-8 for proper care may help ensure compliance with prescribed therapy.

Periodic medical check-ups are necessary; all scheduled appointments should be kept. The doctor should be notified if any of the problems listed in Box 19-9 occur. Furthermore, the patients should be encouraged to call the nurse or physician with any questions.

BOX 19–8

Guidelines for Patients With Venous Disease (With/Without Ulcers)

HYGIENE

Check skin daily. Keep skin in healthy condition. Watch for:
- Cracking
- Breakdown
- Change in color/temperature

If skin is dry, use moisturizing lotion:
- Not for use on open wounds

Wash daily:
- Use mild soap.
- Lukewarm water (body temperature).
- Avoid soaking legs in tub.

Wear clean stockings daily.
Use antifungal powder in shoes if feet are moist.
Consult physician for any problems/concerns.
With venous ulcers:
- Cover dressings prior to bathing.
- Sponge bathe to prevent excessive moisture.

INJURY PREVENTION

Avoid bumping, cutting, bruising legs.
Do not go barefoot.
Avoid shaving legs with razors.
Avoid using pillows under knees.
Avoid:
- Excess heat/cold
- Harsh chemicals
- Hair remover creams

Test bath water with hands not toes.

ACTIVITY

Exercise regularly:
- Even in bed with foot flexing
- Swimming
- Walking
- Cycling

Avoid excess activity that makes legs swell.
No long periods of standing/sitting:
- If one must stand still, exercise legs during that time.

Automobile trips:
- Stop every 2 hours to exercise legs.

Leg elevation:
- Decreases swelling
- Several times a day for 10-15 minutes
- Always at night by 6 inches
  - Blocks under foot of bed

ELASTIC SUPPORT

Always wear stocking while awake.
Apply first thing in the morning.
Wash with mild soap and reuse.
Discard and replace when elasticity is lost.
If using elastic bandages:
  - Wrap from toe to below knee.
  - Overlap edges.
  - Wrap snugly.

GENERAL

No smoking.
Nutrition:
- Maintain well-balanced diet.
- Reduce sodium.
  - ↓fluid retention
- Avoid overeating.
  - ↓weight on legs
- Follow high-fiber diet.
  - ↓straining with bowel movement
  - ↓pressure on veins
  - Main sources:
    - Raw fruits
    - Vegetables
      - Corn
      - Celery
      - Beans
    - Whole grains

CLOTHING

Do not wear constricting garments.
Wear well-fitting shoes.
Always wear socks with shoes to prevent blisters.
Slowly break in new shoes.
If feet are swollen:
- Wear slipper or wide shoe.

BOX 19–9

Medical Follow-Up/Physician Notification

Sudden weight gain or swelling of the feet, ankles, or legs
Increase or decrease in temperature of the leg
Unusual color, amount, or odor of drainage from the wound
Increase in inflammation, redness, tenderness, or pain in the leg
Inability to move the legs without pain
The color of the foot becomes pale
Skin breakdown occurs
Fever >100°F

SUMMARY

Although chronic venous disease symptoms have been documented for centuries, management has not changed dramatically until recently. The mainstays of therapy remain elevation and compression to reduce tissue edema. When one or more of the complications of venous disease does occur, the most conservative yet effective measures should be attempted first. If these are to no avail, there are several operative and interventional therapies available that have been shown to be effective in properly selected patients. Nurses play a major role in the care of the patient with chronic venous disease.

REFERENCES

1. Browse NL, Burnand KG, Irvine AT et al: *Diseases of the veins,* ed 2, London, 1999, Arnold.
2. White JV, Katz ML, Cisek P et al: Venous outflow of the leg: anatomy and physiologic mechanism of the plantar venous plexus, *J Vasc Surg* 24:819-824, 1996.
3. Nicolaides AN, Hussein MK, Szendro G et al: The relation of venous ulceration with ambulatory venous pressure measurements, *J Vasc Surg* 17:414-419, 1993.
4. Gourdin FW, Smith JG Jr: Etiology of venous ulceration, *South Med J* 86:1142-1146, 1993.
5. Cockett FB, Thomas ML: The iliac compression syndrome, *Br J Surg* 52:816-821, 1965.
6. Cockett FB, Thomas ML, Negus D: Iliac vein compression: its relation to iliofemoral thrombosis and the post-thrombotic syndrome, *BMJ* 2:14-19, 1967
7. McMurrich JP: The occurrence of congenital adhesions in the common iliac veins, and their relation to thrombosis of the femoral and iliac veins, *Am J Med Sci* 135:342-346, 1908.
8. Lawrence PF, Gaznak CE: Epidemiology of chronic venous insufficiency. In Ballard JL, Bergan JJ, eds: *Chronic venous insufficiency: diagnosis and treatment,* London, 2000, Springer-Verlag, pp 3-8.
9. Plate G, Brodin L, Eklof B et al: Physiologic and therapeutic aspects in congenital vein valve aplasia of the lower limb, *Ann Surg* 198:229-233, 1983.
10. Clarke H, Smith SR, Vasdekis SN et al: Role of venous elasticity in the development of varicose veins, *Br J Surg* 76:577-580, 1989.
11. O'Donnell JF Jr: Chronic venous insufficiency: an overview of epidemiology, classification, and anatomic considerations, *Semin Vasc Surg* 1:60-65, 1988.
12. Sandri JL, Barros FS, Pontes S et al: Diameter-reflux relationship in perforating veins of patients with varicose veins, *J Vasc Surg* 30:867-875, 1990.
13. Dale WA, Cranley JJ, DeWeese JA et al: Symposium: management of varicose veins, *Contemp Surg* 6:86-124, 1975.
14. Browse NL, Burnand, KG: The cause of venous ulceration, *Lancet* 2:243-245, 1982.
15. Peyton B, Rohrer MJ et al: Patients with venous stasis ulceration have increased monocyte-platelet aggregation, *J Vasc Surg* 27:1109-1116, 1998.
16. Pappas PJ, Duran WN, Hobson RW: Pathology and cellular physiology of chronic venous insufficiency. In Gloviczki P, Yao JST, eds: *Handbook of venous disorders*, ed 2, London, 2001, Arnold, pp 58-67.
17. Wokalek H, Vanscheidt W, Martay K et al: Morphology and localization of sunburst varicosities: an electron microscopic and morphometric study, *J Dermatol Surg Oncol* 15:149-154, 1989.
18. Lalka SG: Autogenous venous bypass grafts for chronic iliac or infrainguinal venous occlusive disease. In Gloviczki P, Yao JST, eds: *Handbook of venous disorders*, ed 2, London, 2001, Arnold, pp 362-373.

19. Dalsing MC: Tutorial 20: venous valvular insufficiency: pathophysiology and treatment options. In Tretotola SO, Savaders SJ, Durham JD, eds: *Venous interventions*, Fairfax, VA, 1995, The Society of Cardiovascular and Interventional Radiologists, pp 225-238.
20. Killewich LA, Martin R, Cramer M et al: Pathophysiology of venous claudication, *J Vasc Surg* 1:507-511, 1984.
21. Labropoulos N, Volteas M, Leon M et al: The role of venous outflow obstruction in patients with chronic venous dysfunction, *Arch Surg* 132:46-51, 1997.
22. Beebe HG, Bergan JJ, Bergqvist D et al: Classification and grading of chronic venous disease in the lower limbs: a consensus statement, *Int Angiol* 14(2):197-201, 1995.
23. Rutherford RB, Robert B, Padberg FT Jr et al: Venous severity scoring: an adjunct to venous outcome assessment, *J Vasc Surg* 31(6):1307-1312, 2000.
24. Raju S: New approaches to the diagnosis and treatment of venous obstruction, *J Vasc Surg* 4:42, 1986.
25. Bays RA, Healy DA, Atnip RG et al: Validation of air plethysmography, photoplethysmography, and duplex ultrasonography in the evaluation of severe venous stasis, *J Vasc Surg* 20:721-727, 1994.
26. Araki CT, Hobson RW II: Indirect noninvasive tests (plethysmography). In Gloviczki P, Yao JST, eds: *Handbook of venous disorders*, ed 2, London, 2001, Arnold, pp 104-109.
27. Mattos MA, Summer DS: Direct noninvasive tests (Duplex scan) for the evaluation of chronic venous obstruction and valvular incompetence. In Gloviczki P, Yao JST, eds: *Handbook of venous disorders*, ed 2, London, 2001, Arnold, pp 120-131.
28. Kistner RL, Feuier EB, Randhawn F et al: A method of performing descending venography, *J Vasc Surg* 4:464-468, 1986.
29. LaBerge JM, Callen PW: Tutorial 17: diagnosis of deep venous thrombosis. In Tretotola SO, Savaders SJ, Durham JD, eds: *Venous interventions*, Fairfax, VA, 1995, The Society of Cardiovascular and Interventional Radiologists, pp 190-201.
30. Erickson CA, Lanza DJ, Karp DL et al: Healing of venous ulcers in an ambulatory care program: the roles of chronic venous insufficiency and patient compliance, *J Vasc Surg* 22:629-636, 1995.
31. Nicoloff AD, Moneta GL, Porter JM: Compression treatment of chronic venous insufficiency. In Gloviczki P, Yao JST, eds: *Handbook of venous disorders*, ed 2, London, 2001, Arnold, pp 303-308.
32. Villavicencio JL: Sclerotherapy guidelines. In Gloviczki P, Yao JST, eds: *Handbook of venous disorders*, ed 2, London, 2001, Arnold, pp 253-266.
33. Neglen P, Einarsson E, Eklof B: The functional long-term value of different types of treatment for saphenous vein incompetence, *J Cardiovasc Surg* 34:295-301, 1993.
34. Raju S, Owen S, Neglen P: Reversal of abnormal lymphoscintigraphy after placement of venous stents for correction of associated venous obstruction, *J Vasc Surg* 34:779-784, 2001.
35. Raju S, Owens S, Neglen P: The clinical impact of iliac venous stents in the management of chronic venous insufficiency, *J Vasc Surg* 35:8-15, 2002.
36. Neglen P, Raju S: Balloon dilation and stenting of chronic iliac vein obstruction: technical aspects and early clinical outcome, *J Endovasc Ther* 7(2):79-93, 2000.
37. Heniford BT, Senler SO, Olsofka JM et al: May-Thurner syndrome: management by endovascular surgical techniques, *Ann Vasc Surg* 12:482-486, 1998.
38. Padberg FT Jr, Pappas PJ, Araki CT et al: Hemodynamic and clinical improvement after superficial vein ablation in primary combined venous insufficiency with ulceration, *J Vasc Surg* 26:169-171, 1997.
39. Chandler JG, Pichot O, Sessa C et al: Treatment of primary venous insufficiency by endovenous saphenous vein obliteration, *Vasc Surg 3* 4:201-209, 2000.
40. Spitz GA, Braxton JM: Outpatient's varicose vein surgery with transilluminated powered phlebectomy. *Proceedings from the American Venous Forum, twelfth annual meeting*, Phoenix, Ariz, Feb 2-6, 2000.
41. Larson RA, Toftgren EP, Myers TT et al: Long-term results after vein surgery: study of 1000 cases after 10 years, *Mayo Clin Proc* 49:114, 1974.
42. Keith LM Jr, Smead WL: Saphenous vein stripping and its complications, *Surg Clin North Am* 63: 1303-1312, 1983.
43. Ramsheyi A, Soury P, Saliou C et al: Inadvertant arterial injury during saphenous vein stripping: three cases and therapeutic strategies, *Arch Surg* 133:1120-1123, 1998.
44. Seror P: Sural nerve neuropathy (external saphenous) linked to a disease of the small saphenous vein, *J Mal Vasc* 25:128-131, 2000.
45. DePalma RG: Management of incompetent perforators: conventional techniques. In Gloviczki P, Yao JST, eds: *Handbook of venous disorders*, ed 2, London, 2001, Arnold, pp 384-390.
46. Gloviczki P, Bergan JJ, Menawat SS et al: Safety, feasibility, and early efficacy of subfascial endoscopic perforator surgery: a preliminary report from the North American registry, *J Vasc Surg* 25:94-105, 1997.

47. Gloviczki P, Bergan JJ, Rhodes JM et al: Mid-term results of endoscopic perforator vein interruption for chronic venous insufficiency: lessons learned from the North American subfascial endoscopic perforator surgery registry. The North American Study Group, *J Vasc Surg* 2 9:489-502, 1999.
48. Schmeller W, Gaber Y: Surgical removal of ulcer and lipodermatosclerosis followed by split-skin grafting (shave therapy) yields good long-term results in "non-healing" venous leg ulcers, *Acta Derm Venereol* 80:267-271, 2000.
49. Falanga V, Sabolinski M: A bilayered living skin construct accelerates complete closure of hard to heal venous ulcers, *Wound Repair Regen* 7(4):201-207, 1999.
50. Raju S, Hardy JD: Technical options in venous valve reconstruction, *Am J Surg* 173:301-307, 1997.
51. Nachreiner RD, Bhuller AS, Dalsing MC: Surgical repair of incompetent venous valves. In Gloviczki P, Yao JST, eds: *Handbook of venous disorders*, ed 2, London, 2001, Arnold, pp 329-335.
52. Masuda EM, Kistner RL: Long-term results of venous valve reconstruction: a four- and twenty-one-year follow-up, *J Vasc Surg* 19:391-403, 1994.
53. Raju S, Fredericks R: Valve reconstruction procedures for non-obstructive venous insufficiency: rationale, techniques, and results in 107 procedures with two-to-eight year follow up, *J Vasc Surg* 7:301-310, 1988.
54. Raju S, Fredericks RK, Neglen PN et al: Durability of venous valve reconstruction techniques for "primary" and postthrombotic reflux, *J Vasc Surg* 23:357-367, 1996.
55. Raju S: Venous insufficiency of the lower limb and stasis ulceration: changing concepts and management, *Ann Surg* 197:688-697, 1983.
56. Bry JDL, Muto PA, O'Donnell TF: The clinical and hemodynamic results after axillary-to-popliteal vein valve transplantation, *J Vasc Surg* 21:110-119, 1995.
57. Burkhart HM, Fath SW, Dalsing MC et al: Experimental repair of venous valvular insufficiency using a cryopreserved venous valve allograft aided by a distal arteriovenous fistula, *J Vasc Surg* 26:817-822, 1997.
58. Dalsing MC, Raju S, Wakefield TW et al: A multicenter, phase I evaluation of cryopreserved venous valve allografts for the treatment of chronic deep venous insufficiency, *J Vasc Surg* 30:854-866, 1999.
59. Dalsing, MC, Sawchuck AD, Lalka SG et al: An early experience with endovascular venous valve transplantation, *J Vasc Surg* 24:903-905, 1996.
60. Vein hopes: interventional alternative to surgery possible, *Interventional News,* p 1, April-June 2001.

PART FIVE

SPECIFIC PROBLEMS

20

Vascular Access

JOAN JACOBSEN

Nurses have a unique role in the management of vascular access, including maintenance of access, patient education, and prevention of complications. Nurses collaborate with members of other disciplines involved in the care of these patients; they may include vascular surgeons, interventional radiologists, pharmacists, nephrologists, and oncologists.

This chapter discusses two major areas: access for dialysis and central venous access devices (CVADs) that have their tips in the central vena cava. Dialysis access focuses on hemodialysis treatment for the patient experiencing renal failure. The chapter excludes discussion of peripheral intravenous access intended for short-term duration. This chapter emphasizes the adult patient population with special consideration of children addressed as appropriate. Nursing management of both dialysis access and CVADs is discussed.

ACCESS FOR DIALYSIS

Treatment of Renal Failure

Hemodialysis is the most commonly employed modality of therapy for patients with end-stage renal disease (ESRD).[1] The population of dialysis patients has been increasing at a rate of 10 percent per year.[2] Elders are the fastest growing age group within the ESRD population. ESRD is generally characterized by an insidious deterioration in renal function that allows for advance planning with long-term vascular access (i.e., arteriovenous [AV] fistula) for the provision of hemodialysis. Dialysis catheters are an integral part of the delivery of hemodialysis but should be considered a bridge to more permanent forms of dialysis access in most patients.[3] The presence of certain physiologic abnormalities may necessitate emergency dialysis. Trauma patients may be treated with continuous arteriovenous hemofiltration that is performed via large-bore arterial and venous catheters, usually in the femoral vessels.[4] This bedside modality is used to treat patients with refractory fluid overload, complicated acute renal failure, and acid-base and electrolyte derangements, and for those in whom conventional hemodialysis is contraindicated.[5]

Planning for Dialysis Access

Vascular access surgery is often performed well in advance of its anticipated need, allowing 6-12 weeks for adequate dilation and thickening of the vein wall before the fistula is cannulated. Preoperative assessment involves careful evaluation of upper-extremity pulses and venous anatomy (Box 20-1). Efforts should be made to preserve the access vessels (Table 20-1) primarily by avoiding venipuncture in the nondominant arm beginning in the earliest stages of renal failure.[6] Iatrogenic destruction of suitable peripheral veins in a hospital environment reduces the possibility of the procedure of choice, an endogenous AV fistula in the nondominant upper extremity. Approximately one half of patients referred for primary access procedures should be suitable for direct fistula at the wrist if these vessels have been preserved.[7]

In devising a strategy for long-term hemodialysis access, one must consider not only the complexity and patency of the procedure but also the potential impact on a future access

BOX 20–1

Planning for Hemodialysis Access

Preservation of primary access vessels
Allen test (see Figure 4-3)
Impact on future access procedures
Preoperative tests (duplex scan, venogram, or computed tomography [CT] scan)
Radial and ulnar pulse assessment
Collateral circulation evaluation

procedure. As a general principle, distal sites are selected first, providing a long vein segment for cannulation and preserving proximal sites for future access procedures. The chosen site should allow for ease of access for cannulation and should be positioned to ensure patient comfort during hemodialysis.[7]

Maintenance of adequate vascular access requires the prospective identification of anatomic lesions that result in access thrombosis, the most common cause of failure with access fistula. Before creating a radiocephalic fistula, the radial and ulnar pulses are palpated. Doppler systolic pressures at the wrist are obtained if the surgeon remains uncertain as to their adequacy. In addition, the Allen test (see Figure 4-3) is performed to determine the ability of the ulnar artery to perfuse the hand if the radial artery should thrombose or be ligated subsequent to fistula creation. For patients who have had repeated failures of dialysis access or a history of multiple central venous catheterizations, preoperative tests may include a duplex scan, a venogram, or a contrast enhanced spiral computed tomography (CT) scan.[8] Careful preoperative evaluation of the potential collateral circulation of the limb is done to predict and prevent ischemia; such evaluation is especially crucial with the diabetic and peripheral vascular disease (PVD) population.[9]

Primary Arteriovenous Fistulae

A primary AV fistula directly connects an artery and a vein via an anastomosis. The endogenous AV fistula remains the standard method of achieving long-term vascular access for hemodialysis purposes. The creation of an AV fistula requires a good inflow artery as well as a satisfactory outflow vein.[8] Best results are achieved by anastomosing the radial artery to the cephalic vein at the wrist (known as the Brescia-Cimino fistula). The Brescia-Cimino fistula was introduced in 1966 and remains the gold standard for hemodialysis access.[8] Preferences for the radiocephalic fistula are based on factors such as superior long-term patency rates, lower incidence and ease of managing infectious complications, and a decreased incidence of other complications such as aneurysm formation.[10]

Lack of a suitable native vessel limits the creation of a primary AV fistula. Constructing a Brescia-Cimino wrist fistula may be precluded by the presence of atherosclerotic changes in the radial artery, thrombosis of the cephalic vein, or a cephalic vein that is small, fragile, or too thin-walled to adequately mature and sustain multiple needle punctures. Veins smaller than 3 mm and arteries smaller than 1.5 mm are less likely to succeed in AV fistulae.[8] As the proportion of elderly and diabetic patients entering hemodialysis centers increases, the proportion of patients with arterial and venous anatomy suitable for endogenous fistula construction is decreasing.[11] In the geriatric population, superficial veins become more tortuous

TABLE 20–1 Primary Access Vessels

Arteries	Veins
Radial	Cephalic
Brachial	Cubital fossa veins (basilic, antecubital, and cephalic)

and the incidence of atherosclerosis increases, making vascular access more difficult to achieve and maintain once hemodialysis is initiated and the access is cannulated.[12]

Other anatomic possibilities for AV fistulae include connecting the ulnar artery to basilic vein and brachial artery to basilic or cephalic vein (Box 20-2). The latter provides a long segment of vein for cannulation and is a reasonable site for primary access if the forearm vessels are unsuitable. The brachial artery to the basilic or cephalic vein also offers an ideal option after late failure of a forearm fistula. Patency rates of these veins compare with or are superior to those used for radiocephalic fistulae.

If no upper-extremity vessels are suitable for access, use of a lower-extremity fistula is possible. However, because of a significantly higher complication rate (most notably infection), lower-extremity fistulae are of little value except for young children or for patients in whom repeated infections preclude the use of the upper extremities.

Venous anatomy is assessed by observation and manual palpation or by engorging veins using a tourniquet or blood pressure cuff inflated below systolic pressure. Once the veins are adequately visualized, they are marked with an indelible pen to facilitate their location in the operating room. Local anesthesia is often sufficient for creating a fistula at the wrist or antecubital fossa. If a more proximal procedure is anticipated, brachial or axillary nerve block or general anesthesia is used. However, general anesthesia may depress cardiac output and reduce fistula flow, while brachial or supraclavicular regional anesthesia may increase arterial blood flow with peripheral vasodilation.[8]

In the operating room, the entire arm is prepared, allowing for use of a more proximal artery and vein if the distal vessels are inadequate. The skin is incised, and the artery and vein are localized. Various anastomotic connections between vessels are possible (Fig. 20-1); in each, the artery and vein are surgically connected. Each type of anastomosis has inherent advantages and disadvantages that are outlined in Table 20-2.

After the artery and vein are sutured and before the incision is closed, a thrill should be easily palpable over the anastomosis and within the proximal vein segment. The presence of a strong arterial pulse without a thrill suggests outflow obstruction in the vein that requires surgical correction to prevent fistula thrombosis. The proximal vein is inspected and may be probed with a Fogarty embolectomy catheter or carefully dilated. If attempts at correction do not produce a thrill, creation of another fistula is considered.

After surgical formation of a fistula, arterial pressure is transmitted directly into the adjoining vein, which dilates and develops a hypertrophied muscular wall amenable to repeated needle puncture (Fig. 20-2). This process, referred to as arterialization or maturation, typically occurs over 2 to 6 months. Ideally, the fistula should not be used before 4 weeks of maturation because premature cannulation is often associated with hematoma formation and early thrombosis.[8]

Graft Fistula

An AV bridge or graft fistula communicates between an artery and vein resulting from a conduit anastomosed separately to each vessel. A graft fistula is considered when an endogenous fistula cannot be constructed or fails. Successful primary AV fistula in the dominant arm is

BOX 20–2

Primary Upper-Extremity Arteriovenous Fistula Sites

MOST PREFERRED SITE (NONDOMINANT ARM BEFORE DOMINANT ARM)
Radial artery to cephalic vein at wrist (Brescia-Cimino fistula)

ALTERNATE CHOICES (NONDOMINANT ARM BEFORE DOMINANT ARM)
Ulnar artery to basilic vein
Brachial artery to basilic or cephalic vein

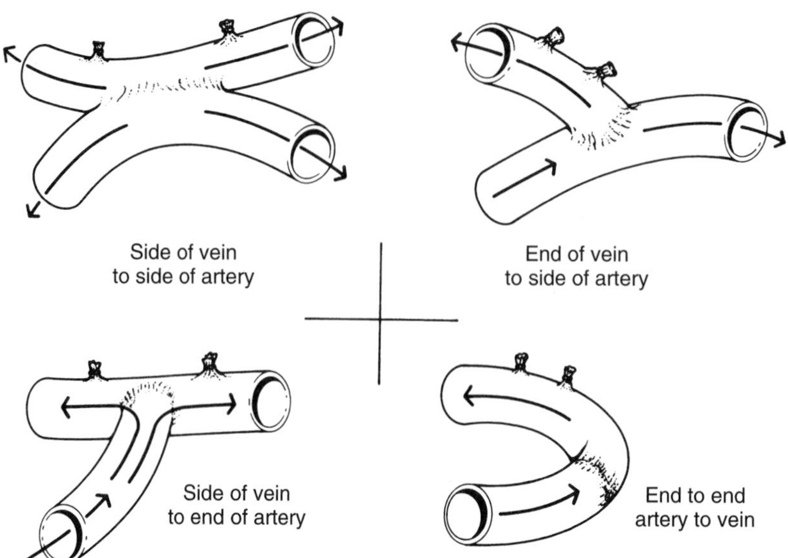

FIG. 20–1. The four major types of arteriovenous anastomoses commonly constructed between the radial artery and the cephalic vein at the wrist. (Modified from Fernanco ON: Arteriovenous fistulas by direct anastomosis. In Wilson SE, Owen ML, eds: *Vascular access surgery,* Chicago, 1980, Year Book.)

preferred over a synthetic graft bridge fistula in the nondominant arm. The patient population for graft fistula is usually elderly and anemic, and up to 50 percent are diabetic.[1]

A graft fistula can be formed between most superficial arteries and veins of acceptable size (Fig. 20-3). Arm placement of synthetic graft fistula is preferred, usually between the radial artery and the cephalic or basilic vein in the antecubital fossa. Placement is either done through a straight (distal radial artery to basilic vein) or loop (brachial artery to basilic vein) configuration. After insertion, graft fistulae are easily palpated and punctured. However, use of a graft fistula should be avoided for several weeks to allow the graft material to incorporate into surrounding tissues and to minimize the risk of extravasation from the graft when the needles are removed. A synthetic graft fistula may be used in 2 weeks. Since polytetrafluoroethylene (PTFE) was introduced in 1976, it has become the most commonly used material in the construction of graft fistulae.[8] PTFE grafts are more prone to infection and thrombosis than endogenous AV fistulae.[13] Patency rates of PTFE grafts at 1 year generally exceed 70 percent.[14]

TABLE 20–2 Types of Arteriovenous Anastomoses

Type	Advantages	Disadvantages
Side of artery to side of vein	Technically easiest to construct; highest flow rate	No major disadvantages
End of artery to side of vein (ligation of distal artery)	Limited flow turbulence; less likelihood of arterial "steal"	Lower flow rate than side to side
Side of artery to end of vein (ligation of distal artery and vein)	Highest proximal venous flow; minimal distal venous tension	Technically more difficult to construct than other types of fistula
End of artery to end of vein (ligation of distal artery and vein)	Least likelihood of arterial "steal" and venous hypertension	Lower flow rate of four types

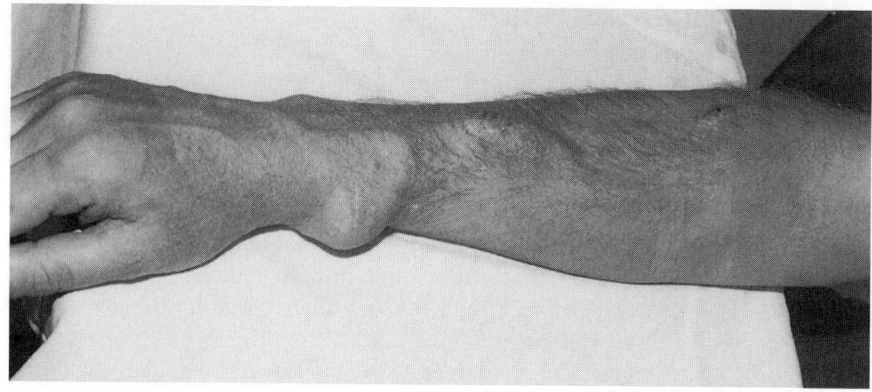

FIG. 20–2. Photograph depicting mature, arterialized fistula. (Courtesy James O. Menzoian, MD, Boston, Mass.)

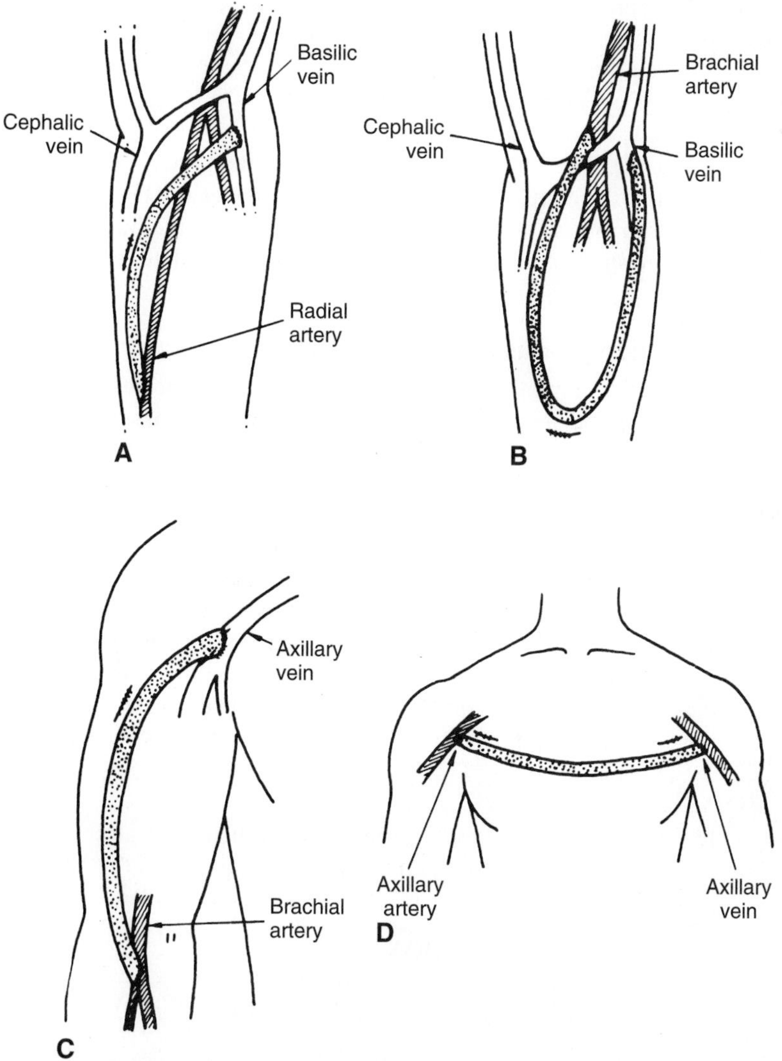

FIG. 20–3. Bridge fistulae of the upper extremity. **A,** Straight graft between radial artery and basilic vein. **B,** Loop graft between brachial artery and basilic vein. **C,** Straight graft between brachial artery and axillary vein. **D,** Straight graft between axillary artery and contralateral axillary vein. (From Bennion RS, Wilson SE: Hemodialysis and vascular access. In Moore WS, ed: *Vascular surgery: a comprehensive review,* Philadelphia, 1991, WB Saunders.)

Physiology of Arteriovenous Fistulae

The local, systemic, and hemodynamic effects of surgically created AV fistulae vary, depending on the nature of the fistula (i.e., acute vs. chronic), the anatomic configuration, and location of the vascular tree (i.e., proximal vs. distal vessels). With all fistulae, the direction of blood flow in the artery and vein proximal to the fistulous connection is normal. Most fistulae created for therapeutic use have a diameter greater than 75 percent of the proximal arterial lumen, resulting in backflow of the blood in the distal artery toward the fistula and retrograde flow in the distal vein away from the fistula. Venous hypertension may develop in the limb distal to the fistula because of this reversal in flow. In addition, as the fistula matures over the ensuing 4 to 6 weeks, the vein thickens and dilates, leading to valvular incompetence, further increasing distal venous pressure.

When a fistulous opening is created, there is a fall in peripheral vascular resistance (PVR) because arterial flow is shunted directly into a vein, bypassing the usual arteriole-capillary-venule circuit. This fall in PVR is compensated for by an increase in cardiac output that increases flow through the fistula. Although proximal venous outflow is also increased, significant central venous pressure elevation normally does not occur because of the large capacity of venous vessels. Flow rates in fistulae created between small-caliber arteries (i.e., radial, tibial) and adjacent veins vary from 150-600 ml/minute, whereas larger-caliber fistulae (i.e., axillary, femoral) have flow rates of 800-1600 ml/minute.[15]

In addition to these hemodynamic alterations, several histologic changes develop as a result of creating a fistula. The smooth muscle of the proximal artery hypertrophies, dilates, and elongates. With time, the muscle layer atrophies and the artery becomes aneurysmal. In the venous limb, smooth muscle and fibrous tissue increase. Eventually, the vein may develop atherosclerosis. The vein also elongates and continues to dilate for up to 8 months postoperatively.

Complications of Endogenous and Prosthetic Fistulae

The surgical risk involved in managing hemodialysis access has increased as the age of dialysis patients and number and significance of comorbid conditions has increased.[8] The ability of nephrologists, dialysis staff, and vascular surgeons to establish and maintain adequate vascular access plays a major role in the morbidity and mortality associated with chronic long-term hemodialysis patients. Patients undergoing chronic hemodialysis are most frequently hospitalized to manage complications of dialysis access (Box 20-3). Among those hemodialysis patients older than 65 years of age, there are more vascular access–related hospital admissions than any other age group, accounting for 24 percent of all hospital admissions compared with less than 19 percent of those younger than 65 years.[12] The endogenous radiocephalic AV fistula is associated with a fairly high early failure rate of 10-15 percent.[14] However, the long-term success rate for AV fistulae is 75 percent patency at 4 years.[8] A discussion of the most common complications of chronic hemodialysis access follows.

Thrombosis

Thrombosis is the most common complication of an AV fistula or graft. The incidence of thrombosis depends on the type of fistula, the diameter and quality of the artery and vein, the

BOX 20–3

Complications of Endogenous and Prosthetic Fistulae Access

- Thrombosis
- Congestive heart failure
- Infection
- Distal ischemia
- Distal venous hypertension
- Neuropathy
- Aneurysm formation

site of the AV anastomosis, the materials used, and the technical skills of the surgeon.[16] Eighty to 90 percent of graft thrombosis is due to stenosis at the venous anastomosis.[8] Thrombosis occurring within 1 month of vascular access placement is often due to technical errors in fistula construction or premature use.[11]

Maintaining vascular access patency is an ongoing challenge. Late thrombosis of AV fistulae is often due to venous fibrosis and stenosis secondary to repeated venipuncture. This fibrotic process may be detected early if increasing pressure is noted in the venous return line during dialysis, suggesting outflow obstruction. Color Doppler evaluation may be used to identify venous stenosis.[8] Increased venous pressure warrants an angiogram that may define the area of obstruction. Chronic fibrosis is usually limited to the venous anastomosis and can often be corrected surgically by local endarterectomy or patch angioplasty.

Late thrombosis of a prosthetic graft is usually due to obstruction at the site of venous outflow. An average of 30 to 40 percent of AV grafts have a thrombotic event during the first year.[8] As with endogenous fistulae, angiography is indicated if function is inadequate. This study may detect a number of surgically correctable problems, including technical anastomotic errors, thrombus within the graft, or extrinsic graft compression within the subcutaneous tunnel. Forty percent of thrombosed graft fistulae can be salvaged with surgical thrombectomy and/or revision. The remaining 60 percent require construction of a new fistula.[14] Implantation of a new graft or fistula has a greater likelihood of achieving long-term patency than does a declotting procedure.

About 20 percent of dialysis access thromboses occur in the absence of an identifiable anatomic lesion.[11] Episodic hypotension and hypercoagulable states may be reasons for thrombosis of dialysis grafts.[8] Specifically, considering the elderly patient's propensity for lower diastolic pressure, careful blood pressure monitoring of elders to prevent hypotensive episodes during and immediately after the dialysis treatment becomes more important. The frail elderly person must perfuse the access in order for it to remain patent and prevent system problems. Accordingly, volume replacement may be indicated for some hypotensive geriatric patients.[12] Additionally, prolonged compression of the fistula during sleep may lead to markedly decreased fistula flow and subsequent thrombosis.

Interventional procedures such as angioplasty in conjunction with thrombolysis may be an effective alternative to surgical thrombectomy. Retrospective studies have found that thrombolysis was initially successful with thrombotic lesions in 60 to 90 percent of cases.[16] Contraindications to thrombolytic therapy of a clotted access graft include suspected graft infection, as well as contraindication to anticoagulant/fibrinolytic therapy or severe allergy to angiographic contrast material (because repeat angiograms are necessary to determine the efficacy of treatment).

Percutaneous transluminal angioplasty (PTLA) also provides a nonsurgical alternative for access grafts that are failing because of arterial anastomotic and venous outflow stenosis. However, restenosis occurs frequently with patency varying between 25 and 50 percent after 6 months.[17,18] Most restenosis can be successfully treated by repeat angioplasty.[11] Long-term patency following multiple angioplasty procedures may be equivalent to that of surgically revised fistulae. However, comparison of long-term patency rates after revascularization is difficult due to trends in surgical reporting.[19] The benefit of successful angioplasty and repeated angioplasty procedures is prolonging the usable life of the original fistula without extending it farther up the arm with a surgical procedure. Mizumoto et al[20] reported the development of directional atherectomy (DA) as a therapeutic modality for vascular access stenosis. An atherectomy device may be used to remove stenotic tissue, which may prolong the period before restenosis. Therapeutic alternatives such as PTLA or DA are methods available as outpatient procedures and do not preclude surgical revision later.[20]

Infection

After thrombosis, infection is the next most common complication of vascular access surgery, particularly for AV grafts.[13,21] Reported national infection rates for local and bacteremic infections are 1-4 percent for endogenous fistulae and 11-20 percent for AV grafts.[22] Infection is a frequent cause of hospitalization in hemodialysis patients.[23] The primary etiology of infection is access manipulation through needle puncture or secondary surgical procedures.[16] Infection may prematurely end the function of endogenous or prosthetic fistulae. The routine use of perioperative antibiotics has helped to decrease the incidence of infections. The most common infecting organism is *Staphylococcus aureus*.[8] Forty to 60 percent of hemodialysis patients carry *S. aureus* in their nares.[22] Administration of preoperative antibiotics against *S. aureus* decreases the risk of perioperative graft infection.

Local signs and symptoms of infection include cellulitis over the graft, purulent drainage from a puncture site, and the presence of an inflammatory pseudoaneurysm near the prosthetic graft anastomosis. Systemic manifestations include leukocytosis, fever, malaise, and positive blood cultures. In bacteremic patients, appropriate intravenous antibiotic therapy is used to combat the specific organism(s) isolated.

Bonomo et al[13] studied the risk factors associated with endogenous and PTFE graft fistulae. In their study, patients with PTFE grafts were 7.8 times more likely to develop an access infection than patients with endogenous AV fistulae. The risk of an infection for PTFE grafts increased 1.5 times with each graft revision. An infection of a bridge fistula frequently requires removal of the prosthetic material, ligation of the artery and vein, and drainage of any local abscess. If possible, creation of another vascular access site should be delayed until all signs of infection have resolved to minimize the risk of seeding and infecting a new area. Preferably, a different extremity should be used for the new access.

Distal Venous Hypertension

Increased venous pressure may occur in tissues distal to the fistula, resulting in painful swelling of the extremity. In extreme situations, discoloration, pigmentation changes, sepsis, and gangrene may develop. This problem may worsen as the fistula matures and valvular incompetence develops. Treatment options include ligating the fistula and using the other arm for access, angioplasty, surgically bypassing the venous lesion, or ligating the vein just distal to the fistula.[8]

Side-to-side AV fistula or subclavian vein stenosis are the two most common causes of venous hypertension. Subclavian vein stenoses usually are a consequence of subclavian venous cannulas placed for hemodynamic monitoring, short- and long-term provision of parenteral nutrition and other intravenous agents, placement of pacemaker wires, and acute hemodialysis leading to the rise of subclavian venous thrombosis.[16] There is a 10 percent risk of subclavian venous thrombosis with placement of a catheter in the subclavian vein vs. 2.3 percent risk for internal jugular position.[24] This is why subclavian vein cannulation should be avoided and the jugular vein used instead for acute hemodialysis access.[8,25] The Dialysis Outcomes Quality Initiative (DOQI) guidelines strongly recommend avoidance of the subclavian vein unless no other option exists or unless the ipsilateral extremity can no longer be used for permanent dialysis access.[26]

Aneurysm Formation

Dilation or true aneurysm formation of the central venous limb of an endogenous fistula often requires no treatment and actually may increase the ease of cannulation. These aneurysms can remain stable for many years.[6] Surgical intervention should be considered, however, if the overlying skin is thin and rupture threatens or if a thrombus within the aneurysmal segment impairs blood flow or makes needle insertion difficult. True aneurysms of prosthetic graft fistulae usually occur as a result of repeated cannulation in the same area. Dilation of the entire graft may also occur secondary to degeneration of the prosthetic material.

False aneurysms or pseudoaneurysms rarely occur with endogenous fistulae. The incidence increases with prosthetic graft fistulae. Pseudoaneurysm formation occurs in focal regions subjected to repeated needle punctures in certain PTFE cannulation sites, as well as following use of oversized needles and use of improper technique of graft puncture at hemodialysis.[27] A pseudoaneurysm is repaired by excision of the damaged graft segment and replacement with an interposing segment of PTFE.

Congestive Heart Failure

Right heart strain or congestive heart failure (CHF) secondary to therapeutic fistulae is exceedingly rare, even with rapid flow rates. Congestive heart failure may occur when fistula flow increases cardiac output as little as 20 percent.[15] However, venous return to the heart increases considerably when a large proximal artery is connected directly to an adjacent vein. The heart compensates by increasing heart rate, stroke volume, and cardiac output as necessary to maintain fistula flow.

Surgical revision of the fistula may be necessary if CHF develops subsequent to fistula maturation and does not respond to conventional medical therapy. The fistula may be banded with a circumferential extrinsic Teflon cuff to decrease flow through the graft. Unfortunately, decreased flow may result in thrombosis, requiring creation of a new fistula.

Distal Ischemia

Distal arterial insufficiency may develop as a consequence of excessive flow through a fistula, resulting in reversed flow in the distal artery toward the fistula. Reversed flow is sometimes seen with side-to-side fistulae at the wrist. This alteration in the direction of flow has been labeled "steal." When it is of sufficient magnitude and cannot be compensated by collateral flow, it results in ischemic manifestations.[9]

The "steal" syndrome rarely produces clinically significant symptoms. About 10 percent of hemodialysis patients may complain of coolness, some numbness, and pain during dialysis.[9] The problem is self-correcting, and symptoms resolve in 1 or 2 months. The majority of patients affected with distal ischemia are diabetics who have severe obstructive disease of the arteries distal to the brachial artery and poor collateral circulation.[16] The "steal" may be corrected by ligating the artery (usually the radial) just distal to the fistula, ligating the fistula entirely, or reducing the diameter of the arterial anastomosis.[8]

Neuropathy

A small number of patients with radiocephalic fistulae report carpal tunnel symptoms (i.e., numbness in the distribution of the median nerve).[14] Nerve conduction studies can confirm or discount the diagnosis. It is theorized that tissue edema and median nerve compression may result from venous hypertension. It is also thought that nerve ischemia may result from arterial "steal" syndrome. Some patients with intolerable symptoms have been managed by the conventional surgical division of the carpal ligament to relieve median nerve compression.

Percutaneous Venous Cannulation

Indications for percutaneous catheter hemodialysis include:

- Acute renal failure requiring a limited number of treatments
- Chronic renal failure in the immediate postoperative period after surgical creation of an internal fistula (to allow for "maturation" of fistula)
- Fistulae that have thrombosed in patients with renal transplant
- Urgent need for transfer from peritoneal dialysis because of complications (i.e., severe peritonitis, abdominal complications, or catheter dysfunction)
- Acute exogenous poisoning
- Physiologic abnormalities, including hyperkalemia, pulmonary edema in the presence of oliguria, metabolic acidosis, severe neurologic symptoms, or pericarditis

During hemodialysis, blood is removed from the cannulated vein, circulated through the dialyzer, and returned to the patient either via a peripheral vein or through the second lumen of a double-lumen catheter. Central venous dialysis catheters are associated with a high rate of failure.[28] However, these may be a regular access choice in a selected patient population (e.g., children) with no inherent thrombotic tendency and no other option available for long-term hemodialysis.[29]

Jugular and Subclavian Vein Access

If an acute dialysis catheter is required, it is placed in a jugular vein rather than the subclavian. Subclavian vein catheters are associated with a 50 percent incidence of large vein stenosis and thrombosis.[6] The long-term complications of subclavian vein thrombosis can impair venous drainage of potential later sites for chronic dialysis. For jugular vein insertion, Forauer and Glockner[30] evaluated the significance of internal jugular vein ultrasound findings in planning vascular access procedures. Their results supported ultrasound examination of the internal jugular vein prior to dialysis catheter placement; three fourths of patients with sonographic abnormalities required a change in access approach.

To catheterize central veins percutaneously, the patient is placed supine in Trendelenburg's position (which dilates the vein and minimizes risk of an embolism) with head rotated to the opposite side. The skin is disinfected, and a local anesthetic is administered. For a noncuffed dialysis catheter, a guidewire is introduced through the lumen of a large-bore needle into the central vein. The noncuffed dialysis catheter is passed over the guidewire and can be used immediately. A chest radiograph is done before dialysis treatment is initiated.

Rigid noncuffed dialysis catheters may be placed at the bedside and can be used for several weeks to months. Permanently implanted dialysis catheters with Dacron cuffs are designed for long-term use, up to several years. The technique for placing a cuffed catheter is similar to that of noncuffed catheters. However, cuffed catheters are usually placed in a patient in an operating room or a radiology suite. Interventional radiologists are taking an increasingly active role in dialysis catheter insertion.[3,31] Radiologic placement of long-term dialysis catheters resulted in substantial savings over surgical placement in a study by Noh et al.[32] The use of fluoroscopy with insertion is recommended because it facilitates the proper placement of the permanently implanted dialysis catheter.[8] Dialysis catheters are kept patent between treatments by filling with heparinized saline solution and clamping or by intermittent flushing with the same solution.

Femoral Access

During femoral vein catheter insertion, the patient lies supine with the leg externally rotated and the knee slightly flexed. Elevating the buttocks on a pillow allows fuller extension of the groin crease. The skin around the femoral vein site is shaved, disinfected, and draped. Local anesthetic is administered. After palpating the femoral artery, the physician inserts a 16-gauge cannula at a 45° angle into the femoral vein located approximately 1-2 cm medial to the femoral artery. If the femoral vein is entered, blood should drip freely from the outer tip of the catheter. A guidewire is inserted through the cannula and threaded into the common iliac vein and inferior vena cava (IVC). With the guidewire in place, the cannula is removed and a dialyzing catheter is threaded over the guidewire into the IVC. If blood returns freely, the catheter is connected to the arterial end of the dialyzer and dialysis is begun.

If the femoral vein catheter is left in place, meticulous care of the insertion site with sterile technique is essential. Interim patency is maintained either by instillation of heparinized saline solution and capping or by intermittent irrigation with heparin flush solution.

Complications of central vein catheterization are listed in Table 20-3. Stenosis and thrombosis occur more frequently in noncuffed dialysis catheters left in place longer than 4 weeks. Catheter thrombosis, including venous thrombus and fibrin sheaths, accounts for up to 40 percent of catheter failures.[33] Recombinant tissue plasminogen activator (rt-PA) has been used by Savader et al[34] to treat dialysis catheter–associated fibrin sheaths.

TABLE 20–3 Percutaneous Dialysis Catheter Complications

	Major Complications	Other Complications
Central vein access	Pneumothorax Hemothorax Subcutaneous hematoma	Air embolism Thrombosis Infection
Femoral vein access	Bleeding from puncture site	Thrombosis Infection Arteriovenous (AV) fistula formation Femoral nerve damage

Twenty percent of central venous catheters become colonized, and bacteremia develops in 10 percent of patients.[6] Up to two thirds of infected catheters need to be removed.[33] Sesso et al[35] evaluated the use of a topical antibiotic (mupirocin) at the cannula site after catheter insertion and after each dialysis session and found that mupirocin reduced the risk of *S. aureus* bacteremia in hemodialysis patients. However, mupirocin ointment has also been associated with mupirocin resistance[36] and may affect the integrity of polyurethane catheters.[37]

The most frequent complication with femoral vein cannulation (see Table 20-3) is bleeding from the vein puncture site. Other less frequent complications include femoral vein thrombosis predisposing the patient to the risk of pulmonary embolism; infection; traumatic formation of AV fistulae between the femoral artery and vein, usually resulting from inadvertent puncture of the artery; and femoral nerve damage.

Minimizing the insertion of central venous dialysis catheters while increasing placements of AV fistulae will reduce vascular access–related infections.[21,38] DOQI Vascular Access Guidelines recommend no more than 10 percent of permanent access be in the form of catheters.[26]

Nursing Management of Patients With Hemodialysis Access

Preoperative Considerations

Chronic renal failure is generally an insidious process that allows time for planning and preparation for both psychosocial and physiologic needs. Consideration of hemodialysis as a treatment modality involves a major adjustment in the daily activities of an individual with ESRD. The individual needs information and education about the hemodialysis process (i.e., equipment, fistula formation, etc.), the commitment of time for dialysis, the arrangements for travel to a dialysis center, consideration of other options available for dialysis, and the impact of renal failure related to the patient's perception of health and well-being.

Primary access vessels should not be used for venipuncture, intravenous cannulation, or invasive monitoring lines in patients with acute or progressive renal disease. All involved hospital personnel must be informed of the need to preserve the selected vessels beginning with the earliest indication of renal failure.[7] Posting a sign over the patient's bed can inform other providers of the need to preserve vessels. Adequate hydration, weight control, hypertension treatment, avoidance of smoking, and control of local dermatitis or cellulitis are all measures that may help increase the chance of being able to perform and maintain an endogenous AV fistula at the wrist.[7]

Perioperative Considerations

Dialysis patients have certain particular needs when they come to the operating room. The perioperative nurse should first note the cause of the patient's renal failure. A patient with newly diagnosed renal failure will have different needs than a patient with chronic renal failure who has had multiple access operations. To provide optimal nursing care, it is essential that the nurse be sensitive to the patient's level of acceptance of his or her disease.[39] Other areas that need to be assessed include (1) the ability of the patient to lie still during the vascular access procedure under local anesthesia, (2) the ability of the patient to follow directions and cooperate during the procedure, and (3) the impact of positioning requirements on the patient's skin integrity.

Postoperative Considerations

Postoperative nursing management after creation of an AV fistula includes elevating the patient's operative arm on a pillow or with a sling for 24 hours to minimize the development of upper-extremity edema. Some swelling nearly always occurs but resolves in several weeks.

The dressing is checked frequently for excessive bleeding. The initial dressing is left intact overnight unless excessive bleeding occurs. Once the initial dressing is removed, the surgical incision is inspected for evidence of infection, including erythema, warmth, excessive tenderness, and drainage. Any suspicion of infection should be reported to the surgeon.

Assessment of adequate fistula function includes palpation for a thrill that is generated as high-pressure arterial blood flows into a contiguous vein. Also, a bruit should be audible on auscultation over the venous limb with a stethoscope. The absence of these finding suggests thrombosis and should be reported to the surgeon. Constricting dressings and blood pressure cuffs on the operative arm are avoided because they restrict venous flow.

Before discharge, the patient is taught the following:

- Avoid wearing tight clothing, hanging things over the arm, or carrying heavy objects so the blood can flow freely through the fistula.
- Check blood flow through the fistula several times daily by feeling for a thrill or listening for a bruit. Report loss of thrill or bruit to the physician or nurse immediately.
- After the sutures are removed, keep the area over the fistula clean and dry. Apply lotion to keep skin moisturized.
- Exercise the operative arm by squeezing a rubber ball or lifting a 1-pound weight (soup can) for 10-15 minutes several times daily to promote enlargement of the vein.
- Elevate the arm for 1-2 days to reduce edema and pain.
- Report any redness, swelling, excessive tenderness, or drainage to the physician or nurse immediately.
- Bathing, swimming, and other similar activities can be safely resumed several weeks after surgery.

Continuing Care

Highly functional AV fistulae and dialysis catheters are the patient's avenue to adequate and optimal dialytic therapy. To achieve long-term success with vascular access, a team approach is needed. This team includes the patient, family/support system, nursing staff, nephrologist, radiologist, and the vascular access surgeon. Once the vascular surgeon successfully creates a primary or graft fistula, the dialysis staff must monitor the access site and correctly care for it. For example, dialysis nurses who cannulate fistulae may observe changes in the extremity (e.g., pain, pallor, swelling, an altered dialysis flow, or a decreased bruit) indicating a possible impending stenosis.[37] Technique and the method of needle placement in the fistula are major factors in achieving the optimal flow rate, maintaining the fistula site for future use, and avoiding gross disfigurement of the fistula limb.[40]

A dialysis nurse performs 64 needle cannulations in a typical workweek and 1248 cannulations in 1 year. Needle cannulation experience increases quickly as a dialysis nurse is prepared and completes 1 year of work; however, clinical expertise may take a longer time. Bacterial contamination of the vascular access and subsequent infection may occur because of poor needle cannulation technique.[41] Two methods of arterial needle insertion (Fig. 20-4) are performed: antegrade cannulation (in the direction of blood flow, pointing toward the venous anastomosis) and retrograde cannulation (toward the arterial anastomosis of the access). There is little evidence that either technique is preferable, and both have their benefits.[42]

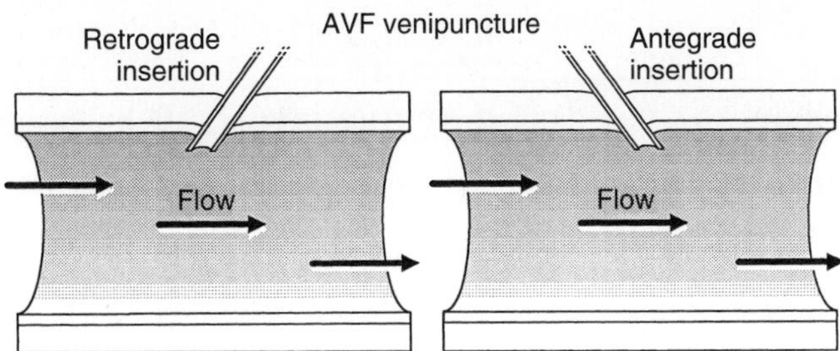

FIG. 20–4. Retrograde and antegrade puncture of an arterialized vein.

It is important to rotate needle cannulation sites to prevent compromise of both skin and vascular access integrity.[41] For each year on dialysis, the patient undergoes 312 needle cannulations. Dialysis staff need to educate patients concerning rotation of needle sites. Patient resistance to needle rotation is only natural. Patient-preferred sites generally have been used repetitively, form scar tissue, and offer little discomfort. Finally, assessment of the patient for the presence or absence of vascular access infection should be done before every dialysis treatment. The use of strict aseptic technique by the nursing staff providing vascular access care is essential; adherence to this standard decreases the risk of bacterial contamination of the access during the dialysis procedure.[39]

CENTRAL VENOUS ACCESS DEVICES

Use of Central Venous Access Devices

The CVADs discussed in this chapter include peripherally inserted central catheters (PICCs), tunneled catheters, and subcutaneous access ports. The availability of dependable long-term venous access is an important consideration in the provision of chemotherapy, total parenteral nutrition (TPN), or long-term antibiotic therapy. In the United States, an estimated 5 million central venous catheters are placed per year.[43] For patients requiring frequent or continuous access, a PICC or tunneled catheter is preferable.[44] Subcutaneous access ports are used for patients who require long-term, intermittent vascular access.

The increased use of CVADs is consistent with "patient-focused" care trends. These devices offer many benefits to patients (Box 20-4). With the development of the tunneled Broviac catheter in 1973, patients are discharged to home or alternate settings with CVADs in place.[46]

The selection of the appropriate CVAD is best made as an interdisciplinary decision. The Centers for Disease Control and Prevention (CDC) recommend that the CVAD product and insertion technique and site with the lowest risk of complications for the type and duration of therapy should be part of the criteria for CVAD selection.[43] Other factors that require consideration are listed in Box 20-5. The type of therapy determines the type of access needed. For example, central venous access with the tip in the superior vena cava is required for hyperalimination[49] and is highly recommended for irritating, sclerosing, or vesicant agents

BOX 20–4

Benefits of Central Venous Access Devices

Conducive to self-care
Decrease in nosocomial infections
Elimination of multiple venipunctures in management of long-term therapies[45]
Use in non–acute care settings, e.g., patient homes
Outpatient procedure for placement

BOX 20–5

Factors to Consider for Appropriate CVAD Selection

SAFETY CONSIDERATIONS[47,48]	PATIENT CHARACTERISTICS
Length and diameter of catheter	Competency level
Number of lumens	Manual dexterity
Use of Dacron cuff	Visual acuity
Type of therapy	Home environment
	Caregiver support
	Elderly or pediatric patient
	Cosmetic appearance concerns
	Anxiety with needle stick into port

because of the rapid dilution of the infusate.[50,51] In addition, the blood vessel needs to be large enough and have adequate flow to support the required therapy.[52] For central venous catheters, the Intravenous Nurses Society (INS) Standards of Practice state the smallest gauge and shortest length to accommodate the prescribed therapy should be considered with catheter selection.[53]

Patient characteristics requiring consideration are also included in Box 20-5. Support systems available for use of the CVAD in a home setting need careful assessment. Support systems include the availability of home nursing and proximity of follow-up care.[46] The patient provides input into the selection of an appropriate device. Issues for the patient to consider include cosmetic appearance, concerns with activity or work limitations, anxiety with a needle stick into a port, site care, and catheter flushing requirements.[50,52]

Cost is also a factor in the choice of appropriate CVAD. The expense of initial insertion of a nontunneled device may be less than an implanted port; however, if the device is used longer than 6 months, the port may be more economical when considering maintenance costs.

Polyurethanes, silicone elastomer (Silastic), and elastomeric hydrogel are the most frequently used materials in the manufacture of CVADs.[47] Rather than acting as passive conduits, the biomaterials used in CVADs elicit active responses from both the host and the endogenous microflora of the host. These interactive responses are involved in the most common complications of venous access: infection, inflammation (phlebitis), and thrombosis.[54] For example, the use of polyvinyl catheters has been identified as a predisposing factor for catheter-related infections.[55] Research continues in the development of new biomaterials and antimicrobial agents to improve the microenvironment of the biofilm.

Long-term catheters need to be radiopaque to allow for visualization of the catheter tip on initial insertion or anytime that displacement is suspected. The confirmation of catheter tip by chest radiograph prior to use is recommended in the Standards of Practice of INS[53] and the Access Device Guidelines from the Oncology Nursing Society.[56]

Peripherally Inserted Central Catheters

The Intravenous Nurses Society defines a PICC as a catheter inserted via a peripheral vein with the tip residing in the vena cava.[57] Advantages of a PICC are included in Box 20-6. Comprehensive PICC RN insertion teams include education, early assessment, placement, and postcare management.[58] The Guidelines for the Prevention of Intravascular Catheter-Related Infections from the CDC recommend full barrier precautions (cap, mask, sterile gown, sterile gloves, large sterile drape) during the insertion of CVADs to reduce the incidence of catheter-related blood stream infection.[43]

PICC catheter lumens are external, nontunneled, and may not be sutured. Maintenance care is similar to that of the tunneled central catheters, including site care, flushing, and cap changes. Therefore, self-care abilities or caregiver support are assessed prior to the placement

BOX 20–6

Advantages of Peripherally Inserted Central Catheters

Ease of insertion without local or general anesthetic
Lack of sutures
Decreased potential of infection
Decreased risk of pneumothorax, hemothorax, air embolism
Placement in nonsurgical setting
Placement by nonphysician providers, including registered nurses

of a PICC. For patients who participate in frequent exercise or strenuous manual work or who have active children, a PICC may not be the best device because of the increased risk of dislodgment or limitation of the upper extremity.[48] Because the catheter lumen is external, body image issues also need to be addressed.

PICCs are a good selection for patients who have or have had chest injury, radical neck dissection, radiation fibrosis within the chest, fungating chest tumor, or neck veins that cannot be cannulated, or are malnourished or physically unable to undergo a surgical procedure.[48] PICCs can be used for patients who have limited peripheral access.[57] Hagle, McDonagh, and Rapp[59] suggested that a PICC should not be considered a "last resort" but rather a "first choice" for patients with poor peripheral veins. PICCs should be used for patients who need several weeks or months of treatment. For example, adults with osteomyelitis require a minimum of 14-19 catheter changes during a standard 6- to 8-week antibiotic course using peripheral intravenous therapy.[59] These individuals are candidates for a PICC. Currently, it is not known if there are limits for the length of time that a single PICC may be used. The INS position paper for PICCs indicates that consideration may be given to leaving a PICC in place for up to 1 year.[57]

PICCs are not effective for rapid, large-volume infusions.[48] Also, small-gauge PICCs are not recommended for blood sampling because of the propensity for catheter collapse. Blood sampling needs an 18-gauge or larger catheter.[59]

After insertion, a chest radiograph confirms the location of the catheter tip. A measurement of the amount of catheter left externally is recorded. The extruding catheter is measured at subsequent dressing changes to monitor for possible dislodgment.[60] When the external catheter length changes, the tip location also changes and the appropriateness of the infusion medium must be evaluated.[59] The catheter may be trimmed so that the tip lies in the proximal segment of the axillary vein. This placement, called peripherally inserted catheter (PIC) or a midline catheter, does not require a postprocedure radiograph. PICCs may be removed by registered nurses. Extreme care must be taken with removal to maintain catheter integrity for the entire length. After removal, the length of the catheter is measured and compared with the documented length.[61]

Tunneled Catheters

Tunneled catheters are recommended for patients requiring prolonged administration of chemotherapeutic agents, antibiotics, or TPN. Tunneled catheters have many benefits, including (1) insertion can be done as an outpatient procedure, (2) catheters can remain in place indefinitely, (3) tunneling helps secure the catheter in position, (4) the separation of the exit site from the entry site reduces risk of infection, and (5) they do not require a needle stick.[50] Tunneled catheters are beneficial for patients in whom port placement would be impractical, such as obese or chronically thrombocytopenic patients.[45]

These one- to three-lumen catheters have external parts; therefore, body image needs to be considered when discussing tunneled catheters as an option for long-term vascular access. Catheter care and maintenance also need to be considered, including procedures for site care, flushing, and cap changes.

Traditionally, tunneled catheters have been inserted in the operating room. However, interventional radiologists are taking a greater role in the insertion of CVADs.[43,44] The subclavian and jugular veins are the most popular routes for establishing central venous access. The catheters are tunneled subcutaneously to an exit site on the chest wall some distance from the entry into the subclavian or external jugular vein (Fig. 20-5). The catheter is advanced into the superior vena cava or right atrium.

Certain conditions such as superior vena cava syndrome, neck or mediastinal tumor, bilateral radical neck resection, an infected median sternotomy, torso burns, or trauma may preclude cannulation of the neck or chest.[62] In such cases, the femoral vein provides an alternate insertion site, and the catheter is advanced into the inferior vena cava. A primary concern with long-term femoral vein catheterization is the presumed increase in the risk of bacteremia compared with lines at other sites because of the proximity to the perineum. Goldstein, Weber, and Sheridan[63] cite a catheter-related sepsis rate of only 4.9 percent for femoral vein access in pediatric patients with burns, which compares favorably with results ranging from 2 to 13 percent obtained with catheters at other sites.

Both Broviac and Hickman catheters have a Dacron felt cuff 30 cm from the Luer-Lok end, allowing fibrous tissue ingrowth of the cuff to provide a barrier to the migration of bacteria from the skin into the venous system.[64] After placement, radiographs are used to confirm proper positioning of the catheter tip. These catheters are heparinized and capped with Luer-Lok caps or may be used immediately. An occlusive gauze or transparent dressing is used over the exit site until the wound has healed.

Subcutaneous Access Ports

With venous access ports, a catheter is attached to a plastic or metal port and both lie completely beneath the skin (Fig. 20-6). The port consists of a dense, resealable silicone septum overlying a small reservoir body of plastic, rubber, or metal. The port lies perpendicular to the skin. The advantages of implanted ports include greater freedom of activity, less maintenance, superior cost-effectiveness, and better cosmetic acceptability as compared with external devices.[45] The minimal care requirements and subcutaneous placement make the venous access port an excellent long-term access option for the elderly or pediatric population. Ports are the only CVADs that are completely protected and cannot be pulled out. However, access-

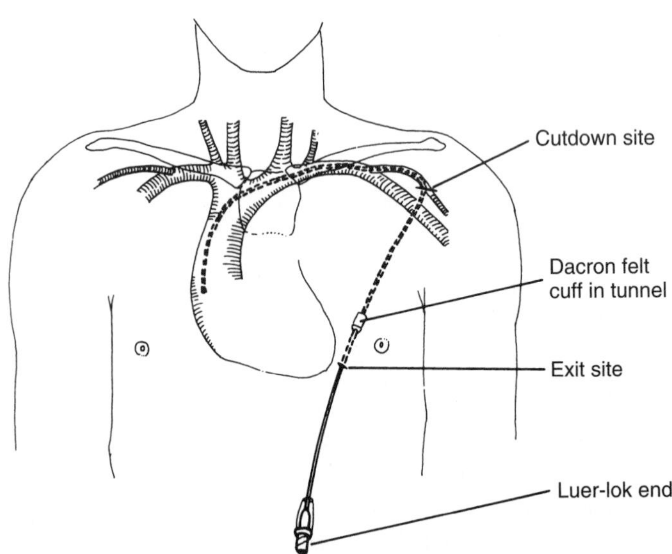

FIG. 20–5. Diagrammatic representation of Broviac catheter in proper position, with tip in right atrium. (From Bennion RS, Wilson SE: Hemodialysis and vascular access. In Moore WS, ed: *Vascular surgery: a comprehensive review,* Philadelphia, 1991, WB Saunders.)

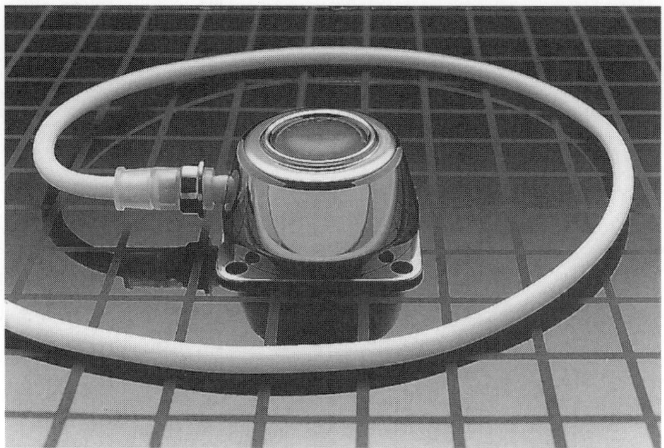

FIG. 20–6. Port-A-Cath implantable venous access system. (Copyright Pharmacia Deltec, Inc., St Paul, Minn.)

ing the port requires a needle stick. Individuals undergoing treatments that cause prolonged myelosuppression should not use port access.[48]

Ports for venous access are generally implanted in the infraclavicular fossa. Mid-arm to upper-arm placement of peripheral ports is an alternative when arm veins are still intact or when implantation in the neck or chest is inadvisable.[65] Peripheral arm port devices are much smaller in all dimensions than the conventional chest port (Fig. 20-7). Arm port devices should be placed in the nondominant arm whenever possible.[66]

The technique for insertion of access ports is similar to that for tunneled catheters. A catheter cut to the appropriate length is advanced into the superior vena cava. A port is then attached and sutured into the subcutaneous pocket. The port is accessed by percutaneous insertion of specially designed noncoring needles, which allows the septum to reseal when the needle is withdrawn (Fig. 20-8).

An alternative to surgically placed central venous access is placement of chest wall ports and arm ports in radiology suites by interventional radiologists. Advantages of interventional radiologic port placement include timeliness, decreased cost, and use of image-guided techniques that support a highly successful procedure rate while minimizing procedural complications.[66-69] A greater than 50 percent cost reduction and comparable infection rates of 4-16 percent support nonsurgical port placement.[70]

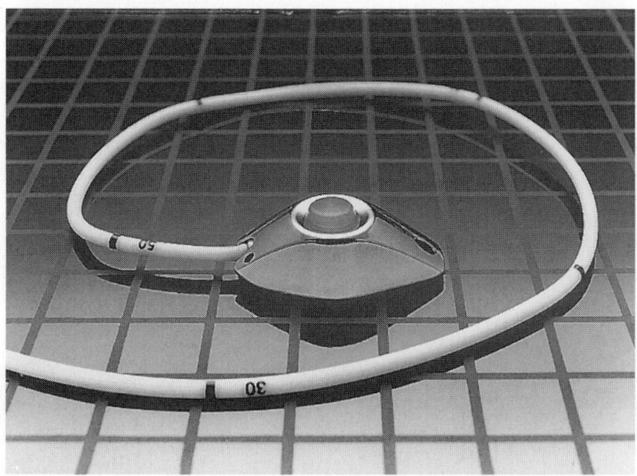

FIG. 20–7. P.A.S. Port implantable peripheral venous access system. (Copyright Pharmacia Deltec, Inc., St Paul, Minn.)

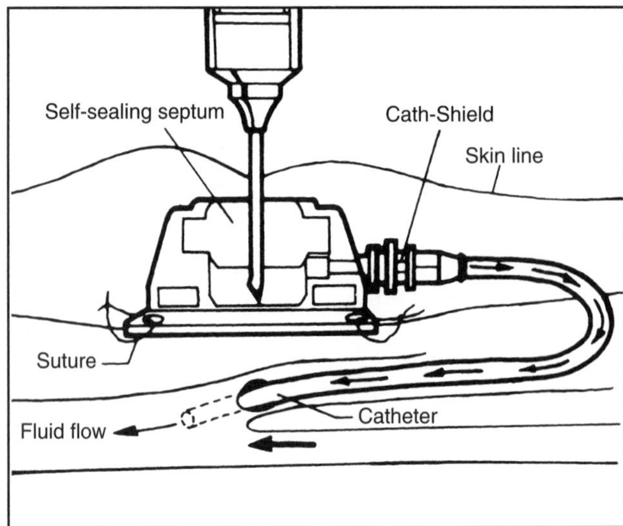

FIG. 20–8. Diagrammatic representation of subcutaneous venous access port (Port-A-Cath), showing perpendicular needle insertion. (Copyright Pharmacia Deltec, Inc., St Paul, Minn.)

Insertion of a totally implantable subcutaneous port in the upper body may be difficult or contraindicated in some clinical situations. Multiple previous placements of catheters to the great vessels of the upper part of the body may further complicate permanent access to those veins. Difficult or contraindicated subclavian or jugular vein access is a clinical situation that can occur in approximately 8 percent of overall long-term port placements. Bertoglio et al[71] evaluated the feasibility of femoral percutaneous port access as an alternative to accessing the subclavian or jugular veins. They concluded that the percutaneous femoral route should be considered a safe alternative.

General Management Principles of Central Venous Access Devices

Flushing

Flushing requirements vary with each device. Flushing CVADs is the primary method used to prevent thrombotic catheter occlusions by cleansing their internal diameters of fibrin buildup and debris.[72] Macklin[73] suggested using a pulsating motion to create enough turbulence to allow the solution to "scrub" the catheter wall. Regardless of which CVAD is being flushed, a low pressure should be used.[74] Excessive pressure, especially when using syringes of 3 ml or less, can cause catheter fracture.[75] Catheter fracture is the complete or partial breakage that occurs internally that may result in the migration of a catheter fragment.

Needleless injection systems can be problematic because of the propensity of blood and injection solution to mix in the catheter cap "dead space."[76] Consequently, the need to maintain positive pressure is of critical importance. Flushing with positive pressure prevents the reflux of blood into the cannula[74] and possible clot development. To achieve positive pressure when flushing, close the clamp on the catheter while maintaining pressure on the syringe plunger or withdraw the syringe tip from the injection cap while injecting the last 0.2 to 0.5 ml of flush solution.[72] INS recommends a flushing volume of heparinized saline solution equal to two times the internal volume of the catheter and a concentration of heparin that will not alter the patient's clotting factors.[74]

A study reported by Mayo et al[77] identified that Groshong catheter valves can allow blood to enter the catheter lumen. When the lumens were flushed weekly with saline, the refluxed blood clotted and adhered to the intraluminal catheter surface, causing obstruction. When heparinized saline flushes were used, blood still occasionally refluxed into the catheters, but the incidence of adherent clots was significantly less. The authors also cited financial advantages for using heparinized saline flush solution vs. using thrombolytic agents when the catheter occludes.

Dressings/Care of Exit Site

Dressing type, frequency of care, and frequency of insertion site assessments remain unresolved issues. Using antimicrobial ointments after cleansing the exit site remains controversial also. Dressings may consist of sterile gauze and tape covering, a transparent semipermeable membrane, or a highly permeable transparent membrane. Using the Center for Advanced Nursing Practice Evidence-Based Practice Model, one organization implemented a hospital-wide CVAD dressing recommendation that used a split transparent dressing with gauze for 48 hours as the initial dressing and a split transparent dressing without gauze after 48 hours.[78] This "best practice" change demonstrated a substantial cost savings for the hospital. Guidelines from the CDC recommend that gauze dressings should be changed every 2 days and transparent dressings may be changed every 7 days for short-term central catheter sites.[43] The CDC also recommends replacing dressings used in tunneled or implanted central catheter sites no more than once per week until the insertion site has healed.

Blood Withdrawals

Several techniques can be used to obtain blood samples, including discarding, reinfusing, or mixing; or a Vacutainer or a syringe can be used. The most commonly reported procedure in the adult population is the discard method.[48] The amount discarded varies from 3 to 10 ml. Blood is withdrawn and discarded, the sample is collected, and the CVAD is flushed with normal saline.

Blood samples used for coagulation studies should be drawn peripherally because heparin adheres to the internal catheter lumen. A study reported by Mayo et al[79] confirmed the difficulty in obtaining reliable coagulation tests with blood samples drawn through tunneled central catheters that have been flushed with heparin. Even after 25 ml of blood is discarded, the difference between the activated partial thromboplastin time (APTT) of catheter blood and peripheral blood was statistically significant, reflecting trace amounts of heparin. However, it is important to differentiate between statistical and clinical significance. Test results from catheter blood that fall into the higher end of normal could be considered clinically reliable even if they are slightly higher than results from peripheral blood. When the objective is to confirm that a patient has normal coagulation tests before an invasive procedure, this would be acceptable. If the results are needed to monitor anticoagulant therapy or to evaluate a coagulopathy, then peripheral blood should be used for sampling.

Clamping

Tunneled and nontunneled catheters have open tips except for the Groshong catheter. Therefore, these external catheter lumens need to be clamped when not being used to prevent blood from backing up into the catheter. The Groshong catheter has a solid blunt tip with a three-position valve on the side (Fig. 20-9). Providing positive pressure into a Groshong catheter opens the valve to allow fluid infusion; significant negative pressure opens its valve inward, allowing blood aspiration. When pressures are equalized, the valve is closed. As a result, the Groshong catheter does not need to be clamped.[59]

Complications of Central Venous Access Devices

There are several potential complications related to placement and maintenance of CVADs (Box 20-7). The risk of developing complications is an important issue for several reasons, including obtaining adequate informed consent prior to placement. Patients must be apprised of the possible problems associated with placement and use of the devices. Central venous catheterization in pediatric patients has a similar complication rate as in adult patients.[80,81]

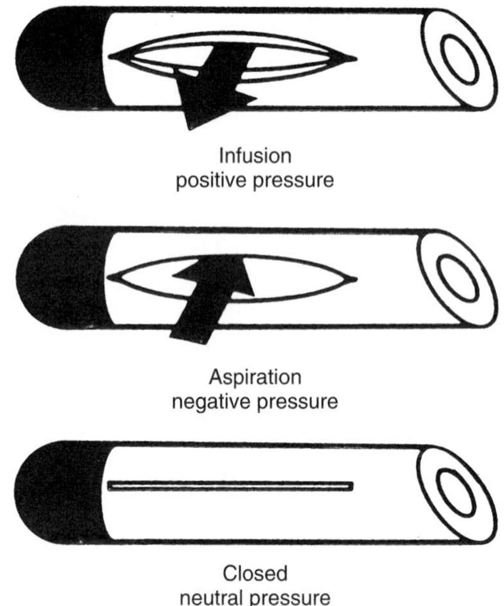

FIG. 20–9. Tip of the Groshong catheter illustrating the unique valve. (Courtesy Bard Access Systems, Inc., Salt Lake City, Utah.)

Early complications (see Box 20-7) of percutaneous catheterization are most often related to technique. The most important predictor of complications associated with insertion is experience of the practitioner inserting the device.

Infection

Infection is the most common and problematic complication of CVADs. A poor outcome with treatment for CVAD infection can be life threatening.[64] The risk of infection is increased the longer a catheter remains in place; this risk is considered cumulative and increases with time.[85] Additional lumens per catheter also increase the risk of infection due to the increased manipulation of the system.[53,56] Much of the risk of infection of a percutaneous central catheter relates to the manner used to insert the catheter. Similar infection rates of 4-6 percent occur whether the CVAD is placed in the operating room or radiology suite.[44] The risk for significant colonization of the catheter may be related to the commutative experience of the physician inserting the catheter.[86] Research continues with products to reduce CVAD-related infections. For example, preparation of central venous sites with 2 percent chlorhex-

BOX 20–7

Complications of Central Venous Access Devices

EARLY COMPLICATIONS[82]
Pneumothorax
Venous or arterial injury
Lymphatic fistulae
Neurologic injury
Cardiac dysrhythmia
Improper catheter placement

COMMON COMPLICATIONS
Infection (may require CVAD removal)[83]
Occlusion

LESS COMMON COMPLICATIONS[84]
Catheter pinch-off and fracture
Catheter malposition and migration
Cardiac perforation
Extravasation
Breakage
Defective devices

idine gluconate has been shown to lower blood stream infection rates compared to site preparation with 10 percent povidone-iodine or 70 percent alcohol.[87] Similarly, a chlorhexidine-impregnated sponge (Biopatch) placed over the site of CVADs reduced the risk of catheter colonization and infection in a multicenter study.[88]

Infections may be local or systemic. Local infections occur at the site where the device exits the body (exit site), along the subcutaneous tunnel of catheters, and in the port pocket of implanted ports. Systemic infection (catheter-related blood stream infection) is confirmed when the same organism is isolated from a culture of a catheter segment and peripheral blood with no clinical evidence of any other apparent source.[43] An episode of local catheter-related infection adds an additional cost of $400, while a catheter-related blood stream infection can add $6000 to $9700 in additional cost.[89] Even without the additional cost, catheter-related blood stream infections are particularly troublesome because of the dramatic morbidity and a case fatality rate of 14 percent.[86]

The most common cause of exit site infections is *Staphylococcus epidermidis*.[85] Other organisms with exit site infections, such as *S. aureus*, *Pseudomonas* species, and *Mycobacterium* species, may be difficult to eradicate.[64] Exit site infection treatment includes increasing the frequency of local exit site care with the addition of topical antibiotic ointment for the short-term.

Prevention of local infection centers on catheter care that in many instances is done by the patient. Ray[55] identifies two important preventative measures to decrease the risk of catheter-related infections: proper access of the CVAD during use and routine catheter injection cap changes. Therefore, patient education should include access techniques and cap changes along with handwashing, aseptic technique, thorough site care, and daily assessment. Another method of prevention is the use of antimicrobial-coated catheters that have been shown to decrease the rate of catheter-associated infections.[89]

Treatment of CVAD infection depends on several factors, including (1) the causative organism, (2) extent of infection, (3) type of device, and (4) physical condition of the patient.[55] Many exit site infections of tunneled catheters can be treated successfully with antibiotic therapy and do not require catheter removal. However, salvaging the CVAD with a catheter-related blood stream infection requires careful observation and prompt decision making about antibiotic therapy options.[64] Coagulase-negative staphylococci, *S. aureus*, aerobic gram-negative bacilli, and *Candida albicans* most commonly cause catheter-related blood stream infections.[90] The salvage of an infected subcutaneous port is more difficult, with the majority requiring removal.[91] A major controversy regarding treatment of CVAD-related infection is whether to remove the device. Most clinicians agree the CVAD should be removed when the signs and symptoms of septicemia persist despite antibiotic therapy or the causative organism is fungi.[64]

Occlusion

Occlusion occurs in all catheter types and is the second most common problem associated with CVADs.[45] There may be several variables related to venous thrombogenicity, including catheter diameter, catheter tip placement, normal physiologic response to access device insertion, left-sided catheter placement, and hypercoagulability associated with certain malignancies.[45,75]

Causes of catheter obstruction are mechanical, nonthrombotic, or thrombotic. Clamped or kinked intravenous (IV) tubing, a tight suture at the catheter exit site, improper catheter tip placement, or catheter kinking or compression may cause mechanical obstructions. Nonthrombotic occlusions are generally related to precipitates (medication or TPN) or lipid residue from TPN.[75] To restore patency of occluded catheters from medication precipitate, hydrochloric acid or sodium bicarbonate have been used depending on the pH of the medication that precipitated.[73,76,92] Hydrochloric acid has also been used to restore patency in catheters occluded with crystallized calcium phosphate from TPN.[93] The appropriate solution is instilled and allowed to dwell inside the line for 20 minutes and is then withdrawn. Lipid residue from TPN may be dissolved in some cases with a 70 percent solution of ethanol.[93] Caution should be taken in using any of these investigative therapies for obstruction.[75] Causes of thrombotic occlusions are listed in Table 20-4. Ninety-five percent of catheter occlusions are related to thrombotic causes.[94]

An occlusion may be classified as either total occlusion or partial occlusion. Resistance when attempting to flush the device, the inability to infuse fluids, and no blood return on aspiration are indicative of a total occlusion.[94] A partial occlusion or persistent withdrawal occlusion is a relatively frequent complication. In this instance there is sluggish or absent blood withdrawal from a CVAD even though fluids may be easily infused.[75,76] There may also be a "positional blood draw"; when a patient changes position or performs Valsalva's maneuver, blood can be aspirated. A fibrin sheath is generally the reason for a partial occlusion. Fibrin sheaths have been reported as early as 24 hours after device insertion and will develop in virtually all catheters left in place for more than 1 week.[95] The sheath eventually covers the catheter tip, acting as a one-way valve or flap.

Hadaway[76] recommends that a careful assessment of events preceding the occlusion should be done prior to using any solution to restore patency in a catheter. Areas to assess are listed in Box 20-8. Blood-clotted catheters can usually be cleared via gentle flushing with solution of a thrombolytic agent. The use of a 1-ml syringe to instill thrombolytic treatment in a totally occluded line is not recommended. Excessive force in flushing the catheter with a 1-ml syringe can result in rupture and/or embolization of the clot. Therefore, a syringe of 5-ml or greater is recommended to inject thrombolytic treatment.[75] If catheter patency is not restored after the prescribed procedure has been followed, the physician should be notified because another cause of occlusion may exist.

Other Complications

Other complications that occur rarely include catheter pinch-off and fracture, catheter malposition and migration, cardiac perforation, extravasation, and device breakage.[85] Catheter pinch-off is the anatomic, mechanical compression of a catheter as it passes between the clavicle and first rib of the costoclavicular space. Two studies have documented a 1.1 percent incidence rate for the pinch-off syndrome.[76] Pinch-off syndrome is the most common cause of catheter fracture when subclavian access is used. Pinch-off is not usually discovered until catheter fracture occurs and interventional radiology is used to retrieve catheter fragments.[44] Catheter migration indicates malposition of a catheter that at one time used to be in the proper location. There is increased risk of catheter migration if the catheter is short or the tip is in the innominate vein or at the junction of innominate vein and superior vena cava.[96] Cardiac perforation may occur during insertion or as a late complication because of catheter migration into the heart.[84] Extravasation is primarily associated with needle dislodgment from implanted ports; backtracking of fluid resulting from a partially or totally occluded catheter may also cause it.[45,95] If there is a sheath solidly encasing a CVAD from its tip to its venous entry point, fluid exiting the lumen may flow retrograde and backtrack along the outside of the catheter. Incidence of extravasation secondary to fibrin sheath formation ranges from 1.2 to 2.6 percent.[95] The most commonly reported cause of breakage is catheter rupture

TABLE 20–4 Causes of Thrombotic Occlusions

Type of Occlusion	Description
Intraluminal blood clot	Thrombus in the internal lumen of the catheter.
Fibrin sheath	Formed around distal tip, causing retrograde flow or fibrin deposit at distal end that allows instillation of fluids but aspiration obstruction.
Mural thrombus	Intima irritation by the catheter leads to catheter adherence to vein wall and venous thrombosis.
Portal reservoir occlusion	Accumulation of fibrin or precipitates in portal reservoir.

BOX 20–8

Assessment of CVAD Occlusion Prior to Catheter Clearance Treatment[76]

Formulation of all solutions being infused
All medications given through the CVAD for past 24 hours
Amount and time of flushing procedures
Alterations to resistance from position changes
Length of time catheter has been in place
Any patient activity
Details about onset of occlusion problem

CVAD, Central venous access device.

caused by forceful flushing.[84] Many of the above problems require removal of the catheter. This presents a serious problem for individuals with limited access choices.

Nursing Management of Patients With Central Venous Access Devices

Preoperative Interventions

Prior to the insertion of a CVAD, accurate assessment of the patient and significant other's ability to manage the care and maintenance of the device is critical. Components of this assessment include manual dexterity, visual acuity, cognitive ability, and willingness to participate with the management of the CVAD. Methods for improving compliance behavior for patients with access devices include encouraging participation in treatment decisions from the time of diagnosis and selection of an access device; reinforcing education on care of the access device; exploring the patient's perception of disease and treatment; and incorporating support from the family, community, and health care professionals.[97] Patients who need a CVAD frequently have cancer or other debilitating chronic illnesses. The health care team needs to consider the trajectory of the illness in the plan of care for managing the device.

Postoperative Interventions

Nursing management of CVADs focuses on maintaining CVAD patency and preventing systemic infections.[78] For patients undergoing insertion of tunneled catheters or subcutaneous infusion ports, broad-spectrum antibiotics should be administered prophylactically immediately before and for 24 hours after placement to minimize the risk of infection. With use of aseptic technique, the catheter or port should be aspirated and irrigated with heparinized saline solution to assure adequate patency. If the CVAD is to be used for continuous infusions, the use of an electronic infusion device is recommended as the standard of practice.[98]

Patient education for self-care is an important independent function of professional nursing practice. Patients need to be empowered as active partners in their care. They should be provided with the opportunity to develop the ability to take control of the use and care of their access devices. Knowing and using the proper techniques for CVAD care reduce the risk of infection or other complications.[45,46] Care and maintenance of the CVAD are important aspects of patient teaching; the signs and symptoms of complications must also be taught to patients.[51] In the present environment of health care with shortened lengths of stay in hospitals and limited time that nurses have to accomplish essential care, practicing nurses employed in hospitals cannot be held entirely responsible for all patient education. However, the information provided to patients and caregivers regarding care of the CVAD should be consistent across settings.[46] Therefore coordination of efforts needs to extend beyond the hospital into clinics, doctor offices, and community agencies. Collaboration between agencies to standardize practices, such as developing a "troubleshooting" guide for both patients and providers, can prevent or reduce access device complications.[97]

Frequently, nurses have the primary responsibility of venous access devices in hospitals, outpatient clinics, or during home health visits. Consequently, nurses are the health care professionals most likely to be first in assessing and initiating treatment of infections in patients with CVADs.[64] Additionally, nurses need to understand the mechanisms and diagnoses of catheter-related occlusion and thrombosis in order to initiate appropriate treatment in a timely manner.[75]

SUMMARY

The steadily increasing number and greater life expectancy of patients requiring maintenance hemodialysis, and the broadened indications for long-term vascular access to treat other medical problems, continue to challenge the expertise and creativity of vascular surgeons, interventional radiologists, nephrologists, pharmacists, and nurses. Nurses need to keep pace with advancements in vascular access procedures, as nurses provide an essential role in patient preparations, maintenance of functional access sites, and prevention and early detection of complications, which might obviate the need for further access procedures. In addition, nurses need to take advantage of opportunities to participate in the research to design and develop new access device and maintenance care products.

REFERENCES

1. Davidson IJA: Vascular access surgery—general considerations. In Davidson IJA, ed: *On call in vascular access*, Austin, Tex, 1996, Landes, pp 1-10.
2. Agoda L, Eggers P: Renal replacement therapy in the United States: data from the United States renal data system, *Am J Kidney Dis* 25:119-133, 1995.
3. Trerotola SO: Hemodialysis catheter placement and management, *Radiology* 215:651-658, 2000.
4. Tominage GT, Ingegno M, Ceralgi C et al: Vascular complications of continuous arteriovenous hemofiltration in trauma patients, *J Trauma* 35:285-289, 1993.
5. Johnson CL, Hiatt JR: Vascular access for trauma, emergency surgery, and critical care. In Wilson SW, ed: *Vascular access: principles and practice*, St Louis, 1996, Mosby, pp 67-78.
6. Monas D: Vascular access. In Davies AH, Beard JD, Wyatt MO, eds: *Essential vascular surgery*, London, 1999, WB Saunders, pp 376-384.
7. White GH: Planning and patient assessment for vascular access surgery. In Wilson SE, ed: *Vascular access: principles and practice*, St Louis, 1996, Mosby, pp 6-11.
8. Gelabert H, Freischlag JA: Hemodialysis access. In Rutherford RB, ed: *Vascular surgery*, ed 5, Philadelphia, 2000, WB Saunders, pp 1466-1477.
9. Haimov M, Schanzer H, Skladani M: Pathogenesis and management of upper-extremity ischemia following angioaccess surgery, *Blood Purif* 14:350-354, 1996.
10. Fernando HC, Fernando ON: Arteriovenous fistulas by direct anastomosis for hemodialysis access. In Wilson SE, ed: *Vascular access: principles and practice*, St Louis, 1996, Mosby, pp 129-136.
11. Berkoben M, Schwab SJ: Maintenance of permanent hemodialysis vascular access patency, *ANNA J* 22: 17-24, 1995.
12. Culp K, Taylor L, Hulme PA: Geriatric hemodialysis patients: a comparative study of vascular access, *ANNA J* 23:583-592, 1996.
13. Bonomo RA, Rice D, Whalen C et al: Risk factors associated with permanent access-site infections in chronic hemodialysis patients, *Infect Control Hosp Epidemiol* 19:643-646, 1998.
14. Wilson SE: Vascular interposition (bridge fistulas) for hemodialysis. In Wilson SE, ed: *Vascular access: principles and practice*, St Louis, 1996, Mosby, pp 157-169.
15. Gordon IL: Physiology of the arteriovenous fistula. In Wilson SE, ed: *Vascular access: principles and practice*, St Louis, 1996, Mosby, pp 29-41.
16. Kafie FE, Wilson SE: Complications of vascular access surgery. In Yao JST, Pierce WH, eds: *Techniques in vascular and endovascular surgery*, Stamford, Conn, 1998, Appleton & Lange, pp 539-552.
17. Bitar G, Yang S, Badosa F: Balloon versus patch angioplasty as an adjuvant treatment to surgical thrombectomy of hemodialysis grafts, *Am J Surg* 175:140-142, 1997.
18. Goodwin S, Arora L, Razavi M et al: Dialysis access graft thombolysis: randomized study of pulse-spray versus continuous urokinase infusion, *Cardiovasc Intervent Radiol* 21:135-137, 1998.

19. Kumpe DA, Durham JD, Mann DJ: Thrombolysis and percutaneous transluminal angioplasty. In Wilson SE, ed: *Vascular access: principles and practice*, St Louis, 1996, Mosby, pp 239-261.
20. Mizumoto D, Watanabe Y, Kumon S et al: The treatment of chronic hemodialysis vascular access by directional artherectomy, *Nephron* 74:45-52, 1996.
21. Nassar GM, Ayus JC: Infectious complications of the hemodialysis access, *Kidney Int* 60(1):1-13, 2001.
22. Stevenson KB, Adcox MJ, Mallea MC et al: Standardized surveillance of hemodialysis access infections: 18-month experience at an outpatient, multifacility hemodialysis center, *Infect Control Hosp Epidemiol* 21:200-203, 2000.
23. Ready AR, Buckels JAC: Management of infection: vascular access surgery in hemodialysis. In Wilson SE, ed: *Vascular access: principles and practice*, St Louis, 1996, Mosby, pp 198-211.
24. Kearns PJ, Coleman S, Wehner JH: Complications of long arm-catheters: a randomized trial of central vs peripheral tip locations, *JPEN J Parenter Enteral Nutr* 20(1):20-24, 1996.
25. Kingdon EJ, Holt SG, Davar J et al: Arterial thrombus and central venous dialysis catheters, *Am J Kidney Dis* 38:631-639, 2001.
26. Schwab SJ, Besarab A, Beathard G et al: NKF-DOQI clinical practice guidelines for vascular access: National Kidney Foundation-Dialysis Outcomes Quality Initiative, *Am J Kidney Dis* 30(suppl 3): S150-S191, 1997.
27. Back MR, White RA: The biologic response of prosthetic dialysis grafts. In Wilson SE, ed: *Vascular access: principles and practice*, St Louis, 1996, Mosby, pp 137-149.
28. Swartz RD, Boyer CL, Messana JM: Central venous catheters for maintenance hemodialysis: a cautionary approach, *Adv Ren Replace Ther* 4:275-285, 1997.
29. Sharma A, Zilleruelo G, Abitbol C et al: Survival and complications of cuffed catheters in children on chronic hemodialysis, *Pediatr Nephrol* 13:245-248, 1999.
30. Forauer AR, Glockner JF: Importance of U.S. findings in access planning during jugular vein hemodialysis catheter placements, *J Vasc Interv Radiol* 11:233-238.
31. Docktor BL, Sadler DJ, Gray RR et al: Radiologic placement of tunneled central catheters: rates of success and of immediate complications in a large series, *AJR Am J Roentgenol* 173:457-460, 1999.
32. Noh HM, Kaufman JA, Rhea JT et al: Cost comparison of radiologic versus surgical placement of long-term hemodialysis catheters, *AJR Am J Roentgenol* 172:673-675, 1999.
33. Trerotola SO: Hemodialysis catheter placement and management, *Radiology* 215:651-658, 2000.
34. Savader SJ, Ehrman KO, Porter DJ et al: Treatment of hemodialysis catheter-associated fibrin sheaths by rt-PA infusion: critical analysis of 124 procedures, *J Vasc Interv Radiol* 12:711-715, 2001.
35. Sesso R, Barbosa D, Leme IL et al: *Staphylococcus aureus* prophylaxis in hemodialysis patients using central venous catheter: effect of mupirocin ointment, *J Am Soc Nephrol* 9:1085-1092, 1998.
36. Zakrzewska-Bode A, Muytjens HL, Liem KD et al: Mupirocin resistance in coagulase-negative staphylococci, after topical prophylaxis for the reduction of colonization of central venous catheters, *J Hosp Infect* 31:189-193, 1995.
37. Rao SP, Oreopoulos DG: Unusual complications of a polyurethane PD catheter, *Perit Dial Int* 17:410-412, 1997.
38. Butterly DW, Schwab SJ: Dialysis access infections, *Curr Opin Nephrol Hypertens* 9:631-635, 2000.
39. MacVittie BA: *Vascular surgery*, St Louis, 1998, Mosby.
40. Stansfield G: Cannulation of arteriovenous fistulae, *Nurs Times* 83:38-39, 1987.
41. Thomas-Hawkins C: Nursing interventions related to vascular access infections, *Adv Renal Replace Ther* 3:218-221, 1996.
42. Hartigan MF: Vascular access and nephrology nursing practice: existing views and rationales for change, *Adv Renal Replace Ther* 1:155-162, 1994.
43. Blum AS: The role of the interventional radiologist in central venous access, *J Intraven Nurs* 22(6S): S32-S39, 1999.
44. O'Grady NP, Alexander M, Dellinger EP et al: *Draft guideline for the prevention on intravascular catheter-related infections*, 2001, www.cdc.gov/ncidod/hip/iv.htm.
45. Dearborn P, DeMuth JS, Requarth AB et al: Nurse and patient satisfaction with three types of venous access devices, *Oncol Nurs Forum* 24:34S-40S, 1997.
46. Fitzpatrick LM: Care and management issues regarding central venous access devices in the home and long-term care setting, *J Intraven Nurs* 22(6S):S40-S45, 1999.
47. Hadaway LC: Comparison of vascular access devices, *Semin Oncol Nurs* 11(3):154-166, 1995.
48. Winslow MN, Trammell L, Camp-Sorrell D: Selection of vascular access devices and nursing care, *Semin Oncol Nurs* 11(3):167-173, 1995.
49. Intravenous Nurses Society: Infusion nursing standards of practice: parenteral infusion, *J Intraven Nurse* 23(6S):S69-S70, 2000.

50. Sansivero GE, Barton-Burke M: Chemotherapy administration: general principles for vascular access. In Barton-Burke M, Wilkes GM, Ingwersen KC, eds: *Cancer chemotherapy: a nursing process approach*, Boston, 2001, Jones & Bartlett.
51. Cole D: Selection and management of central venous access devices in the home setting, *J Intraven Nurs* 22:315-319, 1999.
52. Sansivero GE: Venous anatomy and physiology: considerations for vascular access device placement and function, *J Intraven Nurs* 21(5S):S107-S114, 1998.
53. Intravenous Nurses Society: Infusion nursing standards of practice: catheter placement, *J Intraven Nurse* 23(6S):S42-S43.
54. D'Amelio LF, Greco RS: Biologic properties of venous access devices. In Wilson SE, ed: *Vascular access: principles and practice*, St Louis, 1996, Mosby, pp 42-53.
55. Ray CE: Infection control principles and practices in the care and management of central venous access devices, *J Intraven Nurs* 22(6S):S18-S25, 1999.
56. Oncology Nursing Society: Access device guidelines: recommendations for nursing practice and education, Pittsburgh, 1996, Oncology Nursing Press.
57. Intravenous Nurses Society: Position paper: peripherally inserted central catheters, *J Intraven Nurse* 4:172-174, 1997.
58. Crawford M, Saukup SM, Woods SS et al: Peripherally inserted central catheter program, *Nurs Clin North Am* 35:349-359, 2000.
59. Hagle ME, McDonagh JM, Rapp CJ: Patients with long-term vascular access devices: care and complications, *Orthop Nurs* 13(5):41-52, 1994.
60. Sansivero GE: Taking care of PICCs, *Nursing* 27(5):28, 1997.
61. Intravenous Nurses Society: Infusion nursing standards of practice: catheter removal, *J Intraven Nurse* 23(6S):S50-S51, 2000.
62. Wickham RS: Advances in venous access devices and nursing management strategies, *Nurs Clin North Am* 25:345-364, 1990.
63. Goldstein AM, Weber JM, Sheridan RL: Femoral venous access is safe in burned children: an analysis of 224 catheters, *J Pediatr* 130:442-446, 1997.
64. Jones GR: A practical guide to evaluation and treatment of infections in patients with central venous catheters, *J Intraven Nurs* 21(5S):S135-S142, 1998.
65. Lilienberg A, Bengtsson M, Starkhammer H: Implantable devices for venous access: nurses' and patients' evaluation of three different port systems, *J Adv Nurs* 19:21-28, 1994.
66. Kaufman JA, Salaminpour H, Gellar SC et al: Long-term outcomes of radiologically placed arm ports, *Radiology* 201:725-730, 1996.
67. Simpson KR, Hovsepian DM, Picus D: Interventional radiologic placement of chest wall ports: results and complications in 161 consecutive placements, *J Vasc Interv Radiol* 8:189-195, 1997.
68. Hills JR, Cardella JF, Cardella K et al: Experience with 100 consecutive central venous access arm ports placed by interventional radiologists, *J Vasc Interv Radiol* 8:983-989, 1997.
69. Funaki B, Szymski GX, Hackworth CA et al: Radiologic placement of subcutaneous infusion chest ports for long-term central venous access, *AJR Am J Roentgenol* 169:1431-1434, 1997.
70. Foley MJ: Radiologic placement of long-term central venous peripheral access ports (PAS port): results in 150 patients, *J Vasc Interv Radiol* 6:255-262, 1995.
71. Bertoglio S, DiSomma C, Meszaros P et al: Long-term central venous access in cancer patients, *Eur J Surg Oncol* 22:162-165, 1996.
72. Hadaway LC: Flushing to reduce central catheter occlusions, *Nursing* 20(10):74, 2000.
73. Macklin D: How to manage PICCs, *Am J Nurs* 97(9):26-33, 1997.
74. Intravenous Nurses Society: Infusion nursing standards of practice: flushing, *J Intraven Nurse* 23(6S): S53-S54, 2000.
75. Bagnall-Reeb H: Diagnosis of central venous device occlusion: implications for nursing practice, *J Intraven Nurs* 21(5S):S115-S121, 1998.
76. Hadaway LC: Major thrombotic and nonthrombotic complications: loss of patency, *J Intraven Nurs* 21(5S):S142-S160, 1998.
77. Mayo DJ, Horne MK, Summers BL et al: The effects of heparin flush on patency of the Groshong catheter: a pilot study, *Oncol Nurs Forum* 23:1401-1405, 1996.
78. Woods SS, Nass Y, Deisch P: Selection and implementation of a transparent dressing for central vascular access devices, *Nurs Clin North Am* 35:385-393, 2000.
79. Mayo DJ, Dimond EP, Kramer W et al: Discard volumes necessary for clinically useful coagulation studies from heparinized Hickman catheters, *Oncol Nurs Forum* 23:671-675, 1996.

80. Skudal D, Horak E, Maurer K et al: Complications of percutaneous insertion of Hickman catheters in children, *J Pediatr Surg* 34:1510-1513, 1999.
81. Johnson EM, Saltzman DA, Suh G et al: Complications and risks of central venous catheter placement in children, *Surgery* 124:911-916, 1998.
82. Hye RJ, Stabile BE: Complications of percutaneous vascular access procedures and their management. In Wilson SE, ed: *Vascular access: principles and practices*, St Louis, 1996, Mosby, pp 91-103.
83. Hoch JR: Management of the complications of long-term venous access, *Semin Vasc Surg* 10(3):135-143, 1997.
84. Ingle RJ: Rare complications of vascular access devices, *Semin Oncol Nurs* 11:184-193, 1995.
85. Masoorli S: Managing complications of central venous access devices, *Nursing* 27(8):59-63, 1997.
86. Farr BM: Understaffing: a risk factor for infection in the era of downsizing? *Infect Control Hosp Epidemiol* 17:147-149, 1996.
87. Maki DG, Ringer M, Alvarado CJ: Prospective ramdomised trial of povidone-iodine, alcohol, and chlorhexidine for prevention of infection associated with central venous and arterial catheters, *Lancet* 338:339-343, 1991.
88. Maki DG, Mermel LA, Klugar D et al: The efficacy of a chlorhexidine impregnated sponge (Biopatch) for the prevention of intravascular catheter-related infection—a prospective randomized controlled multicenter study. In *Proceedings of Interscience Conference on Antimicrobial Agents and Chemotherapy*, Toronto, Ontario, Canada, 2000.
89. Saint S, Veenstra DL, Lipsky BA: The clinical and economic consequences of nosocomial central venous catheter-related infection: are antimicrobial catheters useful? *Infect Control Hosp Epidemiol* 21:375-380, 2000.
90. Mermel LA, Farr BM, Scherertz RJ et al: Guidelines for the management of intravascular catheter-related infections, *Infect Control Hosp Epidemiol* 22:222-242, 2001.
91. Barnes JR, Lucas N, Broadwater JR et al: When should the "infected" subcutaneous infusion reservoir be removed? *Am Surg* 62:203-206, 1996.
92. Kupensky DR: Use of hydrochloric acid to restore patency in an occluded implantable port: a case report, *J Intraven Nurs* 18:198-201, 1995.
93. Pennington CR, Pithie AD: Ethanol lock in the management of catheter occlusion, *J Parenter Enterol Nutr* 11:507-508, 1987.
94. Krzywda EA: Predisposing factors, prevention, and management of central venous catheter occlusions, *J Intraven Nurs* 22(6S):S11-S17, 1999.
95. Mayo DR, Pearson DC: Chemotherapy extravasation: a consequence of fibrin sheath formation around venous access devices, *Oncol Nurs Forum* 22:675-680, 1995.
96. Collin GR, Ahmadinejad AS, Misse E: Spontaneous migration of subcutaneous central venous catheters, *Am Surg* 63:322-326, 1997.
97. McDermott MK: Patient education and compliance issues associated with access devices, *Semin Oncol Nurs* 11:221-226, 1995.
98. Intravenous Nurses Society: Infusion nursing standards of practice: flow-control devices, *J Intraven Nurs* 23(6S):S34-S35, 2000.

21

Lower-Extremity Amputation From Arterial Occlusive Disease

MARK HUANG □ TODD KUIKEN

Approximately 125,000 lower-extremity amputations involving the foot or a more proximal level occur each year.[1] In patients older than 45, the majority of these amputations are due to diabetes and peripheral arterial occlusive disease. Approximately 50-70 percent of all lower-extremity amputations involve persons diagnosed with diabetes mellitus.[2,3]

Regardless of the etiology, amputation remains a source of significant physical and psychologic trauma in individuals facing limb loss. While patients and physicians alike may consider amputation a failure of medical and surgical management, it is a reconstructive surgery that is essential to maximize the patient's function and quality of life. Rehabilitation and medical management are critical components that help in the recovery process.

The vascular surgery nurse plays a crucial role with these patients. The nurse is often responsible for getting the entire rehabilitation process started; he or she is the first clinician to work with the patient on mobility issues and is frequently responsible for calling in other team members. The nurse generally spends more time with the patient than any other medical professional, allowing him or her to form a special bond with the patient, to gauge the patient's emotional status, and to provide psychologic support to patients and their families. The nurse is responsible for implementing the pain treatment program, which is essential for a successful rehabilitation program. Finally, the nurse is an important educator for the patient and his or her family. Rehabilitation is as much an educational process as it is a treatment plan.

INDICATIONS FOR AMPUTATION

There are many indications for amputation such as trauma, tumors, and congenital abnormalities. The focus of this chapter are the sequelae of peripheral arterial occlusive disease and diabetes. The majority of scenarios leading to amputation begin when patients suffer trauma that results in an ulcer on the affected limb. This is frequently footwear-related, followed by ulceration and faulty wound healing.[4] Diabetics are at high risk of developing new ulcers due to the sequelae of diabetes such as peripheral neuropathy and accelerating arterial occlusive disease. Ischemic ulceration often precedes gangrene. Both of these conditions can be painful, debilitating, and limb threatening. The primary indication for amputation in the majority of non–insulin-dependent diabetes cases is gangrene.[5]

Infections in the patient with diabetes or arterial occlusive disease can contribute to amputation. Infections of the foot progress quickly due to little resistance from ischemic tissues. The diabetic foot is especially vulnerable to infection of all types: local, diffuse (cellulitis), and necrotizing. Uncontrolled sepsis, as in "gas" gangrene (*Clostridium* infection), is an indication for immediate amputation to preserve life. Intravenous antibiotic therapy combined with early debridement of all dead or infected tissue is essential to preserve as much viable tissue as possible.

Ischemic rest pain may be an indication for surgery. It is characterized by severe burning pain in the toes and forefoot that is intensified by elevation and often relieved by dependency.

The pain may wake the patient from a sound sleep and becomes progressively more constant and severe. Rest pain is an indication for amputation when revascularization is not possible and pain cannot be controlled by any other means. Ischemic rest pain can also occur in a residual limb, necessitating revision to a higher level.

Some patients require amputation when revascularization originally performed for relief of claudication has failed. Vascular patients often have multiple procedures, including bypass surgery, angioplasty, and thrombolytic therapy, before an amputation is the only remaining option. Prior arterial surgery had been performed on up to a third of the limbs requiring amputation.[6]

Acute arterial thrombosis or embolism can result in massive muscle necrosis. Because collateral vessels have not yet developed, severe ischemia ensues within hours. There is rapid progression of symptoms (pain, pallor, pulselessness, paresthesias, paralysis, and poikilothermia), edema of the muscles within the fascial sheath (compartment syndrome) secondary to ischemia or reperfusion, and the development of systemic toxicity with renal failure. Amputation is usually necessary.

In summary, major lower-limb amputation is indicated in limb- or life-threatening situations after careful consideration of the risks and benefits of all available alternatives.

SELECTION OF AMPUTATION LEVEL

The quality and type of amputation performed greatly affect the overall outcome of the patient. It is important to consider all the factors affecting the patient's function when determining amputation level. These include tissue viability, biomechanics of the residual limb, prosthetic options, gait dynamics, and cosmesis. The objective of preoperative evaluation is to determine the level at which healing will occur and maximal function is restored after removal of all dead or infected tissue. Preservation of tissue is balanced with restoration of function because higher amputations result in increased morbidity and mortality as well as decreased rehabilitation potential. Prediction of healing requires careful evaluation of all factors that affect wound healing, including surgical technique, postoperative care, nutritional status, and arterial circulation, particularly tissue perfusion.

The earliest attempts to judge the appropriate level of amputation focused on the presence of palpable pulses, angiographic findings, skin color and temperature, character and location of pain, and, most notably, the presence of incisional skin bleeding at the time of surgery. Various diagnostic methods exist to help determine the level at which healing will occur. These include Doppler pressure measurements, pulse volume recordings, photoplethysmographic pressures, laser Doppler blood flow studies, xenon-133 skin blood flow studies, and transcutaneous oxygen determinations. However, these tests have not been consistently more reliable than clinical judgment in predicting wound healing at a given level.[7,8] Most surgeons use a combination of objective data and assessment of the appearance of the tissues at the time of surgery, particularly bleeding, to decide on the site of amputation.

TYPES OF AMPUTATION

Amputations are classified according to the level and type of operative procedure. Closed amputation is the most commonly used technique when amputations are necessitated by arterial disease. The incision is made through presumably healthy tissues, and skin flaps are shaped for primary (sutured) closure. Open amputations are performed only in instances of severe trauma or overwhelming infection. This allows appropriate drainage and observation of the wound. Guillotine amputation is an open procedure in which all the tissues are cut at the same level through a circular incision. Today, guillotine amputation is reserved for extremely ill patients who require quick control of rapidly spreading infection such as gas gangrene. At a later date, a closed amputation is performed at a higher level.

Toe amputations are probably the most common amputations performed. This is a very successful amputation level as there is minimal impairment and the patient can be expected to have a normal gait without the use of a prosthesis. With ray amputations, the length of the foot is still preserved and normal gait mechanics can be expected. A total-contact shoe insert will also help to distribute pressure throughout the remaining foot, preventing plantar surface callous formation and pressure sores.

The transmetatarsal amputation is also a very successful amputation level (Fig. 21-1). Although the patient can walk without the use of a prosthesis, gait mechanics are abnormal. The foot is shortened; therefore, toe-off is reduced, the stride is shortened, and drop-off in the gait on the amputated side is seen. A total-contact foot orthosis with soft toe filler and a three-quarter length carbon-fiber footplate is required to protect the foot, restore the functional foot length, and normalize gait mechanics.

Although more proximal foot amputation such as tarsometatarsal (Lisfranc) amputation and the transtarsal (Chopart) amputation may be performed, these are problematic for several reasons. The remaining foot is so short that there is no effective lever arm. The remaining ankle is essentially useless. These level amputations lead to equinovarus deformities and anterior bony prominences that are painful and prone to skin breakdown. Another problem with midfoot amputations is that they are very difficult to fit with a good orthosis. Due to these difficulties, midfoot amputations are usually not performed.

The ankle disarticulation, or Syme's amputation, has a number of advantages and disadvantages. The primary advantages are that there is a long residual limb and an end weight-bearing surface. However, ambulation without a prosthesis is usually limited to short distances with an awkward and inefficient gait pattern. Typically, most Syme's amputees do not ambulate without a prosthesis. The main disadvantages are the poor prosthetic cosmesis and difficulty in prosthetic fitting. The distal residual limb is quite bulbous because the malleoli are still in place. The prosthesis must accommodate this bulbous end, and the resulting prosthesis is bulky, fairly heavy, and has poor cosmesis. There is also little room left for a prosthetic foot with the Syme's amputation. These shortcomings should be discussed with patients before surgery so that they have appropriate expectations. The Syme's amputation is worth consideration in a well-perfused limb. However, if there are concerns about wound healing or progression of arterial occlusive disease, these risks may outweigh its advantages.

The transtibial or below-knee amputation is the most common major amputation of the lower extremity.[9] A standard transtibial amputation as advocated by Burgess[10] is performed one third of the way down the tibia. At this length, the bulk of the posterior compartment muscles are available for a flap, and they provide good soft tissue coverage over the distal tibia. The goal of surgery should be a cylindrically shaped residual limb; bulbous residual limbs delay fitting with prosthesis. Long transtibial amputations are sometimes performed to give patients a longer lever arm and more surface area for load distribution.[11] However, no functional muscle attachments are saved with a long transtibial amputation, and it is

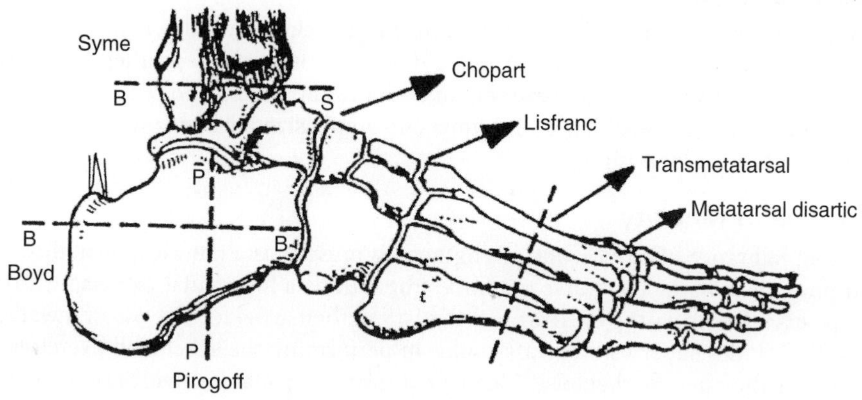

FIG. 21–1. Types of foot amputations.

associated with multiple complications.[12,13] Furthermore, the residual limb is often bony, which makes prosthetic fitting more difficult.[14] Thus, a standard-length transtibial amputation (35-50 percent of tibial length) is strongly recommended as the procedure of choice at this level.

The transtibial amputation is often the easiest to fit with a prosthetic device.[15] Therefore, it is routine to attempt a transtibial amputation when a major amputation is indicated if there is a reasonable chance for healing. Some clinical situations contraindicate a primary transtibial approach. The presence of ulcers, gangrene, or infection extending to the midcalf precludes healing at this level. A severely contracted knee has great potential for nonhealing because of the difficulty with positioning the residual limb to promote healing. Each case must be determined individually because of the importance of preserving the knee.

The knee disarticulation is an uncommon amputation that is performed on about 1 percent of patients.[9] Wearing a prosthetic socket over the long, bulbous residual limb is cosmetically undesirable and can make it difficult for the patient to sit in tight spaces such as cars, church pews, and public transportation. However, the knee disarticulation does have some important advantages over a transfemoral amputation. It is an end weight-bearing amputation and is generally a stronger residual limb.

For the transfemoral amputation, stabilizing the femur with maximal femur length is the primary surgical goal. Myodesis (suturing muscle to bone) of the adductor magnus and the quadriceps to the femur followed by myoplasty of the hamstrings is recommended.[16] Myoplasty alone is inadequate; this does not restore normal muscle length nor does it allow for adequate control of the femur. The femur is too mobile within the residual limb, the distal femur can be a focus of excessive pressure causing pain, and the transfer of energy into the prosthesis is probably compromised. These patients have more difficulty with prosthetic ambulation. The amounts of energy required for ambulation increase dramatically with this level amputation.

PREOPERATIVE MANAGEMENT

The primary goals of the presurgical period are patient assessment, optimal medical management, pain control, psychologic support, and introduction to a rehabilitation program.

Diabetic Control

Many individuals with amputation have diabetes as a concomitant medical condition. Good control of diabetes is difficult when a patient has a significant infection, is under significant stress, or is not eating regularly. These conditions are frequently present in the patient facing amputation; therefore, utilization of an endocrinologist or a diabetes clinical nurse specialist is recommended.

Avoidance of Trauma

For the patient with arterial occlusive disease, further skin breakdown may necessitate a higher level of amputation or may introduce infection to a noninfected leg before surgery. Educating the patient about skin inspection of both the amputated and remaining leg, as well as patient positioning for avoidance of trauma, are emphasized. The main goal is prevention of contralateral lower limb injury.

Preservation of Mobility

Maintaining full range of motion and strengthening muscles is a joint responsibility of nursing and physical therapy. The nurse reinforces the rationale for regular exercise, particularly "push-up" exercises from the chair or bed that strengthen arms for the use of a walker. The nurse's role includes supervision or assistance in performing the scheduled exercises as recommended by the physical therapist. The patient needs to remain active, particularly if there is a prolonged hospitalization.

Prevention of Venous Thrombosis

Patients who are immobilized, obese, aged, hypercoagulable, or who have a previous history of venous thrombosis are at increased risk of deep venous thrombosis and pulmonary embolism. Because venous stasis is the primary mechanism, a program of regular exercise of the lower extremities is recommended. Subcutaneous low-dose heparin or intermittent compression devices are also effective and are indicated when the patient cannot exercise independently.

Promotion of Nutrition

The frail elderly patient or the diabetic patient with sepsis is often at risk for anemia, malnutrition, immunosuppression, and debilitation. Poor nutrition, reflected by an albumin level of less than 3.5 g/dl, severely impairs wound healing. Nutritionists are essential for evaluating the patient's nutritional status, setting goals, determining food preferences, and suggesting supplements. The nurse supervises adequate intake of the recommended diet and oral supplements when ordered. Monitoring the patient's weight on a regular basis is indicated. Serum prealbumin and transferrin levels are also important nutritional markers.

Pain Control

Good perioperative pain control is essential for the patient facing limb loss. Beyond patient comfort, good pain control is necessary to minimize the patient's stress and allow the patient to participate in a rehabilitation program, and it may help prevent chronic pain syndromes.[17] Uncontrolled pain impairs postoperative healing and immune functions.[18,19] The nurse's role should be frequent monitoring and assessment of pain through standardized scales such as a visual analogue scale or verbal Likert scales. Communication with the physicians and pharmacists is vital so that proper adjustments may be made for the patient's analgesic regimen.

The mainstay of perioperative pain control treatment is opioid therapy. Oral narcotics are usually sufficient. If needed, there should be no hesitation to use more aggressive pain control measures, including transdermal, subcutaneous, intramuscular, or intravenous narcotics. A scheduled dose of a long-acting agent is recommended so that the patient has consistent pain relief combined with the availability as needed (prn) of a shorter-acting "rescue" medicine. It is helpful to schedule a sufficient dose of analgesia prior to therapies so that the patient can fully participate in these therapies. Monitoring for side effects due to narcotics is also important as the elderly are at risk for adverse reaction such as lethargy, confusion, and constipation. Patient-controlled analgesia (PCA) systems are useful for severe pain or episodic pain in the perioperative period. These systems provide a continuous infusion of analgesic with the ability of the patient to employ a supplemental dose as needed. As a result, PCA systems provide excellent analgesia and can reduce some of the patient's stress or fear related to pain.

As a complement or alternative to opioid analgesia, continuous regional nerve blocks can also be used for perioperative pain control and even surgical anesthesia.[20] The tip of a fine catheter is guided to near the sciatic nerve using electrical stimulation. Once the catheter tip is in place, a long-acting anesthetic such as bupivacaine can be dosed. The catheter can be left in place, and regular dosing of the anesthetic provides excellent pain control in the limb. This technique allows the systemic side effects of narcotics to be avoided. Furthermore, the patient is not continuously connected by lines to an external apparatus, which facilitates mobility and participation in therapies. However, care must be taken to avoid displacement of the indwelling catheter. Prolonged epidural anesthesia can be useful but is somewhat controversial.[21,22]

Psychologic Support

Psychologic assessment and support for the patient facing limb loss should be a high priority. In addition to the obvious functional consequences of limb loss, amputation results in disfigurement, leading to a negative body image and potential loss of social acceptance.

Grief associated with these losses is expected. Nurses are adept at recognizing the stages of grief: denial, anger, bargaining, depression, and acceptance. The nursing focus at this point is best directed toward establishing a trusting relationship with the patient and family. Active listening is critical. Discussion about the patient's life, work, family, and values may provide the background information to explain the patient's feelings. The patient's specific fears should be identified so that appropriate information may be provided. The most common fears are experiencing pain, dying, and losing independence. Another fear is the reaction of others to the change in body image. Reassurance should be given that these fears are normal.

Assessment of the patient's expectations and goals is also important. Patients and their families tend to overestimate the functional impairment associated with lower-extremity amputation. Frequently, patients fear that they will never be able to walk again after amputation; far less accomplish more demanding tasks at work or in play. Amputees can do very well functionally. Several studies indicate that over 80% of amputees will be able to successfully walk with a prosthesis,[23-25] and this is consistent with our experience. The patient's long-term goals should be identified, and a comprehensive rehabilitation program should be outlined to achieve these goals. Obviously, a patient needs to learn how to stand and walk before he or she can attempt higher activity such as running or other sports. However, recognizing that these higher functions are legitimate goals and that the rehabilitation team will help them achieve these goals is reassuring and empowering for patients.

The nurse should reassure the patient that the surgical procedure itself is short and, unless there are complications, does not require transfer to an intensive care unit postoperatively. Most patients are out of bed within 24-48 hours and discharged to a rehabilitation facility or home within 3-7 days. Describing the rehabilitation process in detail and educating the patients about prosthetics can help to allay their fear of the unknown. Providing patients with educational literature and websites can be a valuable resource to patients and their families (Box 21-1).

Finally, it is important to discuss phantom limb sensation and phantom limb pain with the patient prior to surgery. The patient needs to be told to expect these odd sensations in the missing limb after surgery and realize that they are anticipated. Ideally, evaluation and treatment of the patient by a psychologist should be performed before the surgery to help prepare the patient for amputation emotionally and identify patients who are at higher risk for psychologic problems following amputation.

Functional Rehabilitation

Rehabilitation of the lower limb amputee should begin as soon as amputation is being considered. This can be a very valuable time to introduce the rehabilitation team and proactively start a functional rehabilitation program. Early involvement with rehabilitation professionals such as the physiatrist before surgery may help educate patients as to their anticipated progress and functional outcomes. Consulting the physical and occupational therapists early helps to prepare patients for what may happen during the therapy session and begin to address the baseline functional status prior to rehabilitation. It is often easier to stretch out a tight or contracted joint using the entire limb length before the amputation than it is after surgery when the limb is shortened and tender. Good progress can also be made conditioning remaining limb segments, increasing endurance, improving transfers, and training the patient in one-legged gait with an assistive device. This can reduce or even eliminate the need for inpatient rehabilitation after the amputation.

POSTOPERATIVE MANAGEMENT

The main focus of the vascular surgery nurse is on residual limb care, pain assessment, psychologic adjustment, remobilization of the patient, and prevention of complications (Box 21-2) following amputation surgery.

BOX 21–1

Educational Resources Available for Amputees

BOOKLETS

Below-Knee Amputation: A Guide for Rehabilitation.
T. Kuiken, M. Edwards, and N. Micelli, 2002, Rehabilitation Institute of Chicago.

First Step: A Guide for Adapting to Limb Loss.
2000, Amputee Coalition of America, National Limb Loss Information Center.

For the New Amputee.
N. Broyles, 1991, Amputee Coalition of America, National Limb Loss Information Center.

Patient Care Booklet for Above-Knee Amputees.
D.G. Shurr, 1999, American Academy of Orthotists and Prosthetists.

Patient Care Booklet for Below-Knee Amputees.
J.E. Uellendahl, 1999, American Academy of Orthotists and Prosthetists.

Pre-Prosthetic Care for Above-Knee Amputees.
J.O. Helminski, 1993, Rehabilitation Institute of Chicago.

Pre-Prosthetic Care for Below-Knee Amputees.
J.O. Helminski, 1993, Rehabilitation Institute of Chicago.

Survivor's Guide.
United Amputee Services Association, Inc., 1992, Amputee Coalition of America, National Limb Loss Information Center.

You Have a Choice: Improving Outcomes in O&P.
M.P. Novotny and J.W. Michael.

BOOKS

Challenged by Amputation: Embracing a New Life.
Carol S. Wallace, 1995, Inclusion Concepts Publishing House.

Conditioning With Physical Disabilities.
Kevin F. Lockette, PT, CSCS, and Ann M. Keyes, PT, CSCS, 1994.

Coping With Being Physically Challenged.
Linda Le Ratto, MEd, 1991, The Rosen Publishing Group.

Coping With Limb Loss.
Ellen Winchell, PhD, 1995, Avery Publishing Group.

One Step at a Time: A Young Woman's Struggle to Walk Again.
Lenor Madruga, 1979

The Novel Approach to Sexuality and Disability.
Georgie Maxfield, 1996.

When You Can't Come Back.
Dave Dravecky and Jan Dravecky with Ken Gire, 1992, Zondervan Publishing House.

You're Not Alone.
John Sabolich, CPO, 1993, Sabolich Prosthetic & Research Center.

WEBSITES

Amputee Coalition of America: www.amputee-coalition.org
National Center on Physical Activity and Disability: www.ncpad.org
Disabled Sports USA: www.dsusa.org
O&P Athletic Fund: www.opaaf@opoffice.org
Challenged Athletes Foundation: www.challengedathletes.org

Wound Care

Wound healing is dependent upon adequate tissue perfusion, wound care, and nutrition. Since most amputation wounds are primary surgical wounds, the care is straightforward. The limb should be washed on a daily basis with normal saline or even soap and water. Dressings should be kept clean and changed regularly. Antiseptic agents such as iodine solutions or hydrogen peroxide will inhibit wound healing and should be avoided unless there are signs of infection. In vascular patients, some wound margin necrosis may develop. These fragile

BOX 21–2

Complications Following Amputation Surgery

Venous thrombosis/pulmonary embolus
Delayed wound healing
Wound dehiscence
Bleeding/hematoma formation
Infection
Limb contractures
Phantom pain/residual limb pain
Myocardial infarction
Congestive heart failure
Ileus/constipation
Delirium/encephalopathy
Cerebrovascular accident

wounds should be monitored closely, kept clean, and protected from trauma that could cause dehiscence. Once the nonviable tissue is clearly demarcated, debridement can be considered. Good nutrition must be encouraged and supported with supplements when necessary. Eneroth[26] found that when supplementary nutrition was give to malnourished patients, twice as many patients healed their residual limb wounds compared to those who did not receive supplements.

Care of the residual limb includes other assessments and interventions. Bleeding immediately postoperatively may occur. Drainage areas are marked on dressings, which are reinforced as needed. In the later postoperative period, a hematoma or frank oozing may occur, resulting in delayed wound healing. Pain, pallor, poor capillary refill, petechiae, cyanosis along the incision, or diffuse mottling of the limb is indicative of ischemia. A severely ischemic residual limb may require additional surgical procedures. Erythema, purulent drainage, or elevated temperature may indicate a wound infection. Minor redness at suture sites may be normal inflammation. Redness and tenderness at the distal part of a transtibial limb may be related to constant knee flexion that presses the limb tip into the mattress.

Edema Control

Reducing postsurgical edema quickly is important to promote wound healing and minimize postoperative pain. Postsurgical edema can stretch a surgical wound and compromise wound healing. Swelling and a bulbous shape to the residual limb also interfere with fitting of a prosthesis and can slow the patient's functional recovery. Although dry sterile dressings are a common means of wound coverage and allow easy access, they offer no control of edema.

Swelling needs to be minimized with an effective compressive dressing. Several edema control systems are used. The most commonly used treatment is elastic wraps on the residual limb. Although elastic wraps can provide effective compression, they need to be applied with good technique and should be changed every 4 hours to maintain consistent compression. Most surgeons leave the first wrap on for 24-48 hours. Effective wrapping provides the tightest compression distally. Figure-of-eight turns encourage proper limb shape and proximal joint extension (Figs. 21-2 and 21-3). The key to successful residual limb care with an elastic bandage is even compression. The ideal wrapping technique avoids circular turns and is without wrinkles. This can be difficult and time consuming for a patient or even the health care team to accomplish. Furthermore, if elastic wraps are applied incorrectly or they are displaced in the normal course of a patient moving around, they can turn into tourniquets, causing pressure wounds and even limb ischemia. Therefore, we do not recommend the use of elastic wrapping as a standard compression system.

Elastic socks (i.e., stump shrinkers) or elastic stockinettes are the preferred soft dressings to be used for compression. Elastic stockinettes (e.g., Compressogrip) can be applied in multiple layers to give graded and increasing compression toward the end of the residual limb (Fig. 21-4). They are easy to don without the need for frequent reapplication and stay on well for most transtibial amputees. For the transfemoral amputee, a waist belt must be included as wraps tend to slide off the conical shaped residual limb (Fig. 21-5).

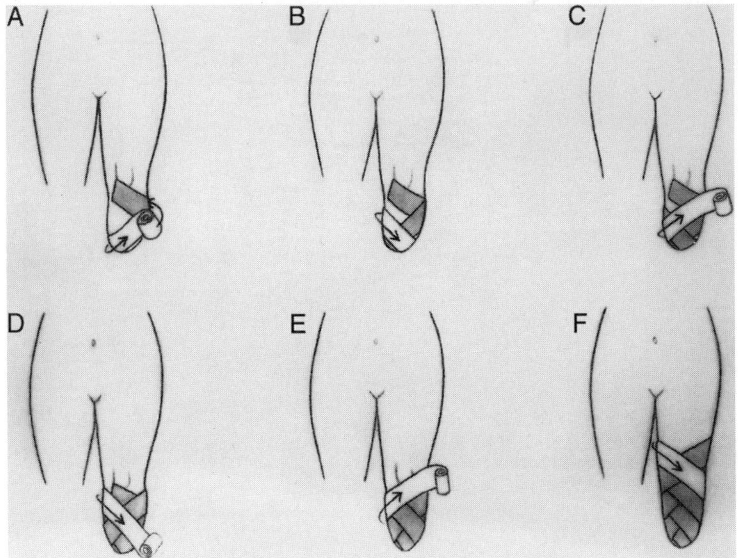

FIG. 21–2. Elastic wrapping of the transtibial residual limb.

Prosthetic elastomeric liners are also being used as compression socks for edema reduction in amputees[27] (Fig. 21-6). They can provide good compression. Some are fairly thick and probably lend some protection to the residual limb. Due to their suction fit, they can be used on the transfemoral amputee without a waist belt. Bony prominences should be closely monitored with any elastic dressing. Pressure can be concentrated on protruding bony areas, leading to skin breakdown. Areas of careful monitoring include the tibial crest and distal tibia in transtibial amputees and the distal femur in transfemoral amputees.

The use of rigid dressings is recommended for transtibial amputees. Rigid dressings help protect the residual limb from inadvertent trauma such as a fall.[28] They provide good compression to minimize edema, and the cast can be conformed to minimize pressure over bony prominences. Weight bearing can also be started through the rigid dressing to help desensitize the limb and build tolerance to pressure. A nonremovable rigid dressing is a cast that is applied over the fully extended residual limb up to the midthigh. This also helps to prevent

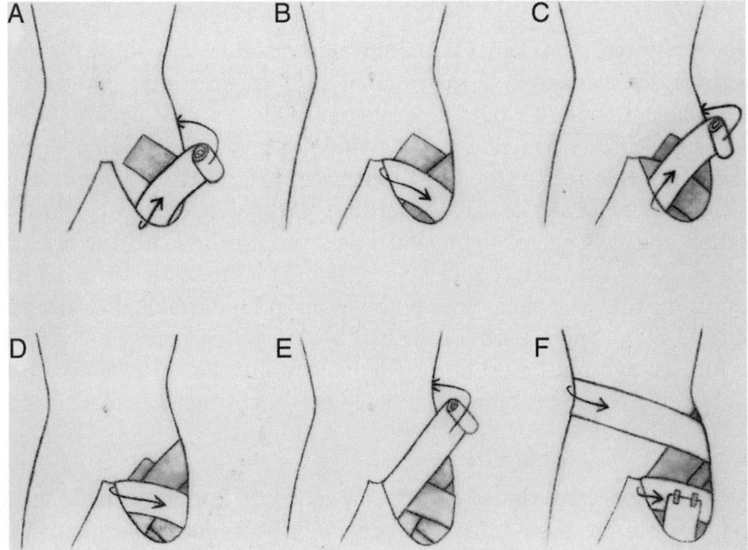

FIG. 21–3. Elastic wrapping of the transfemoral residual limb.

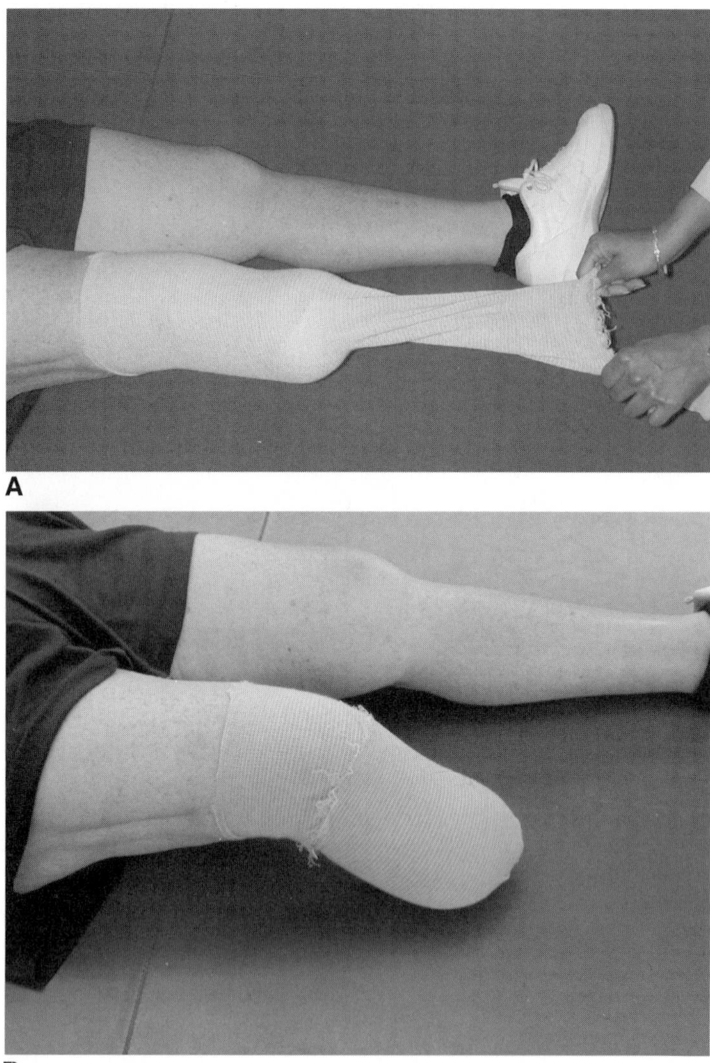

FIG. 21–4. Use of elastic stockinette for the transtibial residual limb. **A,** Place just over half of the length on the limb, and twist one-half turn. **B,** Pull second half over leg to provide two layers of compression.

knee flexion contractures. However, a nonremovable cast does not allow for wound inspection or massage for desensitization of the residual limb except at cast changes.

A rigid removable dressing (RRD)[29] is a custom-made cast that covers the residual limb up to the knee (Fig. 21-7). It is held in place with either elastic stockinette or with a thigh cuff. As the limb shrinks, socks are added underneath the RRD to keep it snug. Shrinker socks and elastic stockinette can be used under the RRD as well. The RRD allows for frequent wound inspection and massage of the residual limb. It also helps to teach patients how to adjust sock ply (i.e., the number of socks worn)—a necessary skill for using most types of prostheses. Our protocol has been to start with a nonrigid removable dressing applied in the operating room. This dressing is used for the first 3-6 days then changed to a rigid removable dressing. The RRD is used until most of the edema is resolved and the wound is well healed. If more than 12-15 ply of sock is required to keep the RRD snug, a new RRD is made.

Pain Issues

Good pain control must be continued postoperatively. It is important that consideration be given to the etiology of the pain. Initially, a generalized residual limb pain is expected secondary to the surgical incision and postoperative edema. This is due to nerve fiber damage and ongoing stimulation of the nerves in the residual limb. This acute pain usually subsides

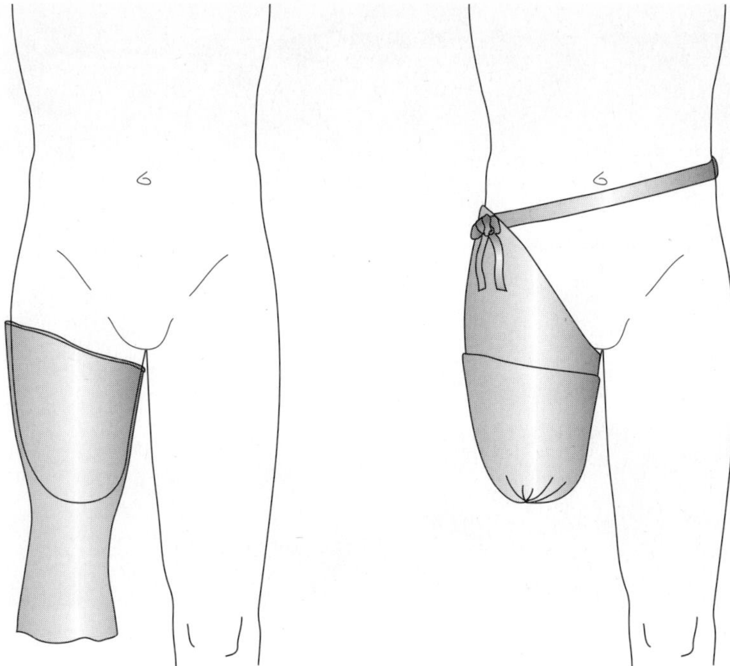

FIG. 21–5. Use of elastic stockinette for transfemoral residual limb. Large stockinette is applied over limb and folded over after twisting one-half turn. The stockinette is then tied onto a waist belt made out of roll of gauze or small-diameter stockinette.

fairly rapidly, and intravenous or intramuscular narcotics can usually be discontinued within 2-3 days. Scheduled doses of oral narcotics should be continued and weaned slowly so that the patient continues to receive adequate pain control, especially during therapy when the patient is more active. Limb swelling compresses and stretches inflamed tissues, including nociceptive fibers, and contributes to postoperative pain. Good limb compression can significantly reduce postoperative edema and pain.

Desensitization techniques should be added to the treatment plan. Patients should be instructed to massage and tap their residual limb within a day or two of surgery. The massage and tapping can be performed through any soft dressing. This gentle stimulation can help to reduce residual limb pain by closing the "pain gate,"[17] and it gives patients a technique for

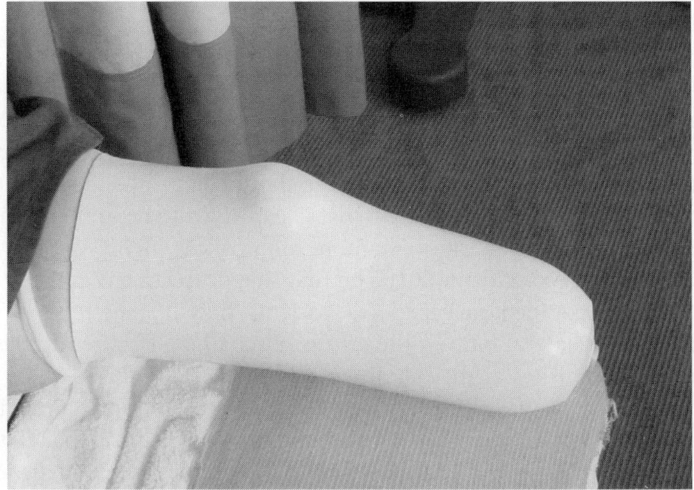

FIG. 21–6. Elastomeric liner for a transtibial amputee.

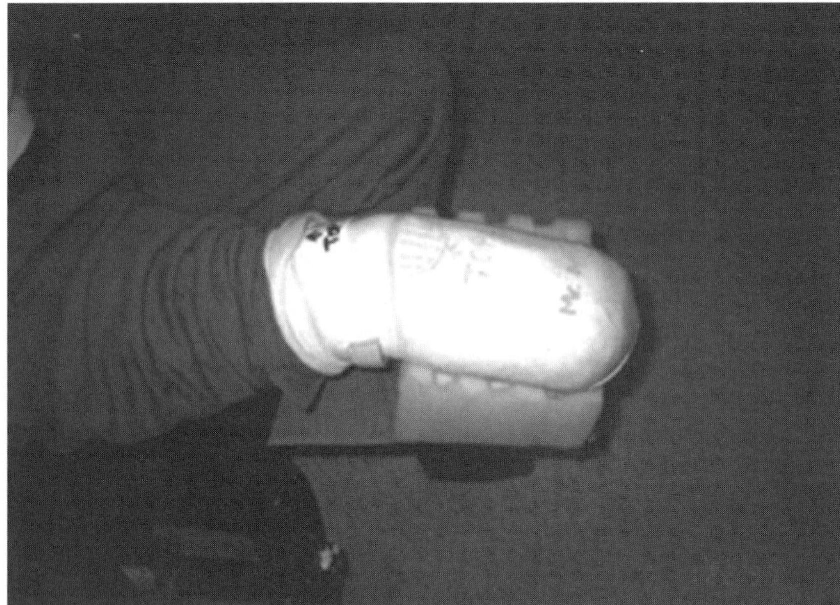

FIG. 21–7. Rigid removable dressing (RRD) for transtibial amputee. RRD is suspended on residual limb with supracondylar cuff.

controlling their pain themselves. Furthermore, self-massage forces patients to attend to their amputation; this can help with their new body image and psychologic adjustment to limb loss.

When generalized residual limb pain does not subside as expected, the patient should be re-evaluated. Wound infection or abscess needs to be ruled out. Continued limb ischemia is possible in patients with arterial occlusive disease and/or diabetes. Poor skin color is often apparent, and frequently the residual limb pain is dependent on the limb's position. In these cases, re-evaluation of arterial blood flow needs to be considered. Over the course of weeks, ischemic pain will often resolve as swelling goes down, the circulation remodels with the decreased distal tissue load, and the limb heals. Sometimes reamputation to a higher level is required. During the interim, the patient needs to continue to receive adequate analgesia, which can be difficult. The patient, the family, and the entire medical team need to be made aware of the plan to wait and see if the residual limb is salvageable.

Phantom limb sensation and phantom limb pain occur to at least some extent in most amputees. Phantom limb sensations are nonpainful "feelings" (cortical sensory illusions) in the part of the limb that is missing. They are perceived in many different ways and are frequently described as tingling, pins and needles, itching, feeling like the foot is asleep, feeling like the toes are moving, or a feeling that the limb is in an awkward position. It is important to ask the patient if the phantom limb sensations are "bothersome." Many times patients will have phantom limb sensations that they do not consider "painful"; however, these sensations can be very annoying, uncomfortable, or interfere with sleep. Phantom limb sensation that is interfering with sleep or diminishing quality of life should be treated like phantom limb pain.

Phantom limb pain is a neuropathic pain that is perceived to be in the portion of the limb that was amputated. The description of phantom limb pain is highly variable: sharp, shooting, electric, stabbing, burning, cramping. The first line of treatment is the use of desensitization techniques as described earlier. Some patients find it beneficial to perform these techniques on the contralateral limb in the area of discomfort. Frequently, patients feel that phantom limb pain diminishes as they start using a prosthesis.

If desensitization techniques are insufficient or the phantom limb pain is interfering significantly with sleep, then pharmacologic treatment should be considered. The two primary categories of medicines used to treat chronic phantom limb phenomenon are antidepressants and anticonvulsants (Table 21-1). Antidepressants have several advantages in addition to

TABLE 21–1 Medication for Phantom Limb Pain

Medication	Mechanism of Action	Primary Side Effects	Cost
ANTIDEPRESSANTS			
Mirtazapine	++ Adrenergic ++ Serotonergic	++ Weight gain + Drowsiness	$$$
Amitriptyline	++ Adrenergic +++ Serotonergic	++ Weight gain ++ Drowsiness +++ Dry mouth	$
Nortriptyline	++ Adrenergic + Serotonergic	+ Weight gain + Drowsiness ++ Dry mouth	$
Doxepin	+ Adrenergic +++ Serotonergic	++ Weight gain +++ Drowsiness +++ Dry mouth	$
Trazodone	++ Serotonergic	++ Drowsiness	$$
ANTICONVULSANTS			
Gabapentin	GABAergic	Drowsiness, ataxia	$$$$
Topiramate	GABAergic Sodium channel blocker Non-NMDA antagonist	Drowsiness, weight loss	$$$$$
Carbamazepine	Membrane stabilization	Drowsiness, aplastic anemia, agranulocytosis	$
Phenytoin	Membrane stabilization	Drowsiness, ataxia, gingivitis	$

NMDA, N-methyl-D-aspartate.

pain control. Obviously, they can also treat depression—a common problem in new amputees. They generally have anxiolytic effects and, some being sedative, can improve sleep. Finally, they are convenient as they are usually taken just once a day. Tricyclic antidepressants have the most anecdotal and empiric support, and they are relatively inexpensive. However, they have undesirable anticholinergic side effects. Mirtazapine is a newer antidepressant with fewer side effects that is useful for the treatment of phantom limb syndrome. A number of anticonvulsants have been used to treat phantom limb pain. Gabapentin is now the most widely used anticonvulsant for the treatment of neuropathic pain syndromes. Side effects are nominal and include sedation and impaired cognition. When needed, the anticonvulsants can be used in combination with the antidepressants or with each other to maximize relief from phantom limb pain. This must be done in a thoughtful fashion to employ complementary mechanisms.

Other nonpharmacologic treatments should also be considered for the treatment of phantom limb syndrome. Stress-relaxation techniques and biofeedback can be helpful in diminishing phantom limb pain. Hypnosis can be used to help a patient "relax" a cramped-feeling phantom limb or move a malpositioned phantom limb.

While the causal relationship between phantom limb pain and amputation is obvious, it is important to remember that other conditions can cause pain in a phantom limb. In trauma patients, proximal nerve injury, plexopathy, radiculopathy, and occult fractures can generate referred pain down the leg even if it has been amputated. Similarly, referred leg pain from knee arthritis, hip arthritis, and spinal stenosis can be mistaken for phantom limb pain. These diagnoses must be considered and will clearly require different treatment plans.

Psychologic Adjustment

The emotional impact of limb loss is devastating, and it is frequently underestimated by health care professionals. Grieving over the loss of one's limb is necessary, and a brief reactive depression is expected. Amputees are at high risk of developing more severe psychologic problems. The incidence of depression is estimated to be 21-35 percent for people with limb loss.[30] Posttraumatic stress disorder (PTSD) is a recognized complication after traumatic amputation, but frequently goes untreated. Nontraumatic amputees can also develop anxiety disorders from the stress related to limb loss.

Nurses are in a unique position to be able to monitor patients' emotional adjustment due to the amount of contact time they have with patients. Patients should be questioned about their mood, appetite, weight changes, quality of sleep, and the occurrence of nightmares. Any correlation between patients' perceived stress level and their pain should be explored. Sometimes adjustment issues will not become problematic until shock/denial diminishes and time passes. Therefore, continued monitoring by the nursing staff is necessary. Chaplain services are an important resource to be used as many patients may find coping through religious or spiritual avenues. Nurses can provide psychologic adjustment in other ways; encouragement about prognosis, providing educational materials, and incorporation of the patient's specific goals into the rehabilitation plan are important. Emphasizing gains made in therapy is also reassuring. Early discussions about prosthetic options with patients will allow them to become involved in the decision-making process about prosthetic components. This not only educates the patient and optimizes the prosthetic prescription, it also helps to empower the patient and give him or her a sense of control.

If resources allow, patients should be encouraged to have an evaluation by an experienced psychologist; it is an important investment in their mental health. This evaluation should include an assessment of mood, pain, other stressors, coping skills, past psychologic problems, alcohol/drug use, body imagine issues, and sexuality. When clinical depression, anxiety disorders, or adjustment disorders are identified, a comprehensive treatment plan should be initiated, including cognitive-behavioral psychotherapy and pharmacotherapy as needed.

Peer counseling and amputee support groups are another important emotional support mechanism. Amputee participation in support groups promotes self-preservation, social acceptance, intimacy, self-expression, and achievement. Acceptance of the amputation can influence the level of activity of the lower-extremity amputee.[31] New amputees learn about circumstances of other amputees (i.e., same etiology, concerns and fears, and initial problems of pain, movement, and body image). Amputee support groups also provide opportunities to obtain resource information such as available community services, possible home adaptations, and the process of rehabilitation. Role models promote independence and share information about organizations that support independent activities such as fishing and golfing. Family participation in the support group activities is also encouraged. The Amputee Coalition of America has a national peer network, provides peer counselor training sessions, and lists amputee support groups by region.

An important component of an organized amputee support group is peer visitation. Amputees participating in a peer visitation program make hospital visits to individuals preoperatively and provide support to new amputees and their families after the surgery. Training for amputees to function as a peer visitor is beneficial and recommended. A successful support group develops a sense of "group ownership" with its participants. Group members gradually become less dependent on the facilitator and other professionals who are involved in the support group. Concurrently, successful support group members initiate plans for activities and use of facilitators and other care providers as resources. Such behaviors reflect successful adjustment to amputation experiences.

Nurses have opportunities to assist with the development of amputee support groups. Because nurses support a holistic approach to care, they are most appropriate to facilitate amputee support groups. Initially, the need for a support group within the institution or community should be assessed. Opportunities for collaboration would typically include physical therapists, occupational therapists, orthotists, prosthetists, chaplains, social workers, psychologists, and patient and family educators.

Functional Rehabilitation

Early rehabilitation management is critical in the postoperative period. Consultation with physiatry, physical therapy, and occupational therapy should begin on the first postoperative day, if not already initiated. Therapy staff will work on a variety of areas such as self-care, bed mobility, transfers, wheelchair skills, ambulation, as well as patient and family teaching. Amputee rehabilitation principles include proper positioning, initiation of range of motion, early mobilization, and evaluation for durable medical equipment and adaptive devices.

Patients should be educated in proper positioning. Common contractures on the amputated side include hip flexion, hip abduction, hip external rotation, and knee flexion. When resting in bed, flexion of the knee and external rotation of the hip is avoided. The residual limb is elevated for only the first[24] postoperative hours. Pillows should not be placed under the knee to prevent knee flexion contractures or between the legs to prevent hip abduction contractures. Patients should be instructed to lie prone several times a day for 10-15 minutes at a time to prevent hip flexion contractures. Individuals who cannot tolerate prone positioning may lie supine on a mat while performing hip extension exercises on their affected limb. Dangling the residual limb over the side of the bed or wheelchair in transtibial amputees should be avoided. In the case of transtibial amputation, a knee extension board (Fig. 21-8) can be fitted underneath the wheelchair or chair to promote knee extension and help prevent dependent edema. The board is usually a sliding board or even a plywood board with distal padding. If knee flexion contractures are of great concern while the patient is in bed, use of a knee immobilizer can maintain knee extension.

Range of motion of the affected limb is an important adjunct to positioning. Active range of motion, strengthening, and conditioning exercises are done slowly three or four times each day. Strengthening of muscles that oppose the common sites of contraction is important; emphasis of exercise on knee and hip extension can help prevent contracture. While supine, adduction and abduction is done at the hip; the knee is flexed and extended; and thighs and buttocks are lifted off the bed. Other important muscles groups include the hip adductors and abductors. Arm strengthening and conditioning is necessary as patients are increasingly reliant on their arms to assist with mobility. Specific exercises include strengthening of wrist and elbow extensors, scapular stabilizers, and latissimus dorsi for use of crutches or a walker.

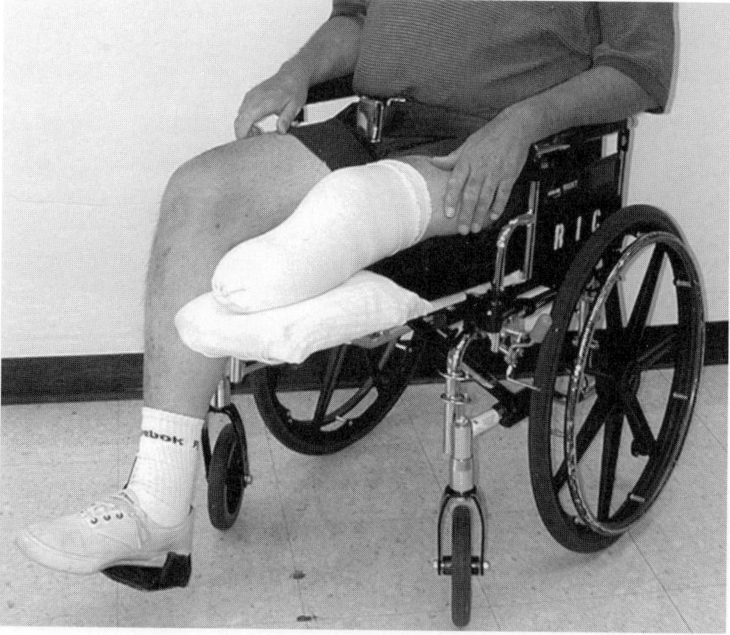

FIG. 21–8. Knee extension board to prevent flexion contracture in transtibial amputee.

Initiation of aerobic exercise is needed to increase endurance and cardiovascular fitness. Upper body ergometry and exercise groups are two examples of aerobic exercise. Adherence to cardiac precautions is important given the high incidence of concomitant cardiovascular disease in individuals with peripheral arterial occlusive disease.

Early mobilization helps to facilitate functional improvements and reduce complications such as pneumonia, thromboembolism, residual limb edema, infection, and loss of balance.[32] Usually the first activities include bed mobility, transfers, and mobilization to a chair or wheelchair. As the patient progresses, the focus should shift to standing and balance exercises in the parallel bars as well as hopping once strength improves. Use of a walker or crutches is the next step in mobilization with the final interventions focusing on curbs, stairs, floor transfers, and community ambulation. Until long-distance independent ambulation is achieved, the patient may be mobile with a wheelchair. The therapist recommends the appropriate type of wheelchair and teaches the patient and the significant other how to operate it safely. Early weight bearing can begin in the first few days if there are no wound complications. For patients with transmetatarsal and toe amputations, wedge shoes can relieve pressure over the forefoot to minimize weight bearing near the incision site (Fig. 21-9). With rigid dressings, patients can perform light weight bearing through their cast using a strap across their wheelchair (Fig. 21-10). When the patient is up in the parallel bars, weight bearing can be done via a tire jack or adjustable footstool (Fig. 21-11). Immediate postoperative prostheses may also be used for early weight bearing as described below. Inspection after weight bearing is important in monitoring wound tolerance of pressure. This is especially important in individuals with amputation from vascular disease or patients with impaired sensation.

Evaluation for appropriate adaptive equipment and durable medical equipment (DME) is also an important aspect. Adaptive devices such as reachers, long handles, sponges, shoehorns, dressing sticks, and sock aids can be issued as needed to assist with activities of daily living. Long-handled mirrors may also be helpful to allow patients to monitor the status of their residual limb easily. Wheelchairs are usually issued to amputees for household and/or long distance locomotion. When sitting in a wheelchair, the amputee's center of gravity is higher and more posterior. Therefore, rear wheels should be set posterior to the chair back, and antitippers should be placed to minimize the risk of tipping backwards and suffering head injury. This is particularly important for transfemoral and bilateral amputees. Other important DME may include shower bench, raised toilet seat, and shower chair.

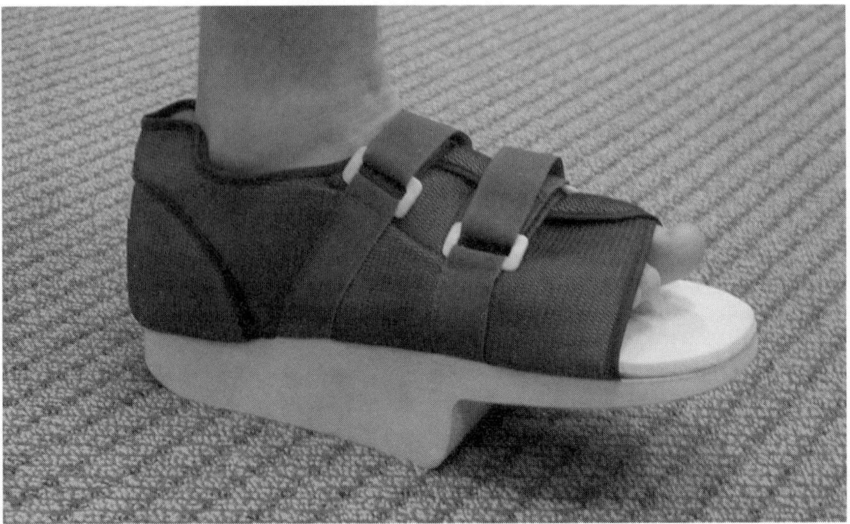

FIG. 21–9. Wedge shoe for the partial foot amputee.

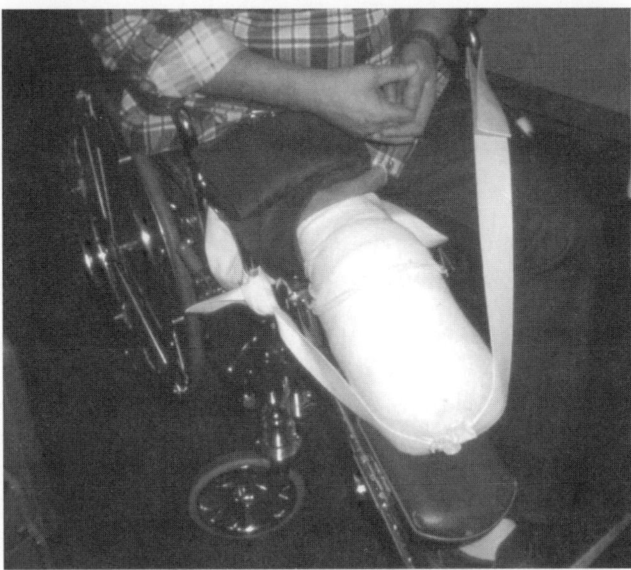

FIG. 21–10. Partial weight bearing with rigid removable dressing on wheelchair strap.

Discharge Planning

Discharge planning should begin on admission. The interdisciplinary team has a responsibility to plan and implement the rehabilitation program and to provide patient education and emotional support until the patient is integrated into the family and community.[33] Variables that impact the length of hospitalization after amputation include comorbidities, status of the incisional wound, presence of postoperative complications, and progress in activities of daily living. Eligibility for support services needs to be considered. The elderly vascular patient is typically on a fixed income with Medicare coverage; however, there may be limitations with Medicare for home care benefits.

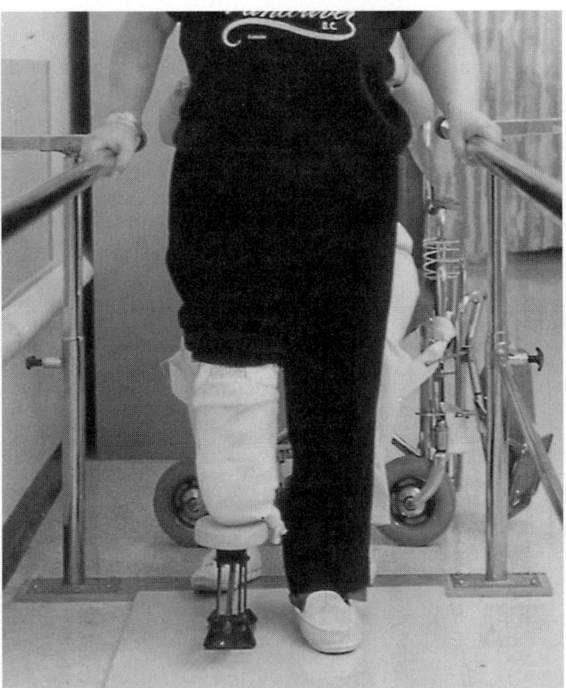

FIG. 21–11. Partial weight bearing with rigid removable dressing on tire jack.

One discharge option is for the patient to go directly home with support services. Prior to discharge, an amputee should be able to transfer from the wheelchair, demonstrate the proposed home exercise program, perform essential activities of daily living independently, and, if possible, safely ambulate short distances independently with a walker or crutches.[34] In this situation, patient teaching is reinforced for a home exercise program, residual limb care, foot care, and medications. Equipment needs are identified in conjunction with rehabilitation therapy staff, and equipment procurement is arranged. Referral to a home health care agency is routine to ease the transition back to normal activities. The home care nurse, occupational therapist, and physical therapist ensure continuity of the rehabilitation plan, monitor the patient's progress, evaluate the home for safety, provide emotional support, and serve as resource personnel. If needed, a home health aide can assist with personal care needs; this provides some relief of caregiver burden to the family.

Another alternative is a direct transfer to an acute rehabilitation center or subacute rehabilitation facility. Patients with amputations can usually be admitted to a rehabilitation unit about 3-7 days after amputation when any drains are out, their pain is under control, and they have the endurance to participate in a comprehensive rehabilitation program. Patients usually stay in an acute rehabilitation facility 1-3 weeks before discharge. Usually, prosthetic fitting is not done in this setting for the vascular patient. Direct transfer to a skilled nursing facility with rehabilitation services for an extended period of time may best serve the needs of patients who have long-term care needs and are unable to live independently. This could be a temporary situation until the residual limb is ready for a prosthesis and would include prosthetic gait training.

Individuals with amputation still drive a car, and most will use a car as their means of transportation in the community. Patients should be referred to the Motor Vehicle Department for information regarding a handicapped person's parking permit and validation of the driving license. This may require a driving test for some amputees. If necessary, the car can be adapted with hand controls. The three major U.S. car manufacturers (GM, Ford, and Chrysler) have programs to support adaptive equipment needed for automobiles and vans.

PROSTHETICS

Candidacy for prosthetic fitting is dependent on several factors such as medical comorbidities, premorbid functional status, age, and cognitive impairment. In a retrospective study by Johnson, Kondqiela, and Gottschalk,[35] the authors concluded that regardless of age, patients with more medical problems had poor ambulation. Thus, age alone should not determine prosthetic rehabilitation.[32] Any person previously walking (or a potential walker) should be considered for a trial of prosthetic fitting.[36] Also, incorporating new skills necessary for using a prosthesis requires the ability to understand and follow instructions. Cognitive abilities such as procedural learning and memory, attention and concentration, and problem solving are skills involved in using and maintaining a prosthesis.[37] Intellectual impairment is a prime cause of failure in rehabilitation programs.[36] If the patient has reliable caregivers who can be trained, they may assist the patient in prosthetic management.

The level of amputation is also important as the energy expenditure required to ambulate per unit distance increases with the level of amputation. Toe and partial foot amputation have very little increased energy expenditure. However, the transtibial amputee expends 25-40 percent more energy than normal individuals; the transfemoral amputee's energy expenditure can be as high as 100 percent above normal.[38] The decision for prosthetic fitting is ideally performed in a multidisciplinary amputee clinic with rehabilitation physicians, therapists, and prosthetists.

Once a patient is deemed a candidate for prosthetic use, the rehabilitation team must determine when to fit with a prosthesis. The residual limb needs to have a cylindrical shape and a good start in healing (although it does not need to be completely healed prior to active prosthetic training). In general, this may take place as early as 3-4 weeks postoperatively in individuals with amputation from arterial insufficiency or up to 6-10 weeks if there is significant eschar or slow wound healing.[39] Full range of motion in the leg is desirable for ambulation with a prosthesis. Other considerations include patient motivation, strength, previous functional level, and the condition of the contralateral leg. Actual prosthetic components and fitting are beyond the scope of this chapter.

Occasionally, patients may be fitted with an immediate postoperative prosthesis (IPOP). IPOPs allow patients to bear some or all of their weight through the residual limb and prosthesis, thus promoting prosthetic ambulation within a few days after surgery (Fig. 21-12). Advocates contend that this allows for decreased edema, prevention of flexion deformities, faster functional recovery, and better psychologic adjustment.[40-42,22] IPOPs have some potential disadvantages that must be considered. Some studies have shown an increase in wound dehiscence and infection with these devices.[43] Frequently, the residual limb is too tender and painful to allow early weight bearing to take full advantage of these devices. The devices are also relatively expensive, and certain models have limited weight-bearing capabilities. Finally, with the nonremovable IPOPs, the patients are unable to inspect or massage their residual limbs.

CONCLUSION

The needs of the amputee patient are complex. The vascular nurse can help coordinate the services of the vascular surgery staff with the rehabilitation team in implementing an effective treatment plan in these patients. With appropriate rehabilitation intervention in the perioperative period, individuals with amputation can maximize their physical and functional potential as well as psychologic adjustment to their limb loss.

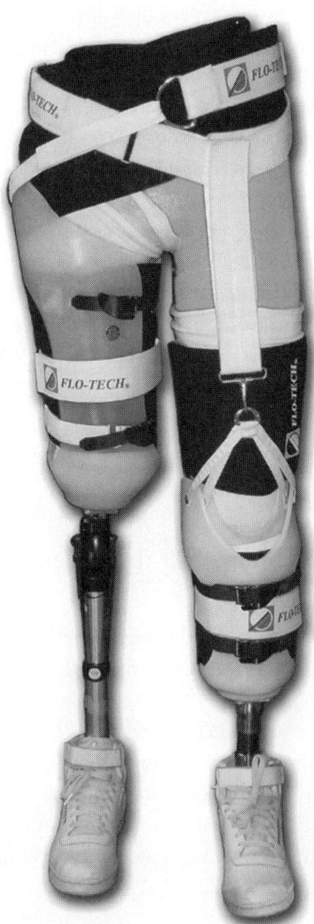

FIG. 21–12. Examples of prefabricated immediate postoperative prostheses. (Courtesy FLO-TECH, Trumansville, New York.)

REFERENCES

1. American Orthotic and Prosthetic Association: *You can make a difference in people's lives: becoming an orthotist or prosthetist*, Alexandria, Va, 1995, Orthotics and Prosthetics National Office.
2. VanHoutum MH, Lavery LA: Outcomes associated with diabetes-related amputations in the Netherlands and in the state of California, USA, *J Intern Med* 240:227-231, 1996.
3. Fylling CP, Knighton DR: Amputation in the diabetic population: incidence, causes, cost, treatment, and prevention, *J Enterostomal Ther* 16:247-255, 1989.
4. Reiber GE: Who is at risk of limb loss and what to do about it? *J Rehabil Res Dev* 31:357-362, 1994.
5. Humphrey LL, Palumbo PJ, Butters MA et al: The contribution of non-insulin dependent diabetes to lower extremity amputation in the community, *Arch Intern Med* 154:885-892, 1994.
6. Hallett JW, Byrne J, Gayari MM et al: Impact of arterial surgery and balloon angioplasty on amputation: a population-based study of 1155 procedures between 1973 and 1992, *J Vasc Surg* 25:29-38, 1997.
7. Bacharach JM, Rooke TW, Osmundson PJ et al: Predictive value of transcutaneous oxygen pressure and amputation success by use of supine and elevation measurements, *J Vasc Surg* 15:558-563, 1992.
8. Dwars BJ, van den Broek TA, Rauwerda JA et al: Criteria for reliable selection of the lowest level of amputation in peripheral vascular disease, *J Vasc Surg* 15:536-542, 1992.
9. Kay HW, Newman JD: Relative incidence of new amputations, *Orthot Prosthet* 29(2):3-16, 1975.
10. Burgess EM, Romano RL: The management of lower extremity amputees using immediate post-surgical prostheses, *Clin Orthop* 57:137-146, 1968.
11. Waters R, Perry J, Antonelli D et al: Energy cost of walking of amputees: the influence of level of amputation, *J Bone Joint Surg* 1:42-46, 1976.
12. Ouriel K, Green RM: Arterial disease. In Schwartz SI, Shires CT, Spencer FC, et al, eds; *Principles of surgery*, ed 7, Philadelphia, 1999, McGraw-Hill, pp 931-1003.
13. Scully SP, Harrelson JM: Amputation and limb substitution. In Sabiston DC, ed: *Textbook of surgery: the biological basis of modern surgical practice*, ed 15, Philadelphia, 1997, WB Saunders, pp 1452-1458.
14. Silver-Thorn MB, Childress DS: Parametric analysis using the finite element method to investigate prosthetic interface stresses for persons with trans-tibial amputation, *J Rehabil Res Dev* 33:227-238, 1996.
15. Houghton AD, Taylor PR, Thurlow S et al: Success rates for rehabilitation of vascular amputees: implications for preoperative assessment and amputation level, *Br J Surg* 79:753-755, 1992.
16. Gottschalk F: Transfemoral amputation. In Bowker JH, Michael JW, eds: *The atlas of limb prosthetics: surgical, prosthetic, and rehabilitation principles*, ed 2, St Louis, 1992, Mosby, pp 509-533.
17. Melzack R, Wall PD: Pain mechanisms: a new theory, *Science* 150:971-979, 1965.
18. Bennet G: Neuropathic pain. In Wall P, Melzack R, eds: *Textbook of pain*, Edinburgh, 1994, Churchill Livingstone, pp 201-224.
19. Devor M: The pathophysiology of damaged peripheral nerves. In Wall P, Melzack R, eds: *Textbook of pain*, Edinburgh, 1994, Churchill Livingstone, pp 79-100.
20. Melzack R: The tragedy of needless pain, *Science* 262:27-33, 1990.
21. Bach S, Noreng MF, Tjellden NU: Phantom limb pain in amputees during the first 12 months following limb amputation, after preoperative lumbar epidural blockade, *Pain* 33:297-301, 1988.
22. Moore WS, Hall AD, Wylie EJ: Below-knee amputation for vascular insufficiency, *Arch Surg* 7:886-893, 1968.
23. Gauthier-Gagnon C, Grise MC, Potvin D: Enabling factors related to prosthetic use by people with transtibial and transfemoral amputation, *Arch Phys Med Rehabil* 80(6):706-713, 1999.
24. Ng D, Berbrayer EK, Hunter GA et al: Transtibial amputation: preoperative vascular assessment and functional outcome, *J Prosthet Orthot* 8(4):123-129, 1996.
25. Pinzur MS, Littooy F, Daniels J et al: Multidisciplinary preoperative assessment and late function in dysvascular amputees, *Clin Orthop* 281:239-243, 1992.
26. Eneroth M: *Improved wound healing in transtibial amputees receiving supplementary nutrition*. Presented at IX World Congress of the International Society of Prosthetics and Orthotics, Amsterdam, Netherlands, June 28-July 3, 1998.
27. Larsson GU: *Post-operative treatment with silicone liner in 176 amputees*. Presented at X World Congress of the International Society of Prosthetics and Orthotics, Glasgow, Scotland, July 1-6, 2001.
28. English R: *Removable rigid dressing for transtibial amputees: a randomized study*. Presented at X World Congress of the International Society of Prosthetics and Orthotics, Glasgow, Scotland, July 1-6, 2001.
29. Wu Y, Keagy RD, Krick HJ et al: An innovative removable rigid dressing technique for below-the-knee amputation, *J Bone Joint Surg Am* 61(5):724-729, 1979.
30. Rybarczyk B, Nicholas JJ, Nyenhuis DL: Coping with a leg amputation: integrating research and clinical practice, *Rehabil Psychol* 42(3):241-256, 1997.

31. Medhat A, Huber PM, Medhat MA: Factors that influence the level of activity in persons with lower extremity amputation, *Rehabil Nurs* 15:13-18, 1990.
32. Cutson TM, Bongiorni D, Michael JW et al: Early management of elderly dysvascular below-knee amputees, *J Prosthet Orthot* 6(3):62-66, 1994.
33. Esquenazi A, Meier RH: Rehabilitation in limb deficiency. IV. Limb amputation, *Arch Phys Med Rehabil* 77:S18-S28, 1996.
34. Andrews KL: Rehabilitation in limb deficiency. III. The geriatric amputee, *Arch Phys Med Rehabil* 77:S14-S17, 1996.
35. Johnson VJ, Kondqiela S, Gottschalk F: Pre- and post-amputation mobility of trans-tibial amputees: correlation to medical problems, age, and mortality, *Prosthet Orthot Int* 19:159-164, 1995.
36. Penington GR: Benefits of rehabilitation in the presence of advanced age or severe disability, *Med J Aust* 157:665-666, 1992.
37. Phillips NA, Mate-Kole C, Kirby RL: Neuropsychological function in peripheral vascular disease amputee patients, *Arch Phys Med Rehabil* 74:1309-1304, 1993.
38. Czerniecki JM. Rehabilitation in limb deficiency. I. Gait and motion analysis, *Arch Phys Med Rehabil* 77:S3-S8, 1996.
39. Leonard JA Jr, Meier RH III: Upper and lower limb prosthetics. In Delisa JA, Gans BM, eds: *Rehabilitation medicine: principles and practice*, ed 3, Philadelphia, 1998, Lippincott-Raven, pp 669-696.
40. Burgess EM, Romano RL, Zettl JH: Amputee management utilizing immediate postsurgical prosthetic fitting, *Prosthet Orthot Int* 3(3):28-37, 1969.
41. Compere CL: Early fitting of prostheses following amputation, *Surg Clin North Am* 48:215-226, 1968.
42. Russek AS: Immediate postsurgical fitting of the lower extremity amputee: research experience with 175 cases, *Med Clin North Am* 53:665-676, 1969.
43. Cohen SI, Goldman LD, Salzman EW et al: The deleterious effects of immediate post-operative prostheses in below knee amputation for ischemic disease, *Surgery* 76:992-1001, 1974.

22

Vascular Trauma

RICHARD R. KEEN

SCOPE OF THE PROBLEM

The effects of trauma on our society are substantial. Trauma remains the leading cause of death for individuals under the age of 40 and the fourth leading cause of death overall.[1] Every year in the United States, approximately 150,000 people die from a traumatic event. Central nervous system trauma and cardiovascular injuries are the number one and number two causes of traumatic deaths in the United States. Furthermore, trauma results in another approximately 400,000 Americans sustaining permanent disability every year. Clearly, the impact on our society in terms of lost productivity, an impaired quality of life, a significant emotional toll, and total health care costs is substantial. These factors bring the total cumulative costs of trauma to our society to over 100 billion dollars per year.[2]

Vascular trauma makes up a major component of all traumatic injuries. Acute and long-term results are optimal when these traumas are treated by experienced surgeons at specialized trauma centers. Regardless of the ability of the surgeon and the appropriate and prompt treatment of these patients, many of these traumatic vascular injuries result in death or serious, permanent disability. On the other hand, cardiovascular injuries also can be the most dramatic injuries that can be successfully treated, in which 100 percent recovery of the patient is possible.

A number of patient issues make nursing of vascular trauma patients especially challenging. First, while vascular problems most commonly are encountered in a mature patient population, the majority of trauma patients are younger, with a median age of only 30 years. Regardless of the cause of the vascular problem and any possible perceived lack of appreciation by the patient, professionalism is essential in the management of all patients with a vascular injury. This person needs the undivided attention of the health care staff.

Second, the traumatic event that brought the patient to the hospital is, by its nature, "unexpected" for both the patient and the staff. This unexpected component increases exponentially the stress level for all parties. Vascular trauma patients are usually completely healthy up until the time of their trauma event, so they are not prepared for the implications of significant medical and nursing care.

Third, things happen very fast. This emergency setting requires a different level of preparedness. If one is not prepared, the urgency and seriousness of the situation can result in adverse outcomes for the patient. For the nurse who is not used to caring for trauma patients, this process can be emotionally and physically draining. All of these stressful factors can make the care of vascular trauma patients very difficult.

The purpose of this chapter is to provide nursing professionals with the information needed to recognize vascular injuries and provide the appropriate care. Vascular nurses play an extremely important role in the excellent outcomes that can occur in these patients.

PRINCIPLES OF TRAUMA

Vascular trauma usually does not occur in isolation. The patients who sustain vascular injuries often incur associated injuries, either in the same or a different body region, that may be even more urgent or life-threatening than the acute vascular problem. The order in which trauma problems are dealt with follows the principles of the "ABCs": airway, breathing, and circulation.

A secure airway is the first problem addressed. If the patient's airway is compromised by unconsciousness, a cervicothoracic injury, or hemodynamic instability, the patient needs either endotracheal intubation or a tracheotomy. This always needs to be the first procedure that is performed.

The next step is to ensure that ventilation is taking place through the secure airway. Besides the ventilation that takes place through an endotracheal tube, ventilation that takes place in the nonintubated patient by the patient's own spontaneous breathing can be supplemented with manual bagging or masking. Supplemental oxygen is provided as necessary to keep the oxygen saturation above 92 percent.

Circulation is addressed only after the airway is secured and ventilation is adequate. The reason for this sequence is that the essential function of our circulatory system is to deliver oxygen and remove carbon dioxide from our bodies. Delivery of oxygen is essential for cell function. Cell death, multisystem organ failure, and patient death will follow without tissue oxygenation. If ventilation and oxygenation are not adequate, little will be accomplished in a trauma patient by controlling hemorrhage or delivery of a circulatory blood volume that is devoid of oxygen.

Circulation consists of two components: tissue perfusion and hemorrhage or bleeding. Two large-bore (14, 16, or 18 gauge) intravenous lines are inserted into the extremities. If the circulatory volume of the trauma victim is compromised, buffered lactated Ringer's intravenous solutions, buffered polymerized starch solutions, or blood products are infused rapidly as circulatory system volume expanders. (Buffered saline products are superior to unbuffered normal saline.) Adequacy of the patient's circulatory volume must be maintained while the source of any bleeding is addressed.

STRATEGIES FOR VASCULAR TRAUMA MANAGEMENT

In the setting of a vascular injury with severe hemorrhage, all attempts are made to stop the bleeding as quickly as possible. For extremity vascular injuries, the best method to control bleeding usually is pressure applied directly to the area that contains the injured vessel. Even if this does not completely stop the bleeding, it will usually slow down the rate of bleeding significantly. This technique involves pushing the base of the palm of a gloved hand directly and forcefully to the area of bleeding. Direct pressure also can be effective for injuries to the neck once the airway is secured. For vascular injuries to the extremities, tourniquets can be used. However, tourniquets should be used only when direct pressure will not control the bleeding and the patient will exsanguinate without the tourniquet. The principle of "life over limb" applies here. Applying a tourniquet not only stops the bleeding but also stops the circulation (the C of the ABCs) and delivery of oxygen to the tissues in that injured extremity. This maneuver of tourniquet application results in warm circulatory arrest to the extremity and can lead to irreversible limb disability after approximately 3 hours.

The acute injuries that are most commonly life threatening are traumas to the head, the chest, the abdomen, and the pelvis. One reason is that direct pressure can be unsuccessful in halting blood loss in these locations. Balloon catheters (such as a large Foley catheter) may be placed into an extraluminal space and help tamponade bleeding in instances when direct pressure is not possible. This technique is used most commonly near the cervicothoracic inlet, where the neck joins the chest. An alternative technique is to insert a gloved finger inside the body cavity through the traumatic wound tract to compress a bleeding vessel against an underlying or overlying bony structure. Examples of this maneuver include compressing the subclavian vessels against the clavicle and compressing the femoral vessels against the pubic bone.

A series of x-ray exams may be essential in delineating the extent of any associated injuries. A chest x-ray is mandatory for evaluating any cervicothoracic trauma (Fig. 22-1). Cervical spine injuries need to be excluded with c-spine x-rays and a computed tomography

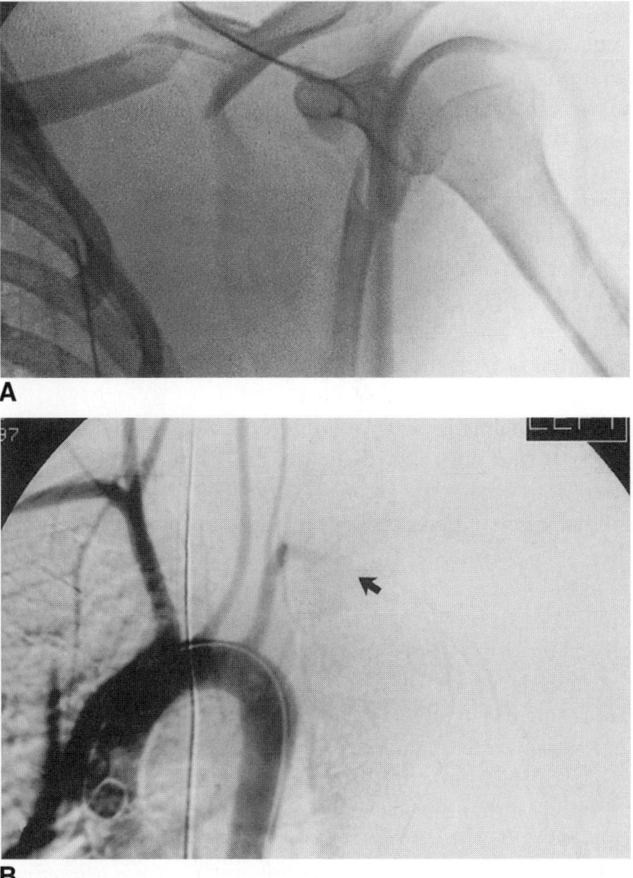

FIG. 22–1. A, Left acromioclavicular dissociation (shoulder-collarbone separation) following a motor vehicle crash. **B,** Upper extremity arteriography demonstrates subclavian artery thrombosis beyond the origin of the left vertebral artery *(arrow)*. The arterial injury was repaired with an interposition saphenous vein graft from the left subclavian artery to the left axillary artery. Left forearm fasciotomy also was performed. A severe concomitant brachial plexus injury limited the functional recovery of the extremity.

(CT) scan if needed as early as possible. An anterior-posterior pelvis x-ray is required to exclude pelvic fractures when this injury is possible.

The neurologic exam is an extremely important component of the initial assessment of the patient with vascular injuries. Both central nervous system deficits due to injuries of the brain or spinal cord and extremity neurologic deficits due to injuries of the nerve roots or peripheral nerves need to be noted. Neurologic injuries accompany nearly 50 percent of all upper-extremity vascular injuries. This is because a large number of upper-extremity nerves, including the brachial plexus and its branches, lie in close proximity to the blood vessels of the upper extremity. A detailed neurologic assessment should be performed if possible before any sedatives or paralytic agents are administered. This exam, which ideally is performed on the initial presentation, should be well documented and include any neurologic deficits. If the extremity neurologic exam cannot be completed because the patient is unconscious, or if no function of the injured extremity is observed, this should be well documented. Examining the unconscious patient who cannot provide a history or specific complaints requires a high level of diligence in order to recognize what could be serious vascular injuries. Thorough documentation can protect the health care provider from subsequent litigation.

Signs of a vascular injury are considered "hard" or "soft." "Hard signs" that provide direct evidence of a significant arterial injury include signs of arterial occlusion (the six Ps: pulseless, polar (cold), pallor, paresthesia, paralysis, and pain), arterial bleeding, rapidly expanding hematoma, and a palpable thrill or audible bruit.

"Soft signs" of an occult vascular injury include ecchymosis, a history of active bleeding at the accident scene, an injury in close proximity to a major vessel, soft tissue swelling or a nonexpanding hematoma, or a neurologic deficit. Soft signs of a vascular injury should not be ignored and classically have been an indication for exclusion arteriography in order to rule out a vascular injury.[3] A potential vascular injury that is not looked for may not be discovered until it presents itself as a catastrophe. Any of these "soft signs" should be documented and, more importantly, the responsible physician notified.

The pulse exam is notable in its propensity for being unreliable and even incorrect. The examiner may feel his or her own pulse rather than that of the patient. A finding of a normal pulse exam only should be noted if the examiner is absolutely sure of these findings. A false-positive pulse exam, where the examiner believes that pulses are present when in fact they are not, will lead to delayed diagnoses, missed vascular injuries, and ultimately, adverse patient outcomes.

A Doppler exam that documents arterial flow in the distal extremity arteries, including the radial, ulnar, dorsal pedal, and posterior tibial arteries, is a more accurate test for assessing the adequacy of the patient's circulation than a pulse exam. This baseline Doppler exam is extremely important for future reference in detecting any changes in the patient's vascular exam. If there is any change in the patient's Doppler exam or pulse exam, a vascular injury, which may have been missed on the initial assessment, now should be suspected and investigated.

All bone fractures need to be diagnosed with x-rays as early as possible. Ideally, these x-rays should be performed prior to transportation of the patient outside the emergency department. When the patient is moved in the setting of unrecognized or unstable extremity fractures, injury can result to any vessels that may lie in close proximity to fractured bones. This outcome is not accepted as it violates the principle of "first do no harm." With both extremity fractures and dislocations, the vascular exam should be noted both before and after the orthopedic reduction. Either splints or extremity traction usually can be applied in the emergency department.

Some vascular injuries are life or limb threatening but not immediately obvious. This includes traumatic rupture of the aorta (Fig. 22-2). The diagnosis of these vascular injuries often is not possible without imaging modalities such as ultrasound, CT scan, and arteriography. For trauma victims, ultrasound can be performed by the physician in the emergency department, but often this test needs to be performed in the radiology suite. The efficacy of this technique in diagnosing vascular injuries is limited by the pain induced by the ultrasound transducer pressed against the body. Patients usually are not very cooperative for duplex scanning in the setting of acute extremity trauma.

Less patient cooperation is needed to complete the imaging tests, CT scan, and arteriography. However, the patient may receive some degree of sedation when undergoing a CT scan or arteriography in the radiology suite. All attempts should be made to stabilize the patient's airway, breathing, and circulation before any diagnostic exams are completed outside the emergency department. If these tests are absolutely essential, and everything has been done to stabilize the patient, then these diagnostic tests should be completed as expeditiously as possible.

CLASSIFICATION AND MECHANISMS OF INJURIES

Vascular injuries can be classified as caused by penetrating, blunt, or iatrogenic trauma. Penetrating trauma consists predominantly of gunshot wounds, shotgun wounds, stab wounds, and impaled objects such as glass and bone fragments. Blunt trauma consists primarily of motor vehicle accidents, pedestrian–motor vehicle collisions, athletic injuries, and falls. Iatrogenic vascular traumas are secondary or incidental injuries resulting from diagnostic or therapeutic procedures. Examples include postcatheterization femoral pseudoaneurysms and dissections.

In major trauma centers in countries such as the United States where firearms are readily available, the majority of vascular injuries are due to penetrating trauma. The approximate fre-

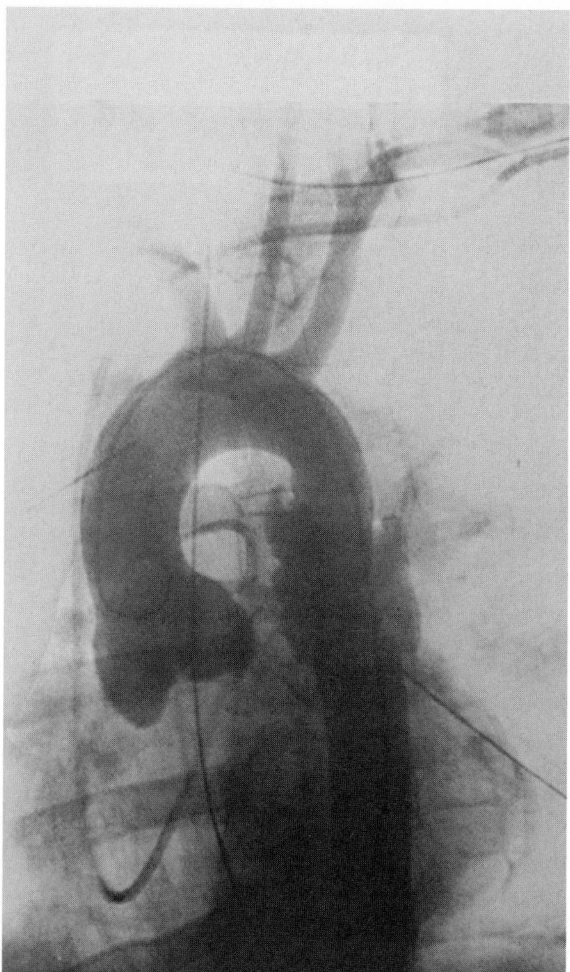

FIG. 22–2. Thoracic aortography demonstrating traumatic rupture of the aorta (TRA). Rapid deceleration injuries cause the internal organs to continue to move forward within the body cavities even after the body has stopped moving. Examples of deceleration injuries include motor vehicle crashes and falls from two or more stories. The thoracic aorta is fixed at the ligamentum arteriosum near the origin of the left subclavian artery. The body stops moving with the rapidly stopping vehicle and when the body hits the ground, but momentum causes the unrestrained descending thoracic aorta to continue to pull forward, causing the thoracic aorta to tear at its fixed location.

quency distribution for the injury mechanism in vascular trauma is 50 percent gunshot wounds, 10 percent stab wounds, 10 percent shotgun wounds, 20 percent blunt injuries, and less than 2 percent iatrogenic injuries.[4,5] A vessel does not need to come into direct contact with the penetrating missile in order to be injured. A "blast effect" can occur, whereby the energy that is released and dissipated from the missile after it enters the tissue causes the vascular injury. Large-caliber, fast-moving missiles deliver greater energy to the tissues and, therefore, cause greater damage than slower-moving, smaller bullets and are more likely to cause blast injuries.

Blunt injuries can be caused by forces that decelerate, crush, stretch, shear, or compress tissues. Just as with penetrating injuries, the amount of energy delivered to the internal tissues in the vicinity of the blood vessel is the critical determinant as to whether a significant vascular injury occurs. As energy is dissipated within the body, the blood vessel can become displaced and the injury occurs. Vascular structures that are attached to musculoskeletal structures, such as the internal carotid artery at the skull base and the thoracic aorta at the ligamentum arteriosum and the diaphragm, or are adjacent to unprotected bony structures, such as the popliteal artery at the knee, are most susceptible to vascular injury due to blunt mechanisms.[6]

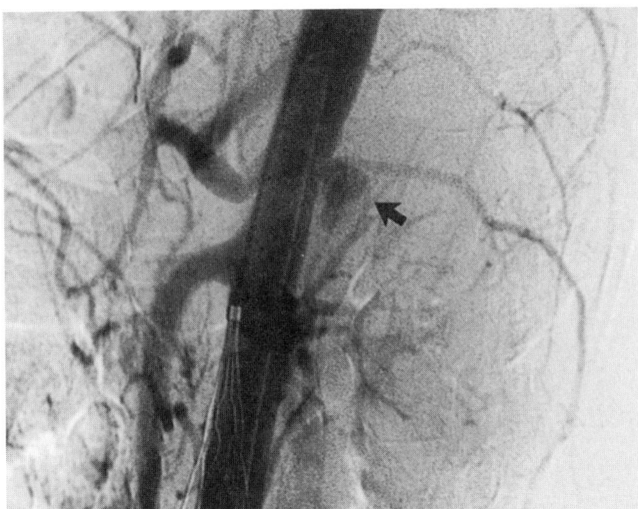

FIG. 22–3. Pseudoaneurysm of the abdominal aorta *(arrow)* seen on abdominal aortography at the level of the celiac artery, secondary to a transabdominal gunshot wound.

The types of vascular injuries include complete or partial transactions, intimal injuries, thromboses, arteriovenous (AV) fistulae, arterial spasm, and pseudoaneurysms (Fig. 22-3). Profound ischemia can be caused by a complete transection of an injured vessel, especially if the trauma has compromised the collateral circulation in the region of the injury. Ischemia can occur as a result of distal embolization of fresh clot that forms in the lumen of the injured vessel. Complete arterial transections do not always result in persistent bleeding. Oftentimes, the transected artery goes into arterial spasm and undergoes thrombosis, which may limit the amount of continued bleeding. Large veins do not have the same degree of circumferential smooth muscle and therefore are unable to go into spasm as their associated arteries do. Large veins are dependent on tamponade and thrombosis to limit continued bleeding following complete transections. Pressure is effective in controlling the bleeding from venous injuries until these injuries can be repaired.

Intimal injuries can be caused either by crushing the vessel with an external force or by stretching of the vessel (Fig. 22-4). These mechanisms are the cause of popliteal artery injuries associated with posterior knee dislocations. Arteriovenous fistulae require simultaneous injuries to arteries and veins that lie in close proximity. AV fistulae usually are seen only with penetrating trauma. Pseudoaneurysms can be asymptomatic and are the most common type of significant missed injury. Intimal injuries, where the outer adventitial strength layer of the artery is spared, can be observed and not treated if the injury involves less than 50 percent of the vessel's circumference.

LOCATION OF INJURIES AND MANAGEMENT

The location of traumatic vascular injuries can be classified as (1) cervicothoracic, (2) abdominal and pelvic, and (3) extremity. For cervicothoracic trauma, the vascular structures that can be involved include the carotid arteries and jugular veins, the great vessels of the chest including the innominate and subclavian arteries and veins, and the intrathoracic aorta and superior vena cava.[7] These injuries are the most life threatening and require immediate operative treatment.

Median sternotomy with or without clavicle resection or neck exploration is the operative approach most favored by experienced vascular trauma surgeons when approaching cervicothoracic vascular trauma. Not all injuries are approached with open operations. Injuries to the vertebral arteries usually are treated with catheter embolization techniques. Associated injuries are common with cervicothoracic trauma and include cervical and thoracic spine

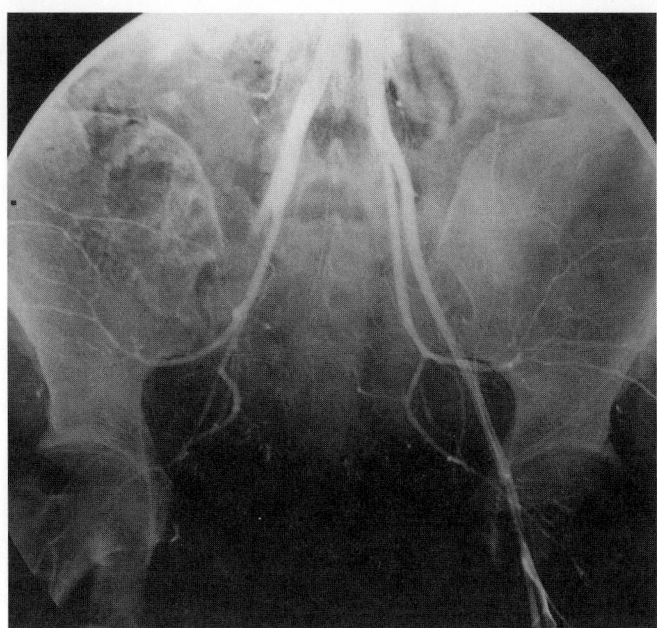

FIG. 22–4. Crush injury to the right iliac artery following a motor vehicle crash. Pelvic arteriography demonstrates complete occlusion of the right external iliac artery due to acute compression and shearing of the external iliac artery at the time of the crash between the victim's seat belt and the pelvic bone.

injuries and injuries to the esophagus, lung, and heart. Cardiac injuries can present as pericardial tamponade (Beck's triad of hypotension, jugular venous distention, and muffled heart sounds) and are treated with pericardiocentesis followed by urgent pericardial window, and direct cardiac repair if indicated.

The intraabdominal vessels that can be injured with abdominal and pelvic trauma include the abdominal aorta and vena cava, the mesenteric arteries and veins, and the iliac arteries and veins. These injuries usually require immediate operative attention via midline celiotomy. Common associated injuries seen with abdominal and pelvic trauma include injuries to the liver, spleen, kidneys, and bowel. Bone injuries include lumbar spine and pelvic fractures. Retroperitoneal hemorrhage associated with pelvic fractures is not always explored in the operating room. Catheter-directed embolization in the angiography suite often is used to control bleeding from internal iliac artery branches that have been injured at the time of the pelvic fracture.

Operative repair of injured upper-extremity and lower-extremity arteries and associated veins is common. In fact, extremity vascular injuries are the most frequent type of traumatic injury seen by vascular nurses.

The type of vascular repair that is performed usually depends upon the location and the extent of the injury. Injuries to vessels that cross a joint, injuries that have an extensive soft tissue component such as shotgun wounds, and gunshot wounds usually require repair with an interposition graft using either a vein interposition graft or a prosthetic conduit. Whenever possible, an autogenous conduit is preferable.[5] Techniques for repair include primary repair, vein or prosthetic patch repair, interposition graft repair with autogenous vein or prosthetic conduit, and more recently, repair with covered stent grafts.[8] Profunda femoral artery injuries often are treated with transcatheter embolization.

Repair of all injured extremity arteries and veins is encouraged unless the extremity is not viable or functional or if the attempted repair could compromise the patient's survival. In these cases, immediate amputation is indicated. The incidence of amputation is greatest following popliteal artery injuries, where the overall rate of limb loss still approaches 10 percent.[6]

Treatment may be region specific. For example, some vascular injuries can be ligated safely, including radial artery injuries and superficial femoral vein injuries. However, other vessels in close proximity, such as the ulnar artery and popliteal vein, must be repaired. Single tibial artery injuries can be ligated. This makes sense since only single vessel perfusion to the foot is adequate for limb survival in elective lower-extremity arterial reconstructions performed for atherosclerosis.

Relatively minor vascular injuries can cause surprisingly serious long-term sequelae. A vascular injury that results in the formation of a hematoma that compresses a susceptible nerve enclosed within the same neurovascular bundle can result in permanent nerve damage if the hematoma is not drained promptly. For example, a hematoma that forms in the axillary sheath following an axillary artery injury can result in nerve compression and permanent damage to the adjacent median or ulnar nerve. In these cases, no hematoma may be evident on physical exam. These patients will present with paresthesias of the hand and weakness of the hand. Prompt operative decompression must be performed for this form of compartment syndrome. Associated neurologic injuries result in an approximately 20 percent incidence of long-term disability following upper-extremity vascular trauma.[9]

Iatrogenic injuries include postcatheterization arterial dissections, arterial infections, femoral artery pseudoaneurysms, and AV fistulae. Covered stents have been used to treat some of these injuries in selected locations, such as the subclavian and iliac arteries.[8]

Femoral artery pseudoaneurysms may be treated in selected cases with the injection of thrombin under duplex ultrasound guidance. This procedure involves inserting a 22-gauge needle on a 3-ml syringe containing 2000 units of thrombin and slowly injecting under direct vision using the duplex scanner in the ultrasound lab. The success rate exceeds 95 percent as long as the neck of the pseudoaneurysm is small (less than 3 mm). This technique of thrombin injection has been demonstrated to be efficacious only for the treatment of arterial pseudoaneurysms caused by arterial punctures. This technique should not be used for the definitive treatment of other types of traumatic arterial pseudoaneurysms.

COMPARTMENT SYNDROME

Compartment syndrome is common following extremity vascular trauma. The most common mechanism involves significant ischemia followed by a period of rapid reperfusion. Compartment syndrome is caused by elevated tissue interstitial pressure, which limits tissue perfusion at a capillary level. An analogy that is useful to explain compartment syndromes and compartmental hypertension is to think of a sink with a plugged drain. Just as water cannot adequately flow (or wash dishes) in a sink with a plugged drain, arterial blood cannot deliver oxygen to tissues if an elevated tissue pressure exceeds the pressure within the tissue capillaries and thereby blocks perfusion at the capillary level by collapsing the capillaries and venules. The result is tissue ischemia even in the setting of a palpable pulse. Phlegmasia cerulea dolens, or venous gangrene due to a deep vein thrombosis (DVT), is in fact a type of compartment syndrome, as is an axillary sheath hematoma or a popliteal fossa hematoma.

Early signs of compartment syndrome include extremity pain and compartment tenderness and pain on passive stretch of the involved compartment. The loss of the arterial pulse is a late finding (sometimes too late) (Box 22-1). Compartment syndromes can present anytime between several hours and several days following the initial ischemia and reperfusion.

BOX 20–1

Signs and Symptoms of Compartment Syndrome

EARLY SIGNS	LATE SIGNS
Pain disproportionate to the injury	Decreased touch sensation
Tenseness or fullness of the compartment	Anesthesia
Pain on passive stretching of the muscle	Loss of pulses
Decreased active motor strength	

The median time at which a compartment syndrome presents is 15 hours after the initial reperfusion.

Following an arterial injury, a neutral limb position (not elevated and not dependent) is most effective in preventing the development of a compartment syndrome. This is distinct from the elevated limb position one utilizes with a DVT and phlegmasia, where the limb should be elevated to enhance venous drainage.

Fasciotomy often is undertaken in the operating room prior to performing the revascularization, as long-term functional results appear to be better when fasciotomy is performed early and frequently.[10] Four-compartment fasciotomies (Fig. 22-5) of the leg require incising the muscle overlying the crural (tibial) arteries of the leg. Fasciotomies sometimes are required to treat compartment syndromes of the forearm and less frequently the thigh. Mannitol given prior to reperfusion and approximately 12 hours later appears to decrease the incidence of postoperative compartment syndrome in patients who have sustained extremity vascular injuries.

CONCLUSION

Vascular trauma results in a distinct and often urgent group of problems that will challenge the vascular nurse. Recognition of the priority in treating associated, often life-threatening problems can have just as important an effect in producing positive long-term outcomes as will the treatment of the vascular injuries themselves. Exemplary nursing care involving accurate assessments, an awareness of complications, and prompt, aggressive interventions has a great impact on achieving successful long-term outcomes.

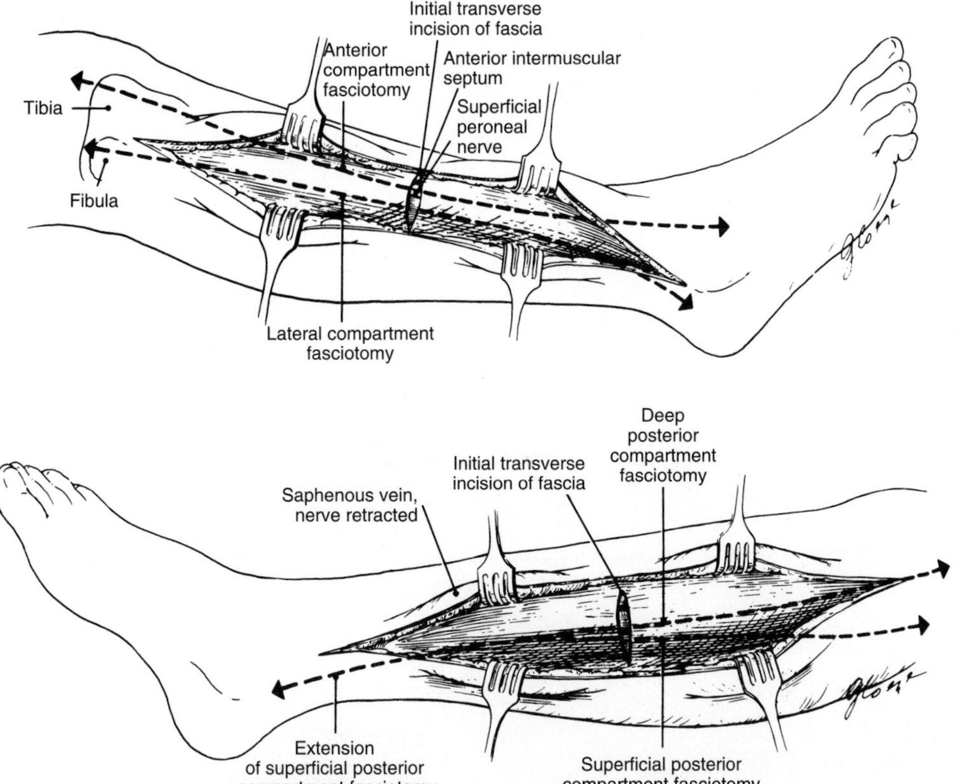

FIG. 22–5. Four-compartment fasciotomy of the right leg using lateral *(top)* and medial *(bottom)* incisions. The soleus muscle must be taken off its insertion on medial tibia in order for the deep posterior compartment to be opened and a complete leg fasciotomy performed. (From Bongard F, Wilson S, Perry M, eds: *Vascular injuries in surgical practice*, Norwalk, Conn, 1991, Appleton & Lange.)

REFERENCES

1. Veise-Berry S, Beachley M: Evolution of the trauma cycle. In Cardona VD, Mason PJB et al, eds: *Trauma nursing: from resuscitation through rehabilitation*, ed 2, Philadelphia, 1994, WB Saunders, pp 2-16.
2. Weigelt JA, Klein JD: Mechanism of injury. In Cardona VD, Hurn PD, Mason PJB et al, eds: *Trauma nursing: from resuscitation through rehabilitation*, ed 2, Philadelphia, 1994, WB Saunders, pp 91-113.
3. Keen JD, Dunne P, Keen RR et al: Proximity arteriography: cost-effectiveness in asymptomatic penetrating extremity trauma, *J Vasc Interv Radiol* 12:813-821, 2001.
4. Keen RR, Meyer JP, Durham JR et al: Autogenous vein graft repair of injured extremity arteries: early and late results with 134 consecutive patients, *J Vasc Surg* 13:664-668, 1991.
5. Hafez HM, Woolgar J, Robbs JV: Lower extremity arterial injury: results in 550 cases and review of risk factors associated with limb loss, *J Vasc Surg* 33:1212-1219, 2001.
6. Keen RR: Posterior approach to popliteal artery injuries. In Pearce WH, Yao JST, eds: *Advances in vascular surgery*, Chicago, 2002, Precept Press, pp 527-538.
7. Keen RR, Cohen MJ, Keen JD: Management of upper extremity trauma. In Pearce WH, Matsumura J, Yao JST, eds: *Trends in vascular surgery*, Chicago, 2002, Precept Press, pp 425-37.
8. DuToit DF, Strauss DC, Blaszcyk M et al: Endovascular treatment of penetrating thoracic outlet injuries, *Eur J Vasc Endovasc Surg* 19:489-495, 2000.
9. Keen RR, Meyer JP, Schuler JJ et al: Early and late results in the treatment of extremity vascular repair: patency, limb salvage, and function. In Flanigan DP, ed: *Civilian vascular trauma*, Philadelphia, 1992, Lea & Febiger, pp 465-472.
10. Lim LT, Michuda MS, Flanigan DP et al: Popliteal artery trauma, *Arch Surg* 115:1307-1313, 1980.

Index

Page numbers followed by "f" denote figures, "t" denote tables, and "b" denote boxes.

C

J

Journal of Vascular Nursing

The Official Publication of the Society for Vascular Nursing

Journal of Vascular Nursing Online includes the text, photographs, illustrations, and tables from each article, with high-resolution detail in formats that download rapidly. Click on a reference, and you will go to that reference. Click again and link to MEDLINE to view the abstract of that reference. Journal of Vascular Nursing Online includes many more reference links and services.

Visit www.jvascnurs.net today!

BUSINESS REPLY MAIL

FIRST-CLASS MAIL PERMIT NO. 7135 ORLANDO FL

POSTAGE WILL BE PAID BY ADDRESSEE

PERIODICALS ORDER FULFILLMENT DEPT
MOSBY
ELSEVIER
6277 SEA HARBOR DRIVE
ORLANDO FL 32821-9918